QUICK LOOK DRUG BOOK

QUICK LOOK DRUG BOOK

1995

Leonard L. Lance, RPh
Senior Editor
Pharmacist
Lexi-Comp Inc.
Hudson, Ohio

Charles Lacy, RPh, PharmD
Editor
Drug Information Pharmacist
Cedars-Sinai Medical Center
Los Angeles, California

Morton P. Goldman, PharmD
Associate Editor
Infectious Diseases Pharmacist
Cleveland Clinic Foundation
Cleveland, Ohio

Williams & Wilkins

BALTIMORE • PHILADELPHIA • HONG KONG
LONDON • MUNICH • SYDNEY • TOKYO

A WAVERLY COMPANY

NOTICE

This handbook is intended to serve the user as a handy quick reference and not as a complete drug information resource. It does not include information on every therapeutic agent available. The publication covers 1344 commonly used drugs and is specifically designed to present certain important aspects of drug data in a more concise format than is generally found in medical literature or product material supplied by manufacturers.

Although great care was taken to ensure the accuracy of the handbook's content when it went to press, the editors, contributors, and publisher cannot be responsible for the continued accuracy of the supplied information due to ongoing research and new developments in the field. Further, the *Quick Look Drug Book* is not offered as a guide to dosing. The reader, herewith, is advised that information shown under the heading **Usual Dosage** is provided only as an indication of the amount of the drug typically given or taken during therapy. Actual dosing amount for any specific drug should be based on an in-depth evaluation of the individual patient's therapy requirement and strong consideration given to such issues as contraindications, warnings, precautions, adverse reactions, along with the interaction of other drugs. The manufacturers most current product information or other standard recognized references should always be consulted for such detailed information prior to drug use.

The editors and contributors have written this book in their private capacities. No official support or endorsement by any federal agency or pharmaceutical company is intended or inferred.

This manual was produced using the FormuLex™ Program —
a complete publishing service of Lexi-Comp Inc.

Lexi-Comp Inc.
1100 Terex Road
Hudson, Ohio 44236
(216) 650-6506

TABLE OF CONTENTS

ABOUT THE AUTHORS

Leonard L. Lance, RPh

Leonard L. (Bud) Lance has been directly involved in the pharmaceutical industry since receiving his bachelor's degree in pharmacy from Ohio Northern University 24 years ago. Upon graduation from ONU, Mr Lance spent four years as a navy pharmacist in various military assignments and was instrumental in the development and operation of the first whole hospital I.V. admixture program in a military (Portsmouth Naval Hospital) facility.

After completing his military service, he entered the retail pharmacy field and has managed both an independent and a home I.V. franchise pharmacy operation. Since the late 1970s Mr Lance has focused much of his interest on using computers to improve pharmacy service and to advance the dissemination of drug information to practitioners and other health care professionals.

As a result of his strong publishing interest, he serves in the capacity of pharmacy editor and technical advisor as well as pharmacy (information) database coordinator for Lexi-Comp. Along with the *Quick Look Drug Book*, he provides technical support to Lexi-Comp's *Drug Information Handbook*, *Pediatric Dosage Handbook*, *Laboratory Test Handbook*, *Diagnostic Procedure Handbook*, *Infectious Diseases Handbook*, *Poisoning & Toxicology Handbook*, and *Geriatric Dosage Handbook* publications. Mr Lance has also assisted approximately 120 major hospitals in producing their own formulary (pharmacy) publications through Lexi-Comp's custom publishing service.

L.L. Lance is a member and past president (1984) of the Summit County Pharmaceutical Association (SCPA). He is also a member of the Ohio Pharmacists Association (OPA), the American Pharmaceutical Association (APhA), and the American Society of Hospital Pharmacists (ASHP).

Charles F. Lacy, PharmD

Dr Lacy received his doctorate from the University of Southern California School of Pharmacy. With over 12 years of clinical experience at one of the nation's largest teaching hospitals, he has developed a reputation as an acknowledged expert in drug information and critical care drug therapy.

In his current capacity as Drug Information specialist at Cedar-Sinai Medical Center in Los Angeles, Dr Lacy plays an active role in the education and training of the medical, pharmacy, and nursing staff. He coordinates the Drug Information Center, the Medical Center's Intern Pharmacist Clinical Training Program, the Department's Continuing Education Program for pharmacists; maintains the Medical Center formulary program; and is editor of the Medical Center's *Drug Formulary Handbook* and the drug information newsletter — *Prescription*.

Presently, Dr Lacy holds teaching affiliations with the University of Southern California School of Pharmacy, the University of California at San Francisco School of Pharmacy, the University of the Pacific School of Pharmacy and the University of Alberta at Edmonton, School of Pharmacy and Health Sciences.

Dr Lacy is an active member of numerous professional associations including the American Society of Hospital Pharmacists (ASHP), the California Society of Hospital Pharmacists (CSHP), and the American College of Clinical Pharmacy (ACCP).

Morton P. Goldman, PharmD

Dr Goldman received his bachelor's degree in pharmacy from the University of Pittsburgh in 1983 and his doctorate from the University of Cincinnati. He completed his residency at the V.A. Medical Center in Cincinnati and subsequently began pharmacy practice at several prominent Cleveland medical centers concentrating in the area of infectious diseases.

In his capacity as infectious disease pharmacist at the Cleveland Clinic Foundation, Dr Goldman is actively involved in the continuing education of the medical and pharmacy staff. He is an editor of the foundation's *Guideline for Antibiotic Use* and has coordinated their Renal Dose Monitoring Program. Dr Goldman has authored numerous journal articles and lectures locally and nationally on the topic of infectious diseases and current drug therapies. He is currently a coauthor of the *Infectious Diseases Handbook* produced by Lexi-Comp Inc. He also provides technical support to Lexi-Comp's *Drug Information Handbook*, *Pediatric Dosage Handbook*, *Poisoning & Toxicology Handbook*, and *Geriatric Dosage Handbook* publications.

Dr Goldman is an active member of the Society of Infectious Disease Pharmacists, American College of Clinical Pharmacy and the American Society of Hospital Pharmacists.

EDITORIAL ADVISORY PANEL

PREFACE

Working with clinical pharmacists, hospital pharmacy and therapeutics committees, and hospital drug information centers, our editors have assisted in developing hospital-specific formulary manuals for major medical institutions in the United States and Canada. These manuals provide pertinent details on medications used within the hospital, office and other clinical settings. The most current information on drugs and medications has been reviewed, coalesced, and cross-referenced to form the *Quick Look Drug Book*.

The Indication/Therapeutic Category Index is an expedient mechanism for locating the medication of choice along with its classification. This index helps the user to, with knowledge of the disease state, identify medications which are most commonly used in treatment. All disease states are cross-referenced to a varying number of medications with the most likely or best medications noted.

All generic and brand names or synonyms appear as individual entries in the alphabetical listing of drugs. Thus, there is no alphabetical index of drugs.

This handbook gives the user quick access to data on 1344 medications. A standard, concise format was developed to ensure consistent presentation of information. Selection of medications included in this handbook was based on an analysis of medications offered in a wide range of hospital formularies.

— L.L. Lance

ACKNOWLEDGMENTS

The *Quick Look Drug Book* exists in its present form as the result of the concerted efforts of many individuals. The publisher and president of Lexi-Comp Inc, Robert D. Kerscher, deserves much credit for bringing the concept of such a book to fruition. His dedication to the project, and his support and development of the many unique and innovative features included in the book, eg, format, internal cross-references and Indication/Therapeutic Category Index, contribute substantially to the content and usefulness of the book.

Other members of the Lexi-Comp staff whose contributions were invaluable and whose patience with the editors' enumerable drafts, revisions, deletions, additions, and enhancements was inexhaustible include: Diane Harbart, MT (ASCP), medical editor; Lynn Coppinger, director of product development; Barbara F. Kerscher, production manager; Alexandra Hart, composition specialist; Jeanne Eads, Beth Daulbaugh, Julie Weekes, and Lisa Leukart, project managers; Jil R. Neuman, and Jacqueline L. Mizer, production assistants; Jeff J. Zaccagnini, Brian B. Vossler, and Jerry Reeves, sales managers; Edmund A. Harbart, vice-president, custom publishing division; and Jack L. Stones, vice-president, reference publishing division. The complex computer programming required for the typesetting of the book was provided by Dennis P. Smithers, Jay L. Katzen, David C. Marcus, Dale Jablonski, and Kenneth J. Hughes, system analysts, under the direction of Thury L. O'Connor, vice-president, and Alan R. Frasz, vice-president, editorial systems.

In addition, sincere appreciation to Vaughn W. Floutz, PhD who served as editorial consultant.

USE OF THE HANDBOOK

The *Quick Look Drug Book* is organized into a drug information section, an appendix, and indication/therapeutic category index.

The drug information section of the handbook, wherein all drugs are listed alphabetically, details information pertinent to each drug. Extensive cross referencing is provided by brand name and synonyms.

Drug information is presented in a consistent format and for quick reference will provide the following:

Generic Name	U.S. adopted name
Pronunciation Guide	
Brand Names	Common trade names
Synonyms	
Therapeutic Category	
Use	Information pertaining to appropriate use of the drug
Usual Dosage	The amount of the drug to be typically given or taken during therapy
Dosage Forms	Information with regard to form, strength and availability of the drug

Appendix

The appendix offers a compilation of tables, guidelines and conversion information which can often be helpful when considering patient care.

Indication/Therapeutic Category Index

This index provides a listing of accepted drugs for various disease states thus focusing attention on selection of medications most frequently prescribed in relation to a clinical diagnosis. Diseases may have other nonofficial drugs for their treatment and this indication/therapeutic category index should not be used by itself to determine the appropriateness of a particular therapy. The listed indications may encompass varying degrees of severity and, since certain medications may not be appropriate for a given degree of severity, it should not be assumed that the agents listed for specific indications are interchangeable. Also included as a valuable reference is each medication's therapeutic category.

SAFE WRITING

Health professionals and their support personnel frequently produce handwritten copies of information they see in print; therefore, such information is subjected to even greater possibilities for error or misinterpretation on the part of others. Thus, particular care must be given to how drug names and strengths are expressed when creating written health care documents.

The following are a few examples of safe writing rules suggested by the Institute for Safe Medication Practices, Inc.*

1. There should be a space between a number and its units as it is easier to read. There should be no periods after the abbreviations mg or mL.

Correct	Incorrect
10 mg	10mg
100 mg	100mg

2. Never place a decimal and a zero after a whole number (2 mg is correct and 2.0 mg is incorrect). If the decimal point is not seen because it falls on a line or because individuals are working from copies where the decimal point is not seen, this causes a tenfold overdose.

3. Just the opposite is true for numbers less than one. Always place a zero before a naked decimal (0.5 mL is correct, .5 mL is **in**correct).

4. Never abbreviate the word "unit." The handwritten U or u, looks like a 0 (zero), and may cause a tenfold overdose error to be made.

5. Q.D. is not a safe abbreviation for once daily, as when the Q is followed by a sloppy dot, it looks like QID which means four times daily.

6. O.D. is not a safe abbreviation for once daily, as it is properly interpreted as meaning "right eye" and has caused liquid medications such as saturated solution of potassium iodide and lugol's solution to be administered incorrectly. There is no safe abbreviation for once daily. It must be written out in full.

7. Do not use chemical names such as 6-mercaptopurine or 6-thioguanine, as 6 fold overdoses have been given when these were not recognized as chemical names. The proper names of these drugs are mercaptopurine or thioguanine.

8. Do not abbreviate drug names (5FC, 6MP, 5-ASA, MTX, HCTZ CPZ, PBZ, etc) as they are misinterpreted and cause error.

9. Do not use the apothecary system or symbols.

10. When writing an outpatient prescription, write a complete prescription. A complete prescription can prevent the prescriber, the pharmacist, and/or the patient from making a mistake and can eliminate the need for further clarification.

---

*From "Safe Writing" by Davis NM, PharmD and Cohen MR, MS, Lecturers and Consultants for Safe Medication Practices, 1143 Wright Drive, Huntingdon Valley, PA 19006. Phone: (215) 947-7566.

The legible prescriptions should contain:

    a.   patient's full name

    b.   for pediatric or geriatric patients: their age (or weight where applicable)

    c.   drug name, dosage form and strength; if a drug is new or rarely prescribed, print this information

    d.   number or amount to be dispensed

    e.   complete instructions for the patient, including the purpose of the medication

    f.   when there are recognized contraindications for a prescribed drug, indicate to the pharmacist that you are aware of this fact (ie, when prescribing a potassium salt for a patient receiving an ACE inhibitor, write "K serum leveling being monitored")

SELECTED REFERENCES

AMA Drug Evaluations Subscription, American Medical Association, Department of Drugs, Division of Drugs and Toxicology, Spring, 1990.

Drug Interaction Facts, St Louis, MO: J.B. Lippincott Co (Facts and Comparisons Division), 1994.

Facts and Comparisons, St Louis, MO: J.B. Lippincott Co (Facts and Comparisons Division), 1994.

Handbook of Nonprescription Drugs, 9th ed, Washington, DC: American Pharmaceutical Association, 1993.

Isada CM, Kasten BL, Goldman MP, et al, *Infectious Diseases Handbook*, 1st ed, Hudson, OH: Lexi-Comp Inc, 1995.

Jacobs DS, DeMott WR, Finley PR, et al, *Laboratory Test Handbook with Key Word Index*, 3rd ed, Hudson, OH: Lexi-Comp Inc, 1994.

Lacy CF, Armstrong LL, Lipsy RJ, and Lance LL, *Drug Information Handbook*, 2nd ed, Hudson, OH: Lexi-Comp Inc, 1994.

Leikin JB and Paloucek FP, *Poisoning & Toxicology Handbook*, 1st ed, Hudson, OH: Lexi-Comp Inc, 1995.

Levin D, *Essentials of Pediatric Intensive Care*, 1st ed, St Louis, MO: Quality Medical Publishing, Inc, 1990.

McEvoy GK and Litvak K, *AHFS Drug Information*, Bethesda, MD: American Society of Hospital Pharmacists, 1994.

Nelson JD, *1991-1992 Pocketbook of Pediatric Antimicrobial Therapy*, 9th ed., Baltimore, MD: Williams & Wilkins, 1991.

Physician's Desk Reference, 49th ed, Oradell, NJ: Medical Economics Books, 1995.

Report of the Committee on Infectious Diseases, American Academy of Pediatrics, 22nd ed, 1991.

Semla TP, Beizer JL, and Higbee MD, *Geriatric Dosage Handbook*, Hudson, OH: Lexi-Comp Inc, 1993.

Taketomo CK, Hodding JH, and Kraus DM, *Pediatric Dosage Handbook*, 2nd ed, Hudson, OH: Lexi-Comp Inc, 1994.

Trissel L, *Handbook of Injectionable Drugs*, 6th ed, Bethesda, MD: American Society of Hospital Pharmacists, 1992.

United States Pharmacopeia Dispensing Information (USP DI), Rockville, MD: United States Pharmacopeial Convention, Inc, 1994.

ALPHABETICAL LISTING
OF DRUGS

A-200™ Pyrinate [OTC] *see* pyrethrins *on page 400*

A and D™ Ointment [OTC] *see* vitamin a and vitamin d *on page 489*

a-ase *see* asparaginase *on page 35*

Abbokinase® Injection *see* urokinase *on page 481*

Abbott HIVAB HIV-1 EIA *see* diagnostic aids (*in vitro*), blood *on page 136*

Abbott HIVAG-1 *see* diagnostic aids (*in vitro*), blood *on page 136*

Abbott HTLV III Confirmatory EIA *see* diagnostic aids (*in vitro*), blood
on page 136

abciximab
Brand Names ReoPro™
Synonyms c7E3
Therapeutic Category Platelet Aggregation Inhibitor
Use Adjunct to percutaneous transluminal coronary angioplasty or atherectomy (PTCA) for the
prevention of acute cardiac ischemic complications in patients at high risk for abrupt closure
of the treated coronary vessel
Usual Dosage I.V.: 0.25 mg/kg bolus followed by an infusion of 10 mcg/minute
Dosage Forms Injection

absorbable cotton *see* cellulose, oxidized *on page 84*

absorbable gelatin sponge *see* gelatin, absorbable *on page 205*

Absorbine Jr.® Antifungal [OTC] *see* tolnaftate *on page 464*

Absorbine® Antifungal [OTC] *see* tolnaftate *on page 464*

Absorbine® Jock Itch [OTC] *see* tolnaftate *on page 464*

Accupril® *see* quinapril hydrochloride *on page 402*

Accusens T® *see* diagnostic aids (*in vitro*), other *on page 137*

Accutane® *see* isotretinoin *on page 254*

acebutolol hydrochloride (a se byoo' toe lole)
Brand Names Sectral"
Therapeutic Category Antiarrhythmic Agent, Class II; Beta-Adrenergic Blocker
Use Treatment of hypertension; ventricular arrhythmias; angina
Usual Dosage Adults: Oral: 400-800 mg/day in 2 divided doses
Dosage Forms Capsule: 200 mg, 400 mg

Acel-Immune® *see* diphtheria, tetanus toxoids, and acellular pertussis vaccine
on page 151

Aceon® *see* perindopril erbumine *on page 358*

Acephen® [OTC] *see* acetaminophen *on this page*

acetaminophen (a seet a min' oh fen)
Brand Names Acephen" [OTC]; Aceta" [OTC]; Apacet® [OTC]; Aspirin Free Anacin® Maxi-
mum Strength [OTC]; Dapa" [OTC]; Dorcol" [OTC]; Feverall™ [OTC]; Genapap® [OTC];
Liquiprin' [OTC]; Myapap" Drops [OTC]; Neopap® [OTC]; Panadol® [OTC]; Redutemp®
[OTC]; Ridenol" [OTC]; Snaplets-FR" Granules [OTC]; Tempra® [OTC]; Tylenol® [OTC];
Uni-Ace' [OTC]
Synonyms apap; n-acetyl-p-aminophenol; paracetamol
Therapeutic Category Analgesic, Non-Narcotic; Antipyretic
Use Treatment of mild to moderate pain and fever; does not have antirheumatic effects

Usual Dosage Oral:
Children: 10-15 mg/kg/dose every 4-6 hours as needed; do **not** exceed 5 doses in 24 hours
Adults: 325-650 mg every 4-6 hours or 1000 mg 3-4 times/day; do **not** exceed 4 g/day
Dosage Forms
Caplet: 160 mg, 325 mg, 500 mg
Drops: 100 mg/mL (15 mL); 120 mg/2.5 mL (35 mL)
Granules, premeasured packs: 80 mg (32s)
Elixir: 120 mg/5 mL (5 mL, 10 mL, 13.5 mL, 25 mL, 27 mL, 120 mL, 480 mL, 3780 mL); 130 mg/5 mL (12.5 mL, 25 mL); 160 mg/5 mL (5 mL, 10 mL, 20 mL, 120 mL, 240 mL, 500 mL, 3780 mL); 325 mg/5 mL (480 mL, 3780 mL)
Liquid, oral: 160 mg/5 mL (2.5 mL, 5 mL, 60 mL, 120 mL, 240 mL, 480 mL); 500 mg/15 mL (240 mL)
Suppository, rectal: 120 mg, 125 mg, 325 mg, 650 mg
Suspension: 100 mg/mL, 160 mg/mL
Tablet: 325 mg, 500 mg, 650 mg
Tablet, chewable: 80 mg, 160 mg

acetaminophen and dextromethorphan (a seet a min' oh fen)
Brand Names Bayer® Select® Chest Cold Caplets [OTC]; Drixoral® Cough & Sore Throat Liquid Caps [OTC]
Therapeutic Category Analgesic, Non-Narcotic; Antipyretic; Antitussive
Use Treatment of mild to moderate pain and fever; symptomatic relief of coughs caused by minor viral upper respiratory tract infections or inhaled irritants; most effective for a chronic nonproductive cough
Usual Dosage Oral:
Children: 10-15 mg/kg/dose every 4-6 hours as needed; do **not** exceed 5 doses in 24 hours
Adults: 325-650 mg every 4-6 hours or 1000 mg 3-4 times/day; do **not** exceed 4 g/day
Dosage Forms
Caplet: Acetaminophen 500 and dextromethorphan hydrobromide 15 mg
Capsule: Acetaminophen 325 and dextromethorphan hydrobromide 15 mg

acetaminophen and aspirin
Brand Names Excedrin®, Extra Strength [OTC]; Gelpirin" [OTC]; Goody's" Headache Powders
Therapeutic Category Analgesic, Non-Narcotic; Antipyretic
Use Relief of mild to moderate pain
Usual Dosage Adults: Oral: 1-2 tablets every 2-6 hours as needed for pain
Dosage Forms
Powder: Acetaminophen 250 mg and aspirin 520 mg with caffeine 32.5 mg per dose
Tablet: Acetaminophen 125 mg and aspirin 240 mg with caffeine 32 mg; acetaminophen 250 mg and aspirin 250 mg with caffeine 65 mg

acetaminophen and codeine
Brand Names Capital® and Codeine; CodAphen®; Margesic" No. 3; Tylenol" With Codeine
Synonyms codeine and acetaminophen
Therapeutic Category Analgesic, Narcotic; Antipyretic
Use Relief of mild to moderate pain
Usual Dosage Doses should be adjusted according to severity of pain and response of the patient. Adult doses of 60 mg codeine and higher fail to give commensurate relief of pain but merely prolong analgesia and are associated with an appreciably increased incidence of side effects. Oral:

Children:
Analgesic: 0.5-1 mg codeine/kg/dose every 4-6 hours
Acetaminophen: 10-15 mg/kg/dose every 4 hours up to a maximum of 2.6 g/24 hours for children <12 years
3-6 years: 5 mL 3-4 times/day as needed of elixir
7-12 years: 10 mL 3-4 times/day as needed of elixir
>12 years: 15 mL every 4 hours as needed of elixir

Adults:
Antitussive: Based on codeine (15-30 mg/dose) every 4-6 hours
(Continued)
3

acetaminophen and codeine *(Continued)*

Analgesic: Based on codeine (30-60 mg/dose) every 4-6 hours
1-2 tablets every 4 hours to a maximum of 12 tablets/24 hours
Dosage Forms
Capsule:
#2: Acetaminophen 325 mg and codeine phosphate 15 mg
#3: Acetaminophen 325 mg and codeine phosphate 30 mg
#4: Acetaminophen 325 mg and codeine phosphate 60 mg
Elixir: Acetaminophen 120 mg and codeine phosphate 12 mg per 5 mL with alcohol 7% (C-V)
Suspension, oral, alcohol free: Acetaminophen 120 mg and codeine phosphate 12 mg per 5 mL (C-V)
Tablet: Acetaminophen 500 mg and codeine phosphate 30 mg; acetaminophen 650 mg and codeine phosphate 30 mg
Tablet:
#1: Acetaminophen 300 mg and codeine phosphate 7.5 mg
#2: Acetaminophen 300 mg and codeine phosphate 15 mg
#3: Acetaminophen 300 mg and codeine phosphate 30 mg
#4: Acetaminophen 300 mg and codeine phosphate 60 mg

acetaminophen and diphenhydramine

Brand Names Arthritis Foundation® Nighttime [OTC]; Excedrin® P.M. [OTC]; Midol® PM [OTC]
Therapeutic Category Analgesic, Non-Narcotic; Antipyretic
Use Relief of mild to moderate pain; sinus headache
Dosage Forms
Caplet:
Excedrin® P.M.: Acetaminophen 500 mg and diphenhydramine citrate 30 mg
Arthritis Foundation® Nighttime, Midol® PM: Acetaminophen 500 mg and diphenhydramine 25 mg
Liquid (wild berry flavor) (Excedrin® P.M.): Acetaminophen 1000 mg and diphenhydramine hydrochloride 50 mg per 30 mL (180 mL)

acetaminophen and hydrocodone *see* hydrocodone and acetaminophen

on page 230

acetaminophen and isometheptene mucate

Brand Names Midrin®
Therapeutic Category Analgesic, Non-Narcotic; Antimigraine Agent; Antipyretic
Use Relief of migraine and tension headache
Usual Dosage Adults: Oral: 2 capsules at first sign of headache, followed by 1 capsule every 60 minutes until relieved, up to 5 capsules in a 12-hour period
Dosage Forms Capsule: Acetaminophen 326 mg and isometheptene mucate 65 mg with dichloralphenazone 100 mg

acetaminophen and oxycodone *see* oxycodone and acetaminophen

on page 342

acetaminophen and phenyltoloxamine

Brand Names Percogesic® [OTC]
Therapeutic Category Analgesic, Non-Narcotic; Antipyretic
Use Relief of mild to moderate pain
Usual Dosage Adults: Oral: 1-2 tablets every 4 hours
Dosage Forms Tablet: Acetaminophen 325 mg and phenyltoloxamine citrate 30 mg

acetaminophen, chlorpheniramine, and pseudoephedrine

Brand Names Alka-Seltzer® Plus Cold Liqui-Gels Capsules [OTC]; Aspirin-Free Bayer® Select® Allergy Sinus Caplets [OTC]; Sinutab® Tablets [OTC]
Therapeutic Category Analgesic, Non-Narcotic; Antihistamine/Decongestant Combination; Antipyretic

Use Temporary relief of sinus symptoms

Usual Dosage Adults: Oral: 2 tablets every 6 hours

Dosage Forms

Caplet: Acetaminophen 500 mg, chlorpheniramine hydrochloride 2 mg, and pseudoephedrine hydrochloride 30 mg

Capsule: Acetaminophen 250 mg, chlorpheniramine hydrochloride 2 mg, and pseudoephedrine hydrochloride 30 mg

Tablet: Acetaminophen 325 mg, chlorpheniramine hydrochloride 2 mg, and pseudoephedrine hydrochloride 30 mg

Aceta® [OTC] *see* acetaminophen *on page 2*

Acetasol® HC Otic *see* acetic acid, propanediol diacetate, and hydrocortisone *on next page*

acetazolamide (a set a zole' a mide)

Brand Names Dazamide®; Diamox®

Therapeutic Category Anticonvulsant, Miscellaneous; Carbonic Anhydrase Inhibitor; Diuretic, Carbonic Anhydrase Inhibitor

Use Lower intraocular pressure to treat glaucoma, also as a diuretic, adjunct treatment of refractory seizure and acute altitude sickness

Usual Dosage

Children:

Glaucoma:

Oral: 8-30 mg/kg/day divided every 6-8 hours

I.M., I.V.: 20-40 mg/kg/day divided every 6 hours

Edema: Oral, I.M., I.V.: 5 mg/kg or 150 mg/m^2 once every day or every other day

Epilepsy: Oral: 8-30 mg/kg/day in 2-4 divided doses, not to exceed 1 g/day

Adults:

Glaucoma:

Oral: 250 mg 1-4 times/day or 500 mg sustained release capsule twice daily

I.M., I.V.: 250-500 mg, may repeat in 2-4 hours

Edema: Oral, I.M., I.V.: 250-375 mg once daily

Epilepsy: Oral: 8-30 mg/kg/day in 1-4 divided doses

Altitude sickness: Oral: 250 mg every 8-12 hours

Dosage Forms

Capsule, sustained release: 500 mg

Injection: 500 mg/5 mL

Tablet: 125 mg, 250 mg

acetic acid

Brand Names VóSol® Otic

Synonyms ethanoic acid

Therapeutic Category Antibacterial, Otic; Antibacterial, Topical

Use Continuous or intermittent irrigation of the bladder; treatment of superficial bacterial infections of the external auditory canal and vagina

Usual Dosage

Irrigation: For continuous irrigation of the urinary bladder with 0.25% acetic acid irrigation, the rate of administration will approximate the rate of urine flow; usually 500-1500 mL/24 hours; for periodic irrigation of an indwelling urinary catheter to maintain patency, approximately 50 mL of 0.25% acetic acid irrigation is required. (Note dosage of an irrigating solution depends on the capacity or surface area of the structure being irrigated.)

Otic: Insert saturated wick, keep moist 24 hours; remove wick and instill 5 drops 3-4 times/day

Dosage Forms Solution:

Irrigation: 0.25% (1000 mL)

Otic: Acetic acid 2% in propylene glycol (15 mL, 30 mL, 60 mL)

acetic acid, propanediol diacetate, and hydrocortisone
Brand Names Acetasol® HC Otic; VōSol® HC Otic
Therapeutic Category Otic Agent, Anti-infective
Use Treatment of superficial infections of the external auditory canal caused by organisms susceptible to the action of the antimicrobial, complicated by inflammation
Usual Dosage Adults: Otic: Instill 4 drops in ear(s) 3-4 times/day
Dosage Forms Solution, otic: Acetic acid 2%, propylene glycol diacetate 3%, and hydrocortisone 1% (10 mL)

acetohexamide (a set oh hex' a mide)
Brand Names Dymelor®
Therapeutic Category Antidiabetic Agent; Hypoglycemic Agent, Oral; Sulfonylurea Agent
Use Adjunct to diet for the management of mild to moderately severe, stable, noninsulin-dependent (type II) diabetes mellitus
Usual Dosage Adults: Oral: 250 mg to 1.5 g/day in 1-2 divided doses
Dosage Forms Tablet: 250 mg, 500 mg

acetohydroxamic acid (a see' toe hye drox am ik)
Brand Names Lithostat®
Synonyms aha
Therapeutic Category Urinary Tract Product
Use Adjunctive therapy in chronic urea-splitting urinary infection
Usual Dosage Oral:
Children: Initial: 10 mg/kg/day
Adults: 250 mg 3-4 times/day for a total daily dose of 10-15 mg/kg/day
Dosage Forms Tablet: 250 mg

acetophenazine maleate (a set oh fen' a zeen)
Brand Names Tindal®
Therapeutic Category Antipsychotic Agent
Use Management of manifestations of psychotic disorders
Usual Dosage Adults: Oral: 20 mg 3 times/day up to 40-80 mg/day
Hospitalized schizophrenic patients may require doses as high as 400-600 mg/day
Dosage Forms Tablet: 20 mg

acetoxymethylprogesterone see medroxyprogesterone acetate on page 283

acetylcholine chloride (a se teel koe' leen)
Brand Names Miochol®
Therapeutic Category Cholinergic Agent, Ophthalmic; Ophthalmic Agent, Miotic
Use Produce complete miosis in cataract surgery, keratoplasty, iridectomy and other anterior segment surgery where rapid miosis is required
Usual Dosage Adults: 0.5-2 mL of 1% injection (5-20 mg) instilled into anterior chamber before or after securing one or more sutures
Dosage Forms Powder, intraocular: 1:100 [10 mg/mL] (2 mL, 15 mL)

acetylcysteine (a se teel sis' tay een)
Brand Names Mucomyst®; Mucosol®
Therapeutic Category Antidote, Acetaminophen; Mucolytic Agent
Use Adjunctive therapy in patients with abnormal or viscid mucous secretions in acute and chronic bronchopulmonary diseases, pulmonary complications of surgery and cystic fibrosis; diagnostic bronchial studies; antidote for acute acetaminophen toxicity
Usual Dosage
Acetaminophen poisoning: Children and Adults: Oral: 140 mg/kg followed by 17 doses of 70 mg/kg every 4 hours or until acetaminophen assay reveals nontoxic levels; repeat dose if emesis occurs within 1 hour of administration

Inhalation: Acetylcysteine 10% and 20% solution (Mucomyst®) (Dilute with water):
  Infants: 2 mL of 5% solution until nebulized given 3-4 times/day
  Children: 3-5 mL of 5% to 10% solution until nebulized given 3-4 times/day
  Adolescents: 5-10 mL of 5% to 10% solution until nebulized given 3-4 times/day
  Note: Patients should receive an aerosolized bronchodilator 10-15 minutes prior to ace-
  tylcysteine

Meconium Ileus equivalent: Children and Adults: 100-200 mL of 5% to 10% solution by irrigation or orally
Dosage Forms Solution, as sodium: 10% [100 mg/mL] (4 mL, 10 mL, 30 mL); 20% [200 mg/
mL] (4 mL, 10 mL, 30 mL, 100 mL)

acetylsalicylic acid see aspirin on page 35
Aches-N-Pain® [OTC] see ibuprofen on page 240
Achromycin® Ophthalmic see tetracycline on page 451
Achromycin® Topical see tetracycline on page 451
Achromycin® V Oral see tetracycline on page 451
aciclovir see acyclovir on this page
acidulated phosphate fluoride see fluoride on page 196
Aclovate® Topical see alclometasone dipropionate on page 11
act see dactinomycin on page 124
Actagen-C® see triprolidine, pseudoephedrine, and codeine on page 475
Actagen® [OTC] see triprolidine and pseudoephedrine on page 474
acth see corticotropin on page 115
Acthar® see corticotropin on page 115
Actidose-Aqua® [OTC] see charcoal on page 86
Actidose® With Sorbitol [OTC] see charcoal on page 86
Actifed® [OTC] see triprolidine and pseudoephedrine on page 474
Actifed® With Codeine see triprolidine, pseudoephedrine, and codeine
  on page 475
Actigall™ see ursodiol on page 482
Actimmune® see interferon gamma-1b on page 248
Actinex® see masoprocol on page 280
actinomycin d see dactinomycin on page 124
Activase® Injection see alteplase, recombinant on page 14
activated carbon see charcoal on page 86
activated charcoal see charcoal on page 86
activated dimethicone see simethicone on page 423
activated ergosterol see ergocalciferol on page 169
activated methylpolysiloxane see simethicone on page 423
ACT® [OTC] see fluoride on page 196
Acular® Ophthalmic see ketorolac tromethamine on page 258
Acutrim® Precision Release® [OTC] see phenylpropanolamine hydrochloride
  on page 365
acv see acyclovir on this page
acycloguanosine see acyclovir on this page

acyclovir (ay sye' kloe ver)
  Brand Names Zovirax® Injection; Zovirax® Oral; Zovirax® Topical
  Synonyms aciclovir; acv; acycloguanosine
  Therapeutic Category Antiviral Agent, Oral; Antiviral Agent, Parenteral; Antiviral Agent,
  Topical
  (Continued)

acyclovir *(Continued)*

Use Treatment of initial and prophylaxis of recurrent mucosal and cutaneous herpes simplex (HSV-1 and HSV-2) infections; herpes simplex encephalitis; herpes zoster; genital herpes infection; and varicella-zoster infections in immunocompromised patients

Usual Dosage

Neonates HSV infection: I.V.: 1500 mg/m^2/day divided every 8 hours or 30 mg/kg/day divided every 8 hours for 10-14 days

Children and Adults: I.V.:

Mucocutaneous HSV infection: 750 mg/m^2/day divided every 8 hours or 15 mg/kg/day divided every 8 hours for 5-10 days

HSV encephalitis: 1500 mg/m^2/day divided every 8 hours or 30 mg/kg/day divided every 8 hours for 10 days

Varicella-zoster virus infection: 1500 mg/m^2/day divided every 8 hours or 30 mg/kg/day divided every 8 hours for 5-10 days

Adults:

Oral: Initial: 200 mg every 4 hours while awake (5 times/day); prophylaxis: 200 mg 3-4 times/day or 400 mg twice daily. Prophylaxis of varicella or herpes zoster in HIV positive patients: 400 mg 5 times/day

Topical: $^1/_2$" ribbon of ointment every 3 hours (6 times/day)

Herpes zoster in immunocompromised patients:

Children: Oral: 250-600 mg/m^2/dose 4-5 times/day

Adults: Oral: 800 mg every 4 hours (5 times/day) for 7-10 days

Children and Adults: I.V.: 7.5 mg/kg/dose every 8 hours

Varicella-zoster infections: Oral:

Children: 10-20 mg/kg/dose (up to 800 mg) 4 times/day

Adults: 600-800 mg/dose 5 times/day for 7-10 days or 1000 mg every 6 hours for 5 days

Prophylaxis of bone marrow transplant recipients: Children and Adults: I.V.:

Autologous patients who are HSV seropositive: 150 mg/m^2/dose every 12 hours; with clinical symptoms of herpes simplex: 150 mg/m^2/dose every 8 hours

Autologous patients who are CMV seropositive: 500 mg/m^2/dose every 8 hours; for clinically symptomatic CMV infection, ganciclovir should be used in place of acyclovir

Dosage Forms

Capsule: 200 mg

Injection: 500 mg (10 mL); 1000 mg (20 mL)

Ointment, topical: 5% [50 mg/g] (3 g, 15 g)

Suspension, oral (banana flavor): 200 mg/5 mL

Tablet: 400 mg, 800 mg

Adagen™ *see* pegademase bovine *on page 351*

Adalat® *see* nifedipine *on page 328*

Adalat® CC *see* nifedipine *on page 328*

adamantanamine hydrochloride *see* amantadine hydrochloride *on page 17*

Adapin® Oral *see* doxepin hydrochloride *on page 157*

Adeflor® *see* vitamin, multiple (pediatric) *on page 491*

adenine arabinoside *see* vidarabine *on page 487*

Adenocard® *see* adenosine *on this page*

adenosine (a den' oh seen)

Brand Names Adenocard"

Synonyms 9-beta-D-ribofuranosyladenine

Therapeutic Category Antiarrhythmic Agent, Miscellaneous

Use Treatment of paroxysmal supraventricular tachycardia (PSVT). Orphan drug for treatment of brain tumors in conjunction with BCNU.

Usual Dosage

Children: Initial dose: Rapid I.V.: 0.05 mg/kg; if not effective within 2 minutes, increase dose in 0.05 mg/kg increments every 2 minutes to a maximum dose of 0.25 mg/kg or until termination of PSVT; median dose required: 0.15 mg/kg; do not exceed adult doses

Adults: Rapid I.V. push: 6 mg, if the dose is not effective within 1-2 minutes, a rapid I.V. dose of 12 mg may be given; may repeat 12 mg bolus if needed
Dosage Forms Injection, preservative free: 3 mg/mL (2 mL)

Adipex-P® *see* phentermine hydrochloride *on page 363*

Adlone® Injection *see* methylprednisolone *on page 300*

adr *see* doxorubicin hydrochloride *on page 157*

Adrenalin® *see* epinephrine *on page 167*

adrenaline *see* epinephrine *on page 167*

adrenocorticotropic hormone *see* corticotropin *on page 115*

Adriamycin PFS™ *see* doxorubicin hydrochloride *on page 157*

Adriamycin RDF™ *see* doxorubicin hydrochloride *on page 157*

Adrucil® Injection *see* fluorouracil *on page 198*

adsorbent charcoal *see* charcoal *on page 86*

Adsorbocarpine® Ophthalmic *see* pilocarpine *on page 369*

Adsorbonac® Ophthalmic [OTC] *see* sodium chloride *on page 426*

Advance® *see* diagnostic aids (*in vitro*), urine *on page 137*

Advil® [OTC] *see* ibuprofen *on page 240*

Aeroaid® [OTC] *see* thimerosal *on page 456*

AeroBid®-M Oral Aerosol Inhaler *see* flunisolide *on page 195*

AeroBid® Oral Aerosol Inhaler *see* flunisolide *on page 195*

Aerolate III® *see* theophylline *on page 453*

Aerolate JR® *see* theophylline *on page 453*

Aerolate SR® S *see* theophylline *on page 453*

Aeroseb-Dex® *see* dexamethasone *on page 131*

Aerosporin® Injection *see* polymyxin b sulfate *on page 376*

AeroZoin® [OTC] *see* benzoin *on page 49*

Afrinol® [OTC] *see* pseudoephedrine *on page 397*

Afrin® Nasal Solution [OTC] *see* oxymetazoline hydrochloride *on page 343*

Aftate® [OTC] *see* tolnaftate *on page 464*

AgNO₃ *see* silver nitrate *on page 422*

aha *see* acetohydroxamic acid *on page 6*

ahf *see* antihemophilic factor (human) *on page 29*

A-hydroCort® *see* hydrocortisone *on page 232*

Airet® *see* albuterol *on next page*

Akarpine® Ophthalmic *see* pilocarpine *on page 369*

AKBeta® Ophthalmic *see* levobunolol hydrochloride *on page 264*

AK-Chlor® Ophthalmic *see* chloramphenicol *on page 88*

AK-Con® Ophthalmic *see* naphazoline hydrochloride *on page 319*

AK-Dex® *see* dexamethasone *on page 131*

AK-Dilate® Ophthalmic Solution *see* phenylephrine hydrochloride *on page 364*

AK-Fluor® Injection *see* fluorescein sodium *on page 196*

AK-Homatropine® Ophthalmic *see* homatropine hydrobromide *on page 226*

Akineton® *see* biperiden hydrochloride *on page 54*

AK-Mycin® *see* erythromycin, topical *on page 172*

AK-Nefrin® Ophthalmic Solution *see* phenylephrine hydrochloride *on page 364*

Akne-Mycin® *see* erythromycin, topical *on page 172*

AK-Pentolate® *see* cyclopentolate hydrochloride *on page 120*

AK-Poly-Bac® Ophthalmic *see* bacitracin and polymyxin b *on page 43*

AK-Pred® Ophthalmic *see* prednisolone *on page 383*

AK-Spore H.C.® Otic *see* neomycin, polymyxin b, and hydrocortisone *on page 323*

AK-Spore® Ophthalmic Solution *see* neomycin, polymyxin b, and gramicidin *on page 322*

AK-Sulf® Ophthalmic *see* sodium sulfacetamide *on page 431*

AK-Taine® Ophthalmic *see* proparacaine hydrochloride *on page 392*

AKTob® Ophthalmic *see* tobramycin *on page 462*

AK-Tracin® Ophthalmic *see* bacitracin *on page 42*

AK-Trol® Ophthalmic *see* neomycin, polymyxin b, and dexamethasone *on page 322*

Ala-Cort® *see* hydrocortisone *on page 232*

Ala-Quin® Topical *see* clioquinol and hydrocortisone *on page 106*

Ala-Scalp® *see* hydrocortisone *on page 232*

Alazide® *see* hydrochlorothiazide and spironolactone *on page 229*

Alazine® Oral *see* hydralazine hydrochloride *on page 228*

Albalon-A® Ophthalmic *see* naphazoline and antazoline *on page 318*

Albalon® Liquifilm® Ophthalmic *see* naphazoline hydrochloride *on page 319*

Albuminar® *see* albumin human *on this page*

albumin human

Brand Names Albuminar®; Albunex®; Albutein®; Buminate®; Plasbumin®

Therapeutic Category Blood Product Derivative; Plasma Volume Expander

Use Plasma volume expansion and maintenance of cardiac output in the treatment of certain types of shock or impending shock

Usual Dosage 5% should be used in hypovolemic patients; 25% should be used in patients in whom fluid and sodium intake must be minimized

Children: Emergency initial dose: 25 g; nonemergencies: 25% to 50% of the adult dose

Adults: Depends on condition of patient, usual adult dose is 25 g; no more than 250 g should be administered within 48 hours

Hypoproteinemia: I.V.: 0.5-1 g/kg/dose; repeat every 1-2 days as calculated to replace on-going losses

Hypovolemia: I.V.: 0.5-1 g/kg/dose; repeat as needed; maximum dose: 6 g/kg/day

Dosage Forms Injection: 5% [50 mg/mL] (5 mL, 10 mL, 20 mL, 50 mL, 250 mL, 500 mL, 1000 mL); 25% [250 mg/mL] (10 mL, 20 mL, 50 mL, 100 mL)

Albunex® *see* albumin human *on this page*

Albutein® *see* albumin human *on this page*

albuterol (al byoo' ter ole)

Brand Names Airet®; Proventil®; Ventolin®; Volmax®

Synonyms salbutamol

Therapeutic Category Adrenergic Agonist Agent; Beta-2-Adrenergic Agonist Agent; Bronchodilator

Use Bronchodilator in reversible airway obstruction due to asthma or COPD

Usual Dosage

Oral:

2-6 years: 0.1-0.2 mg/kg/dose 3 times/day; maximum dose not to exceed 12 mg/day (divided doses)

6-12 years: 2 mg/dose 3-4 times/day; maximum dose not to exceed 24 mg/day (divided doses)

>12 years: 2-4 mg/dose 3-4 times/day; maximum dose not to exceed 32 mg/day (divided doses)

Inhalation MDI: 90 mcg/spray:
<12 years: 1-2 inhalations 4 times/day using a tube spacer
≥12 years: 1-2 inhalations every 4-6 hours

Exercise-induced bronchospasm: 2 inhalations 15 minutes before exercising

Inhalation: Nebulization: 2.5 mg = 0.5 mL of the 0.5% inhalation solution to be diluted in 1-2.5 mL of NS
<5 years: 1.25-2.5 mg every 4-6 hours as needed
>5 years: 2.5-5 mg every 4-6 hours

Dosage Forms
Aerosol, oral: 90 mcg/spray [200 inhalations] (17 g)
Capsule, microfine, for inhalation, as sulfate (Rotacaps®): 200 mcg
Solution, inhalation, as sulfate: 0.083% (3 mL); 0.5% (20 mL)
Syrup, as sulfate (strawberry flavor): 2 mg/5 mL (480 mL)
Tablet, as sulfate: 2 mg, 4 mg
Tablet, extended release (Volmax®): 4 mg, 8 mg

Alcaine® Ophthalmic *see* proparacaine hydrochloride *on page 392*

alclometasone dipropionate (al kloe met' a sone)
Brand Names Aclovate® Topical
Therapeutic Category Corticosteroid, Topical (Low Potency)
Use Inflammation of corticosteroid-responsive dermatosis
Usual Dosage Topical: Apply a thin film to the affected area 2-3 times/day
Dosage Forms
Cream: 0.05% (15 g, 45 g)
Ointment, topical: 0.05% (15 g, 45 g)

alcohol, ethyl
Brand Names Lavacol® [OTC]
Synonyms ethanol
Therapeutic Category Intravenous Nutritional Therapy; Pharmaceutical Aid
Use Topical anti-infective; pharmaceutical aid; as an antidote for ethylene glycol overdose; as antidote for methanol overdose
Usual Dosage I.V. doses of 100-125 mg/kg/hour to maintain blood levels of 100 mg/dL are recommended after a loading dose of 0.6 g/kg; maximum dose: 400 mL of a 5% solution within 1 hour
Dosage Forms
Injection, absolute: 2 mL
Liquid, topical, denatured: 70% (473 mL)
Solution, inhalation: 20%, 40%

Alconefrin® Nasal Solution [OTC] *see* phenylephrine hydrochloride *on page 364*

Aldactazide® *see* hydrochlorothiazide and spironolactone *on page 229*

Aldactone® *see* spironolactone *on page 434*

aldesleukin (al des loo' kin)
Brand Names Proleukin®
Synonyms interleukin-2
Therapeutic Category Antineoplastic Agent, Miscellaneous; Biological Response Modulator
(Continued)

11

aldesleukin *(Continued)*

Use Primarily investigated in tumors known to have a response to immunotherapy, such as melanoma and renal cell carcinoma; has been used in conjunction with LAK cells, TIL cells, IL-1, and interferon

Usual Dosage Adults: Metastatic renal cell carcinoma: Treatment consists of two 5-day treatment cycles separated by a rest period; 600,000 units/kg (0.037 mg/kg)/dose administered every 8 hours by a 15-minute I.V. infusion for a total of 14 doses; following 9 days of rest, the schedule is repeated for another 14 doses, maximum: 28 doses/course

Dosage Forms Powder for injection, lyophilized: 22 x 10^6 units [18 million units/mL- 1.1 mg/mL]

Aldoclor® *see* chlorothiazide and methyldopa *on page 92*

Aldomet® *see* methyldopa *on page 298*

Aldoril® *see* methyldopa and hydrochlorothiazide *on page 299*

alendronate *(a len' droe nate)*

Brand Names Fosamax®

Therapeutic Category Antidote, Hypercalcemia; Biphosphonate Derivative

Use Symptomatic treatment of Paget's disease and heterotopic ossification due to spinal cord injury or after total hip replacement, hypercalcemia associated with malignancy

Alersule Forte® *see* chlorpheniramine, phenylephrine and methscopolamine *on page 95*

Aleve® **[OTC]** *see* naproxen *on page 319*

Alfenta® **Injection** *see* alfentanil hydrochloride *on this page*

alfentanil hydrochloride *(al fen' ta nill)*

Brand Names Alfenta® Injection

Therapeutic Category Analgesic, Narcotic

Use Analgesia; analgesia adjunct; anesthetic agent

Usual Dosage Doses should be titrated to appropriate effects; wide range of doses is dependent upon desired degree of analgesia/anesthesia

Children <12 years: Dose not established

Adults: For anesthesia of ≤30 minutes: Initial (induction): 8-20 mcg/kg, then 3-5 mcg/kg/dose or 0.5-1 mcg/kg/minute for maintenance; total dose: 8-40 mcg/kg; higher doses used for longer anesthesia required procedures

Dosage Forms Injection, preservative free: 500 mcg/mL (2 mL, 5 mL, 10 mL, 20 mL)

Alferon® **N** *see* interferon alfa-n3 *on page 247*

alglucerase *(al glue' cir race)*

Brand Names Ceredase® Injection

Synonyms glucocerebrosidase

Therapeutic Category Enzyme, Glucocerebrosidase

Use Orphan drug for treatment of Gaucher's disease

Usual Dosage Usually administered as a 20-60 units/kg I.V. infusion given with a frequency ranging from 3 times/week to once every 2 weeks

Dosage Forms Injection: 10 units/mL (5 mL); 80 units/mL (5 mL)

alimenazine tartrate *see* trimeprazine tartrate *on page 472*

Alkaban-AQ® *see* vinblastine sulfate *on page 487*

Alka-Mints® **[OTC]** *see* calcium carbonate *on page 66*

Alka-Seltzer® Plus Cold Liqui-Gels Capsules [OTC] *see* acetaminophen, chlorpheniramine, and pseudoephedrine *on page 4*

Alkeran® *see* melphalan *on page 285*

Allbee® With C [OTC] *see* vitamin b complex with vitamin c *on page 490*

Aller-Chlor® Oral [OTC] *see* chlorpheniramine maleate *on page 95*

Allerest® 12 Hour Capsule [OTC] *see* chlorpheniramine and phenylpropanolamine *on page 94*

Allerest® 12 Hour Nasal Solution [OTC] *see* oxymetazoline hydrochloride *on page 343*

Allerest® Eye Drops [OTC] *see* naphazoline hydrochloride *on page 319*

Allerfrin® [OTC] *see* triprolidine and pseudoephedrine *on page 474*

Allerfrin® w/Codeine *see* triprolidine, pseudoephedrine, and codeine *on page 475*

Allergan® Ear Drops *see* antipyrine and benzocaine *on page 30*

AllerMax® Oral [OTC] *see* diphenhydramine hydrochloride *on page 149*

Allerphed® [OTC] *see* triprolidine and pseudoephedrine *on page 474*

allopurinol (al oh pure' i nole)
Brand Names Lopurin®; Zyloprim®
Therapeutic Category Uric Acid Lowering Agent; Uricosuric Agent
Use Prevention of attack of gouty arthritis and nephropathy; also used to treat secondary hyperuricemia which may occur during treatment of tumors or leukemia; to prevent recurrent calcium oxalate calculi
Usual Dosage Oral:
Children: 10 mg/kg/day in 2-3 divided doses or 200-300 mg/m^2/day in 2-4 divided doses, maximum: 600 mg/24 hours
  Alternative:
    <6 years: 150 mg/day in 3 divided doses
    6-10 years: 300 mg/day in 2-3 divided doses
Children >10 years and Adults: Daily doses >300 mg should be administered in divided doses
  Myeloproliferative neoplastic disorders: 600-800 mg/day in 2-3 divided doses for prevention of acute uric acid nephropathy for 2-3 days starting 1-2 days before chemotherapy
  Gout: 200-300 mg/day (mild); 400-600 mg/day (severe)
  Maximum dose: 800 mg/day
Dosage Forms Tablet: 100 mg, 300 mg

Alomide® Ophthalmic *see* lodoxamide tromethamine *on page 271*

Alophen Pills® [OTC] *see* phenolphthalein *on page 362*

alpha₁-PI *see* alpha₁-proteinase inhibitor (human) *on this page*

alpha₁-proteinase inhibitor (human)
Brand Names Prolastin® Injection
Synonyms alpha₁-PI
Therapeutic Category Antitrypsin Deficiency Agent
Use Congenital alpha₁-antitrypsin deficiency
Usual Dosage Adults: I.V.: 60 mg/kg once weekly
Dosage Forms Injection, preservative free: ≥20 mg alpha₁-PI/mL (25 mL, 50 mL)

Alphamin® *see* hydroxocobalamin *on page 235*

Alphamul® [OTC] *see* castor oil *on page 78*

AlphaNine® *see* factor ix complex (human) *on page 184*
Alphatrex® *see* betamethasone *on page 52*
Alpidine® *see* apraclonidine hydrochloride *on page 32*

alprazolam (al pray' zoe lam)
Brand Names Xanax⁽ᴿ⁾
Therapeutic Category Antianxiety Agent; Benzodiazepine
Use Treatment of anxiety; adjunct in the treatment of depression; management of panic attacks
Usual Dosage Oral:
Children <18 years: Dose not established

Adults: 0.25-0.5 mg 2-3 times/day, titrate dose upward; maximum: 4 mg/day (anxiety); 10 mg/day (panic attacks)
Dosage Forms
Solution, oral: 0.5 mg/5 mL (2.5 mL, 5 mL, 10 mL, 500 mL); 1 mg/mL (30 mL)
Tablet: 0.25 mg, 0.5 mg, 1 mg, 2 mg

alprostadil (al pross' ta dil)
Brand Names Prostin VR Pediatric⁽ᴿ⁾ Injection
Synonyms pge₁; prostaglandin e₁
Therapeutic Category Prostaglandin
Use Temporary maintenance of patency of ductus arteriosus in neonates with ductal-dependent congenital heart disease until surgery can be performed. These defects include cyanotic (eg, pulmonary atresia, pulmonary stenosis, tricuspid atresia, Fallot's tetralogy, transposition of the great vessels) and acyanotic (eg, interruption of aortic arch, coarctation of aorta, hypoplastic left ventricle) heart disease.
Usual Dosage I.V. continuous infusion into a large vein, or alternatively through an umbilical artery catheter placed at the ductal opening: 0.05-0.1 mcg/kg/minute with therapeutic response, rate is reduced to lowest effective dosage; with unsatisfactory dose, rate is increased gradually; maintenance: 0.01-0.4 mcg/kg/minute

PGE₁ is usually given at an infusion rate of 0.1 mcg/kg/minute, but it is often possible to reduce the dosage to $\frac{1}{2}$ or even $\frac{1}{10}$ without losing the therapeutic effect.
Dosage Forms Injection: 500 mcg/mL (1 mL)

Alramucil® [OTC] *see* psyllium *on page 398*
Altace™ Oral *see* ramipril *on page 406*

alteplase, recombinant (al' te place)
Brand Names Activase⁽ᴿ⁾ Injection
Synonyms tissue plasminogen activator, recombinant; t-pa
Therapeutic Category Thrombolytic Agent
Use Management of acute myocardial infarction for the lysis of thrombi in coronary arteries; management of acute massive pulmonary embolism (PE) in adults
Usual Dosage
Coronary artery thrombi:
Total dose of 100 mg given as 60 mg over the first hour (of which 6-10 mg is used over first 1-2 minutes), 20 mg over the second hour, and 20 mg over the third hour
Adults <65 kg: Total dose of 1.25 mg/kg given as 0.75 mg/kg over the first hour, 0.25 mg/kg over the second hour, and 0.25 mg/kg over the third hour

Acute pulmonary embolism: 100 mg over 2 hours
Dosage Forms Powder for injection, lyophilized: 20 mg [11.6 million units] (20 mL); 50 mg [29 million units] (50 mL)

ALternaGEL® [OTC] *see* aluminum hydroxide *on next page*

altretamine (al tret' a meen)
Brand Names Hexalen®
Synonyms hexamethylmelamine
Therapeutic Category Antineoplastic Agent, Alkylating Agent
Use Palliative treatment of persistent or recurrent ovarian cancer
Usual Dosage Adults: Oral: 260 mg/m^2/day (4 divided doses after meals and at bedtime) for 14 or 21 consecutive days in a 28-day cycle
Dosage Forms Capsule: 50 mg

Alu-Cap® [OTC] *see* aluminum hydroxide *on this page*

Aludrox® [OTC] *see* aluminum hydroxide and magnesium hydroxide *on next page*

aluminum acetate and acetic acid
Brand Names Otic Domeboro®
Therapeutic Category Otic Agent, Anti-infective
Use Treatment of superficial infections of the external auditory canal
Usual Dosage Otic: Instill 4-6 drops in ear(s) every 2-3 hours
Dosage Forms Solution, otic: Aluminum acetate 10% and acetic acid 2% (60 mL)

aluminum acetate and calcium acetate
Brand Names Bluboro® [OTC]; Domeboro® [OTC]; Pedi-Boro® [OTC]
Therapeutic Category Topical Skin Product
Use Astringent wet dressing for relief of inflammatory conditions of the skin and to reduce weeping that may occur in dermatitis
Usual Dosage Topical: Soak affected area in the solution 2-4 times/day for 15-30 minutes or apply wet dressing soaked in the solution 2-4 times/day for 30-minute treatment periods; rewet dressing with solution every few minutes to keep it moist
Dosage Forms
Powder, to make topical solution: 1 packet/pint of water [1:40 solution]
Tablet, effervescent: 1 tablet/pint [1:40 dilution]

aluminum carbonate
Brand Names Basaljel® [OTC]
Therapeutic Category Antacid
Use Hyperacidity; hyperphosphatemia
Usual Dosage Adults: Oral:
Antacid: 2 tablets/capsules or 10 mL of suspension every 2 hours, up to 12 times/day
Hyperphosphatemia: 2 tablets/capsules or 12 mL of suspension with meals
Dosage Forms
Capsule: Equivalent to 500 mg aluminum hydroxide
Suspension: Equivalent to 400 mg/5 mL aluminum hydroxide
Tablet: Equivalent to 500 mg aluminum hydroxide

aluminum chloride hexahydrate
Brand Names Drysol™
Therapeutic Category Topical Skin Product
Use Astringent in the management of hyperhidrosis
Usual Dosage Adults: Topical: Apply at bedtime
Dosage Forms Solution, topical: 20% in SD alcohol 40 (35 mL, 37.5 mL)

aluminum hydroxide
Brand Names ALternaGEL® [OTC]; Alu-Cap® [OTC]; Alu-Tab® [OTC]; Amphojel® [OTC]; Dialume® [OTC]; Nephrox Suspension [OTC]
Therapeutic Category Antacid; Antidote, Hyperphosphatemia
Use Hyperacidity; hyperphosphatemia
(Continued)

aluminum hydroxide *(Continued)*
Usual Dosage Oral:
Peptic ulcer disease:
Children: 5-15 mL/dose every 3-6 hours or 1 and 3 hours after meals and at bedtime
Adults: 15-45 mL every 3-6 hours or 1 and 3 hours after meals and at bedtime

Prophylaxis against gastrointestinal bleeding:
Infants: 2-5 mL/dose every 1-2 hours
Children: 5-15 mL/dose every 1-2 hours
Adults: 30-60 mL/dose every hour
Titrate to maintain the gastric pH >5

Hyperphosphatemia:
Children: 50 mg to 150 mg/kg/24 hours in divided doses every 4-6 hours, titrate dosage to maintain serum phosphorus within normal range
Adults: 500-1800 mg, 3-6 times/day, between meals and at bedtime

Antacid: Adults: 30 mL 1 and 3 hours postprandial and at bedtime
Dosage Forms
Capsule: 475 mg, 500 mg
Gel: 600 mg/5 mL (360 mL)
Suspension, oral: 320 mg/5 mL (500 mL)
Tablet: 300 mg, 500 mg, 600 mg

aluminum hydroxide and magnesium carbonate
Brand Names Gaviscon® Liquid [OTC]
Therapeutic Category Antacid
Use Temporary relief of symptoms associated with gastric acidity
Usual Dosage Adults: Oral: 15-30 mL 4 times/day after meals and at bedtime
Dosage Forms Liquid: Aluminum hydroxide 95 mg and magnesium carbonate 358 mg (15 mL)

aluminum hydroxide and magnesium hydroxide
Brand Names Aludrox™ [OTC]; Maalox® [OTC]; Maalox® Therapeutic Concentrate [OTC]
Synonyms magnesium hydroxide and aluminum hydroxide
Therapeutic Category Antacid
Use Antacid, hyperphosphatemia in renal failure
Usual Dosage Adults: Oral: 5-10 mL or 1-2 tablets 4-6 times/day, between meals and at bedtime; may be used every hour for severe symptoms
Dosage Forms
Suspension:
Aludrox™: Aluminum hydroxide 307 mg and magnesium hydroxide 103 mg per 5 mL
Maalox™: Aluminum hydroxide 225 mg and magnesium hydroxide 200 mg per 5 mL
High potency (Maalox™ TC): Aluminum hydroxide 600 mg and magnesium hydroxide 300 mg per 5 mL
Tablet, chewable (Maalox™): Aluminum hydroxide 600 mg and magnesium hydroxide 300 mg

aluminum hydroxide and magnesium trisilicate
Brand Names Gaviscon®-2 Tablet [OTC]; Gaviscon® Tablet [OTC]
Therapeutic Category Antacid
Use Temporary relief of hyperacidity
Usual Dosage Adults: Oral: Chew 2-4 tablets 4 times/day or as directed by physician
Dosage Forms Tablet, chewable:
Gaviscon™: Aluminum hydroxide 80 mg and magnesium trisilicate 20 mg
Gaviscon™-2: Aluminum hydroxide 160 mg and magnesium trisilicate 40 mg

aluminum hydroxide, magnesium hydroxide, and simethicone
Brand Names Di-Gel™ [OTC]; Gelusil™ [OTC]; Maalox® Plus [OTC]; Mylanta® [OTC]; Mylanta™-II [OTC]
Therapeutic Category Antacid; Antiflatulent

Use Temporary relief of hyperacidity associated with gas; may also be used for indications associated with other antacids

Usual Dosage Adults: 15-30 mL or 2-4 tablets 4-6 times/day between meals and at bedtime; may be used every hour for severe symptoms

Dosage Forms
Liquid:
Gelusil", Mylanta": Aluminum hydroxide 200 mg, magnesium hydroxide, 200 mg, and simethicone 25 mg per 5 mL
Maalox" Plus: Aluminum hydroxide 225 mg, magnesium hydroxide 200 mg, and simethicone 25 mg per 5 mL (30 mL, 180 mL)
Mylanta"-II: Aluminum hydroxide 400 mg, magnesium hydroxide 400 mg, and simethicone 40 mg per 5 mL (150 mL, 360 mL)
Tablet, chewable:
Mylanta®: Aluminum hydroxide 200 mg, magnesium hydroxide 200 mg, and simethicone 20 mg
Mylanta®-II: Aluminum hydroxide 400 mg, magnesium hydroxide 400 mg, and simethicone 40 mg

aluminum phosphate

Brand Names Phosphaljel® [OTC]
Therapeutic Category Electrolyte Supplement, Oral
Use Reduce fecal excretion of phosphates
Usual Dosage Adults: Oral: 15-30 mL every 2 hours between meals
Dosage Forms Suspension, oral: 233 mg/5 mL

aluminum sucrose sulfate, basic see sucralfate on page 438

Alupent® see metaproterenol sulfate on page 290

Alu-Tab® [OTC] see aluminum hydroxide on page 15

amantadine hydrochloride (a man' ta deen)

Brand Names Symadine®; Symmetrel®
Synonyms adamantanamine hydrochloride
Therapeutic Category Anti-Parkinson's Agent; Antiviral Agent, Oral
Use Symptomatic and adjunct treatment of parkinsonism; also used in prophylaxis and treatment of influenza A viral infection
Usual Dosage
Children:
1-9 years: 4.4-8.8 mg/kg/day in 1-2 divided doses to a maximum of 150 mg/day
9-12 years: 100-200 mg/day in 1-2 divided doses
After first influenza A virus vaccine dose, amantadine prophylaxis may be administered for up to 6 weeks or until 2 weeks after the second dose of vaccine
Adults:
Parkinson's disease: 100 mg twice daily
Influenza A viral infection: 200 mg/day in 1-2 divided doses
Prophylaxis: Minimum 10-day course of therapy following exposure or continue for 2-3 weeks after influenza A virus vaccine is given
Elderly patients should take the drug in 2 daily doses rather than a single dose to avoid adverse neurologic reactions
Dosage Forms
Capsule: 100 mg
Syrup: 50 mg/5 mL (480 mL)

Amaphen® see butalbital compound on page 63

ambenonium chloride (am be noe' nee um)

Brand Names Mytelase® Caplets®
Therapeutic Category Cholinergic Agent
Use Treatment of myasthenia gravis
(Continued)

ambenonium chloride *(Continued)*
Usual Dosage Adults: Oral: 5-25 mg 3-4 times/day
Dosage Forms Tablet: 10 mg

Ambenyl® Cough Syrup *see bromodiphenhydramine and codeine on page 58*
Ambi 10® [OTC] *see benzoyl peroxide on page 50*
Ambien™ *see zolpidem tartrate on page 496*

amcinonide *(am sin' oh nide)*
Brand Names Cyclocort® Topical
Therapeutic Category Corticosteroid, Topical (Medium/High Potency)
Use Relief of the inflammatory and pruritic manifestations of corticosteroid-responsive dermatoses
Usual Dosage Adults: Topical: Apply in a thin film 2-3 times/day
Dosage Forms
Cream: 0.1% (15 g, 30 g, 60 g)
Lotion: 0.1% (20 mL, 60 mL)
Ointment, topical: 0.1% (15 g, 30 g, 60 g)

Amcort® *see triamcinolone on page 467*
Amen® Oral *see medroxyprogesterone acetate on page 283*
Americaine® [OTC] *see benzocaine on page 48*
Amesec® [OTC] *see aminophylline, amobarbital, and ephedrine on page 20*
A-methaPred® Injection *see methylprednisolone on page 300*
amethocaine hydrochloride *see tetracaine hydrochloride on page 450*
amethopterin *see methotrexate on page 295*
amfepramone *see diethylpropion hydrochloride on page 143*
Amgenal® Cough Syrup *see bromodiphenhydramine and codeine on page 58*
Amicar® *see aminocaproic acid on next page*
Amidate® Injection *see etomidate on page 183*

amikacin sulfate *(am i kay' sin)*
Brand Names Amikin® Injection
Therapeutic Category Antibiotic, Aminoglycoside
Use Treatment of documented gram-negative enteric infection resistant to gentamicin and tobramycin; documented infection of mycobacterial organisms susceptible to amikacin
Usual Dosage I.M., I.V.:
Neonates:
<1200 g, 0-4 weeks: 7.5 mg/kg/dose every 12 hours
Postnatal age <7 days:
1200-2000 g: 7.5 mg/kg/dose every 12 hours
>2000 g: 10 mg/kg/dose every 12 hours
Postnatal age >7 days:
1200-2000 g: 7 mg/kg/dose every 8 hours
>2000 g: 7.5-10 mg/kg/dose every 8 hours

Infants and Children: 15-20 mg/kg/day divided every 8 hours

Adults: 15 mg/kg/day divided every 8-12 hours
Dosage Forms Injection: 50 mg/mL (2 mL, 4 mL); 250 mg/mL (2 mL, 4 mL)

Amikin® Injection *see amikacin sulfate on this page*

amiloride and hydrochlorothiazide
Brand Names Moduretic®
Synonyms hydrochlorothiazide and amiloride
Therapeutic Category Diuretic, Combination
Use Antikaliuretic diuretic, antihypertensive
Usual Dosage Adults: Oral: Initial: 1 tablet daily, then may be increased to 2 tablets/day if needed; usually given in a single dose
Dosage Forms Tablet: Amiloride hydrochloride 5 mg and hydrochlorothiazide 50 mg

amiloride hydrochloride (a mill' oh ride)
Brand Names Midamor®
Therapeutic Category Diuretic, Potassium Sparing
Use Counteract potassium loss induced by other diuretics in the treatment of hypertension or edematous conditions including CHF, hepatic cirrhosis and hypoaldosteronism; usually used in conjunction with a more potent diuretic such as thiazides or loop diuretics
Usual Dosage Oral:
Children: Although safety and efficacy have not been established by the FDA in children, a dosage of 0.625 mg/kg/day has been used in children weighing 6-20 kg

Adults: 5-10 mg/day (up to 20 mg)
Dosage Forms Tablet: 5 mg

2-amino-6-mercaptopurine *see* thioguanine *on page 456*
aminobenzylpenicillin *see* ampicillin *on page 26*

aminocaproic acid (a mee noe ka proe' ik)
Brand Names Amicar®
Therapeutic Category Hemostatic Agent
Use Treatment of excessive bleeding from fibrinolysis
Usual Dosage In the management of acute bleeding syndromes, oral dosage regimens are the same as the I.V. dosage regimens in adults and children

Chronic bleeding: Oral, I.V.: 5-30 g/day in divided doses at 3- to 6-hour intervals

Acute bleeding syndrome:
Children: Oral, I.V.: 100 mg/kg or 3 g/m^2 during the first hour, followed by continuous infusion at the rate of 33.3 mg/kg/hour or 1 g/m^2/hour; total dosage should not exceed 18 g/m^2/24 hours
Adults:
Oral: For elevated fibrinolytic activity, give 5 g during first hour, followed by 1-1.25 g/hour for approximately 8 hours or until bleeding stops
I.V.: Give 4-5 g in 250 mL of diluent during first hour followed by continuous infusion at the rate of 1-1.25 g/hour in 50 mL of diluent, continue for 8 hours or until bleeding stops
Dosage Forms
Injection: 250 mg/mL (20 mL, 96 mL, 100 mL)
Syrup (raspberry flavor): 250 mg/mL (480 mL)
Tablet: 500 mg

Amino-Cerv™ Vaginal Cream *see* urea *on page 480*

aminoglutethimide (a mee noe gloo teth' i mide)
Brand Names Cytadren®
Therapeutic Category Antiadrenal Agent; Antineoplastic Agent, Adjuvant
Use Suppression of adrenal function in selected patients with Cushing's syndrome; also used successfully in postmenopausal patients with advanced breast carcinoma and in patients with metastatic prostate carcinoma
Usual Dosage Adults: Oral: 250 mg every 6 hours may be increased to a total of 2 g/day; give in divided doses, 2-3 times/day to reduce incidence of nausea and vomiting
Dosage Forms Tablet: 250 mg

Amino-Opti-E® Oral [OTC] *see* vitamin e *on page 490*
Aminophyllin® *see* aminophylline *on this page*

aminophylline (am in off' i lin)
Brand Names Aminophyllin®; Phyllocontin®; Somophyllin®; Truphylline®
Synonyms theophylline ethylenediamine
Therapeutic Category Antiasthmatic; Bronchodilator; Theophylline Derivative
Use Bronchodilator in reversible airway obstruction due to asthma or COPD; for neonatal idiopathic apnea/bradycardia spells
Usual Dosage All dosages based upon **aminophylline**
Neonates: Apnea of prematurity:
Loading dose: 5 mg/kg for one dose
Maintenance: I.V.:
0-24 days: Begin at 2 mg/kg/day divided every 12 hours and titrate to desired levels and effects
>24 days: 3 mg/kg/day divided every 12 hours; increased dosages may be indicated as liver metabolism matures (usually >30 days of life); monitor serum levels to determine appropriate dosages
Theophylline levels should be initially drawn after 3 days of therapy; repeat levels are indicated 3 days after each increase in dosage or weekly if on a stabilized dosage

Treatment of acute bronchospasm:
Loading dose (in patients not currently receiving aminophylline or theophylline): 6 mg/kg (based on aminophylline) given I.V. over 20-30 minutes; administration rate should not exceed 25 mg/minute (aminophylline)

Approximate I.V. maintenance dosages are based upon **continuous infusions**; bolus dosing (often used in children <6 months of age) may be determined by multiplying the hourly infusion rate by 24 hours and dividing by the desired number of doses/day
Infants 6 weeks to 6 months: 0.5 mg/kg/hour
Children:
6 months to 1 year: 0.6-0.7 mg/kg/hour
1-9 years: 1-1.2 mg/kg/hour
12-16 years: 0.7 mg/kg/hour
9-12 years and young adult smokers: 0.9 mg/kg/hour
Adults (healthy, nonsmoking): 0.7 mg/kg/hour
Elderly and patients with cor pulmonale with congestive heart failure or liver failure: 0.25 mg/kg/hour
Dosage should be adjusted according to serum level measurements during the first 12- to 24-hour period. Avoid using suppositories due to erratic, unreliable absorption.
Rectal: Adults: 500 mg 3 times/day
Dosage Forms
Injection, I.V.: 25 mg/mL (10 mL, 20 mL)
Liquid, oral: 105 mg/5 mL (240 mL)
Suppository, rectal (Truphylline®): 250 mg, 500 mg
Tablet: 100 mg, 200 mg
Tablet, controlled release [12 hours] (Phyllocontin®): 225 mg

aminophylline, amobarbital, and ephedrine
Brand Names Amesec® [OTC]
Therapeutic Category Antiasthmatic; Bronchodilator
Use Symptomatic relief of asthma
Usual Dosage Adults: Oral: 1 capsule every 6 hours
Dosage Forms Capsule: Aminophylline 130 mg, amobarbital 24 mg, and ephedrine sulfate 24 mg

aminosalicylate sodium (a mee noe sal i sill' ik)
Brand Names Sodium P.A.S.
Therapeutic Category Antitubercular Agent; Nonsteroidal Anti-Inflammatory Agent (NSAID), Oral

Use Treatment of tuberculosis with combination drugs
Usual Dosage Oral:
  Children: 150-300 mg/kg/day in 3-4 equally divided doses
  Adults: 150 mg/kg/day in 2-3 equally divided doses (usually 12-14 g/day)
Dosage Forms Tablet: 500 mg

aminosalicylic acid
Brand Names Paser®
Therapeutic Category Antitubercular Agent; Nonsteroidal Anti-Inflammatory Agent (NSAID), Oral
Use Treatment of tuberculosis with combination drugs
Usual Dosage Oral: Sprinkle on acidic drink/food 3 times daily
Dosage Forms Granules: 4 g per packet

aminosalicylate sodium *see* para-aminosalicylate sodium *on page 348*

5-aminosalicylic acid *see* mesalamine *on page 289*

amiodarone hydrochloride (a mee' oh da rone)
Brand Names Cordarone®
Therapeutic Category Antiarrhythmic Agent, Class III
Use Management of resistant, life-threatening ventricular arrhythmias unresponsive to conventional therapy with less toxic agents; has also been used for treatment of supraventricular arrhythmias unresponsive to conventional therapy
Usual Dosage Children <1 year should be dosed as calculated by body surface area
  Children: Loading dose: 10-15 mg/kg/day or 600-800 mg/1.73 m²/day for 4-14 days or until adequate control of arrhythmia or prominent adverse effects occur (this loading dose may be given in 1-2 divided doses/day); dosage should then be reduced to 5 mg/kg/day or 200-400 mg/1.73 m²/day given once daily for several weeks; if arrhythmia does not recur reduce to lowest effective dosage possible; usual daily minimal dose: 2.5 mg/kg; maintenance doses may be given for 5 of 7 days/week.

  Adults: Ventricular arrhythmias: 800-1600 mg/day in 1-2 doses for 1-3 weeks, then 600-800 mg/day in 1-2 doses for 1 month; maintenance: 400 mg/day; lower doses are recommended for supraventricular arrhythmias, usually 100-400 mg/day
Dosage Forms Tablet: 200 mg

Ami-Tex LA® *see* guaifenesin and phenylpropanolamine *on page 215*

Amitone® [OTC] *see* calcium carbonate *on page 66*

amitriptyline and chlordiazepoxide
Brand Names Limbitrol®
Synonyms chlordiazepoxide and amitriptyline
Therapeutic Category Antidepressant, Tricyclic; Antipsychotic Agent
Use Treatment of moderate to severe anxiety and/or agitation and depression
Usual Dosage Oral: Initial dose: 3-4 tablets in divided doses; this may be increased to 6 tablets/day as required; some patients respond to smaller doses and can be maintained on 2 tablets
Dosage Forms Tablet:
  5-12.5: Amitriptyline hydrochloride 12.5 mg and chlordiazepoxide 5 mg
  10-25: Amitriptyline hydrochloride 25 mg and chlordiazepoxide 10 mg

amitriptyline and perphenazine
Brand Names Etrafon®; Triavil®
Synonyms perphenazine and amitriptyline
Therapeutic Category Antidepressant, Tricyclic; Benzodiazepine
(Continued)

21

amitriptyline and perphenazine *(Continued)*
Use Treatment of patients with moderate to severe anxiety and depression
Usual Dosage Oral: 1 tablet 2-4 times/day
Dosage Forms Tablet:
  2-10: Amitriptyline hydrochloride 10 mg and perphenazine 2 mg
  4-10: Amitriptyline hydrochloride 10 mg and perphenazine 4 mg
  2-25: Amitriptyline hydrochloride 25 mg and perphenazine 2 mg
  4-25: Amitriptyline hydrochloride 25 mg and perphenazine 4 mg
  4-50: Amitriptyline hydrochloride 50 mg and perphenazine 4 mg

amitriptyline hydrochloride (a mee trip' ti leen)
Brand Names Elavil®; Endep®; Enovil®
Therapeutic Category Antidepressant, Tricyclic
Use Treatment of various forms of depression, often in conjunction with psychotherapy; as an analgesic for certain chronic and neuropathic pain, migraine prophylaxis
Usual Dosage
Children <12 years: Not recommended

Adolescents: Oral: Initial: 25-50 mg/day; may give in divided doses; increase gradually to 100 mg/day in divided doses

Adults:
  Oral: 30-100 mg/day single dose at bedtime or in divided doses; dose may be gradually increased up to 300 mg/day; once symptoms are controlled, decrease gradually to lowest effective dose
  I.M.: 20-30 mg 4 times/day
Dosage Forms
Injection: 10 mg/mL (10 mL)
Tablet: 10 mg, 25 mg, 50 mg, 75 mg, 100 mg, 150 mg

amlodipine (am loe' di peen)
Brand Names Norvasc™
Therapeutic Category Calcium Channel Blocker
Use Treatment of hypertension and angina
Usual Dosage Oral: Adults: 2.5-10 mg once daily
Dosage Forms Tablet: 2.5 mg, 5 mg, 10 mg

ammonia spirit, aromatic
Brand Names Aromatic Ammonia Aspirols®
Therapeutic Category Respiratory Stimulant
Use Respiratory and circulatory stimulant, treatment of fainting
Usual Dosage Used as "smelling salts" to treat or prevent fainting
Dosage Forms
Inhalant, crushable glass perles: 0.33 mL, 0.4 mL
Solution: 30 mL, 60 mL, 120 mL

ammonium chloride
Therapeutic Category Metabolic Alkalosis Agent; Urinary Acidifying Agent
Use Diuretic or systemic and urinary acidifying agent; treatment of hypochloremic states
Usual Dosage The following equations represent different methods of correction utilizing either the serum HCO_3^-, the serum Cl^- or the base excess

Correction of refractory hypochloremic metabolic alkalosis: Dose mEq = 0.5 (L/kg) x wt (kg) x [serum HCO_3-24] mEq/L; give $\frac{1}{2}$ to $\frac{2}{3}$ of the calculated dose, then re-evaluate

Correction of hypochloremia: mEq NH_4Cl = 0.2 L/kg x wt x [103 - serum Cl^-] mEq/L, give $\frac{1}{2}$ to $\frac{2}{3}$ of calculated dose, then re-evaluate

Correction of alkalosis: mEq NH_4Cl = 0.3 L/kg x wt (kg) x base excess (mEq/L), give $\frac{1}{2}$ to $\frac{2}{3}$ of calculated dose, then re-evaluate

Children: Oral, I.V.: 75 mg/kg/day in 4 divided doses for urinary acidification; maximum daily dose: 6 g

Adults:
Oral: 2-3 g every 6 hours
I.V.: 1.5 g/dose every 6 hours
Dosage Forms
Injection: 26.75% [5 mEq/mL] (20 mL)
Tablet: 500 mg
Tablet, enteric coated: 500 mg

ammonium lactate see lactic acid with ammonium hydroxide on page 261
Amnipaque® see radiological/contrast media (non-ionic) on page 406

amobarbital (am oh bar' bi tal)
Brand Names Amytal®
Synonyms amylobarbitone
Therapeutic Category Barbiturate; Hypnotic; Sedative
Use
Oral: Hypnotic in short-term treatment of insomnia, to reduce anxiety and provide sedation preoperatively
I.M., I.V.: Used to control status epilepticus or acute seizure episodes; also used in catatonic, negativistic, or manic reactions and in "Amytal® Interviewing" for narcoanalysis
Usual Dosage
Children: Oral:
Insomnia: 2 mg/kg or 70 mg/m^2/day in 4 equally divided doses
Hypnotic: 2-3 mg/kg

Adults:
Insomnia: Oral: 65-200 mg at bedtime
Sedation: Oral: 30-50 mg 2-3 times/day
Preanesthetic: Oral: 200 mg 1-2 hours before surgery
Hypnotic:
Oral: 65-200 mg at bedtime
I.M.: 65-500 mg, should not exceed 500 mg
I.V.: 65-500 mg, should not exceed 1000 mg
Dosage Forms
Capsule, as sodium: 65 mg, 200 mg
Powder: 15 g, 30 g
Powder for injection, as sodium: 250 mg, 500 mg
Tablet: 30 mg, 50 mg, 100 mg

amobarbital and secobarbital
Brand Names Tuinal®
Synonyms secobarbital and amobarbital
Therapeutic Category Barbiturate; Hypnotic
Use Short-term treatment of insomnia
Usual Dosage Adults: Oral: 1-2 capsules at bedtime
Dosage Forms Capsule:
100: Amobarbital 50 mg and secobarbital 50 mg
200: Amobarbital 100 mg and secobarbital 100 mg

amoxapine (a mox' a peen)
Brand Names Asendin®
Therapeutic Category Antidepressant, Tricyclic
Use Treatment of neurotic and endogenous depression and mixed symptoms of anxiety and depression
(Continued)

amoxapine *(Continued)*

Usual Dosage Oral (once symptoms are controlled, decrease gradually to lowest effective dose):

Children: Not established in children <16 years

Adolescents: Initial: 25-50 mg/day; increase gradually to 100 mg/day; may give as divided doses or as a single dose at bedtime

Adults: Initial: 25 mg 2-3 times/day, if tolerated, dosage may be increased to 100 mg 2-3 times/day; may be given in a single bedtime dose when dosage <300 mg/day

Maximum daily dose:
Outpatient: 400 mg
Inpatient: 600 mg

Dosage Forms Tablet: 25 mg, 50 mg, 100 mg, 150 mg

amoxicillin and clavulanate potassium *see* amoxicillin and clavulanic acid
on this page

amoxicillin and clavulanic acid

Brand Names Augmentin®
Synonyms amoxicillin and clavulanate potassium
Therapeutic Category Antibiotic, Penicillin
Use Infections caused by susceptible organisms involving the lower respiratory tract, otitis media, sinusitis, skin and skin structure, and urinary tract
Usual Dosage Oral:
Children <40 kg: 20-40 mg (amoxicillin component)/kg/day in divided doses every 8 hours
Children >40 kg and Adults: 250-500 mg every 8 hours; maximum dose: 2 g/day
Dosage Forms
Suspension, oral (banana flavor):
125: Amoxicillin trihydrate 125 mg and clavulanic acid 31.25 mg per 5 mL (75 mL, 150 mL)
250: Amoxicillin trihydrate 250 mg and clavulanic acid 62.5 mg per 5 mL (75 mL, 150 mL)
Tablet:
250: Amoxicillin trihydrate 250 mg and clavulanic acid 125 mg
500: Amoxicillin trihydrate 500 mg and clavulanic acid 125 mg
Tablet, chewable:
125: Amoxicillin trihydrate 125 mg and clavulanic acid 31.25 mg
250: Amoxicillin trihydrate 250 mg and clavulanic acid 62.5 mg

amoxicillin trihydrate *(a mox i sill' in)*

Brand Names Amoxil®; Biomox®; Polymox®; Trimox®; Wymox®
Synonyms amoxycillin; *p*-hydroxyampicillin
Therapeutic Category Antibiotic, Penicillin
Use Infections caused by susceptible organisms involving the respiratory tract, otitis media, sinusitis, skin, and urinary tract; prophylaxis of bacterial endocarditis
Usual Dosage Oral:
Children: 25-50 mg/kg/day in divided doses every 8 hours
Uncomplicated gonorrhea: ≥2 years: 50 mg/kg plus probenecid 25 mg/kg in a single dose; do not use this regimen in children <2 years of age, probenecid is contraindicated in this age group
SBE prophylaxis: 50 mg/kg 1 hour before procedure and 25 mg/kg 6 hours later; not to exceed adult dosage

Adults: 250-500 mg every 8 hours; maximum dose: 2-3 g/day
Uncomplicated gonorrhea: 3 g plus probenecid 1 g in a single dose
Endocarditis prophylaxis: 3 g 1 hour before procedure and 1.5 g 6 hours later
Dosage Forms
Capsule: 250 mg, 500 mg
Powder for oral suspension: 125 mg/5 mL (5 mL, 80 mL, 100 mL, 150 mL, 200 mL); 250 mg/5 mL (5 mL, 80 mL, 100 mL, 150 mL, 200 mL)
Powder for oral suspension, drops: 50 mg/mL (15 mL, 30 mL)
Tablet, chewable: 125 mg, 250 mg

Amoxil® *see* amoxicillin trihydrate *on previous page*

amoxycillin *see* amoxicillin trihydrate *on previous page*

amphetamine sulfate (am fet' a meen)
Synonyms racemic amphetamine sulfate

Therapeutic Category Amphetamine; Central Nervous System Stimulant, Amphetamine

Use Narcolepsy; exogenous obesity; abnormal behavioral syndrome in children (minimal brain dysfunction); attention deficit hyperactive disorder (ADHD)

Usual Dosage Oral:
Narcolepsy:
Children:
6-12 years: 5 mg/day, increase by 5 mg at weekly intervals
>12 years: 10 mg/day, increase by 10 mg at weekly intervals
Adults: 5-60 mg/day in divided doses

Minimal brain dysfunction: Children:
3-5 years: 2.5 mg/day, increase by 2.5 mg at weekly intervals
>6 years: 5 mg/day, increase by 5 mg at weekly intervals

Short-term adjunct to exogenous obesity: Children >12 years and Adults: 10 mg or 15 mg long-acting capsule daily, up to 30 mg/day; or 5-30 mg/day in divided doses (immediate release tablets only)

Dosage Forms Tablet: 5 mg, 10 mg

ampho *see* amphotericin B *on this page*

Amphojel® [OTC] *see* aluminum hydroxide *on page 15*

amphotericin B (am foe ter' i sin)
Brand Names Fungizone®

Synonyms ampho

Therapeutic Category Antifungal Agent, Systemic; Antifungal Agent, Topical

Use Treatment of severe systemic infections and meningitis caused by susceptible fungi; fungal peritonitis; irrigant for bladder fungal infections; and topically for cutaneous and mucocutaneous candidal infections

Usual Dosage The minimum dilution for amphotericin B infusions is 0.1 mg/mL for peripheral lines and 1 mg/mL for central lines

Infants and Children:
Test dose: I.V.: 0.1 mg/kg/dose to a maximum of 1 mg; infuse over 30-60 minutes. If the test dose is tolerated, the initial therapeutic dose is 0.25 mg/kg. The daily dose can then be gradually increased, usually in 0.25 mg/kg increments on each subsequent day until the desired daily dose is reached.
Maintenance dose: 0.25-1 mg/kg/day given once daily; infuse over 2-6 hours. Once therapy has been established, amphotericin B can be administered on an every other day basis at 1-1.5 mg/kg/dose.
I.T.: 25-100 mcg every 48-72 hours; increase to 500 mcg as tolerated

Adults:
Test dose: I.V.: 1 mg infused over 20-30 minutes. Institute therapy with 0.25 mg/kg administered over 2-6 hours; the daily dose can be gradually increased on subsequent days to the desired level.
Maintenance dose: I.V.: 0.25-1 mg/kg/day or 1.5 mg/kg every other day; do not exceed 1.5 mg/kg/day. If the test dose is tolerated, the initial therapeutic dose is 0.25 mg/kg. The daily dose can then be gradually increased, usually in 0.25 mg/kg increments on each subsequent day until the desired daily dose is reached.
Duration of therapy varies with nature of infection: Histoplasmosis, *Cryptococcus*, or blastomycosis may be treated with total dose of 2-4 g
I.T.: 25-300 mcg every 48-72 hours; increase to 500 mcg to 1 mg as tolerated

Children and Adults:
Bladder irrigation: 50 mg/day in 1 L of sterile water irrigation solution instilled over 24 hours for 2-7 days or until cultures are clear

(Continued)

amphotericin B *(Continued)*

Dialysate: 1-2 mg/L of peritoneal dialysis fluid either with or without low-dose I.V. amphotericin B (a total dose of 2-10 mg/kg given over 7-14 days)

Topical: Apply to affected areas 2-4 times/day for 1-4 weeks of therapy depending on nature and severity of infection

Dosage Forms
Cream: 3% (20 g)
Lotion: 3% (30 mL)
Ointment, topical: 3% (20 g)
Powder for injection, lyophilized: 50 mg

ampicillin (am pi sill' in)

Brand Names Marcillin™; Omnipen®; Omnipen®-N; Polycillin®; Polycillin-N®; Principen®; Totacillin™; Totacillin™-N

Synonyms aminobenzylpenicillin

Therapeutic Category Antibiotic, Penicillin

Use Treatment of susceptible bacterial infections

Usual Dosage
Neonates: I.M., I.V.:
Postnatal age <7 days:
<2000 g: 50 mg/kg/day in 2 divided doses; meningitis: 100 mg/kg/day in 2 divided doses
>2000 g: 75 mg/kg/day in 3 divided doses; meningitis: 150 mg/kg/day in 3 divided doses
Postnatal age >7 days:
<2000 g: 75 mg/kg/day in 3 divided doses; meningitis: 150 mg/kg/day in 3 divided doses
>2000 g: 100 mg/kg/day in 4 divided doses; meningitis: 200 mg/kg/day in 4 divided doses

Infants and Children:
Oral: 50-100 mg/kg/day divided every 6 hours; maximum dose: 2-3 g/day
I.M., I.V.: 100-200 mg/kg/day in 4-6 divided doses; meningitis: 200-400 mg/kg/day in 4-6 divided doses; maximum dose: 12 g/day

Adults:
Oral: 250-500 mg every 6 hours
I.M., I.V.: 8-12 g/day in 4-6 divided doses

Dosage Forms
Capsule, as anhydrous: 250 mg, 500 mg
Capsule, as trihydrate: 250 mg, 500 mg
Powder for injection, as sodium: 125 mg, 250 mg, 500 mg, 1 g, 2 g, 10 g
Powder for oral suspension, as trihydrate: 125 mg/5 mL (5 mL unit dose, 80 mL, 100 mL, 150 mL, 200 mL); 250 mg/5 mL (5 mL unit dose, 80 mL, 100 mL, 150 mL, 200 mL); 500 mg/5 mL (5 mL unit dose, 100 mL)
Powder for oral suspension, drops, as trihydrate: 100 mg/mL (20 mL)

ampicillin and probenecid

Brand Names Polycillin-PRB™; Proampacin®

Therapeutic Category Antibiotic, Penicillin

Use Uncomplicated infections caused by susceptible strains of *Neisseria gonorrhoeae* in adults

Usual Dosage Administer the entire contents of bottle as a single one time dose

Dosage Forms Powder for oral suspension: Ampicillin 3.5 g and probenecid 1 g per bottle

ampicillin sodium and sulbactam sodium

Brand Names Unasyn™

Synonyms sulbactam and ampicillin

Therapeutic Category Antibiotic, Penicillin

Use Treatment of susceptible bacterial infections involved with skin and skin structure, intra-abdominal infections, gynecological infections; spectrum is that of ampicillin plus organisms producing beta-lactamases such as *S. aureus*, *H. influenzae*, *E. coli*, *Klebsiella*, *Acinetobacter*, *Enterobacter* and anaerobes

Usual Dosage Not FDA approved for children <12 years of age

Unasyn® (ampicillin/sulbactam) is a combination product. Each 3 g vial contains 2 g of ampicillin and 1 g of sulbactam. Sulbactam has very little antibacterial activity by itself, but effectively extends the spectrum of ampicillin to include beta-lactamase producing strains that are resistant to ampicillin alone. Therefore, dosage recommendations for Unasyn® are based on the ampicillin component.

Children: I.M., I.V.: 100-200 mg ampicillin/kg/day divided every 6 hours; maximum dose: 8 g ampicillin/day

Adults: I.M., I.V.: 1-2 g ampicillin every 6-8 hours; maximum dose: 8 g ampicillin/day

Dosage Forms Powder for injection: 1.5 g [ampicillin sodium 1 g and sulbactam sodium 0.5 g]; 3 g [ampicillin sodium 2 g and sulbactam sodium 1 g]

amrinone lactate (am' ri none)

Brand Names Inocor®

Therapeutic Category Adrenergic Agonist Agent

Use Treatment of low cardiac output states (sepsis, congestive heart failure); adjunctive therapy of pulmonary hypertension; normally prescribed for patients who have not responded well to therapy with digitalis, diuretics, and vasodilators

Usual Dosage Dosage is based on clinical response. **Note:** Dose should not exceed 10 mg/kg/24 hours.

Neonates: 0.75 mg/kg I.V. bolus over 2-3 minutes followed by maintenance infusion 3-5 mcg/kg/minute; I.V. bolus may need to be repeated in 30 minutes

Children: 0.75 mg/kg I.V. bolus over 2-3 minutes followed by maintenance infusion 5-10 mcg/kg/minute; I.V. bolus may need to be repeated in 30 minutes

Adults: 0.75 mg/kg I.V. bolus over 2-3 minutes followed by maintenance infusion of 5-10 mcg/kg/minute

Dosage Forms Injection: 5 mg/mL (20 mL)

Amvisc® *see* sodium hyaluronate *on page 428*

amyl nitrite

Synonyms isoamyl nitrite

Therapeutic Category Vasodilator, Coronary

Use Coronary vasodilator in angina pectoris; an adjunct in treatment of cyanide poisoning; also used to produce changes in the intensity of heart murmurs

Usual Dosage 1-6 inhalations from 1 capsule are usually sufficient to produce the desired effect

Dosage Forms Inhalant, crushable glass perles: 0.18 mL, 0.3 mL

amylobarbitone *see* amobarbital *on page 23*

Amytal® *see* amobarbital *on page 23*

Anabolin® Injection *see* nandrolone *on page 318*

Anacin® [OTC] *see* aspirin *on page 35*

Anadrol® *see* oxymetholone *on page 344*

Anafranil® *see* clomipramine hydrochloride *on page 107*

Ana-Kit® *see* insect sting kit *on page 245*

Anamine T.D.® *see* chlorpheniramine and pseudoephedrine *on page 94*

Anaprox® *see* naproxen *on page 319*

Anaspaz® *see* hyoscyamine sulfate *on page 239*

ALPHABETICAL LISTING OF DRUGS

Anatrast® *see* radiological/contrast media (ionic) *on page 404*

Anatuss® **[OTC]** *see* guaifenesin, phenylpropanolamine, and dextromethorphan *on page 217*

Anbesol® **Maximum Strength [OTC]** *see* benzocaine *on page 48*

Ancef® *see* cefazolin sodium *on page 79*

Ancobon® *see* flucytosine *on page 194*

Andro-Cyp® **Injection** *see* testosterone *on page 449*

Andro/Fem® **Injection** *see* estradiol and testosterone *on page 174*

Android® *see* methyltestosterone *on page 301*

Andro® **Injection** *see* testosterone *on page 449*

Andro-L.A.® **Injection** *see* testosterone *on page 449*

Androlone®**-D Injection** *see* nandrolone *on page 318*

Androlone® **Injection** *see* nandrolone *on page 318*

Andronate® **Injection** *see* testosterone *on page 449*

Andropository® **Injection** *see* testosterone *on page 449*

Anectine® **Chloride Injection** *see* succinylcholine chloride *on page 437*

Anectine® **Flo-Pack**® *see* succinylcholine chloride *on page 437*

Anergan® **Injection** *see* promethazine hydrochloride *on page 390*

Anestacon® *see* lidocaine hydrochloride *on page 267*

aneurine hydrochloride *see* thiamine hydrochloride *on page 455*

Anexsia® *see* hydrocodone and acetaminophen *on page 230*

Angio Conray® *see* radiological/contrast media (ionic) *on page 404*

Angiovist® *see* radiological/contrast media (ionic) *on page 404*

anisotropine methylbromide (an iss oh troe' peen)
Therapeutic Category Anticholinergic Agent; Antispasmodic Agent, Gastrointestinal
Use Adjunctive treatment of peptic ulcer
Usual Dosage Adults: Oral: 50 mg 3 times/day
Dosage Forms Tablet: 50 mg

anisoylated plasminogen streptokinase activator complex *see* anistreplase *on this page*

anistreplase (a niss' tre place)
Brand Names Eminase®
Synonyms anisoylated plasminogen streptokinase activator complex; apsac
Therapeutic Category Thrombolytic Agent
Use Management of acute myocardial infarction (AMI) in adults; lysis of thrombi obstructing coronary arteries, reduction of infarct size; and reduction of mortality associated with AMI
Usual Dosage Adults: I.V.: 30 units injected over 2 5 minutes as soon as possible after onset of symptoms
Dosage Forms Powder for injection, lyophilized: 30 units

Anoquan® *see* butalbital compound *on page 63*

Ansaid® **Oral** *see* flurbiprofen sodium *on page 200*

ansamycin *see* rifabutin *on page 411*

Answer® *see* diagnostic aids (*in vitro*), urine *on page 137*

Answer® **Ovulation** *see* diagnostic aids (*in vitro*), urine *on page 137*

Answer® **Plus** *see* diagnostic aids (*in vitro*), urine *on page 137*

Antabuse® *see* disulfiram *on page 152*

Antazoline-V® Ophthalmic *see* naphazoline and antazoline *on page 318*

Anthra-Derm® *see* anthralin *on this page*

anthralin (an' thra lin)

Brand Names Anthra-Derm®; Drithocreme®; Dritho-Scalp®
Synonyms dithranol
Therapeutic Category Antipsoriatic Agent, Topical; Keratolytic Agent
Use Treatment of psoriasis
Usual Dosage Adults: Topical: Apply in a thin film at bedtime
Dosage Forms
Cream: 0.1% (50 g, 65 g); 0.2% (65 g); 0.25% (50 g); 0.4% (65 g); 0.5% (50 g); 1% (50 g, 65 g)
Ointment, topical: 0.1% (42.5 g); 0.25% (42.5 g); 0.4% (60 g); 0.5% (42.5 g); 1% (42.5 g)

AntibiOtic® Otic *see* neomycin, polymyxin b, and hydrocortisone *on page 323*

antidigoxin fab fragments *see* digoxin immune fab (ovine) *on page 145*

antidiuretic hormone *see* vasopressin *on page 484*

antihemophilic factor (human) (an tee hee moe fill' ik)

Brand Names Hemofil® M; Humate-P®; Kōate®-HP; Kōate®-HS; KoGENate®; Monoclate-P®; Profilate® OSD
Synonyms ahf; factor viii
Therapeutic Category Antihemophilic Agent; Blood Product Derivative
Use Management of hemophilia A in patients whom a deficiency in factor VIII has been demonstrated
Usual Dosage I.V.: Individualize dosage based on coagulation studies performed prior to and during treatment at regular intervals. One AHF unit is the activity present in 1 mL of normal pooled human plasma; dosage should be adjusted to actual vial size currently stocked in the pharmacy.

Hospitalized patients: 20-50 units/kg/dose; may be higher for special circumstances; dose can be given every 12-24 hours and more frequently in special circumstances

Formula to approximate percentage increase in plasma antihemophilic factor:
Units required = desired level increase (desired level - actual level) x plasma volume (mL)
Total blood volume (mL blood/kg) = 70 mL/kg (adults); 80 mL/kg (children).
Plasma volume = total blood volume (mL) x [1 - Hct (in decimals)]
ie, for a 70 kg adult with a Hct = 40% : plasma volume = [70 kg x 70 mL/kg] x [1 - 0.4] = 2940 mL

To calculate number of units of factor VIII needed to increase level to desired range (highly individualized and dependent on patient's condition):
Number of units = desired level increase [desired level - actual level] x plasma volume (in mL)
ie, for a 100% level in the above patient who has an actual level of 20% the number of units needed = [1 (for a 100% level) - 0.2] x 2940 mL = 2352 units
Dosage Forms Injection: Single-dose vials with varied units; 10 mL, 20 mL, 30 mL

antihemophilic factor (recombinant)

Brand Names Bioclate®; Hexlixate®; Recombinate®
Therapeutic Category Antihemophilic Agent
Use Management of hemophilia A in patients whom a deficiency in factor VIII has been demonstrated
Usual Dosage I.V.: Individualize dosage based on coagulation studies performed prior to and during treatment at regular intervals. One AHF unit is the activity present in 1 mL of normal pooled human plasma; dosage should be adjusted to actual vial size currently stocked in the pharmacy.
(Continued)

29

antihemophilic factor (recombinant) *(Continued)*

Hospitalized patients: 20-50 units/kg/dose; may be higher for special circumstances; dose can be given every 12-24 hours and more frequently in special circumstances

Formula to approximate percentage increase in plasma antihemophilic factor:

Units required = desired level increase (desired level - actual level) x plasma volume (mL)

Total blood volume (mL blood/kg) = 70 mL/kg (adults); 80 mL/kg (children).

Plasma volume = total blood volume (mL) x [1 - Hct (in decimals)]

ie, for a 70 kg adult with a Hct = 40% : plasma volume = [70 kg x 70 mL/kg] x [1 - 0.4] = 2940 mL

To calculate number of units of factor VIII needed to increase level to desired range (highly individualized and dependent on patient's condition):

Number of units = desired level increase [desired level - actual level] x plasma volume (in mL)

ie, for a 100% level in the above patient who has an actual level of 20% the number of units needed = [1 (for a 100% level) - 0.2] x 2940 mL = 2352 units

Dosage Forms Injection: 250 units, 500 units, 1000 units

Antihist-1® [OTC] *see* clemastine fumarate *on page 104*

anti-inhibitor coagulant complex

Brand Names Autoplex T®; Feiba VH Immuno®

Therapeutic Category Hemophilic Agent

Use Patients with factor VIII inhibitors who are to undergo surgery or those who are bleeding

Usual Dosage Dosage range: 25-100 factor VIII correctional units per kg depending on the severity of hemorrhage

Dosage Forms Injection:

Autoplex T®, with heparin 2 units: Each bottle is labeled with correctional units of Factor VIII

Feiba VH Immuno®, heparin free: Each bottle is labeled with correctional units of Factor VIII

Antilirium® Injection *see* physostigmine *on page 368*

Antiminth® [OTC] *see* pyrantel pamoate *on page 399*

antipyrine and benzocaine

Brand Names Allergan® Ear Drops; Auralgan®; Auroto®; Otocalm® Ear

Synonyms benzocaine and antipyrine

Therapeutic Category Otic Agent, Analgesic; Otic Agent, Cerumenolytic

Use Temporary relief of pain and reduction of inflammation associated with acute congestive and serous otitis media, swimmer's ear, otitis externa; facilitates ear wax removal

Usual Dosage Otic: Fill ear canal; moisten cotton pledget, place in external ear, repeat every 1-2 hours until pain and congestion is relieved; for ear wax removal instill drops 3-4 times/day for 2-3 days

Dosage Forms Solution, otic: Antipyrine 5.4% and benzocaine 1.4% (10 mL, 15 mL)

antirabies serum, equine origin

Synonyms ars

Therapeutic Category Serum

Use Rabies prophylaxis

Usual Dosage I.M.: 1000 units/55 lb in a single dose, infiltrate up to 50% of dose around the wound

Dosage Forms Injection: 125 units/mL (8 mL)

Antispas® Injection *see* dicyclomine hydrochloride *on page 142*

antithrombin III

Brand Names ATnativ®; Thrombate® III

Therapeutic Category Blood Product Derivative

Use Agent for hereditary antithrombin III deficiency

Usual Dosage After first dose of antithrombin III, level should increase to 120% of normal; thereafter maintain at levels >80%. Generally, achieved by administration of maintenance doses once every 24 hours; initially and until patient is stabilized, measure antithrombin III level at least twice daily, thereafter once daily and always immediately before next infusion.

Initial dosage (units) = [desired AT-III level % - baseline AT-III level %] x body weight (kg) divided by 1%/units/kg

Measure antithrombin III preceding and 30 minutes after dose to calculate *in vivo* recovery rate; maintain level within normal range for 2-8 days depending on type of surgery or procedure

Dosage Forms Powder for injection: 500 units (50 mL)

Anti-Tuss® Expectorant [OTC] *see* guaifenesin *on page 213*

antivenin, black widow spider (equine)
Synonyms black widow spider antivenin (*Latrodectus mactans*); *Latrodectus mactans* antivenin
Therapeutic Category Antivenin
Use Treat patients with symptoms of black widow spider bites
Usual Dosage
Children <12 years (severe or shock): I.V.: 2.5 mL in 10-50 mL over 15 minutes
Children and Adults: I.M.: 2.5 mL
Dosage Forms Powder for injection: 6000 antivenin units (2.5 mL)

antivenin polyvalent (*Crotalidae*)
Synonyms crotaline antivenin, polyvalent; north and south American antisnake-bite serum; pit vipers antivenin; snake (pit vipers) antivenin
Therapeutic Category Antivenin
Use Neutralization of the venoms of North and South America Crotalids: rattlesnake, copperhead, cottonmouth, tropical moccasins, fer-de-lance, bushmaster
Usual Dosage Initial intradermal sensitivity test. The entire initial dose of antivenin should be administered as soon as possible to be most effective (within 4 hours after the bite).
Children and Adults: I.V.: Minimal envenomation: 20-40 mL; moderate envenomation: 50-90 mL; severe envenomation: 100-150 mL
Additional doses of antivenin is based on clinical response to the initial dose. If swelling continues to progress, symptoms increase in severity, hypotension occurs, or decrease in hematocrit appears, an additional 10-50 mL should be administered.
For I.V. infusion: 1:1-1:10 dilution of reconstituted antivenin in normal saline or D_5W should be prepared. Infuse the initial 5-10 mL of diluted antivenin over 3-5 minutes monitoring closely for signs of sensitivity reactions.
Dosage Forms Injection: Lyophilized serum, diluent (10 mL); one vacuum vial to yield 10 mL of serum

antivenin (*Micrurus fulvius*)
Synonyms north American coral snake antivenin
Therapeutic Category Antivenin
Use Neutralize the venom of Eastern coral snake and Texas coral snake but not neutralize venom of Arizona or Sonoran coral snake
Usual Dosage I.V.: 3-5 vials by slow injection
Dosage Forms Injection: One vial antivenin and one vial diluent

Antivert® *see* meclizine hydrochloride *on page 282*
Antrizine® *see* meclizine hydrochloride *on page 282*
Anturane® *see* sulfinpyrazone *on page 441*
Anucort-HC® Suppository *see* hydrocortisone *on page 232*

Anuprep HC®️ Suppository *see* hydrocortisone *on page 232*

Anusol®️ HC-1 [OTC] *see* hydrocortisone *on page 232*

Anusol®️ HC-2.5% [OTC] *see* hydrocortisone *on page 232*

Anusol-HC®️ Suppository *see* hydrocortisone *on page 232*

Anxanil®️ *see* hydroxyzine *on page 237*

Apacet®️ [OTC] *see* acetaminophen *on page 2*

apap *see* acetaminophen *on page 2*

Apatate®️ [OTC] *see* vitamin b complex *on page 490*

Aphrodyne™️ *see* yohimbine hydrochloride *on page 493*

A.P.L.®️ *see* chorionic gonadotropin *on page 101*

Aplisol®️ *see* tuberculin tests *on page 477*

appg *see* penicillin g procaine, aqueous *on page 354*

apraclonidine hydrochloride (a pra kloe' ni deen)
    Brand Names Alpidine®️; Iopidine®️
    Therapeutic Category Alpha-2-Adrenergic Agonist Agent, Ophthalmic
    Use Prevention and treatment of postsurgical intraocular pressure elevation
    Usual Dosage Ophthalmic: Instill 1 drop in operative eye 1 hour prior to laser surgery, second drop in eye upon completion of procedure
    Dosage Forms Solution, ophthalmic: 0.5% (5 mL); 1% (0.1 mL, 0.25 mL)

Apresazide®️ *see* hydralazine and hydrochlorothiazide *on page 228*

Apresoline®️ Injection *see* hydralazine hydrochloride *on page 228*

Apresoline®️ Oral *see* hydralazine hydrochloride *on page 228*

Aprodine®️ [OTC] *see* triprolidine and pseudoephedrine *on page 474*

Aprodine®️ w/C *see* triprolidine, pseudoephedrine, and codeine *on page 475*

aprotinin
    Brand Names Trasylol®️
    Therapeutic Category Hemostatic Agent
    Use Reduction or prevention of blood loss in patients undergoing coronary artery bypass surgery when a high index of suspicion of excessive bleeding potential exists; this includes open heart reoperation, pre-existing coagulopathy, operations on the great vessels, and patients whose religious beliefs prohibit blood transfusions
    Usual Dosage
    Test dose: **All** patients should receive a 1 mL I.V. test dose at least 10 minutes prior to the loading dose to assess the potential for allergic reactions

    Regimen A:
        2 million units (280 mg) loading dose I.V. over 20-30 minutes
        2 million units (280 mg) into pump prime volume
        500,000 units/hour (70 mg/hour) I.V. during operation

    Regimen B:
        1 million units (140 mg) loading dose I.V. over 20-30 minutes
        1 million units (140 mg) into pump prime volume
        250,000 units/hour (35 mg/hour) I.V. during operation
    Dosage Forms Injection: 1.4 mg/mL [10,000 units/mL] (100 mL, 200 mL)

apsac *see* anistreplase *on page 28*

Aquacare®️ Topical [OTC] *see* urea *on page 480*

Aquachloral®️ Supprettes®️ *see* chloral hydrate *on page 87*

AquaMEPHYTON®️ Injection *see* phytonadione *on page 368*

Aquaphor® Antibiotic Topical [OTC] *see* bacitracin and polymyxin b *on page 43*

Aquaphyllin® *see* theophylline *on page 453*

Aquasol A® [OTC] *see* vitamin a *on page 489*

Aquasol E® Oral [OTC] *see* vitamin e *on page 490*

Aquatag® *see* benzthiazide *on page 50*

AquaTar® [OTC] *see* coal tar *on page 110*

Aquatensen® *see* methylclothiazide *on page 297*

Aquazide-H® *see* hydrochlorothiazide *on page 229*

aqueous procaine penicillin g *see* penicillin g procaine, aqueous *on page 354*

Aquest® *see* estrone *on page 175*

ara-a *see* vidarabine *on page 487*

arabinosylcytosine *see* cytarabine hydrochloride *on page 123*

ara-c *see* cytarabine hydrochloride *on page 123*

Aralen® Phosphate *see* chloroquine phosphate *on page 91*

Aralen® Phosphate With Primaquine Phosphate *see* chloroquine and primaquine *on page 91*

Aramine® *see* metaraminol bitartrate *on page 291*

Arcet® *see* butalbital compound *on page 63*

Arduan® *see* pipecuronium bromide *on page 370*

Aredia™ *see* pamidronate disodium *on page 345*

Arfonad® Injection *see* trimethaphan camsylate *on page 472*

Argesic®-SA *see* salsalate *on page 417*

arginine hydrochloride (ar' ji neen)
Brand Names R-Gene®
Therapeutic Category Metabolic Alkalosis Agent
Use Pituitary function test (growth hormone); management of severe, uncompensated, metabolic alkalosis (pH $\geq$7.55) **after** optimizing therapy with Na$^+$ and K$^+$ supplements
Usual Dosage I.V.:
Growth hormone reserve test:
  Children: 500 mg/kg over 30 minutes
  Adults: 300 mL

Note: Arginine hydrochloride should never be used as an alternative to chloride supplementation but used in the patient who is unresponsive to sodium chloride or potassium chloride supplementation.

Metabolic alkalosis: Children and Adults:
  Acid required (mEq) =
    [0.2 (L/kg) x wt (kg)] x [103 - serum <1] mEq/L **or**
    0.3 (L/kg) x wt (kg) x base excess (mEq/L) **or**
    0.5 (L/kg) x wt (kg) x [serum HCO$_3$ - 24] mEq/L
  Give $\frac{1}{2}$ to $\frac{2}{3}$ of calculated dose and re-evaluate

Children: 500 mg/kg/dose administered over 30 minutes

Adults: 30 g administered at a constant rate over 30 minutes
Dosage Forms Injection: 10% [100 mg/mL = 950 mOsm/L] (500 mL)

8-arginine vasopressin *see* vasopressin *on page 484*

Argyrol® S.S. 20% *see* silver protein, mild *on page 423*

Aristocort® Forte *see* triamcinolone *on page 467*

Aristocort® Intralesional Suspension *see* triamcinolone *on page 467*

Aristocort® **Tablet** *see* triamcinolone *on page 467*

Aristospan® *see* triamcinolone *on page 467*

Arm-a-Med® **Isoetharine** *see* isoetharine *on page 251*

Arm-a-Med® **Isoproterenol** *see* isoproterenol *on page 253*

Arm-a-Med® **Metaproterenol** *see* metaproterenol sulfate *on page 290*

Armour® **Thyroid** *see* thyroid *on page 459*

Aromatic Ammonia Aspirols® *see* ammonia spirit, aromatic *on page 22*

Arrestin® *see* trimethobenzamide hydrochloride *on page 472*

ars *see* antirabies serum, equine origin *on page 30*

Artane® *see* trihexyphenidyl hydrochloride *on page 471*

Artha-G® *see* salsalate *on page 417*

Arthritis Foundation® **Nighttime [OTC]** *see* acetaminophen and diphenhydramine *on page 4*

Arthritis Foundation® **Pain Reliever [OTC]** *see* aspirin *on next page*

Arthritis Foundation® **Ibuprofen [OTC]** *see* ibuprofen *on page 240*

Arthropan® **[OTC]** *see* choline salicylate *on page 100*

Articulose-50® **Injection** *see* prednisolone *on page 383*

artificial tears

Brand Names Isopto" Plain [OTC]; Isopto" Tears [OTC]; Tearisol® [OTC]
Synonyms polyvinyl alcohol
Therapeutic Category Ophthalmic Agent, Miscellaneous
Use Ophthalmic lubricant; for relief of dry eyes and eye irritation
Usual Dosage Ophthalmic: Use as needed to relieve symptoms, 1-2 drops into eye(s) 3-4 times/day
Dosage Forms Solution: 15 mL with dropper

asa *see* aspirin *on next page*

A.S.A. [OTC] *see* aspirin *on next page*

5-asa *see* mesalamine *on page 289*

Asacol® **Oral** *see* mesalamine *on page 289*

ascorbic acid (a skor' bik)

Brand Names Ascorbicap" [OTC]; C-Crystals" [OTC]; Cecon® [OTC]; Cevalin® [OTC]; Ce-Vi-Sol" [OTC]; Dull-C" [OTC]; Flavorcee" [OTC]; Vita-C" [OTC]
Synonyms vitamin c
Therapeutic Category Urinary Acidifying Agent; Vitamin, Water Soluble
Use Prevention and treatment of scurvy; urinary acidification; dietary supplementation; prevention and decreasing the severity of colds
Usual Dosage Oral, I.M., I.V., S.C.:
Children:
Scurvy: 100-300 mg/day in divided doses for at least 2 weeks
Urinary acidification: 500 mg every 6-8 hours
Dietary supplement: 35-45 mg

Adults:
Scurvy: 500-1000 mg for at least 2 weeks
Urinary acidification: 4-12 g/day in 3-4 divided doses
Dietary supplement: 50-60 mg/day
Prevention and treatment of cold: 1-3 g/day
Dosage Forms
Capsule, timed release: 500 mg

Crystals: 4 g/teaspoonful (100 g, 500 g); 5 g/teaspoonful (180 g)
Injection: 250 mg/mL (2 mL, 30 mL); 500 mg/mL (2 mL, 50 mL)
Liquid, oral: 35 mg/0.6 mL (50 mL)
Lozenges: 60 mg
Powder: 4 g/teaspoonful (100 g, 500 g)
Solution, oral: 100 mg/mL (50 mL)
Syrup: 500 mg/5 mL (5 mL, 10 mL, 120 mL, 480 mL)
Tablet: 25 mg, 50 mg, 100 mg, 250 mg, 500 mg, 1000 mg
Tablet:
    Chewable: 100 mg, 250 mg, 500 mg
    Timed release: 500 mg, 1000 mg, 1500 mg

ascorbic acid and ferrous sulfate *see* ferrous salt and ascorbic acid
on page 190

Ascorbicap® [OTC] *see* ascorbic acid *on previous page*

Ascriptin® [OTC] *see* aspirin *on this page*

Asendin® *see* amoxapine *on page 23*

Asmalix® *see* theophylline *on page 453*

asn-ase *see* asparaginase *on this page*

asparaginase (a spare' a ji nase)
Brand Names Elspar®
Synonyms a-ase; asn-ase; colaspase
Therapeutic Category Antineoplastic Agent, Miscellaneous
Use Treatment of acute lymphocytic leukemia, lymphoma
Usual Dosage Refer to individual protocols; the manufacturer recommends performing intradermal sensitivity testing before the initial dose

Children and Adults:
    I.M. (preferred route): 6000 units/m^2 3 times/week for 3 weeks for combination therapy
    I.V.: 1000 units/kg/day for 10 days for combination therapy or 200 units/kg/day for 28
        days if combination therapy is inappropriate
Dosage Forms Injection: 10,000 units/vial

Aspergum® [OTC] *see* aspirin *on this page*

aspirin (as' pir in)
Brand Names Anacin® [OTC]; Arthritis Foundation® Pain Reliever [OTC]; A.S.A. [OTC]; Ascriptin® [OTC]; Aspergum® [OTC]; Bayer® Aspirin [OTC]; Bayer® Buffered Aspirin [OTC]; Bayer® Low Adult Strength [OTC]; Bufferin® [OTC]; Easprin®; Ecotrin® [OTC]; Empirin® [OTC]; Extra Strength Bayer® Enteric 500 Aspirin [OTC]; Gensan® [OTC]; Halfprin® 81 [OTC]; Measurin® [OTC]; St. Joseph® Adult Chewable Aspirin [OTC]; ZORprin®
Synonyms acetylsalicylic acid; asa
Therapeutic Category Analgesic, Non-Narcotic; Anti-inflammatory Agent; Antiplatelet Agent; Antipyretic; Nonsteroidal Anti-Inflammatory Agent (NSAID), Oral; Salicylate
Use Treatment of mild to moderate pain, inflammation and fever; may be used as a prophylaxis of myocardial infarction and transient ischemic attacks (TIA)
Usual Dosage
Children:
    Analgesic and antipyretic: Oral, rectal: 10-15 mg/kg/dose every 4-6 hours
    Anti-inflammatory: Oral: Initial: 60-90 mg/kg/day in divided doses; usual maintenance: 80-
        100 mg/kg/day divided every 6-8 hours; monitor serum concentrations
    Kawasaki disease: Oral: 100 mg/kg/day divided every 6 hours; after fever resolves: 8-10
        mg/kg/day once daily; monitor serum concentrations

Adults:
    Analgesic and antipyretic: Oral, rectal: 325-1000 mg every 4-6 hours up to 4 g/day
(Continued)

aspirin *(Continued)*

Anti-inflammatory: Oral: Initial: 2.4-3.6 g/day in divided doses; usual maintenance: 3.6-5.4 g/day; monitor serum concentrations

Transient ischemic attack: Oral: 1.3 g/day in 2-4 divided doses

Myocardial infarction prophylaxis: 160-325 mg/day

Dosage Forms

Capsule: 356.4 mg and caffeine 30 mg

Suppository, rectal: 60 mg, 120 mg, 125 mg, 130 mg, 195 mg, 200 mg, 300 mg, 325 mg, 600 mg, 650 mg, 1.2 g

Tablet: 65 mg, 75 mg, 81 mg, 325 mg, 500 mg

Tablet: 400 mg and caffeine 32 mg

Tablet:

Buffered: 325 mg and magnesium-aluminum hydroxide 150 mg; 325 mg, magnesium hydroxide 75 mg, aluminum hydroxide 75 mg, buffered with calcium carbonate; 325 mg and magnesium-aluminum hydroxide 75 mg

Chewable: 81 mg

Controlled release: 800 mg

Delayed release: 81 mg

Enteric coated: 81 mg, 325 mg, 500 mg, 650 mg, 975 mg

Gum: 227.5 mg

Timed release: 650 mg

aspirin and codeine

Brand Names Empirin" With Codeine

Synonyms codeine and aspirin

Therapeutic Category Analgesic, Narcotic; Antipyretic

Use Relief of mild to moderate pain

Usual Dosage Oral:

Children:

Aspirin: 10 mg/kg/dose every 4 hours

Codeine: 0.5-1 mg/kg/dose every 4 hours

Adults: 1-2 tablets every 4-6 hours as needed for pain

Dosage Forms Tablet:

#2: Aspirin 325 mg and codeine phosphate 15 mg

#3: Aspirin 325 mg and codeine phosphate 30 mg

#4: Aspirin 325 mg and codeine phosphate 60 mg

aspirin and meprobamate

Brand Names Equagesic"

Synonyms meprobamate and aspirin

Therapeutic Category Skeletal Muscle Relaxant, Long Acting

Use Adjunct to treatment of skeletal muscular disease in patients exhibiting tension and/or anxiety

Usual Dosage Oral: 1 tablet 3-4 times/day

Dosage Forms Tablet: Aspirin 325 mg and meprobamate 200 mg

Aspirin Free Anacin® Maximum Strength [OTC] *see* acetaminophen *on page 2*

Aspirin-Free Bayer® Select® Allergy Sinus Caplets [OTC] *see* acetaminophen, chlorpheniramine, and pseudoephedrine *on page 4*

astemizole (a stem' mi zole)

Brand Names Hismanal"

Therapeutic Category Antihistamine

Use Perennial and seasonal allergic rhinitis and other allergic symptoms including urticaria

Usual Dosage Oral:

Children:

<6 years: 0.2 mg/kg/day

6-12 years: 5 mg/day

Children > 12 years and Adults: 10-30 mg/day; give 30 mg on first day, 20 mg on second day, then 10 mg/day in a single dose
Dosage Forms Tablet: 10 mg

AsthmaHaler® *see* epinephrine *on page 167*
AsthmaNefrin® [OTC] *see* epinephrine *on page 167*
Astramorph™ PF Injection *see* morphine sulfate *on page 311*
Atarax® *see* hydroxyzine *on page 237*

atenolol (a ten' oh lole)
Brand Names Tenormin®
Therapeutic Category Antianginal Agent; Beta-Adrenergic Blocker
Use Treatment of hypertension, alone or in combination with other agents; also used in management of angina pectoris; selective inhibitor of beta$_1$-adrenergic receptors; post myocardial infarction patients; acute alcohol withdrawal
Usual Dosage
Oral:
Children: 1-2 mg/kg/dose given daily
Adults: 50-100 mg/dose given daily

I.V.: Adults: For early treatment of myocardial infarction: 5 mg slow I.V. over 5 minutes; may repeat in 10 minutes; if both doses are tolerated, may start oral atenolol 50 mg every 12 hours;

Postmyocardial infarction:
Oral: Follow with 100 mg/day or 50 mg twice daily for 6-9 days postmyocardial infarction
I.V.: Administer as soon as possible 5 mg over 5 minutes; follow with 5 mg I.V. 10 minutes later
Dosage Forms
Injection: 0.5 mg/mL (10 mL)
Tablet: 25 mg, 50 mg, 100 mg

atenolol and chlorthalidone
Brand Names Tenoretic®
Therapeutic Category Antihypertensive, Combination
Use Treatment of hypertension with a cardioselective beta blocker and a diuretic
Usual Dosage Adults: Oral: Initial: One (50) tablet once daily, then individualize dose until optimal dose is achieved
Dosage Forms Tablet:
50: Atenolol 50 mg and chlorthalidone 25 mg
100: Atenolol 100 mg and chlorthalidone 25 mg

atg *see* lymphocyte immune globulin, antithymocyte globulin (equine) *on page 275*
Atgam® *see* lymphocyte immune globulin, antithymocyte globulin (equine) *on page 275*
Ativan® *see* lorazepam *on page 273*
ATnativ® *see* antithrombin III *on page 30*

atovaquone (a toe' va kwone)
Brand Names Mepron®
Therapeutic Category Antiprotozoal
Use Acute oral treatment of mild to moderate *Pneumocystis carinii* pneumonia (PCP) in patients who are intolerant to co-trimoxazole
Usual Dosage Adults: Oral: 750 mg 3 times/day with food for 21 days
Dosage Forms Tablet, film coated: 250 mg

Atozine® *see* hydroxyzine *on page 237*

atracurium besylate (a tra kyoo' ree um)
Brand Names Tracrium™
Therapeutic Category Neuromuscular Blocker Agent, Nondepolarizing; Skeletal Muscle Relaxant
Use Ease endotracheal intubation as an adjunct to general anesthesia and to relax skeletal muscle during surgery or mechanical ventilation; does not appear to have a cumulative effect on the duration of blockade; does not relieve pain
Usual Dosage I.V.:
Children 1 month to 2 years: 0.3-0.4 mg/kg initially followed by maintenance doses of 0.08-0.1 mg/kg as needed to maintain neuromuscular blockade

Children >2 years to Adults: 0.4-0.5 mg/kg then 0.08-0.1 mg/kg every 20-45 minutes after initial dose to maintain neuromuscular block

Continuous infusion: 0.4-0.8 mg/kg/hour
Dosage Forms Injection: 10 mg/mL (5 mL, 10 mL)

Atromid-S® *see* clofibrate *on page 107*
Atropair® Ophthalmic *see* atropine sulfate *on this page*
atropine and diphenoxylate *see* diphenoxylate and atropine *on page 149*
Atropine-Care® Ophthalmic *see* atropine sulfate *on this page*

atropine sulfate (a' troe peen)
Brand Names Atropair™ Ophthalmic; Atropine-Care® Ophthalmic; Atropisol® Ophthalmic; Isopto™ Atropine Ophthalmic; I-Tropine® Ophthalmic; Ocu-Tropine® Ophthalmic
Therapeutic Category Anticholinergic Agent; Anticholinergic Agent, Ophthalmic; Antidote, Organophosphate Poisoning; Antispasmodic Agent, Gastrointestinal; Bronchodilator; Ophthalmic Agent, Mydriatic
Use Preoperative medication to inhibit salivation and secretions; treatment of sinus bradycardia; management of peptic ulcer; treat exercise-induced bronchospasm; antidote for organophosphate pesticide poisoning; used to produce mydriasis and cycloplegia for examination of the retina and optic disk and accurate measurement of refractive errors; uveitis
Usual Dosage
Preanesthesia: I.M., I.V., S.C.:
Infants:
<5 kg: 0.04 mg/kg/dose repeated every 4-6 hours as needed
>5 kg: 0.03 mg/kg/dose repeated every 4-6 hours as needed
Children: 0.01 mg/kg/dose up to a maximum of 0.4 mg/dose; repeat every 4-6 hours as needed
Adults: 0.5 mg/dose repeated every 4-6 hours as needed

Bronchodilation:
Children:
Oral: 0.02 mg/kg/dose 3 times/day
Inhalation: 0.03-0.05 mg/kg/dose 3-4 times/day
Adults: Inhalation: 0.025-0.05 mg/kg/dose over 10 minutes, repeated every 4-5 hours as needed

Cardiopulmonary resuscitation (bradycardia): I.T., I.V.:
Infants: 0.02-0.04 mg/kg/dose; repeat every 2-5 minutes, if needed, up to 2-3 times
Children: 0.01-0.02 mg/kg/dose; repeat every 2-5 minutes, if needed, up to 2-3 times; minimum dose should be 0.1 mg (smaller doses may cause paradoxic bradycardia); maximum total dose is 1 mg (2 mg for adolescents)
Adults: 0.5 mg/dose; repeat every 5 minutes, if needed, up to 2-3 times for a maximum total dose of 2 mg

Organophosphate or carbamate poisoning: I.V.:
Children: 0.02-0.05 mg/kg/dose every 10-20 minutes until atropine effect (dry flushed skin, tachycardia, mydriasis, fever) is observed, then every 1-4 hours to maintain atropine effect for at least 24 hours

Children >12 years and Adults: 1-2 mg/dose every 10-20 minutes until atropine effect (see above) is observed, then 1-3 mg/dose every 1-4 hours, as needed to maintain atropine effect for at least 24 hours

Neuromuscular blockade reversal: I.V.:
Before neostigmine: Give 25-30 mcg/kg (0.025-0.03 mg/kg) 30 seconds before neostigmine (0.07-0.08 mg/kg)
Before edrophonium: 10 mcg/kg (0.01 mg/kg) 30 seconds before edrophonium (1 mg/kg)
Note: May contain benzyl alcohol as a preservative; administration of benzyl alcohol in doses ranging from 99-234 mg/kg has been associated with a fatal gasping syndrome in neonates; clinical signs of this syndrome include metabolic acidosis, hypotension, CNS depression, and cardiovascular collapse

Dosage Forms
Injection: 0.05 mg/mL (5 mL); 0.1 mg/mL (5 mL, 10 mL); 0.3 mg/mL (1 mL, 30 mL); 0.4 mg/mL (1 mL, 20 mL, 30 mL); 0.5 mg/mL (1 mL, 5 mL, 30 mL); 0.8 mg/mL (0.5 mL, 1 mL); 1 mg/mL (1 mL, 10 mL)
Ointment, ophthalmic: 0.5% (3.5 g); 1% (3.5 g)
Solution, ophthalmic: 0.5% (1 mL, 5 mL); 1% (1 mL, 2 mL, 5 mL, 15 mL); 2% (1 mL, 2 mL); 3% (5 mL)
Tablet: 0.4 mg
    Sal-Tropine®: 0.4 mg
Tablet, soluble: 0.4 mg, 0.6 mg

Atropisol® Ophthalmic see atropine sulfate *on previous page*

Atrovent® Aerosol Inhalation see ipratropium bromide *on page 250*

Atrovent® Inhalation Solution see ipratropium bromide *on page 250*

A/T/S® see erythromycin, topical *on page 172*

attapulgite (at a pull' gite)
Brand Names Children's Kaopectate® [OTC]; Diasorb® [OTC]; Kaopectate® Advanced Formula [OTC]; Kaopectate® Maximum Strength Caplets; Rheaban® [OTC]
Therapeutic Category Antidiarrheal
Use Symptomatic treatment of diarrhea
Usual Dosage Oral:
Children:
    <3 years: Not recommended
    3-6 years: 750 mg/dose up to 2250 mg/24 hours
    6-12 years: 1200-1500 mg/dose up to 4500 mg/24 hours

Adults: 1200-1500 mg after each loose bowel movement or every 2 hours; 15-30 mL up to 8 times/day, up to 9000 mg/24 hours
Dosage Forms
Liquid, oral concentrate: 600 mg/15 mL (180 mL, 240 mL, 360 mL, 480 mL); 750 mg/15 mL (120 mL)
Tablet: 750 mg
Tablet, chewable: 300 mg, 600 mg

Attenuvax® see measles virus vaccine, live, attenuated *on page 281*

Augmentin® see amoxicillin and clavulanic acid *on page 24*

Auralate® see gold sodium thiomalate *on page 211*

Auralgan® see antipyrine and benzocaine *on page 30*

auranofin (au rane' oh fin)
Brand Names Ridaura®
Therapeutic Category Gold Compound
Use Management of active stage of classic or definite rheumatoid arthritis in patients that do not respond to or tolerate other agents; psoriatic arthritis
(Continued)

auranofin *(Continued)*
Usual Dosage Oral:
    Children: Initial: 0.1 mg/kg/day divided daily; usual maintenance: 0.15 mg/kg/day in 1-2 divided doses; maximum: 0.2 mg/kg/day in 1-2 divided doses

    Adults: 6 mg/day in 1-2 divided doses; after 3 months may be increased to 9 mg/day in 3 divided doses; if still no response after 3 months at 9 mg/day, discontinue drug
Dosage Forms Capsule: 3 mg [gold 29%]

Aureomycin® *see* chlortetracyline hydrochloride *on page 98*
Auro® Ear Drops [OTC] *see* carbamide peroxide *on page 74*

aurothioglucose (aur oh thye oh gloo' kose)
Brand Names Solganal®
Therapeutic Category Gold Compound
Use Adjunctive treatment in adult and juvenile active rheumatoid arthritis; alternative or adjunct in treatment of pemphigus; for psoriatic patients who do not respond to NSAIDs
Usual Dosage I.M. (doses should initially be given at weekly intervals):
    Children 6-12 years: Initial: 0.25 mg/kg/dose first week; increment at 0.25 mg/kg/dose increasing with each weekly dose; maintenance: 0.75-1 mg/kg/dose weekly not to exceed 25 mg/dose to a total of 20 doses, then every 2-4 weeks

    Adults: 10 mg first week; 25 mg second and third week; then 50 mg/week until 800 mg to 1 g cumulative dose has been given – if improvement occurs without adverse reactions, give 25-50 mg every 2-3 weeks, then every 3-4 weeks
Dosage Forms Suspension, sterile: 50 mg/mL [gold 50%] (10 mL)

Auroto® *see* antipyrine and benzocaine *on page 30*
Autoplex T® *see* anti-inhibitor coagulant complex *on page 30*
AVC™ Vaginal Cream *see* sulfanilamide *on page 441*
AVC™ Vaginal Suppository *see* sulfanilamide *on page 441*
Aveeno® Cleansing Bar [OTC] *see* sulfur and salicylic acid *on page 442*
Aventyl® Hydrochloride *see* nortriptyline hydrochloride *on page 333*
Avitene® *see* microfibrillar collagen hemostat *on page 306*
Axid® *see* nizatidine *on page 331*
Axotal® *see* butalbital compound *on page 63*
Aygestin® *see* norethindrone *on page 332*
Ayr® Nasal [OTC] *see* sodium chloride *on page 426*

azacitidine (ay za sye' ti deen)
Brand Names Mylosar®
Synonyms aza-cr; 5-azacytidine; 5-azc; ladakamycin
Therapeutic Category Antineoplastic Agent, Miscellaneous
Use Refractory acute lymphocytic and myelogenous leukemia
Usual Dosage Children and Adults: I.V.: 200-300 mg/m^2/day for 5-10 days, repeated at 2- to 3-week intervals
Dosage Forms Injection: 100 mg

aza-cr *see* azacitidine *on this page*
Azactam® *see* aztreonam *on next page*
5-azacytidine *see* azacitidine *on this page*

azatadine and pseudoephedrine
Brand Names Trinalin®
Synonyms pseudoephedrine and azatadine
Therapeutic Category Antihistamine/Decongestant Combination

Use Perennial and seasonal allergic rhinitis and other allergic symptoms including urticaria
Usual Dosage Adults: Oral: 1-2 mg twice daily
Dosage Forms Tablet: Azatadine maleate 1 mg and pseudoephedrine sulfate 120 mg

azatadine maleate (a za' ta deen)
Brand Names Optimine®
Therapeutic Category Antihistamine
Use Treatment of perennial and seasonal allergic rhinitis and chronic urticaria
Usual Dosage Children >12 years and Adults: Oral: 1-2 mg twice daily
Dosage Forms Tablet: 1 mg

azathioprine (ay za thye' oh preen)
Brand Names Imuran®
Therapeutic Category Antineoplastic Agent, Adjuvant; Immunosuppressant Agent
Use Adjunct with other agents in prevention of rejection of renal transplants; also used in severe rheumatoid arthritis unresponsive to other agents
Usual Dosage
Children and Adults: Renal transplantation: Oral, I.V.: Initial: 3-5 mg/kg/day; maintenance: 1-3 mg/kg/day

Adults: Rheumatoid arthritis: Oral: 1 mg/kg/day for 6-8 weeks; increase by 0.5 mg/kg every 4 weeks until response or up to 2.5 mg/kg/day I.V. dose is equivalent to oral dose
Dosage Forms
Injection, as sodium: 100 mg (20 mL)
Tablet: 50 mg

5-azc *see* azacitidine *on previous page*

Azdone® *see* hydrocodone and aspirin *on page 230*

azidothymidine *see* zidovudine *on page 494*

azithromycin dihydrate (az ith roe mye' sin)
Brand Names Zithromax™
Therapeutic Category Antibiotic, Macrolide
Use Treatment of adult patients (> 16 years of age) with mild to moderate infections of susceptible strains in upper and lower respiratory tract, skin and skin structure, and sexually transmitted diseases
Usual Dosage Adults: Oral: 500 mg as a single dose on day 1 followed by 250 mg daily on days 2-5 (1.5 g total); the recommended dose for nongonococcal urethritis and cervicitis due to *C. trachomatis* is a single 1 g dose
Dosage Forms Capsule: 250 mg

Azmacort™ *see* triamcinolone *on page 467*

Azo Gantanol® *see* sulfamethoxazole and phenazopyridine *on page 441*

Azo Gantrisin® *see* sulfisoxazole and phenazopyridine *on page 442*

Azo-Standard® *see* phenazopyridine hydrochloride *on page 360*

Azostix® [OTC] *see* diagnostic aids (*in vitro*), blood *on page 136*

azt *see* zidovudine *on page 494*

azthreonam *see* aztreonam *on this page*

aztreonam (az' tree oh nam)
Brand Names Azactam®
Synonyms azthreonam
Therapeutic Category Antibiotic, Miscellaneous
Use Treatment of patients with documented multidrug resistant aerobic gram-negative infection in which beta-lactam therapy is contraindicated; used for urinary tract infection, lower
(Continued)

aztreonam *(Continued)*

respiratory tract infections, septicemia, skin/skin structure infections, intra-abdominal infections, and gynecological infections

Usual Dosage
Neonates: I.M., I.V.:
Postnatal age <7 days:
<2000 g: 60 mg/kg/day in 2 divided doses every 12 hours
>2000 g: 90 mg/kg/day in 3 divided doses every 8 hours
Postnatal age >7 days:
<2000 g: 90 mg/kg/day in 3 divided doses every 8 hours
>2000 g: 120 mg/kg/day in 4 divided doses every 6 hours

Children >1 month: I.M., I.V.: 90-120 mg/kg/day divided every 6-8 hours
Cystic fibrosis: 50 mg/kg/dose every 6-8 hours (ie, up to 200 mg/kg/day); maximum: 6-8 g/day

Adults:
Urinary tract infection: I.M., I.V.: 500 mg to 1 g every 8-12 hours
Moderately severe systemic infections: 1 g I.V. or I.M. or 2 g I.V. every 8-12 hours
Severe systemic or life-threatening infections (especially caused by *Pseudomonas aeruginosa*): I.V.: 2 g every 6-8 hours; maximum: 8 g/day

Dosage Forms Powder for injection: 500 mg (15 mL, 100 mL); 1 g (15 mL, 100 mL); 2 g (15 mL, 100 mL)

Azulfidine® *see* sulfasalazine *on page 441*

Azulfidine® EN-tabs® *see* sulfasalazine *on page 441*

Babee® Teething Lotion [OTC] *see* benzocaine *on page 48*

bac *see* benzalkonium chloride *on page 48*

bacampicillin hydrochloride *(ba kam pi sill' in)*

Brand Names Spectrobid®
Synonyms carampicillin hydrochloride
Therapeutic Category Antibiotic, Penicillin
Use Treatment of susceptible bacterial infections involving the urinary tract, skin structure, upper and lower respiratory tract; activity is identical to that of ampicillin
Usual Dosage Oral:
Children: 25-50 mg/kg/day in divided doses every 12 hours
Adults: 400-800 mg every 12 hours
Dosage Forms
Powder for oral suspension: 125 mg/5 mL [chemically equivalent to ampicillin 87.5 mg per 5 mL] (70 mL)
Tablet: 400 mg [chemically equivalent to ampicillin 280 mg]

Bacid® [OTC] *see* lactobacillus *on page 261*

Baciguent® Topical [OTC] *see* bacitracin *on this page*

Baci-IM® Injection *see* bacitracin *on this page*

bacillus calmette-guérin *see* BCG *on page 45*

bacitracin *(bass i tray' sin)*

Brand Names AK-Tracin® Ophthalmic; Baciguent® Topical [OTC]; Baci-IM® Injection
Therapeutic Category Antibiotic, Miscellaneous; Antibiotic, Ophthalmic; Antibiotic, Topical
Use Treatment of susceptible bacterial infections; due to toxicity risks, systemic and irrigant uses of bacitracin should be limited to situations where less toxic alternatives would not be effective

Usual Dosage Children and Adults (I.M. recommended; **do not administer I.V.**):
Infants:
<2.5 kg: 900 units/kg/day in 2-3 divided doses
>2.5 kg = 1000 units/kg/day in 2-3 divided doses

Children: 800-1200 units/kg/day divided every 8 hours

Adults: 10,000-25,000 units/dose every 6 hours; not to exceed 100,000 units/day

Topical: Apply 1-5 times/day

Ophthalmic ointment: $^1/_4$" to $^1/_2$" ribbon every 3-4 hours to conjunctival sac for acute infections or 2-3 times/day for mild to moderate infections for 7-10 days

Irrigation, solution: 50-100 units/mL in normal saline, lactated Ringer's, or sterile water for irrigation; soak sponges in solution for topical compresses 1-5 times/day or as needed during surgical procedures
Dosage Forms
Injection: 50,000 units
Ointment:
Ophthalmic: 500 units/g (1 g, 3.5 g, 454 g)
Topical: 500 units/g (1.5 g, 3.75 g, 15 g, 30 g, 120 g, 454 g)

bacitracin and polymyxin b
Brand Names AK-Poly-Bac® Ophthalmic; Aquaphor® Antibiotic Topical [OTC]; Polysporin® Ophthalmic; Polysporin® Topical
Therapeutic Category Antibiotic, Ophthalmic; Antibiotic, Topical
Use Treatment of superficial infections caused by susceptible organisms
Usual Dosage
Ophthalmic: Apply $^1/_2$" ribbon to the affected eye(s) every 3-4 hours
Topical: Apply to affected area 1-3 times/day; may cover with sterile bandage if needed
Dosage Forms
Ointment:
Ophthalmic: Bacitracin 500 units and polymyxin b sulfate 10,000 units per g (3.5 g)
Topical: Bacitracin 500 units and polymyxin b sulfate 10,000 units per g (1/32 oz, 15 g, 30 g)
Powder, topical: Bacitracin 500 units and polymyxin b sulfate 10,000 units per g (10 g)

bacitracin, neomycin, and polymyxin b
Brand Names Medi-Quick® Ointment [OTC]; Mycitracin® [OTC]; Neomixin®; Neosporin® Ophthalmic Ointment; Neosporin® Topical Ointment [OTC]; Ocutricin® Topical Ointment; Septa® Ointment [OTC]; Triple Antibiotic®
Therapeutic Category Antibiotic, Ophthalmic; Antibiotic, Topical
Use Helps prevent infection in minor cuts, scrapes and burns; short-term treatment of superficial external ocular infections caused by susceptible organisms
Usual Dosage Children and Adults:
Ophthalmic ointment: Instill into the conjunctival sac one or more times/day every 3-4 hours for 7-10 days
Topical: Apply 1-3 times/day
Dosage Forms Ointment:
Ophthalmic: Bacitracin 400 units, neomycin sulfate 3.5 mg, and polymyxin b sulfate 10,000 units and per g
Topical: Bacitracin 400 units, neomycin sulfate 3.5 mg, and polymyxin b sulfate 5000 units per g

bacitracin, neomycin, polymyxin b, and hydrocortisone
Brand Names Cortisporin® Ophthalmic Ointment; Cortisporin® Topical Ointment
Therapeutic Category Antibiotic, Ophthalmic; Antibiotic, Otic; Antibiotic, Topical; Corticosteroid, Ophthalmic; Corticosteroid, Otic; Corticosteroid, Topical (Low Potency)
Use Prevention and treatment of susceptible superficial topical infections
Usual Dosage
Ophthalmic ointment: Apply $^1/_2$" ribbon to inside of lower lid every 3-4 hours until improvement occurs
(Continued)

43

bacitracin, neomycin, polymyxin b, and hydrocortisone *(Continued)*
Topical: Apply sparingly 2-4 times/day
Dosage Forms Ointment:
Ophthalmic: Bacitracin 400 units, neomycin sulfate 3.5 mg, polymyxin b sulfate 10,000 units, and hydrocortisone 10 mg per g (3.5 g)
Topical: Bacitracin 400 units, neomycin sulfate 3.5 mg, polymyxin b sulfate 10,000 units, and hydrocortisone 10 mg per g (15 g)

baclofen (bak' loe fen)
Brand Names Lioresal®
Therapeutic Category Skeletal Muscle Relaxant
Use Treatment of reversible spasticity associated with multiple sclerosis or spinal cord lesions
Usual Dosage Oral:
Children:
2-7 years: Initial: 10-15 mg/24 hours divided every 8 hours; titrate dose every 3 days in increments of 5-15 mg/day to a maximum of 40 mg/day
≥8 years: Maximum: 60 mg/day in 3 divided doses

Adults: 5 mg 3 times/day, may increase 5 mg/dose every 3 days to a maximum of 80 mg/day; may be necessary to reduce dosage in renal impairment
Dosage Forms
Injection, intrathecal: 0.5 mg/mL (20 mL); 2 mg/mL (5 mL)
Tablet: 10 mg, 20 mg

Bacticort® Otic *see neomycin, polymyxin b, and hydrocortisone on page 323*

Bactocill® Injection *see oxacillin sodium on page 340*

Bactocill® Oral *see oxacillin sodium on page 340*

BactoShield® Topical [OTC] *see chlorhexidine gluconate on page 90*

Bactrim™ *see co-trimoxazole on page 117*

Bactrim™ DS *see co-trimoxazole on page 117*

Bactroban® Nasal Spray *see mupirocin on page 313*

Bactroban® Topical *see mupirocin on page 313*

Baker's P&S Topical [OTC] *see phenol on page 362*

baking soda *see sodium bicarbonate on page 426*

bal *see dimercaprol on page 147*

balanced salt solution
Brand Names BSS® Ophthalmic
Therapeutic Category Ophthalmic Agent, Miscellaneous
Use Intraocular irrigating solution; also used to soothe and cleanse the eye in conjunction with hard contact lenses
Usual Dosage Use as needed for foreign body removal, gonioscopy and other general ophthalmic office procedures
Dosage Forms Ophthalmic:
Drops: 15 mL
Solution, sterile: 500 mL

Baldex® *see dexamethasone on page 131*

BAL in Oil® *see dimercaprol on page 147*

Balnetar® [OTC] *see coal tar, lanolin, and mineral oil on page 110*

Bancap HC® *see hydrocodone and acetaminophen on page 230*

Banophen® Oral [OTC] *see diphenhydramine hydrochloride on page 149*

Banthine® *see methantheline bromide on page 293*

Barbidonna® *see* hyoscyamine, atropine, scopolamine, and phenobarbital *on page 238*

Barbita® *see* phenobarbital *on page 361*

Baricon® *see* radiological/contrast media (ionic) *on page 404*

barium sulfate *see* radiological/contrast media (ionic) *on page 404*

Barobag® *see* radiological/contrast media (ionic) *on page 404*

Baro-CAT® *see* radiological/contrast media (ionic) *on page 404*

Baroflave® *see* radiological/contrast media (ionic) *on page 404*

Barophen® *see* hyoscyamine, atropine, scopolamine, and phenobarbital *on page 238*

Barosperse® *see* radiological/contrast media (ionic) *on page 404*

Bar-Test® *see* radiological/contrast media (ionic) *on page 404*

Basaljel® [OTC] *see* aluminum carbonate *on page 15*

Bayer® Select® Chest Cold Caplets [OTC] *see* acetaminophen and dextromethorphan *on page 3*

Bayer® Aspirin [OTC] *see* aspirin *on page 35*

Bayer® Buffered Aspirin [OTC] *see* aspirin *on page 35*

Bayer® Low Adult Strength [OTC] *see* aspirin *on page 35*

Bayer® Select® Pain Relief Formula [OTC] *see* ibuprofen *on page 240*

BCG

Brand Names TheraCys™; TICE® BCG

Synonyms bacillus calmette-guérin; bcg, intravesical

Therapeutic Category Biological Response Modulator; Vaccine, Live Bacteria

Use BCG vaccine is no longer recommended for adults at high risk for tuberculosis in the United States. BCG vaccination may be considered for infants and children who are skin test-negative to 5 tuberculin units of tuberculin and who cannot be given isoniazid preventive therapy but have close contact with untreated or ineffectively treated active tuberculosis patients or who belong to groups which other control measures have not been successful.

In the United States, tuberculosis control efforts are directed toward early identification, treatment of cases, and preventive therapy with isoniazid.

Usual Dosage Intravesical treatment and prophylaxis for carcinoma *in situ* of the urinary bladder: Begin between 7-14 days after biopsy or transurethral resection. Give a dose of 3 vials of BCG live intravesically under aseptic conditions once weekly for 6 weeks (induction therapy). Each dose (3 reconstituted vials) is further diluted in an additional 50 mL sterile, preservative free saline for a total of 53 mL. A urethral catheter is inserted into the bladder under aseptic conditions, the bladder is drained, and then the 53 mL suspension is instilled slowly by gravity, following which the catheter is withdrawn. If the bladder catheterization has been traumatic, BCG live should not be administered, and there must be a treatment delay of at least 1 week. Resume subsequent treatment; follow the induction therapy by one treatment given 3, 6, 12, 18 and 24 months following the initial treatment.

Dosage Forms Powder for injection, lyophilized:
Connaught Strain (TheraCys™): $3.4 \pm 3 \times 10^8$ CFU equivalent to approximately 27 mg
Tice Strain (TICE® BCG): $1-8 \times 10^8$ CFU equivalent to approximately 50 mg (2 mL)

bcg, intravesical *see* BCG *on this page*

bcnu *see* carmustine *on page 77*

B-D Glucose® [OTC] *see* glucose, instant *on page 209*

Because® [OTC] *see* nonoxynol 9 *on page 331*

beclomethasone dipropionate (be kloe meth' a sone)

Brand Names Beclovent® Oral Inhaler; Beconase AQ® Nasal Inhaler; Beconase® Nasal Inhaler; Vancenase® AQ Inhaler; Vancenase® Nasal Inhaler; Vanceril® Oral Inhaler

Therapeutic Category Anti-inflammatory Agent; Corticosteroid, Inhalant

(Continued)

beclomethasone dipropionate *(Continued)*

Use
Oral inhalation is used for treatment of bronchial asthma in patients who require chronic administration of corticosteroids
Nasal aerosol is used for the symptomatic treatment of seasonal or perennial rhinitis and nasal polyposis

Usual Dosage
Inhalation:
  Children 6-12 years: 1-2 inhalations 3-4 times/day, not to exceed 10 inhalations/day
  Adults: 2-4 inhalations twice daily, not to exceed 20 inhalations/day

Aerosol inhalation (nasal):
  Children 6-12 years: 1 spray each nostril 3 times/day
  Adults: 2-4 sprays each nostril twice daily

Aqueous inhalation (nasal): 1-2 sprays each nostril twice daily

Dosage Forms
Inhalation:
  Nasal (Beconase", Vancenase"): 42 mcg/inhalation [200 metered doses] (16.8 g)
  Oral (Beclovent", Vanceril®): 42 mcg/inhalation [200 metered doses] (16.8 g)
  Spray, aqueous, nasal (Beconase AQ®, Vancenase® AQ): 42 mcg/inhalation [200 metered doses] (25 g)

Beclovent® Oral Inhaler *see* beclomethasone dipropionate *on previous page*

Beconase AQ® Nasal Inhaler *see* beclomethasone dipropionate *on previous page*

Beconase® Nasal Inhaler *see* beclomethasone dipropionate *on previous page*

Beepen-VK® Oral *see* penicillin v potassium *on page 354*

Belix® Oral [OTC] *see* diphenhydramine hydrochloride *on page 149*

belladonna *(bell a don' a)*
Therapeutic Category Anticholinergic Agent; Antispasmodic Agent, Gastrointestinal
Use Decrease gastrointestinal activity in functional bowel disorders and to delay gastric emptying as well as decrease gastric secretion
Usual Dosage Adults: Oral: 0.3-1 mL 3-4 times/day
Dosage Forms Tincture: Belladonna alkaloids (principally hyoscyamine and atropine) 0.3 mg/mL with alcohol 65% to 70% (120 mL, 480 mL, 3780 mL)

belladonna and opium
Brand Names B&O Supprettes®
Synonyms opium and belladonna
Therapeutic Category Analgesic, Narcotic
Use Relief of moderate to severe pain associated with rectal or bladder tenesmus that may occur in postoperative states and neoplastic situations; pain associated with ureteral spasms not responsive to non-narcotic analgesics and to space intervals between injections of opiates
Usual Dosage Rectal:
  Children: Dose not established
  Adults: 1 suppository 1-2 times/day, up to 4 doses/day
Dosage Forms Suppository, rectal:
  #15A: Belladonna extract 15 mg and powdered opium 30 mg (12s)
  #16A: Belladonna extract 15 mg and powdered opium 60 mg (12s)

belladonna, phenobarbital, and ergotamine tartrate
Brand Names Bellergal-S®; Bel-Phen-Ergot S®; Phenerbel-S®
Therapeutic Category Ergot Alkaloid
Use Management and treatment of menopausal disorders, gastrointestinal disorders and recurrent throbbing headache

Usual Dosage Oral: 1 tablet each morning and evening
Dosage Forms Tablet, sustained release: l-alkaloids of belladonna 0.2 mg, phenobarbital 40 mg, and ergotamine tartrate 0.6 mg

Bellergal-S® *see* belladonna, phenobarbital, and ergotamine tartrate *on previous page*
Bel-Phen-Ergot S® *see* belladonna, phenobarbital, and ergotamine tartrate *on previous page*
Bena-D® Injection *see* diphenhydramine hydrochloride *on page 149*
Benadryl® Injection *see* diphenhydramine hydrochloride *on page 149*
Benadryl® Oral [OTC] *see* diphenhydramine hydrochloride *on page 149*
Benadryl® Topical *see* diphenhydramine hydrochloride *on page 149*
Benahist® Injection *see* diphenhydramine hydrochloride *on page 149*
Ben-Aqua® [OTC] *see* benzoyl peroxide *on page 50*

benazepril hydrochloride (ben ay' ze prill)
Brand Names Lotensin®
Therapeutic Category Angiotensin-Converting Enzyme (ACE) Inhibitors
Use Treatment of hypertension, either alone or in combination with other antihypertensive agents
Usual Dosage Adults: Oral: 20-40 mg/day as a single dose or 2 divided doses
Dosage Forms Tablet: 5 mg, 10 mg, 20 mg, 40 mg

bendroflumethiazide (ben droe floo meth eye' a zide)
Brand Names Naturetin®
Therapeutic Category Diuretic, Thiazide
Use Management of mild to moderate hypertension, edema associated with congestive heart failure, pregnancy, or nephrotic syndrome; reportedly does not alter serum electrolyte concentrations appreciably at recommended doses
Usual Dosage Oral:
Children: Initial: 0.1-0.4 mg/kg in 1-2 doses; maintenance dose: 0.05-0.1 mg/kg/day in 1-2 doses

Adults: 2.5-20 mg/day or twice daily in divided doses
Dosage Forms Tablet: 5 mg, 10 mg

Benemid® *see* probenecid *on page 386*
Benoject® Injection *see* diphenhydramine hydrochloride *on page 149*
Benoxyl® *see* benzoyl peroxide *on page 50*

bentiromide (ben teer' oh mide)
Brand Names Chymex®
Synonyms btpaba
Therapeutic Category Diagnostic Agent, Pancreatic Exocrine Insufficiency
Use Screening test for pancreatic exocrine insufficiency
Usual Dosage
Children <12 years: 14 mg/kg followed with 8 oz of water

Children >12 years and Adults: Administer following an overnight fast and morning void, single 500 mg dose and follow with 8 oz of water
Dosage Forms Solution, oral: 500 mg [PABA 170 mg] in propylene glycol 40% (7.5 mL)

Bentyl® Hydrochloride Injection *see* dicyclomine hydrochloride *on page 142*
Bentyl® Hydrochloride Oral *see* dicyclomine hydrochloride *on page 142*
Benylin DM® [OTC] *see* dextromethorphan hydrobromide *on page 135*

Benylin® Cough Syrup [OTC] *see* diphenhydramine hydrochloride *on page 149*

Benylin® Expectorant [OTC] *see* guaifenesin and dextromethorphan *on page 214*

Benzac AC® Gel *see* benzoyl peroxide *on page 50*

Benzac AC® Wash *see* benzoyl peroxide *on page 50*

Benzac W® *see* benzoyl peroxide *on page 50*

benzalkonium chloride (benz al koe' nee um)
Brand Names Benza™ [OTC]; Zephiran® [OTC]
Synonyms bac
Therapeutic Category Antibacterial, Topical
Use Surface antiseptic and germicidal preservative
Usual Dosage Thoroughly rinse anionic detergents and soaps from the skin or other areas prior to use of solutions because they reduce the antibacterial activity of BAC; to protect metal instruments stored in BAC solution, add crushed Anti-Rust Tablets, 4 tablets per quart, to antiseptic solution, change solution at least once weekly; not to be used for storage of aluminum or zinc instruments, instruments with lenses fastened by cement, lacquered catheters or some synthetic rubber goods
Dosage Forms
Concentrate, topical: 17% (500 mL, 4000 mL)
Solution, aqueous: 1:750 (60 mL, 120 mL, 240 mL)
Tincture: 1:750 (30 mL, 960 mL)
Tincture, spray: 1:750 (30 g, 180 g)
Tissue: 1:750 (packets)

Benzamycin® *see* erythromycin and benzoyl peroxide *on page 171*

Benza® [OTC] *see* benzalkonium chloride *on this page*

Benzashave® *see* benzoyl peroxide *on page 50*

benzathine benzylpenicillin *see* penicillin g benzathine *on page 352*

benzathine penicillin g *see* penicillin g benzathine *on page 352*

benzazoline hydrochloride *see* tolazoline hydrochloride *on page 463*

Benzedrex® [OTC] *see* propylhexedrine *on page 395*

benzene hexachloride *see* lindane *on page 269*

benzhexol hydrochloride *see* trihexyphenidyl hydrochloride *on page 471*

benzocaine (ben' zoe kane)
Brand Names Americaine® [OTC]; Anbesol® Maximum Strength [OTC]; Babee® Teething Lotion [OTC]; BiCOZENE® [OTC]; Chiggertox® [OTC]; Dermoplast® [OTC]; Foille Plus® [OTC]; Hurricaine™; Orabase®-B [OTC]; Orabase®-O [OTC]; Orajel® Brace-Aid Oral Anesthetic [OTC]; Orajel® Maximum Strength [OTC]; Orajel® Mouth-Aid [OTC]; Rhulicaine® [OTC]; Rid-A-Pain™ [OTC]; Solarcaine® [OTC]; Unguentine® [OTC]
Synonyms ethyl aminobenzoate
Therapeutic Category Local Anesthetic, Oral; Local Anesthetic, Topical
Use Local anesthetic
Usual Dosage
Gel, cream, ointment: Topical: Apply a small amount on affected area
Otic: Instill 4-5 drops into external ear every 1-2 hours as needed
Spray: Topical: To affected area as needed
Dosage Forms Topical:
Aerosol: 5% (97.5 mL, 105 mL); 20% (20 g, 60 g, 120 g)
Cream: 5% (30 g, 454 g); 6% (28.4 g)
Liquid: With benzyl benzoate and soft soap (30 mL)
Lotion: 8% (90 mL)
Ointment: 5% (3.5 g, 30 g)

benzocaine and antipyrine *see* antipyrine and benzocaine *on page 30*

benzocaine and cetylpyridinium chloride *see* cetylpyridinium chloride and benzocaine *on page 86*

benzocaine, butyl aminobenzoate, tetracaine, and benzalkonium chloride

Brand Names Cetacaine®
Therapeutic Category Local Anesthetic, Topical
Use Topical anesthetic to control pain or gagging
Usual Dosage Topical: Apply to affected area for approximately 1 second or less
Dosage Forms Aerosol: Benzocaine 14%, butyl aminobenzoate 2%, tetracaine 2%, and benzalkonium chloride 0.5% (56 g)

benzocaine, gelatin, pectin, and sodium carboxymethylcellulose

Brand Names Orabase® With Benzocaine [OTC]
Therapeutic Category Local Anesthetic, Topical
Use Topical anesthetic and emollient for oral lesions
Usual Dosage Apply 2-4 times/day
Dosage Forms Paste: Benzocaine 20%, gelatin, pectin, and sodium carboxymethylcellulose (15 g, 5 g)

benzoic acid and salicylic acid

Brand Names Whitfield's Ointment [OTC]
Synonyms salicylic acid and benzoic acid
Therapeutic Category Antifungal Agent, Topical
Use Treatment of athlete's foot and ringworm of the scalp
Usual Dosage Topical: Apply 1-4 times/day
Dosage Forms
Lotion, topical:
Full strength: Benzoic acid 12% and salicylic acid 6% with isopropyl alcohol 70% (240 mL)
Half strength: Benzoic acid 6% and salicylic acid 3% with isopropyl alcohol 70% (240 mL)
Ointment, topical: Benzoic acid 12% and salicylic acid 6% in anhydrous lanolin and petrolatum (30 g, 454 g)

benzoin (ben' zoin)

Brand Names AeroZoin® [OTC]; TinBen® [OTC]; TinCoBen® [OTC]
Synonyms gum benjamin
Therapeutic Category Pharmaceutical Aid; Protectant, Topical
Use Protective application for irritations of the skin; sometimes used in boiling water as steam inhalants for their expectorant and soothing action
Usual Dosage Apply 1-2 times/day
Dosage Forms
Spray, as compound tincture: 40% (105 mL)
Tincture: 79% (480 mL)
Tincture, as compound tincture: 20% (60 mL); 25% (120 mL)

benzonatate (ben zoe' na tate)

Brand Names Tessalon® Perles
Therapeutic Category Antitussive; Local Anesthetic, Oral
Use Symptomatic relief of nonproductive cough
Usual Dosage Oral:
Children <10 years: 8 mg/kg in 3-6 divided doses
Children >10 years and Adults: 100 mg 3 times/day up to 600 mg/day
Dosage Forms Capsule: 100 mg

benzoyl peroxide (ben' zoe ill peer ox' ide)
Brand Names Ambi 10® [OTC]; Ben-Aqua® [OTC]; Benoxyl®; Benzac AC® Gel; Benzac AC® Wash; Benzac W™; Benzashave®; Brevoxyl®; Clear By Design® [OTC]; Clearsil® [OTC]; Dermoxyl™ [OTC]; Desquam-X®; Exact® [OTC]; Loroxide® [OTC]; Neutrogena® Acne Mask [OTC]; Oxy-5® [OTC]; Oxy-5® Tinted [OTC]; PanOxyl® [OTC]; PanOxyl®-AQ; Peroxin A5®; Peroxin A10™; Persa-Gel®; Theroxide® Wash [OTC]; Vanoxide® [OTC]
Therapeutic Category Acne Products; Topical Skin Product
Use Adjunctive treatment of mild to moderate acne vulgaris and acne rosacea
Usual Dosage Children >12 years and Adults: Topical: Apply sparingly 1-3 times/day
Dosage Forms
Cleanser:
Bar: 5% (120 g); 10% (120 g)
Liquid: 5% (120 mL, 150 mL, 240 mL); 10% (120 mL, 150 mL)
Cream: 5% (30 g); 10% (30 g, 45 g)
Gel: 2.5% (45 g, 60 g, 90 g); 5% (45 g, 60 g, 90 g, 120 g); 10% (45 g, 60 g, 90 g, 120 g)
Lotion: 5% (30 mL, 42.5 mL, 60 mL); 5.5% (25 mL); 10% (30 mL, 42.5 mL, 60 mL)
Mask: 5% (60 g)
Shaving cream: 5% (113.4 g); 10% (113.4 g)

benzoyl peroxide and hydrocortisone
Brand Names Vanoxide-HC®
Therapeutic Category Acne Products; Corticosteroid, Topical (Low Potency); Topical Skin Product
Use Treatment of acne vulgaris and oily skin
Usual Dosage Shake well; apply thin film 1-3 times/day, gently massage into skin
Dosage Forms Lotion: Benzoyl peroxide 5% and hydrocortisone alcohol 0.5% (25 mL)

benzphetamine hydrochloride (benz fet' a meen)
Brand Names Didrex®
Therapeutic Category Anorexiant
Use Short-term adjunct in exogenous obesity
Usual Dosage Adults: Oral: 25-50 mg 2-3 times/day, preferably twice daily, midmorning and midafternoon
Dosage Forms Tablet: 25 mg, 50 mg

benzthiazide (benz thye' a zide)
Brand Names Aquatag®; Exna®; Hydrex®; Marazide®; Proaqua®
Therapeutic Category Diuretic, Thiazide
Use Management of mild to moderate hypertension; treatment of edema in congestive heart failure and nephrotic syndrome
Usual Dosage Adults: Oral: 50-200 mg/day
Dosage Forms Tablet: 50 mg

benztropine mesylate (benz' troe peen)
Brand Names Cogentin®
Therapeutic Category Anticholinergic Agent; Anti-Parkinson's Agent
Use Adjunctive treatment of all forms of parkinsonism; also used in treatment of drug-induced extrapyramidal effects (except tardive dyskinesia) and acute dystonic reactions
Usual Dosage Titrate dose in 0.5 mg increments at 5- to 6-day intervals
Extrapyramidal reaction, drug induced: Oral, I.M., I.V.:
Children >3 years: 0.02-0.05 mg/kg/dose 1-2 times/day
Adults: 1-4 mg/dose 1-2 times/day

Parkinsonism: Oral: 0.5-6 mg/day in 1-2 divided doses; if one dose is greater, give at bedtime
Dosage Forms
Injection: 1 mg/mL (2 mL)
Tablet: 0.5 mg, 1 mg, 2 mg

benzylpenicillin benzathine *see* penicillin g benzathine *on page 352*
benzylpenicillin potassium *see* penicillin g, parenteral *on page 353*
benzylpenicillin sodium *see* penicillin g, parenteral *on page 353*

benzylpenicilloyl-polylysine (ben' zil pen i sill' oil polly lie' seen)
Brand Names Pre-Pen®
Synonyms penicilloyl-polylysine; ppl
Therapeutic Category Diagnostic Agent, Penicillin Allergy Skin Test
Use Adjunct in assessing the risk of administering penicillin (penicillin or benzylpenicillin) in adults with a history of clinical penicillin hypersensitivity
Usual Dosage
Use scratch technique with a 20-gauge needle to make 3-5 mm scratch on epidermis, apply a small drop of solution to scratch, rub in gently with applicator or toothpick.

A positive reaction consists of a pale wheal surrounding the scratch site which develops within 10 minutes and ranges from 5-15 mm or more in diameter.

If the scratch test is negative an intradermal test may be performed.
Intradermal test: Use intradermal test with a tuberculin syringe with a 26- to 30-gauge short bevel needle; a dose of 0.01-0.02 mL is injected intradermally. A control of 0.9% sodium chloride should be injected at least 1½" from the PPL test site. Most skin responses to the intradermal test will develop within 5-15 minutes.
(–) = no reaction or increase in size compared to control
(±) = wheal slightly larger with or without erythematous flare and larger than control site
(+) = itching and increase in size of original bleb may exceed 20 mm in diameter
Dosage Forms Injection: 0.25 mL per ampul

bepridil hydrochloride (be' pri dil)
Brand Names Vascor®
Therapeutic Category Antianginal Agent; Calcium Channel Blocker
Use Treatment of chronic stable angina; only approved indication is hypertension, but may be used for congestive heart failure; doses should not be adjusted for at least 10 days after beginning therapy
Usual Dosage Adults: Oral: Initial: 200 mg/day, then adjust dose until optimal response is achieved; maximum daily dose: 400 mg
Dosage Forms Tablet: 200 mg, 300 mg, 400 mg

beractant (ber akt' ant)
Brand Names Survanta®
Synonyms bovine lung surfactant; natural lung surfactant
Therapeutic Category Lung Surfactant
Use Prevention and treatment of respiratory distress syndrome in premature infants
Prophylactic therapy: Body weight <1250 g in infants at risk for developing or with evidence of surfactant deficiency

Rescue therapy: Treatment of infants with RDS confirmed by x-ray and requiring mechanical ventilation
Usual Dosage Intratracheal:
Prophylactic treatment: Give 4 mL/kg as soon as possible; as many as 4 doses may be administered during the first 48 hours of life, no more frequently than 6 hours apart. The need for additional doses is determined by evidence of continuing respiratory distress; if the infant is still intubated and requiring at least 30% inspired oxygen to maintain a PaO_2 ≤80 torr.

Rescue treatment: Give 4 mL/kg as soon as the diagnosis of RDS is made.
Dosage Forms Suspension: Phospholipids 25 mg/mL, suspended in sodium chloride 0.9% (8 mL)

Berocca® *see vitamin b complex with vitamin c and folic acid on page 490*

Berubigen® *see cyanocobalamin on page 119*

Beta-2® *see isoetharine on page 251*

beta-carotene (kare' oh teen)
Brand Names Max-Caro® [OTC]; Provatene® [OTC]; Solatene®
Therapeutic Category Vitamin, Fat Soluble
Use Reduce the severity of photosensitivity reactions in patients with erythropoietic protoporphyria (EPP)
Usual Dosage Oral:
Children <14 years: 30-150 mg/day
Adults: 30-300 mg/day
Dosage Forms Capsule: 15 mg, 30 mg

Betachron E-R® *see propranolol hydrochloride on page 394*

Betadine® [OTC] *see povidone-iodine on page 380*

9-beta-D-ribofuranosyladenine *see adenosine on page 8*

Betagan® Liquifilm® Ophthalmic *see levobunolol hydrochloride on page 264*

Betalin® S *see thiamine hydrochloride on page 455*

betamethasone (bay ta meth' a sone)
Brand Names Alphatrex®; Betatrex®; Beta-Val®; Celestone®; Celestone® Soluspan®; Cel-U-Jec®; Diprolene®; Diprolene® AF; Diprosone®; Maxivate®; Psorion® Cream; Selestoject®; Teladar®; Uticort®; Valisone®
Synonyms flubenisolone
Therapeutic Category Anti-inflammatory Agent; Corticosteroid, Systemic; Corticosteroid, Topical (Medium/High Potency)
Use Inflammatory dermatoses such as seborrheic or atopic dermatitis, neurodermatitis, anogenital pruritus, psoriasis, inflammatory phase of xerosis, late phase of allergic dermatitis or irritant dermatitis
Usual Dosage Children and Adults:
I.M.: Betamethasone sodium phosphate and betamethasone acetate: 0.5-9 mg/day ($\frac{1}{3}$ to $\frac{1}{2}$ of oral dose)
Intrabursal, intra-articular: 0.5-2 mL
Oral: 0.6-7.2 mg/day
Topical: Apply thin film 2-4 times/day
Dosage Forms
Base (Celestone®):
Syrup: 0.6 mg/5 mL
Tablet: 0.6 mg
Benzoate (Uticort®):
Cream, emollient base: 0.025% (60 g)
Gel, topical: 0.025% (15 g, 60 g)
Lotion: 0.025% (60 mL)
Dipropionate (Alphatrex®, Diprosone®, Maxivate®, Teladar®):
Aerosol, topical: 0.1% (85 g)
Cream: 0.05% (15 g, 45 g)
Lotion: 0.05% (20 mL, 30 mL, 60 mL)
Ointment, topical: 0.05% (15 g, 45 g)
Dipropionate (Psorion®):
Cream: 0.05% (15 g, 45 g)
Dipropionate, augmented (Diprolene®, Diprolene® AF):
Cream, emollient base: 0.05% (15 g, 45 g)
Gel, topical: 0.05% (15 g, 45 g)
Lotion: 0.05% (30 mL, 60 mL)
Ointment, topical: 0.05% (15 g, 45 g)

Valerate (Betatrex®, Beta-Val®, Valisone®):
   Cream: 0.01% (15 g, 60 g); 0.1% (15 g, 45 g, 110 g, 430 g)
   Lotion: 0.1% (20 mL, 60 mL)
   Ointment, topical: 0.1% (15 g, 45 g)
   Powder for compounding: 5 g, 10 g
Sodium phosphate (B-S-P®, Selestoject®):
   Injection: Equivalent to 3 mg/mL (5 mL)
Sodium phosphate and acetate (Celestone® Soluspan®):
   Injection, suspension: 6 mg/mL [betamethasone sodium phosphate 3 mg and beta-
      methasone acetate 3 mg per mL] (5 mL)

betamethasone dipropionate and clotrimazole
Brand Names Lotrisone®
Therapeutic Category Antifungal Agent, Topical; Corticosteroid, Topical (Medium/High Po-
   tency)
Use Topical treatment of various dermal fungal infections
Usual Dosage Topical: Apply twice daily
Dosage Forms Cream: Betamethasone dipropionate 0.05% and clotrimazole 1% (15 g, 45 g)

Betapace® Oral see sotalol hydrochloride on page 433

Betapen®-VK Oral see penicillin v potassium on page 354

Betaseron® see interferon beta-1b on page 247

Betatrex® see betamethasone on previous page

Beta-Val® see betamethasone on previous page

betaxolol hydrochloride (be tax' oh lol)
Brand Names Betoptic® Ophthalmic; Betoptic® S Ophthalmic; Kerlone® Oral
Therapeutic Category Beta-Adrenergic Blocker; Beta-Adrenergic Blocker, Ophthalmic
Use Treatment of chronic open-angle glaucoma, ocular hypertension; management of hyper-
   tension
Usual Dosage Adults:
   Ophthalmic: Instill 1 drop twice daily
   Oral: 10 mg/day; may increase dose to 20 mg/day after 7-14 days if desired response is not
      achieved; initial dose in elderly patients: 5 mg/day
Dosage Forms
   Solution, ophthalmic (Betoptic®): 0.5% (2.5 mL, 5 mL, 10 mL)
   Suspension, ophthalmic (Betoptic® S): 0.25% (2.5 mL, 10 mL, 15 mL)
   Tablet (Kerlone®): 10 mg, 20 mg

bethanechol chloride (be than' e kole)
Brand Names Duvoid®; Myotonachol™; Urecholine®
Therapeutic Category Cholinergic Agent
Use Nonobstructive urinary retention and retention due to neurogenic bladder; treatment and
   prevention of bladder dysfunction caused by phenothiazines; diagnosis of flaccid or atonic
   neurogenic bladder
Usual Dosage
   Children:
      Oral:
         Abdominal distention or urinary retention: 0.6 mg/kg/day divided 3-4 times/day
         Gastroesophageal reflux: 0.1-0.2 mg/kg/dose given 30 minutes to 1 hour before each
            meal to a maximum of 4 times/day
      S.C.: 0.15-0.2 mg/kg/day divided 3-4 times/day
   Adults:
      Oral: 10-50 mg 2-4 times/day
      S.C.: 2.5-5 mg 3-4 times/day, up to 7.5-10 mg every 4 hours for neurogenic bladder
(Continued)

bethanechol chloride *(Continued)*
Dosage Forms
Injection: 5 mg/mL (1 mL)
Tablet: 5 mg, 10 mg, 25 mg, 50 mg

Betoptic® Ophthalmic *see* betaxolol hydrochloride *on previous page*

Betoptic® S Ophthalmic *see* betaxolol hydrochloride *on previous page*

Bexophene® *see* propoxyphene and aspirin *on page 394*

Biavax®_{II} *see* rubella and mumps vaccines, combined *on page 415*

Biaxin™ Filmtabs® *see* clarithromycin *on page 104*

Bicillin® C-R 900/300 Injection *see* penicillin g benzathine and procaine combined *on page 353*

Bicillin® C-R Injection *see* penicillin g benzathine and procaine combined *on page 353*

Bicillin® L-A Injection *see* penicillin g benzathine *on page 352*

Bicitra® *see* sodium citrate and citric acid *on page 427*

BiCNU® *see* carmustine *on page 77*

BiCOZENE® [OTC] *see* benzocaine *on page 48*

Bili-Labstix® [OTC] *see* diagnostic aids *(in vitro)*, urine *on page 137*

Bilopaque® *see* radiological/contrast media (ionic) *on page 404*

Biltricide® *see* praziquantel *on page 382*

Biocef *see* cephalexin monohydrate *on page 84*

Bioclate® *see* antihemophilic factor (recombinant) *on page 29*

Biocult-GC® *see* diagnostic aids *(in vitro)*, other *on page 137*

Biomox® *see* amoxicillin trihydrate *on page 24*

Bio-Tab® Oral *see* doxycycline *on page 158*

Biozyme-C® *see* collagenase *on page 114*

biperiden hydrochloride (bye per' i den)
Brand Names Akineton®
Therapeutic Category Anti-Parkinson's Agent
Use Treatment of all forms of Parkinsonism including drug induced type (extrapyramidal symptoms)
Usual Dosage Adults:
Parkinsonism: Oral: 2 mg 3-4 times/day

Extrapyramidal:
Oral: 2-6 mg 2-3 times/day
I.M., I.V.: 2 mg every 30 minutes up to 4 doses or 8 mg/day
Dosage Forms
Injection, as lactate: 5 mg/mL (1 mL)
Tablet, as hydrochloride: 2 mg

biphenabid *see* probucol *on page 387*

bisacodyl (bis a koe' dill)
Brand Names Bisacodyl Uniserts® [OTC]; Bisco-Lax® [OTC]; Carter's Little Pills® [OTC]; Clysodrast™; Dulcagen™ [OTC]; Dulcolax® [OTC]; Fleet® Laxative [OTC]
Therapeutic Category Laxative, Stimulant
Use Treatment of constipation; colonic evacuation prior to procedures or examination
Usual Dosage
Children:
Oral: >6 years: 5-10 mg (0.3 mg/kg) at bedtime or before breakfast

Rectal suppository:
  <2 years: 5 mg as a single dose
  >2 years: 10 mg
Adults:
  Oral: 5-15 mg as single dose (up to 30 mg when complete evacuation of bowel is required)
  Rectal suppository: 10 mg as single dose
  Tannex:
    Enema: 2.5 g in 1000 mL warm water
    Barium enema: 2.5-5 g in 1000 mL barium suspension
    Do not give >10 g within 72-hour period

Dosage Forms
Enema: 10 mg/30 mL
Powder (Clysodrast®): 1.5 mg with tannic acid 2.5 g per packet (25s, 50s)
Suppository, rectal: 10 mg
Suppository, rectal, pediatric: 5 mg
Tablet, enteric coated: 5 mg

Bisacodyl Uniserts® [OTC] *see bisacodyl on previous page*

Bisco-Lax® [OTC] *see bisacodyl on previous page*

bishydroxycoumarin *see dicumarol on page 141*

Bismatrol® [OTC] *see bismuth subsalicylate on this page*

bismuth subsalicylate

Brand Names Bismatrol® [OTC]; Pepto-Bismol® [OTC]
Therapeutic Category Antidiarrheal
Use Symptomatic treatment of mild, nonspecific diarrhea
Usual Dosage Oral:
  Nonspecific diarrhea: Subsalicylate:
    Children: Up to 8 doses/24 hours:
      3-6 years: $\frac{1}{3}$ tablet or 5 mL every 30 minutes to 1 hour as needed
      6-9 years: $\frac{2}{3}$ tablet or 10 mL every 30 minutes to 1 hour as needed
      9-12 years: 1 tablet or 15 mL every 30 minutes to 1 hour as needed
    Adults: 2 tablets or 30 mL every 30 minutes to 1 hour as needed up to 8 doses/24 hours
    Prevention of traveler's diarrhea: 2.1 g/day or 2 tablets 4 times/day before meals and at bedtime
    Subgallate: 1-2 tablets 3 times/day with meals

Dosage Forms
Caplet, swallowable: 262 mg
Liquid: 262 mg/15 mL (120 mL, 240 mL, 360 mL, 480 mL); 524 mg/15 mL (120 mL, 240 mL, 360 mL)
Tablet, chewable: 262 mg

bismuth subgallate

Brand Names Devrom® [OTC]
Therapeutic Category Antidiarrheal
Use Symptomatic treatment of mild, nonspecific diarrhea
Usual Dosage Oral: 1-2 tablets 3 times/day with meals
  Dosing adjustment in renal impairment: Should probably be avoided in patients with renal failure
Dosage Forms Tablet, chewable: 200 mg

bisoprolol and hydrochlorothiazide

Brand Names Ziac™
Therapeutic Category Beta-Adrenergic Blocker; Diuretic, Thiazide
Use Treatment of hypertension
(Continued)

bisoprolol and hydrochlorothiazide *(Continued)*
Usual Dosage Adults: Oral: Dose is individualized, given once daily
Dosage Forms Tablet: Bisoprolol fumarate 2.5 mg and hydrochlorothiazide 6.25 mg; bisoprolol fumarate 5 mg and hydrochlorothiazide 6.25 mg; bisoprolol fumarate 10 mg and hydrochlorothiazide 6.25 mg

bisoprolol fumarate (bis oh' proe lol)
Brand Names Zebeta®
Therapeutic Category Beta-Adrenergic Blocker
Use Treatment of hypertension, alone or in combination with other agents
Usual Dosage Adults: Oral: 5 mg once daily, may be increased to 10 mg, and then up to 20 mg once daily, if necessary; may be given without regard to meals
Dosage Forms Tablet: 5 mg, 10 mg

bistropamide *see* tropicamide *on page 476*

bitolterol mesylate (bye tole' ter ole)
Brand Names Tornalate®
Therapeutic Category Beta-2-Adrenergic Agonist Agent; Bronchodilator
Use Prevent and treat bronchial asthma and bronchospasm
Usual Dosage Children >12 years and Adults:
Bronchospasm: 2 inhalations at an interval of at least 1-3 minutes, followed by a third inhalation if needed
Prevention of bronchospasm: 2 inhalations every 8 hours
Dosage Forms
Aerosol, oral: 0.8% [370 mcg/metered spray, 300 inhalations] (15 mL)
Solution, inhalation: 0.2% (10 mL, 30 mL, 60 mL)

Black Draught® [OTC] *see* senna *on page 420*

black widow spider antivenin (*Latrodectus mactans*) *see* antivenin, black widow spider (equine) *on page 31*

Blenoxane® *see* bleomycin sulfate *on this page*

bleomycin sulfate (blee oh mye' sin)
Brand Names Blenoxane®
Synonyms blm
Therapeutic Category Antineoplastic Agent, Antibiotic
Use Palliative treatment of squamous cell carcinomas, testicular carcinoma and lymphomas
Usual Dosage Refer to individual protocol
Children and Adults:
Test dose for lymphoma patients: I.M., I.V., S.C.: 1-2 units of bleomycin for the first 2 doses; monitor vital signs every 15 minutes; wait a minimum of 1 hour before administering remainder of dose
I.M., I.V., S.C.: 10-20 units/m^2 (0.25-0.5 units/kg) 1-2 times/week in combination regimens
I.V. continuous infusion: 15-20 units/m^2/day for 4-5 days
Adults: Intracavitary injection for pleural effusion: 15-240 units have been given
Dosage Forms Powder for injection: 15 units

Bleph®-10 Ophthalmic *see* sodium sulfacetamide *on page 431*

Blephamide® *see* sodium sulfacetamide and prednisolone *on page 431*

blm *see* bleomycin sulfate *on this page*

Blocadren® Oral *see* timolol maleate *on page 461*

Bluboro® [OTC] *see* aluminum acetate and calcium acetate *on page 15*

Bonine® [OTC] *see* meclizine hydrochloride *on page 282*

boric acid
Brand Names Borofax® Topical [OTC]; Dri-Ear® Otic [OTC]; Swim-Ear® Otic [OTC]
Therapeutic Category Pharmaceutical Aid
Use
Ophthalmic: Mild antiseptic used for inflamed eyelids
Topical ointment: Temporary relief of chapped, chafed, or dry skin, diaper rash, abrasions, minor burns, sunburn, insect bites, and other skin irritations
Usual Dosage Apply to lower eyelid 1-2 times/day
Dosage Forms
Ointment:
Ophthalmic: 5% (3.5 g); 10% (3.5 g)
Topical: 5% (52.5 g); 10% (28 g)
Topical (Borofax®): 5% boric acid and lanolin (1¾ oz)
Solution, otic: 2.75% with isopropyl alcohol (30 mL)

Borofax® Topical [OTC] *see* boric acid *on this page*

B&O Supprettes® *see* belladonna and opium *on page 46*

Botox® *see* botulinum toxin type A *on this page*

botulinum toxin type A (bot' yoo lin num)
Brand Names Botox®
Therapeutic Category Ophthalmic Agent, Toxin
Use Treatment of strabismus and blepharospasm
Usual Dosage
Strabismus: 1.25-5 units (0.05-0.15 mL) injected into any one muscle
Blepharospasm: 1.25-5 units (0.05-0.15 mL) injected into the orbicularis oculi muscle
Dosage Forms Powder for injection, lyophilized, preservative free: *Clostridium botulinum* Toxin type A 100 units

bovine lung surfactant *see* beractant *on page 51*

BQ® Tablet [OTC] *see* chlorpheniramine, phenylpropanolamine, and acetaminophen *on page 96*

Breezee® Mist Antifungal [OTC] *see* miconazole *on page 305*

Breonesin® [OTC] *see* guaifenesin *on page 213*

Brethaire® Inhalation Aerosol *see* terbutaline sulfate *on page 447*

Brethine® Injection *see* terbutaline sulfate *on page 447*

Brethine® Oral *see* terbutaline sulfate *on page 447*

bretylium tosylate (bre til' ee um toss' a late)
Brand Names Bretylol®
Therapeutic Category Antiarrhythmic Agent, Class III
Use Ventricular tachycardia and fibrillation; also used in the treatment of other serious ventricular arrhythmias resistant to lidocaine
Usual Dosage
Children:
I.M.: 2-5 mg/kg as a single dose
I.V.: Initial: 5 mg/kg, then attempt electrical defibrillation; repeat with 10 mg/kg if ventricular fibrillation persists
Maintenance dose: I.M., I.V.: 5 mg/kg every 6-8 hours
Adults:
Immediate life-threatening ventricular arrhythmias; ventricular fibrillation; unstable ventricular tachycardia. **Note**: Patients should undergo defibrillation/cardioversion before and after bretylium doses as necessary.
(Continued)
57

bretylium tosylate *(Continued)*

Initial dose: I.V.: 5 mg/kg (undiluted) over 1 minute; if arrhythmia persists, give 10 mg/kg (undiluted) over 1 minute and repeat as necessary (usually at 15- to 30-minute intervals) up to a total dose of 30 mg/kg

Other life-threatening ventricular arrhythmias:

Initial dose: I.M., I.V.: 5-10 mg/kg, may repeat every 1-2 hours if arrhythmia persist; give I.V. dose (diluted) over 10-30 minutes

Maintenance dose: I.M.: 5-10 mg/kg every 6-8 hours; I.V. (diluted): 5-10 mg/kg every 6 hours; I.V. infusion (diluted): 1-2 mg/minute (little experience with doses >40 mg/kg/day)

Dosage Forms

Injection: 50 mg/mL (10 mL, 20 mL)

Injection, premixed in D_5W: 1 mg/mL (500 mL); 2 mg/mL (250 mL); 4 mg/mL (250 mL, 500 mL)

Bretylol® *see* bretylium tosylate *on previous page*

Brevibloc® Injection *see* esmolol hydrochloride *on page 172*

Brevicon® *see* ethinyl estradiol and norethindrone *on page 178*

Brevital® Sodium *see* methohexital sodium *on page 295*

Brevoxyl® *see* benzoyl peroxide *on page 50*

Brexin® L.A. *see* chlorpheniramine and pseudoephedrine *on page 94*

Bricanyl® Injection *see* terbutaline sulfate *on page 447*

Bricanyl® Oral *see* terbutaline sulfate *on page 447*

British anti-lewisite *see* dimercaprol *on page 147*

Brofed® *see* brompheniramine and pseudoephedrine *on next page*

Bromaline® [OTC] *see* brompheniramine and phenylpropanolamine *on next page*

Bromanate DC® *see* brompheniramine, phenylpropanolamine, and codeine *on page 60*

Bromanate® [OTC] *see* brompheniramine and phenylpropanolamine *on next page*

Bromanyl® Cough Syrup *see* bromodiphenhydramine and codeine *on this page*

Bromarest® [OTC] *see* brompheniramine maleate *on next page*

Bromatapp® [OTC] *see* brompheniramine and phenylpropanolamine *on next page*

Bromfed-PD® *see* brompheniramine and pseudoephedrine *on next page*

bromocriptine mesylate (broe moe krip' teen mess' a late)

Brand Names Parlodel®

Therapeutic Category Anti-Parkinson's Agent; Ergot Alkaloid

Use Treatment of parkinsonism in patients unresponsive or allergic to levodopa; also used in conditions associated with hyperprolactinemia and to suppress lactation

Usual Dosage Oral:

Parkinsonism: 1.25 mg twice daily, increased by 2.5 mg/day in 2- to 4-week intervals (usual dose range: 30-90 mg/day in 3 divided doses)

Hyperprolactinemia and postpartum lactation: 2.5 mg 2-3 times/day

Dosage Forms

Capsule: 5 mg

Tablet: 2.5 mg

bromodiphenhydramine and codeine (brome oh dye fen hye' dra meen)

Brand Names Ambenyl® Cough Syrup; Amgenal® Cough Syrup; Bromanyl® Cough Syrup; Bromotuss® w/Codeine Cough Syrup

Synonyms codeine and bromodiphenhydramine

Therapeutic Category Antihistamine; Cough Preparation

Use Relief of upper respiratory symptoms and cough associated with allergies or common cold

Usual Dosage Oral: 5-10 mL every 4-6 hours

Dosage Forms Liquid: Bromodiphenhydramine hydrochloride 12.5 mg and codeine phosphate 10 mg per 5 mL

Bromotuss® w/Codeine Cough Syrup *see* bromodiphenhydramine and codeine *on previous page*

Bromphen DC® w/Codeine *see* brompheniramine, phenylpropanolamine, and codeine *on next page*

brompheniramine and phenylpropanolamine

Brand Names Bromaline® [OTC]; Bromanate® [OTC]; Bromatapp® [OTC]; Bromphen® Tablet [OTC]; Dimetapp® [OTC]; Dimetapp® Extentabs® [OTC]; E.N.T.®; Myphetapp® [OTC]; Tamine® [OTC]; Vicks® DayQuil® Allergy Relief 12 Hour [OTC]

Synonyms phenylpropanolamine and brompheniramine

Therapeutic Category Antihistamine/Decongestant Combination

Use Temporary relief of nasal congestion, running nose, sneezing, and itchy, watery eyes

Usual Dosage Oral:

Children:

1-6 months: 1.25 mL 3-4 times/day
7-24 months: 2.5 mL 3-4 times/day
2-4 years: 3.75 mL 3-4 times/day
4-12 years: 5 mL 3-4 times/day

Adults: 5-10 mL 3-4 times/day or 1 tablet twice daily

Dosage Forms

Elixir (grape flavor): Brompheniramine maleate 2 mg and phenylpropanolamine hydrochloride 12.5 mg per 5 mL with alcohol 2.3% (5 mL, 120 mL, 240 mL, 480 mL, 3780 mL)
Tablet: Brompheniramine maleate 4 mg and phenylpropanolamine hydrochloride 25 mg
Tablet, sustained release: Brompheniramine maleate 12 mg and phenylpropanolamine hydrochloride 75 mg

brompheniramine and pseudoephedrine

Brand Names Brofed®; Bromfed-PD®; Dallergy-JR®; Dristan® Allergy [OTC]; Respahist®; ULTRAbrom® PD

Therapeutic Category Antihistamine/Decongestant Combination

Use Temporary relief of symptoms of seasonal and perennial allergic rhinitis, and vasomotor rhinitis, including nasal obstruction

Usual Dosage Oral:

Children 6-12 years: 1 capsule every 12 hours
Children >12 years and Adults: 1 or 2 capsules every 12 hours

Dosage Forms

Caplet: Brompheniramine maleate 4 mg and pseudoephedrine hydrochloride 60 mg
Capsule, timed-release: Brompheniramine maleate 6 mg and pseudoephedrine hydrochloride 60 mg
Elixir: Brompheniramine maleate 4 mg and pseudoephedrine hydrochloride 30 mg

brompheniramine maleate (brome fen ir' a meen)

Brand Names Bromarest® [OTC]; Bromphen® Elixir [OTC]; Chlorphed® [OTC]; Cophene-B® Injection; Dehist® Injection; Diamine T.D.® Oral [OTC]; Dimetane® Oral [OTC]; Histaject® Injection; Nasahist B® Injection; ND-Stat® Injection; Oraminic® II Injection; Sinusol-B® Injection; Veltane® Tablet

Synonyms parabromdylamine

Therapeutic Category Antihistamine

Use Perennial and seasonal allergic rhinitis and other allergic symptoms including urticaria

Usual Dosage

Oral:

Children:

<6 years: 0.125 mg/kg/dose given every 6 hours; maximum: 6-8 mg/day
6-12 years: 2-4 mg every 6-8 hours; maximum: 12-16 mg/day

(Continued)

brompheniramine maleate *(Continued)*

Adults: 4 mg every 4-6 hours or 8 mg of sustained release form every 8-12 hours or 12 mg of sustained release every 12 hours; maximum: 24 mg/day

I.M., I.V., S.C.:
Children <12 years: 0.5 mg/kg/24 hours divided every 6-8 hours
Adults: 5-50 mg every 4-12 hours, maximum: 40 mg/24 hours

Dosage Forms
Elixir: 2 mg/5 mL with alcohol 3% (120 mL, 480 mL, 4000 mL)
Injection: 10 mg/mL (10 mL)
Tablet: 4 mg, 8 mg, 12 mg
Tablet, sustained release: 8 mg, 12 mg

brompheniramine, phenylpropanolamine, and codeine

Brand Names Bromanate DC®; Bromphen DC® w/Codeine; Dimetane®-DC; Myphetane DC®; Poly-Histine CS®
Therapeutic Category Antihistamine/Decongestant Combination; Cough Preparation
Use Relief of coughs and upper respiratory symptoms, including nasal congestion, associated with allergy or the common cold
Usual Dosage Oral:
Children:
2-6 years: 2.5 mL every 4 hours
6-12 years: 5 mL every 4 hours

Children >12 years and Adults: 10 mL every 4 hours
Dosage Forms Liquid: Brompheniramine maleate 2 mg, phenylpropanolamine hydrochloride 12.5 mg, and codeine phosphate 10 mg per 5 mL with alcohol 0.95% (480 mL)

Bromphen® Tablet [OTC] *see* brompheniramine and phenylpropanolamine *on previous page*

Bromphen® Elixir [OTC] *see* brompheniramine maleate *on previous page*

Bronchial® *see* theophylline and guaifenesin *on page 454*

Bronitin® *see* epinephrine *on page 167*

Bronkaid® Mist [OTC] *see* epinephrine *on page 167*

Bronkephrine® Injection *see* ethylnorepinephrine hydrochloride *on page 182*

Bronkodyl® *see* theophylline *on page 453*

Bronkometer® *see* isoetharine *on page 251*

Bronkosol® *see* isoetharine *on page 251*

Brontex® Liquid *see* guaifenesin and codeine *on page 214*

Brontex® Tablet *see* guaifenesin and codeine *on page 214*

BSS® Ophthalmic *see* balanced salt solution *on page 44*

btpaba *see* bentiromide *on page 47*

Bucet™ *see* butalbital compound *on page 63*

Bucladin®-S Softab® *see* buclizine hydrochloride *on this page*

buclizine hydrochloride (byoo' kli zeen)

Brand Names Bucladin®-S Softab®
Therapeutic Category Antiemetic; Antihistamine
Use Prevention and treatment of motion sickness; symptomatic treatment of vertigo
Usual Dosage Adults: Oral:
Motion sickness (prophylaxis): 50 mg 30 minutes prior to traveling; may repeat 50 mg after 4-6 hours

Vertigo: 50 mg twice daily, up to 150 mg/day
Dosage Forms Tablet, chewable: 50 mg

budesonide (byoo des' oh nide)
Brand Names Rhinocort®
Therapeutic Category Anti-inflammatory Agent; Corticosteroid, Inhalant
Use Management of symptoms of seasonal or perennial rhinitis in adults and nonallergic perennial rhinitis in adults
Usual Dosage Adults and children ≥6 years of age: 256 mcg daily, given as either 2 sprays in each nostril in the morning and evening or as 4 sprays in each nostril in the morning.
Dosage Forms Aerosol: 32 mcg per actuation (7 g)

Bufferin® [OTC] *see* aspirin *on page 35*

bumetanide (byoo met' a nide)
Brand Names Bumex®
Therapeutic Category Diuretic, Loop
Use Management of edema secondary to congestive heart failure or hepatic or renal disease including nephrotic syndrome; may also be used alone or in combination with antihypertensives in the treatment of hypertension
Usual Dosage
Children:
    <6 months: Dose not established
    >6 months:
        Oral: Initial: 0.015 mg/kg/dose once daily or every other day; maximum dose: 0.1 mg/kg/day
      I.M., I.V.: Dose not established

Adults:
    Oral: 0.5-2 mg/dose (maximum: 10 mg/day) 1-2 times/day
    I.M., I.V.: 0.5-1 mg/dose (maximum: 10 mg/day)
Dosage Forms
Injection: 0.25 mg/mL (2 mL, 4 mL, 10 mL)
Tablet: 0.5 mg, 1 mg, 2 mg

Bumex® *see* bumetanide *on this page*
Buminate® *see* albumin human *on page 10*

bupivacaine hydrochloride (byoo piv' a kane)
Brand Names Marcaine®; Sensorcaine®; Sensorcaine-MPF®
Therapeutic Category Local Anesthetic, Injectable
Use Local anesthetic (injectable) for peripheral nerve block, infiltration, sympathetic block, caudal or epidural block, retrobulbar block
Usual Dosage Dose varies with procedure, depth of anesthesia, vascularity of tissues, duration of anesthesia and condition of patient

Caudal block (with or without epinephrine):
    Children: 1-3.7 mg/kg
    Adults: 15-30 mL of 0.25% or 0.5%

Epidural block (other than caudal block):
    Children: 1.25 mg/kg/dose
    Adults: 10-20 mL of 0.25% or 0.5%

Peripheral nerve block: 5 mL dose of 0.25% or 0.5% (12.5-25 mg); maximum: 2.5 mg/kg (plain); 3 mg/kg (with epinephrine); up to a maximum of 400 mg/day

Sympathetic nerve block: 20-50 mL of 0.25% (no epinephrine) solution
Dosage Forms
Bupivacaine Injection:
    Preservative free: 0.25% [2.5 mg/mL]; 0.5% [5 mg/mL]; 0.75% [7.5 mg/mL]
    With preservative: 0.25% [2.5 mg/mL]; 0.5% [5 mg/mL]

Bupivacaine and Epinephrine [1:200,000] Injection:
    Preservative free: 0.25% [2.5 mg/mL]; 0.5% [5 mg/mL]; 0.75% [7.5 mg/mL]
    With preservative: 0.25% [2.5 mg/mL]; 0.5% [5 mg/mL]
(Continued)

bupivacaine hydrochloride *(Continued)*
Bupivacaine in Dextrose [8.25%] Injection (Spinal):
  Preservative free: 0.75% [7.5 mg/mL]

Buprenex® *see buprenorphine hydrochloride on this page*

buprenorphine hydrochloride (byoo pre nor' feen)
Brand Names Buprenex®
Therapeutic Category Analgesic, Narcotic
Use Management of moderate to severe pain
Usual Dosage Adults: I.M., slow I.V.: 0.3-0.6 mg every 6 hours as needed
Dosage Forms Injection: 0.3 mg/mL (1 mL)

bupropion (byoo proe' pee on)
Brand Names Wellbutrin®
Therapeutic Category Antidepressant
Use Treatment of depression
Usual Dosage Adults: Oral: 100 mg 3 times/day; begin at 100 mg twice daily; may increase to a maximum dose of 450 mg/day
Dosage Forms Tablet: 75 mg, 100 mg

BuSpar® *see buspirone hydrochloride on this page*

buspirone hydrochloride (byoo spye' rone)
Brand Names BuSpar®
Therapeutic Category Antianxiety Agent
Use Management of anxiety
Usual Dosage Adults: Oral: 15 mg/day (5 mg 3 times/day); may increase to a maximum of 60 mg/day
Dosage Forms Tablet: 5 mg, 10 mg

busulfan (byoo sul' fan)
Brand Names Myleran®
Therapeutic Category Antineoplastic Agent, Alkylating Agent
Use Chronic myelogenous leukemia and marrow-ablative conditioning regimens prior to bone marrow transplantation
Usual Dosage Oral (refer to individual protocols):
  Children:
    Remission induction of chronic myelogenous leukemia: 0.06-0.12 mg/kg/day or 1.8-4.6 mg/m^2/day; titrate dose to maintain leukocyte count about 20,000/mm^3
    BMT marrow-ablative conditioning regimen: 1 mg/kg/dose every 6 hours for 16 doses

  Adults: Remission induction of chronic myelogenous leukemia: 4-8 mg/day; maintenance dose: controversial, range from 1-4 mg/day to 2 mg/week
Dosage Forms Tablet: 2 mg

butabarbital sodium (byoo ta bar' bi tal)
Brand Names Butalan®; Buticaps®; Butisol Sodium®
Therapeutic Category Barbiturate; Hypnotic; Sedative
Use Sedative, hypnotic
Usual Dosage
  Children: Preop: 2-6 mg/kg/dose; maximum: 100 mg
  Adults:
    Sedative: 15-30 mg 3-4 times/day

Hypnotic: 50-100 mg
Preop: 50-100 mg 1-1½ hours before surgery
Dosage Forms
Capsule: 15 mg, 30 mg
Elixir, with alcohol 7%: 30 mg/5 mL (480 mL, 3780 mL); 33.3 mg/5 mL (480 mL, 3780 mL)
Tablet: 15 mg, 30 mg, 50 mg, 100 mg

Butalan® *see* butabarbital sodium *on previous page*

butalbital compound (byoo tal' bi tal)
Brand Names Amaphen®; Anoquan®; Arcet®; Axotal®; Bucet™; Endolor®; Esgic®; Esgic-Plus®; Femcet®; Fiorgen PF®; Fioricet®; Fiorinal®; Isocet®; Isollyl Improved®; Lanorinal®; Margesic®; Marnal®; Medigesic®; Phrenilin®; Phrenilin® Forte®; Repan; Sedapap-10®; Tencent™; Tencon®; Triad®; Triaprin®; Two-Dyne®
Therapeutic Category Analgesic, Non-Narcotic; Barbiturate
Use Relief of the symptomatic complex of tension or muscle contraction headache
Usual Dosage Adults: Oral: 1-2 tablets or capsules every 4 hours; not to exceed 6/day
Dosage Forms
Capsule, with acetaminophen:
Amaphen®, Anoquan®, Endolor®, Esgic®, Femcet®, Margesic®, Medigesic®, Repan, Tencet™, Triad®, Two-Dyne®: Butalbital 50 mg, caffeine 40 mg, and acetaminophen 325 mg
Triapin®: Butalbital 50 mg and acetaminophen 325 mg
Phrenilin® Forte®, Tencon®: Butalbital 50 mg and acetaminophen 650 mg
Capsule, with aspirin: (Fiorgen PF®, Fiorinal®, Isollyl Improved®, Lanorinal®, Marnal®): Butalbital 50 mg, caffeine 40 mg, and aspirin 325 mg
Tablet, with acetaminophen:
Arcet®, Esgic®, Fioricet®, Repan: Butalbital 50 mg, caffeine 40 mg, and acetaminophen 325 mg
Bucet™, Sedapap-10®: Butalbital 50 mg and acetaminophen 650 mg
Esgic-Plus®: Butalbital 50 mg, caffeine 40 mg, and acetaminophen 500 mg
Isocet®: Butalbital 50 mg, caffeine 40 mg, and acetaminophen 325 mg
Phrenilin®: Butalbital 50 mg and acetaminophen 325 mg
Tablet, with aspirin:
Axotal®: Butalbital 50 mg and aspirin 650 mg
Fiorinal®, Isollyl Improved®, Lanorinal®, Marnal®: Butalbital 50 mg, caffeine 40 mg, and aspirin 325 mg

butalbital compound and codeine
Brand Names Fiorinal® With Codeine
Synonyms codeine and butalbital compound
Therapeutic Category Analgesic, Narcotic; Barbiturate
Use Mild to moderate pain when sedation is needed
Usual Dosage Oral: 1-2 capsules every 4-6 hours as needed for pain
Dosage Forms Capsule: Butalbital 50 mg, caffeine 40 mg, aspirin 325 mg and codeine phosphate 30 mg

Buticaps® *see* butabarbital sodium *on previous page*
Butisol Sodium® *see* butabarbital sodium *on previous page*

butoconazole nitrate (byoo toe koe' na zole)
Brand Names Femstat®
Therapeutic Category Antifungal Agent, Vaginal
Use Local treatment of vulvovaginal candidiasis
Usual Dosage Adults:
Nonpregnant: 1 applicatorful (~5 g) intravaginally at bedtime for 3 days, may extend for up to 6 days if necessary
(Continued)

butoconazole nitrate (Continued)
Pregnant: **Use only during second or third trimesters**
Dosage Forms Cream, vaginal: 2% with applicator (28 g)

butorphanol tartrate (byoo tor' fa nole)
Brand Names Stadol(R); Stadol(R) NS
Therapeutic Category Analgesic, Narcotic
Use Management of moderate to severe pain
Usual Dosage Adults:
  I.M.: 1-4 mg every 3-4 hours as needed
  I.V.: 0.5-2 mg every 3-4 hours as needed
  Nasal: 1 mg (1 spray in one nostril) initially, allow 60-90 minutes to elapse before deciding
    whether a second 1 mg dose is needed; this 2 dose sequence may be repeated in 3-4
    hours if needed
Dosage Forms
  Injection: 1 mg/mL (1 mL); 2 mg/mL (1 mL, 2 mL, 10 mL)
  Nasal spray: 10 mg/mL [14-15 doses] (2.5 mL)

Byclomine® Injection see dicyclomine hydrochloride on page 142

Bydramine® Cough Syrup [OTC] see diphenhydramine hydrochloride on page 149

c7E3 see abciximab on page 2

c8-cck see sincalide on page 423

Cafatine® see ergotamine derivatives on page 169

Cafergot® see ergotamine derivatives on page 169

Cafetrate® see ergotamine derivatives on page 169

caffeine and sodium benzoate (kaf' een)
Synonyms sodium benzoate and caffeine
Therapeutic Category Diuretic, Miscellaneous
Use Emergency stimulant in acute circulatory failure; as a diuretic; and to relieve spinal punc-
  ture headache
Usual Dosage
  Children: I.M., I.V., S.C.: 8 mg/kg every 4 hours as needed
  Adults: I.M., I.V.: 500 mg, maximum single dose: 1 g
Dosage Forms Injection: Caffeine 125 mg and sodium benzoate 125 mg per mL (2 mL)

caffeine, citrated
Therapeutic Category Central Nervous System Stimulant, Nonamphetamine; Respiratory
  Stimulant
Use Central nervous system stimulant; used in the treatment of idiopathic apnea of prematuri-
  ty. Has several advantages over theophylline in the treatment of neonatal apnea, its half-life
  is about 3 times as long, allowing once daily dosing, drug levels do not need to be drawn at
  peak and trough; has a wider therapeutic window, allowing more room between an effective
  concentration and toxicity.
Usual Dosage Apnea of prematurity: Oral:
  Loading dose: 10-20 mg/kg as caffeine citrate (5-10 mg/kg as caffeine base). If theophylline
    has been administered to the patient within the previous 5 days, a full or modified loading
    dose (50% to 75% of a loading dose) may be given at the discretion of the physician.
  Maintenance dose: 5-10 mg/kg/day as caffeine citrate (2.5-5 mg/kg/day as caffeine base)
    once daily starting 24 hours after the loading dose. Maintenance dose is adjusted based
    on patient's response, (efficacy and adverse effects), and serum caffeine concentrations.
Dosage Forms
  Solution, oral: 20 mg/mL [anhydrous caffeine 10 mg/mL]
  Tablet: 65 mg [anhydrous caffeine 32.5 mg]

Calan® *see* verapamil hydrochloride *on page 486*

Cal Carb-HD® [OTC] *see* calcium carbonate *on next page*

Calcibind® *see* cellulose sodium phosphate *on page 84*

Calci-Chew™ [OTC] *see* calcium carbonate *on next page*

Calciday-667® [OTC] *see* calcium carbonate *on next page*

calcifediol (kal si fe dye' ole)
Brand Names Calderol®
Synonyms 25-d_3; 25-hydroxycholecalciferol; 25-hydroxyvitamin d_3
Therapeutic Category Vitamin D Analog
Use Treatment and management of metabolic bone disease associated with chronic renal failure
Usual Dosage Hepatic osteodystrophy: Oral:
Infants: 5-7 mcg/kg/day

Children and Adults: 20-100 mcg/day or every other day; titrate to obtain normal serum calcium/phosphate levels
Dosage Forms Capsule: 20 mcg, 50 mcg

Calciferol™ Injection *see* ergocalciferol *on page 169*

Calciferol™ Oral *see* ergocalciferol *on page 169*

Calcijex™ *see* calcitriol *on this page*

Calcimar® *see* calcitonin (salmon) *on this page*

Calci-Mix™ [OTC] *see* calcium carbonate *on next page*

Calciparine® *see* heparin *on page 222*

calcipotriene (kal si poe' try een)
Brand Names Dovonex®
Therapeutic Category Antipsoriatic Agent, Topical
Use Treatment of plaque psoriasis
Usual Dosage Apply to skin lesions twice daily
Dosage Forms Ointment, topical: 0.005% (30 g, 60 g, 100 g)

calcitonin (salmon) (kal si toe' nin)
Brand Names Calcimar®; Miacalcin®; Osteocalcin®
Therapeutic Category Antidote, Hypercalcemia
Use Treatment of Paget's disease of bone and as adjunctive therapy for hypercalcemia; also used in postmenopausal osteoporosis
Usual Dosage Dosage for children not established
Hepatic osteodystrophy:
Infants: 5-7 mcg/kg/day
Children and Adults: 20-100 mcg/kg/day or every other day, titrate to obtain normal serum calcium/phosphate levels
Skin test: 1 unit/0.1 mL intracutaneously
Paget's disease: I.M., S.C.: 100 units/day
Postmenopause osteoporosis: I.M., S.C.: 100 units/day
Hypercalcemia: I.M., S.C.: 4 units/kg every 12 hours, may increase to maximum of 8 units/kg every 6 hours
Dosage Forms Injection: 200 units/mL (2 mL)

calcitriol (kal si trye' ole)
Brand Names Calcijex™; Rocaltrol®
Synonyms 1,25 dihydroxycholecalciferol
Therapeutic Category Vitamin D Analog
(Continued)

65

calcitriol *(Continued)*

Use Management of hypocalcemia in patients on chronic renal dialysis; reduce elevated parathyroid hormone levels

Usual Dosage Individualize dosage to maintain calcium levels of 9-10 mg/dL
Renal failure: Oral:
Children: Initial: 15 ng/kg/day; maintenance: 30-60 ng/kg/day
Adults: 0.25 mcg/day or every other day (may require 0.5-1 mcg/day)

Unlabeled dose:
Renal failure: I.V.: Adults: 0.5 mcg (0.01 mcg/kg) 3 times/week; most doses in the range
of 0.5-3 mcg (0.01-0.05 mcg/kg) 3 times/week
Hypoparathyroidism/pseudohypoparathyroidism: Oral:
Children 1-5 years: 0.25-0.75 mcg/day
Children >6 years and Adults: 0.5-2 mcg/day

Dosage Forms
Capsule: 0.25 mcg, 0.5 mcg
Injection: 1 mcg/mL (1 mL); 2 mcg/mL (1 mL)

calcium acetate

Brand Names PhosLo®
Therapeutic Category Calcium Salt
Use Control of hyperphosphatemia in end stage renal failure and does not promote aluminum absorption
Usual Dosage Adults: Oral: 2 tablets with each meal; dosage may be increased to bring serum phosphate value to <6 mg/dL; most patients require 3-4 tablets with each meal
Dosage Forms Elemental calcium listed in brackets
Capsule: 500 mg [125 mg]
Tablet: 250 mg [62.5 mg], 667 mg [169 mg], 1000 mg [250 mg]

calcium carbonate

Brand Names Alka-Mints® [OTC]; Amitone® [OTC]; Cal Carb-HD® [OTC]; Calci-Chew™ [OTC]; Calciday-667® [OTC]; Calci-Mix™ [OTC]; Cal-Plus® [OTC]; Caltrate® 600 [OTC]; Caltrate,® Jr [OTC]; Chooz® [OTC]; Dicarbosil® [OTC]; Equilet® [OTC]; Florical® [OTC]; Gencalc® 600 [OTC]; Mallamint® [OTC]; Nephro-Calci® [OTC]; Os-Cal® 500 [OTC]; Oyst-Cal 500 [OTC]; Oystercal® 500; Rolaids® Calcium Rich [OTC]; Tums® [OTC]; Tums® E-X Extra Strength Tablet [OTC]; Tums® Extra Strength Liquid [OTC]
Therapeutic Category Antacid; Antidote, Hyperphosphatemia; Calcium Salt
Use Antacid and calcium supplement; control of hyperphosphatemia in end stage renal failure and does not promote aluminum absorption
Usual Dosage Dosage is in terms of elemental calcium
Recommended daily allowance (RDA):
<6 months: 360 mg/day
6-12 months: 540 mg/day
1-10 years: 800 mg/day
10-18 years: 1200 mg/day
Adults: 800 mg/day

Hypocalcemia (dose depends on clinical condition and serum calcium level):
Neonates: 50-150 mg/kg/day in 4-6 divided doses; not to exceed 1 g/day
Children: 20-65 mg/kg/day in 4 divided doses
Adults: 1-2 g or more per day
Dosage Forms Elemental calcium listed in brackets
Capsule: 1500 mg [600 mg]
Calci-Mix™: 1250 mg [500 mg]
Florical®: 364 mg [145.6 mg] with sodium fluoride 8.3 mg
Liquid (Tums® Extra Strength): 1000 mg/5 mL (360 mL)
Lozenge (Mylanta® Soothing Antacids): 600 mg [240 mg]
Powder (Cal Carb-HD®): 6.5 g/packet [2.6 g]
Suspension, oral: 1250 mg/5 mL [500 mg]
Tablet: 650 mg [260 mg], 1500 mg [600 mg]

Calciday-667®: 667 mg [267 mg]
Os-Cal® 500, Oyst-Cal® 500, Oystercal® 500: 1250 mg [500 mg]
Cal-Plus®, Caltrate® 600, Gencalc® 600, Nephro-Calci®: 1500 mg [600 mg]
Chewable:
  Alka-Mints®: 850 mg [340 mg]
  Amitone®: 350 mg [140 mg]
  Caltrate,® Jr®: 750 mg [300 mg]
  Calci-Chew™, Os-Cal®: 750 mg [300 mg]
  Chooz®, Dicarbosil®, Equilet®, Tums®: 500 mg [200 mg]
  Mallamint®: 420 mg [168 mg]
  Rolaids® Calcium Rich: 550 mg [220 mg]
  Tums® E-X Extra Strength: 750 mg [300 mg]
  Tums® Ultra®: 1000 mg [400 mg]
Florical®: 364 mg [145.6 mg] with sodium fluoride 8.3 mg

calcium carbonate and simethicone
Brand Names Titralac® Plus Liquid [OTC]
Synonyms simethicone and calcium carbonate
Therapeutic Category Antacid
Use Relief of acid indigestion, heartburn, peptic esophagitis, hiatal hernia, and gas
Usual Dosage Oral: 0.5-2 g 4-6 times/day
Dosage Forms Elemental calcium listed in brackets
Liquid: Calcium carbonate 500 mg [200 mg] and simethicone 20 mg per 5 mL

calcium chloride
Therapeutic Category Calcium Salt; Electrolyte Supplement, Parenteral
Use Cardiac resuscitation when epinephrine fails to improve myocardial contractions, cardiac disturbances of hyperkalemia, hypocalcemia or calcium channel blocking agent toxicity
Usual Dosage I.V.:
Cardiac arrest in the presence of hyperkalemia or hypocalcemia, magnesium toxicity, or calcium antagonist toxicity:
  Infants and Children: 10-20 mg/kg; may repeat in 10 minutes if necessary
  Adults: 1.5-4 mg/kg/dose or 2.5-5 mL/dose every 10 minutes

Hypocalcemia:
  Infants and Children: 10-20 mg/kg/dose, repeat every 4-6 hours if needed
  Adults: 500 mg to 1 g at 1- to 3-day intervals

Exchange transfusion: 0.45 mEq after each 100 mL of blood exchanged I.V.

Hypocalcemia secondary to citrated blood transfusion give 0.45 mEq **elemental** calcium for each 100 mL citrated blood infused

Tetany:
  Infants and Children: 10 mg/kg over 5-10 minutes. May repeat after 6 hours or follow with an infusion with a maximum dose of 200 mg/kg/day
  Adults: 1 g over 10-30 minutes; may repeat after 6 hours
Dosage Forms Elemental calcium listed in brackets
Injection: 10% = 100 mg/mL [27.2 mg/mL] (10 mL)

calcium citrate
Brand Names Citracal® [OTC]
Therapeutic Category Calcium Salt
Use Adjunct in prevention of postmenopausal osteoporosis, treatment and prevention of calcium depletion
Usual Dosage Oral (dosage is in terms of elemental calcium):
Adults: 1-2 g/day

Recommended daily allowance (RDA):
  <6 months: 360 mg/day
(Continued)

67

calcium citrate *(Continued)*

6-12 months: 540 mg/day
1-10 years: 800 mg/day
10-18 years: 1200 mg/day
Adults: 800 mg/day

Dosage Forms Elemental calcium listed in brackets
Tablet: 950 mg [200 mg]
Tablet, effervescent: 2376 mg [500 mg]

Calcium Disodium Versenate® *see* edetate calcium disodium *on page 162*

calcium edta *see* edetate calcium disodium *on page 162*

calcium glubionate (gloo bye' oh nate)

Brand Names Neo-Calglucon® [OTC]
Therapeutic Category Calcium Salt
Use Adjunct in prevention of postmenopausal osteoporosis, treatment and prevention of calcium depletion
Usual Dosage Oral (syrup is a hyperosmolar solution; dosage is in terms of calcium glubionate):

Neonatal hypocalcemia: 1200 mg/kg/day in 4-6 divided doses
Maintenance: Infants and Children: 600-2000 mg/kg/day in 4 divided doses up to a maximum of 9 g/day

Adults: 6-18 g/day in divided doses

Recommended daily allowance (RDA):
<6 months: 360 mg/day
6-12 months: 540 mg/day
1-10 years: 800 mg/day
10-18 years: 1200 mg/day
Adults: 800 mg/day

Dosage Forms Elemental calcium listed in brackets
Syrup: 1.8 g/5 mL [115 mg/5 mL] (480 mL)

calcium gluceptate (gloo sep' tate)

Therapeutic Category Calcium Salt
Use Cardiac disturbances of hyperkalemia; cardiac resuscitation when epinephrine fails to improve myocardial contractions
Usual Dosage I.V.:

Cardiac resuscitation in the presence of hypocalcemia, hyperkalemia, or calcium channel blocker toxicity:
Children: 110 mg/kg/dose or 0.5 mL/kg/dose every 10 minutes
Adults: 5 mL every 10 minutes

Hypocalcemia:
Children: 200-500 mg/kg/day divided every 6 hours
Adults: 500 mg to 1.1 g/dose as needed

Exchange transfusion: 0.45 mEq (0.5 mL) after each 100 mL of blood exchanged

After citrated blood administration: Children and Adults: 0.4 mEq/100 mL blood infused
Dosage Forms Elemental calcium listed in brackets
Injection: 220 mg/mL [18 mg/mL] (5 mL, 50 mL)

calcium gluconate (gloo' koe nate)

Brand Names Kalcinate®
Therapeutic Category Calcium Salt
Use Treatment and prevention of hypocalcemia, treatment of tetany, cardiac disturbances of hyperkalemia, cardiac resuscitation when epinephrine fails to improve myocardial contractions, hypocalcemia, or calcium chemical blocker toxicity

Usual Dosage Dosage is in terms of elemental calcium
Recommended daily allowance (RDA):
    <6 months: 360 mg/day
    6-12 months: 540 mg/day
    1-10 years: 800 mg/day
    10-18 years: 1200 mg/day
    Adults: 800 mg/day

Calcium gluconate electrolyte requirement in newborn period:
    Premature: 200-1000 mg/kg/24 hours
    Term:
        0-24 hours: 0-500 mg/kg/24 hours
        24-48 hours: 200-500 mg/kg/24 hours
        48-72 hours: 200-600 mg/kg/24 hours
        >3 days: 200-800 mg/kg/24 hours

Hypocalcemia:
    I.V.:
        Neonates: 200-400 mg/kg/day as a continuous infusion or in 4 divided doses
        Infants and Children: 200-1000 mg/kg/day as a continuous infusion or in 4 divided
            doses
        Adults: 2-15 g/24 hours as a continuous infusion or in divided doses
    Oral:
        Children: 200-500 mg/kg/day divided every 6 hours
        Adults: 500 mg to 2 g 2-4 times/day

Calcium antagonist toxicity, magnesium intoxication; cardiac arrest in the presence of hyper-
    kalemia or hypocalcemia: I.V.:
        Infants and Children: 100 mg/kg/dose
        Adults: 1-3 g

Tetany: I.V.:
    Neonates: 100-200 mg/kg/dose, may follow with 500 mg/kg/day in 3-4 divided doses or as
        an infusion
    Infants and Children: 100-200 mg/kg/dose over 5-10 minutes; may repeat after 6 hours or
        follow with an infusion of 500 mg/kg/day
    Adults: 1-3 g may be administered until therapeutic response occurs

Cardiac resuscitation: I.V.:
    Infants and Children: 100 mg/kg/dose (1 mL/kg/dose) every 10 minutes
    Adults: 500-800 mg/dose (5-8 mL) every 10 minutes

Hypocalcemia secondary to citrated blood infusion; give 0.45 mEq **elemental** calcium for
    each 100 mL citrated blood infused

Exchange transfusion:
    Neonates: 100 mg/100 mL of citrated blood exchanged
    Adults: 300 mg/100 mL of citrated blood exchanged

Maintenance electrolyte requirements for total parenteral nutrition: I.V.: Daily requirements:
    Adults: 10-20 mEq/1000 kcals/24 hours

Dosage Forms Elemental calcium listed in brackets
Injection: 10% = 100 mg/mL [9 mg/mL] (10 mL, 50 mL, 100 mL, 200 mL)
Tablet: 500 mg [45 mg], 650 mg [58.5 mg], 975 mg [87.75 mg], 1 g [90 mg]

calcium lactate

Therapeutic Category Calcium Salt
Use Adjunct in prevention of postmenopausal osteoporosis, treatment and prevention of calci-
um depletion
Usual Dosage Oral:
    Infants: 400-500 mg/kg/day divided every 4-6 hours
    Children: 500 mg/kg/day divided every 6-8 hours; maximum daily dose: 9 g
    Adults: 1.5-3 g divided every 8 hours
Dosage Forms Elemental calcium listed in brackets
Tablet: 325 mg [42.25 mg], 650 mg [84.5 mg]

calcium leucovorin *see* leucovorin calcium *on page 263*

calcium pantothenate *see* pantothenic acid *on page 348*

calcium phosphate, dibasic
Brand Names Posture" [OTC]
Synonyms dicalcium phosphate
Therapeutic Category Calcium Salt
Use Adjunct in prevention of postmenopausal osteoporosis, treatment and prevention of calcium depletion
Usual Dosage Oral (doses in g of elemental calcium):
Children: 45-65 mg/kg/day
Adults: 1-2 g/day
Dosage Forms Elemental calcium listed in brackets
Tablet, sugar free: 1565.2 mg [600 mg]

calcium polycarbophil (pol ee kar' boe fil)
Brand Names Equalactin® Chewablet Tablet [OTC]; Fiberall® Chewable Tablet [OTC]; Fiber-Con" Tablet [OTC]; Fiber-Lax® Tablet [OTC]; FiberNorm® [OTC]; Konsyl Fiber® [OTC]; Mitrolan" Chewable Tablet [OTC]
Therapeutic Category Antidiarrheal; Laxative, Bulk-Producing
Use Treatment of constipation or diarrhea by restoring a more normal moisture level and providing bulk in the patient's intestinal tract; calcium polycarbophil is supplied as the approved substitute whenever a bulk-forming laxative is ordered in a tablet, capsule, wafer, or other oral solid dosage form
Usual Dosage Oral:
Children:
2-6 years: 500 mg 1-2 times/day, up to 1.5 g/day
6-12 years: 500 mg 1-3 times/day, up to 3 g/day

Adults: 1 g 4 times/day, up to 6 g/day
Dosage Forms Tablet:
Sodium free:
Fiber-Lax", FiberNorm'", Konsyl Fiber": 625 mg
FiberCon": 500 mg
Chewable:
Equalactin", Mitrolan'": 500 mg
Fiberall'": 1250 mg

calcium undecylenate (un de sil len' ate)
Brand Names Caldesene" Powder [OTC]; Cruex® Powder [OTC]; Protectol® Medicated Powder [OTC]
Therapeutic Category Antifungal Agent, Topical
Use Adjunctive therapy in treatment of athlete's foot and ringworm
Usual Dosage Topical: Apply as needed after cleansing and drying area
Dosage Forms Powder, topical:
Caldesene", Cruex": 10% (45 g, 60 g, 120 g)
Protectol" Medicated: 15% (56.7 g)

Caldecort® *see* hydrocortisone *on page 232*

Caldecort® Anti-Itch Spray *see* hydrocortisone *on page 232*

Calderol® *see* calcifediol *on page 65*

Caldesene® Powder [OTC] *see* calcium undecylenate *on this page*

Caldesene® Topical [OTC] *see* undecylenic acid and derivatives *on page 479*

Calm-X® Oral [OTC] *see* dimenhydrinate *on page 147*

Cal-Plus® [OTC] *see* calcium carbonate *on page 66*

Caltrate® 600 [OTC] *see* calcium carbonate *on page 66*

Caltrate,® Jr [OTC] *see* calcium carbonate *on page 66*

Cam-ap-es® *see* hydralazine, hydrochlorothiazide, and reserpine *on page 228*

Campho-Phenique® [OTC] *see* camphor and phenol *on this page*

camphor and phenol
Brand Names Campho-Phenique® [OTC]
Therapeutic Category Topical Skin Product
Use Relief of pain and for minor infections
Usual Dosage Apply as needed
Dosage Forms Liquid: Camphor 10.8% and phenol 4.7%

camphorated tincture of opium *see* paregoric *on page 349*

camphor, menthol and phenol
Brand Names Sarna [OTC]
Therapeutic Category Topical Skin Product
Use Relief of dry, itching skin
Usual Dosage Topical: Apply as needed for dry skin
Dosage Forms Lotion, topical: Camphor 0.5%, menthol 0.5%, and phenol 0.5% in emollient base (240 mL)

Candida albicans (Monilia) (kan' dee daa al' bee kans mo nill' ya)
Brand Names Dermatophytin-O
Synonyms *Monilia* skin test
Therapeutic Category Diagnostic Agent, Fungus
Use Screen for detection of nonresponsiveness to antigens in immunocompromised individuals
Usual Dosage 0.1 mL intradermally, examine reaction site in 24-48 hours; induration of ≥5 mm in diameter is a positive reaction
Dosage Forms Injection:
Intradermal: 1:100 (5 mL)
Scratch: 1:10 (5 mL)

Cankaid® [OTC] *see* carbamide peroxide *on page 74*

cantharidin (can thar' e din)
Brand Names Verr-Canth™
Therapeutic Category Keratolytic Agent
Use Removal of ordinary and periungual warts
Usual Dosage Topical: Apply directly to lesion, cover with nonporous tape, remove tape in 24 hours, reapply if necessary
Dosage Forms Liquid: 0.7% in a film-forming vehicle containing acetone, pyroxylin, castor oil and camphor (7.5 mL)

Cantil® *see* mepenzolate bromide *on page 286*

Capastat® Sulfate *see* capreomycin sulfate *on next page*

Capital® and Codeine *see* acetaminophen and codeine *on page 3*

Capitrol® *see* chloroxine *on page 93*

Capoten® *see* captopril *on next page*

Capozide® *see* captopril and hydrochlorothiazide *on next page*

capreomycin sulfate (kap ree oh mye' sin)
Brand Names Capastat® Sulfate
Therapeutic Category Antibiotic, Miscellaneous; Antitubercular Agent
Use In conjunction with at least one other antituberculosis agent in the treatment of tuberculosis
Usual Dosage Adults: I.M.: 15 mg/kg/day up to 1 g/day for 60-120 days
Dosage Forms Injection: 100 mg/mL (10 mL)

capsaicin (kap say' sin)
Brand Names Capzasin-P® [OTC]; No Pain-HP® [OTC]; R-Gel® [OTC]; Zostrix® [OTC]; Zostrix® HP [OTC]
Therapeutic Category Analgesic, Topical; Topical Skin Product
Use
　Zostrix®: Temporary relief of pain (neuralgia) following herpes zoster infections
　Zostrix® HP: Relief of neuralgias such as diabetic neuropathy and postsurgical pain
Usual Dosage Children >2 years and Adults: Apply to area up to 3-4 times/day only
Dosage Forms
　Cream:
　　Capzasin-P®, Zostrix®: 0.025% (45 g, 90 g)
　　Zostrix® HP: 0.075% (30 g, 60 g)
　Gel (R-Gel®): 0.025% (15 g, 30 g)
　Roll-on (No Pain-HP®): 0.075% (60 mL)

captopril (kap' toe pril)
Brand Names Capoten®
Therapeutic Category Angiotensin-Converting Enzyme (ACE) Inhibitors
Use Management of hypertension and treatment of congestive heart failure; increase circulation in Raynaud's phenomenon; idiopathic edema
Usual Dosage Note: Dosage must be titrated according to patient's response; use lowest effective dose. Oral:

　Neonates: Initial: 0.05-0.1 mg/kg/dose every 8-24 hours; titrate dose up to 0.5 mg/kg/dose given every 6-24 hours

　Infants: Initial: 0.15-0.3 mg/kg/dose; titrate dose upward to maximum of 6 mg/kg/day in 1-4 divided doses; usual required dose: 2.5-6 mg/kg/day

　Children: Initial: 0.5 mg/kg/dose; titrate upward to maximum of 6 mg/kg/day in 2-4 divided doses

　Older Children: Initial: 6.25-12.5 mg/dose every 12-24 hours; titrate upward to maximum of 6 mg/kg/day

　Adolescents and Adults: Initial: 12.5-25 mg/dose given every 8-12 hours; increase by 25 mg/dose to maximum of 450 mg/day

　Note: Smaller dosages given every 8-12 hours are indicated in patients with renal dysfunction. Renal function and leukocyte count should be carefully monitored during therapy.
Dosage Forms Tablet: 12.5 mg, 25 mg, 50 mg, 100 mg

captopril and hydrochlorothiazide
Brand Names Capozide®
Therapeutic Category Antihypertensive, Combination
Use Management of hypertension and treatment of congestive heart failure
Usual Dosage Adults: Oral:
　Hypertension: Initial: 25 mg 2-3 times/day; may increase at 1- to 2-week intervals up to 150 mg 3 times/day (captopril dosages)

　Congestive heart failure: 6.25-25 mg 3 times/day (maximum: 450 mg/day) (captopril dosages)
Dosage Forms Tablet:
　25/15: Captopril 25 mg and hydrochlorothiazide 15 mg

25/25: Captopril 25 mg and hydrochlorothiazide 25 mg
50/15: Captopril 50 mg and hydrochlorothiazide 15 mg
50/25: Captopril 50 mg and hydrochlorothiazide 25 mg

Capzasin-P® [OTC] *see* capsaicin *on previous page*

Carafate® *see* sucralfate *on page 438*

caramiphen and phenylpropanolamine
Brand Names Ordine AT® Extended Release Capsule; Rescaps-D® S.R. Capsule; Tuss-Allergine® Modified T.D. Capsule; Tuss-Genade® Modified Capsule; Tussogest® Extended Release Capsule; Tuss-Ornade® Liquid; Tuss-Ornade® Spansule®
Synonyms phenylpropanolamine and caramiphen
Therapeutic Category Antihistamine/Decongestant Combination
Use Symptomatic relief of cough and nasal congestion associated with the common cold
Usual Dosage Oral:
Children:
2-6 years: $\frac{1}{2}$ teaspoonful every 4 hours
6-12 years: 1 teaspoonful every 4 hours

Children >12 years and Adults: 1 capsule every 12 hours or 2 teaspoonfuls every 4 hours
Dosage Forms
Capsule, timed release: Caramiphen edisylate 40 mg and phenylpropanolamine hydrochloride 75 mg
Liquid: Caramiphen edisylate 6.7 mg and phenylpropanolamine hydrochloride 12.5 mg per 5 mL

carampicillin hydrochloride *see* bacampicillin hydrochloride *on page 42*

carbachol (kar' ba kole)
Brand Names Isopto® Carbachol Ophthalmic; Miostat® Intraocular
Synonyms carbacholine; carbamylcholine chloride
Therapeutic Category Cholinergic Agent, Ophthalmic; Ophthalmic Agent, Miotic
Use Lower intraocular pressure in the treatment of glaucoma; to cause miosis during surgery
Usual Dosage Adults:
Intraocular: 0.5 mL instilled into anterior chamber before or after securing sutures
Ophthalmic: Instill 1-2 drops up to 4 times/day
Dosage Forms Solution:
Intraocular (Miostat®): 0.01% (1.5 mL)
Topical, ophthalmic (Isopto® Carbachol): 0.75% (15 mL, 30 mL); 1.5% (15 mL, 30 mL); 2.25% (15 mL); 3% (15 mL, 30 mL)

carbacholine *see* carbachol *on this page*

carbamazepine (kar ba maz' e peen)
Brand Names Epitol®; Tegretol®
Therapeutic Category Anticonvulsant, Miscellaneous
Use Prophylaxis of generalized tonic-clonic, partial (especially complex partial), and mixed partial or generalized seizure disorder; may be used to relieve pain in trigeminal neuralgia or diabetic neuropathy; has been used to treat bipolar disorders
Usual Dosage Oral (dosage must be adjusted according to patient's response and serum concentrations):

Children:
<6 years: Initial: 5 mg/kg/day; dosage may be increased every 5-7 days to 10 mg/kg/day; then up to 20 mg/kg/day if necessary; administer in 2-4 divided doses/day
6-12 years: Initial: 100 mg twice daily or 10 mg/kg/day in 2 divided doses; increase by 100 mg/day depending upon response; usual maintenance: 15-30 mg/kg/day in 2-4 divided doses/day; maximum: 1000 mg/24 hours

(Continued)

carbamazepine *(Continued)*

Children >12 years and Adults: 200 mg twice daily to start, increase by 200 mg/day at weekly intervals until therapeutic levels achieved; usual dose: 800-1200 mg/day in 3-4 divided
doses; some patients have required up to 1.6-2.4 g/day

Dosage Forms
Suspension, oral (citrus-vanilla flavor): 100 mg/5 mL (450 mL)
Tablet: 200 mg
Tablet, chewable: 100 mg

carbamide *see* urea *on page 480*

carbamide peroxide (kar' ba mide per ox' ide)

Brand Names Auro® Ear Drops [OTC]; Cankaid® [OTC]; Debrox® [OTC]; Gly-Oxide® [OTC];
Murine™ Ear Drops [OTC]; Orajel® Brace-Aid Rinse [OTC]; Proxigel® [OTC]
Synonyms urea peroxide
Therapeutic Category Anti-infective Agent, Oral; Otic Agent, Cerumenolytic
Use Relief of minor inflammation of gums, oral mucosal surfaces and lips including canker
sores and dental irritation; emulsify and disperse ear wax
Usual Dosage Children >12 years and Adults:
Oral: Apply several drops undiluted to affected area of the mouth 4 times/day and at bedtime
for up to 7 days, expectorate after 2-3 minutes; as an adjunct to oral hygiene after brush-
ing, swish 10 drops for 2-3 minutes, then expectorate; gel: massage on affected area 4
times/day
Otic: Instill 5-10 drops twice daily for up to 4 days; keep drops in ear for several minutes by
keeping head tilted or placing cotton in ear
Dosage Forms
Gel, oral (Proxigel®): 11% (36 g)
Solution:
Oral (Cankaid®, Gly-Oxide®, Orajel® Brace-Aid Rinse): 10% in glycerin (15 mL, 22.5 mL,
30 mL, 60 mL)
Otic (Auro® Ear Drops, Debrox®, Murine® Ear Drops): 6.5% in glycerin (15 mL, 30 mL)

carbamylcholine chloride *see* carbachol *on previous page*

carbenicillin (kar ben i sill' in)

Brand Names Geocillin®
Synonyms carindacillin
Therapeutic Category Antibiotic, Penicillin
Use Treatment of serious infections caused by susceptible gram-negative aerobic bacilli or
mixed aerobic-anaerobic bacterial infections and/or urinary tract infections
Usual Dosage Oral:
Children: 30-50 mg/kg/day divided every 6 hours; maximum dose: 2-3 g/day
Adults: 1-2 tablets every 6 hours
Dosage Forms Tablet, film coated: 382 mg

carbidopa (kar bi doe' pa)

Brand Names Lodosyn®
Therapeutic Category Anti-Parkinson's Agent
Use Given with levodopa in the treatment of parkinsonism to enable a lower dosage of the lat-
ter to be used and a more rapid response to be obtained, and to decrease side-effects; for
details of administration and dosage, see Levodopa
Usual Dosage Adults: Oral: 70-100 mg/day; maximum daily dose: 200 mg
Dosage Forms Tablet: 25 mg

carbidopa and levodopa *see* levodopa and carbidopa *on page 265*

carbinoxamine and pseudoephedrine

Brand Names Carbiset® Tablet; Carbiset-TR® Tablet; Carbodec® Syrup; Carbodec® Tablet; Carbodec TR® Tablet; Cardec-S® Syrup; Rondec® Drops; Rondec® Filmtab®; Rondec® Syrup; Rondec-TR®

Therapeutic Category Antihistamine/Decongestant Combination

Use Perennial and seasonal allergic rhinitis and other allergic symptoms including urticaria

Usual Dosage Oral:

Children:

Drops: 1-18 months: 0.25-1 mL 4 times/day

Syrup:

18 months to 6 years: 2.5 mL 3-4 times/day

>6 years: 5 mL 2-4 times/day

Adults:

Liquid: 5 mL 4 times/day

Tablets: 1 tablet 4 times/day

Dosage Forms

Drops: Carbinoxamine maleate 2 mg and pseudoephedrine hydrochloride 25 mg per mL (30 mL with dropper)

Syrup: Carbinoxamine maleate 4 mg and pseudoephedrine hydrochloride 60 mg per 5 mL (120 mL, 480 mL)

Tablet:

Film-coated: Carbinoxamine maleate 4 mg and pseudoephedrine hydrochloride 60 mg

Sustained release: Carbinoxamine maleate 8 mg and pseudoephedrine hydrochloride 120 mg

carbinoxamine, pseudoephedrine, and dextromethorphan

Brand Names Carbodec DM®; Cardec DM®; Pseudo-Car® DM; Rondamine-DM® Drops; Rondec®-DM; Tussafed® Drops

Therapeutic Category Antihistamine/Decongestant Combination; Cough Preparation

Use Relief of coughs and upper respiratory symptoms, including nasal congestion, associated with allergy or the common cold

Usual Dosage

Infants: Drops:

1-3 months: $\frac{1}{4}$ mL 4 times/day

3-6 months: $\frac{1}{2}$ mL 4 times/day

6-9 months: $\frac{3}{4}$ mL 4 times/day

9-18 months: 1 mL 4 times/day

Children $1\frac{1}{2}$ to 6 years: Syrup: 2.5 mL 4 times/day

Children >6 years and Adults: Syrup: 5 mL 4 times/day

Dosage Forms

Drops: Carbinoxamine maleate 2 mg, pseudoephedrine hydrochloride 25 mg, and dextromethorphan hydrobromide 4 mg per mL (30 mL)

Syrup: Carbinoxamine maleate 4 mg, pseudoephedrine hydrochloride 60 mg, and dextromethorphan hydrobromide 15 mg per 5 (120 mL, 480 mL, 4000 mL)

Carbiset® Tablet *see* carbinoxamine and pseudoephedrine *on this page*

Carbiset-TR® Tablet *see* carbinoxamine and pseudoephedrine *on this page*

Carbocaine® Injection *see* mepivacaine hydrochloride *on page 288*

Carbodec DM® *see* carbinoxamine, pseudoephedrine, and dextromethorphan *on this page*

Carbodec® Syrup *see* carbinoxamine and pseudoephedrine *on this page*

Carbodec® Tablet *see* carbinoxamine and pseudoephedrine *on this page*

Carbodec TR® Tablet *see* carbinoxamine and pseudoephedrine *on this page*

carbol-fuchsin solution (kar bol fook' sin)

Synonyms Castellani paint

Therapeutic Category Antifungal Agent, Topical

Use Treatment of superficial mycotic infections

(Continued)

carbol-fuchsin solution *(Continued)*
Usual Dosage Topical: Apply to affected area 2-4 times/day
Dosage Forms Solution: Basic fuchsin 0.3%, boric acid 1%, phenol 4.5%, resorcinol 10%, acetone 5%, and alcohol 10%

carbolic acid *see phenol on page 362*

carboplatin (kar' boe pla tin)
Brand Names Paraplatin®
Synonyms cbdca
Therapeutic Category Antineoplastic Agent, Alkylating Agent
Use Ovarian carcinoma, cervical, small cell lung carcinoma, esophagus, testicular, bladder cancer, mesothelioma, pediatric brain tumors
Usual Dosage I.V. (refer to individual protocols):
Children:
Solid tumor: 560 mg/m^2 once every 4 weeks
Brain tumor: 175 mg/m^2 once weekly for 4 weeks with a 2-week recovery period between courses; dose is then adjusted on platelet count and neutrophil count values

Adults: Single agent: 360 mg/m^2 once every 4 weeks; dose is then adjusted on platelet count and neutrophil count values
Dosage Forms Powder for injection, lyophilized: 50 mg, 150 mg, 450 mg

carboprost tromethamine (kar' boe prost tro meth' a meen)
Formerly Known As Prostin/15M®
Brand Names Hemabate™
Therapeutic Category Abortifacient; Prostaglandin
Use Termination of pregnancy
Usual Dosage I.M.: 250 mcg to start, 250 mcg at 1½-hour to 3½-hour intervals depending on uterine response; a 500 mcg/dose may be given if uterine response is not adequate after several 250 mcg/dose
Dosage Forms Injection: Carboprost 250 mcg and tromethamine 83 mcg per mL (1 mL)

carbose d *see carboxymethylcellulose sodium on this page*

carboxymethylcellulose sodium (kar box ee meth ill sell' yoo lose)
Brand Names Celluvisc® [OTC]
Synonyms carbose d
Therapeutic Category Ophthalmic Agent, Miscellaneous
Use Preservative free artificial tear substitute
Usual Dosage Adults: Ophthalmic: Instill 1-2 drops into eye(s) 3-4 times/day
Dosage Forms Solution, ophthalmic, preservative free: 1% (0.3 mL)

Cardec DM® *see carbinoxamine, pseudoephedrine, and dextromethorphan on previous page*

Cardec-S® Syrup *see carbinoxamine and pseudoephedrine on previous page*

Cardene® *see nicardipine hydrochloride on page 326*

Cardene® SR *see nicardipine hydrochloride on page 326*

Cardilate® *see erythrityl tetranitrate on page 170*

Cardio-Green® *see indocyanine green on page 244*

Cardioquin® *see quinidine on page 403*

Cardizem® CD *see diltiazem hydrochloride on page 146*

Cardizem® Injectable *see diltiazem hydrochloride on page 146*

Cardizem® SR *see* diltiazem hydrochloride *on page 146*

Cardizem® Tablet *see* diltiazem hydrochloride *on page 146*

Cardura® *see* doxazosin mesylate *on page 157*

carindacillin *see* carbenicillin *on page 74*

carisoprodate *see* carisoprodol *on this page*

carisoprodol (kar eye soe proe' dole)
Brand Names Rela®; Sodol®; Soma®; Soma® Compound; Soprodol®; Soridol®
Synonyms carisoprodate; isobamate
Therapeutic Category Skeletal Muscle Relaxant
Use Skeletal muscle relaxant
Usual Dosage Adults: Oral: 350 mg 3-4 times/day; take last dose at bedtime; compound: 1-2 tablets 4 times/day
Dosage Forms Tablet:
  Rela®, Sodol®, Soma®, Soprodol®, Soridol®: 350 mg
  Soma® Compound: Carisoprodol 200 mg and aspirin 325 mg

Carmol-HC® Topical *see* urea and hydrocortisone *on page 480*

Carmol® Topical [OTC] *see* urea *on page 480*

carmustine (kar mus' teen)
Brand Names BiCNU®
Synonyms bcnu
Therapeutic Category Antineoplastic Agent, Alkylating Agent (Nitrosourea)
Use Brain tumors, multiple myeloma and Hodgkin's disease and non-Hodgkin's lymphomas, melanoma, lung cancer
Usual Dosage Children and Adults: I.V. infusion (refer to individual protocols): 75-100 mg/m^2/day for 2 days or 150-200 mg/m^2 every 6 weeks as a single dose or divided into daily injections on 2 successive days; next dose is to be determined based on hematologic response to the previous dose
Dosage Forms Powder for injection: 100 mg/vial packaged with 3 mL of absolute alcohol for use as a sterile diluent

Carnitor® Injection *see* levocarnitine *on page 265*

Carnitor® Oral *see* levocarnitine *on page 265*

carteolol hydrochloride (kar' tee oh lole)
Brand Names Cartrol® Oral; Ocupress® Ophthalmic
Therapeutic Category Beta-Adrenergic Blocker; Beta-Adrenergic Blocker, Ophthalmic
Use Management of hypertension; treatment of increased intraocular pressure
Usual Dosage Adults:
  Oral: 2.5 mg as a single daily dose, with a maintenance dose normally 2.5-5 mg once daily
  Ophthalmic: 1 drop in eye(s) twice daily
Dosage Forms
  Solution, ophthalmic (Ocupress®): 1% (5 mL, 10 mL)
  Tablet (Cartrol®): 2.5 mg, 5 mg

Carter's Little Pills® [OTC] *see* bisacodyl *on page 54*

Cartrol® Oral *see* carteolol hydrochloride *on this page*

casanthranol and docusate *see* docusate and casanthranol *on page 154*

cascara sagrada (kas kar' a)
Therapeutic Category Laxative, Stimulant
Use Temporary relief of constipation; sometimes used with milk of magnesia ("black and white" mixture)
(Continued)

cascara sagrada (Continued)

Usual Dosage Note: Cascara sagrada fluid extract is 5 times more potent than cascara sagrada aromatic fluid extract.

Oral (aromatic fluid extract):
Infants: 1.25 mL/day (range: 0.5-1.5 mL) as needed
Children 2-11 years: 2.5 mL/day (range: 1-3 mL) as needed
Children ≥12 years and Adults: 5 mL/day (range: 2-6 mL) as needed at bedtime (1 tablet as needed at bedtime)

Dosage Forms
Liquid, aromatic fluid extract: 5 mL, 120 mL
Tablet: 325 mg

Castellani paint see carbol-fuchsin solution on page 75

castor oil

Brand Names Alphamul® [OTC]; Emulsoil® [OTC]; Fleet® Flavored Castor Oil [OTC]; Neoloid® [OTC]; Purge® [OTC]
Synonyms oleum ricini
Therapeutic Category Laxative, Stimulant
Use Preparation for rectal or bowel examination or surgery; rarely used to relieve constipation; also applied to skin as emollient and protectant
Usual Dosage Oral:
Castor oil:
Infants <2 years: 1-5 mL or 15 mL/m^2/dose as a single dose
Children 2-11 years: 5-15 mL as a single dose
Children ≥12 years and Adults: 15-60 mL as a single dose

Emulsified castor oil:
Infants: 2.5-7.5 mL/dose
Children <2 years: 5-15 mL/dose
Children 2-11 years: 7.5-30 mL/dose
Children ≥12 years and Adults: 30-60 mL/dose

Dosage Forms
Emulsion, oral:
Alphamul®: 60% (90 mL, 3780 mL)
Emulsoil®: 95% (63 mL)
Fleet® Flavored Castor Oil: 67% (45 mL, 90 mL)
Neoloid®: 36.4% (118 mL)
Liquid, oral:
100% (60 mL, 120 mL, 480 mL)
Purge®: 95% (30 mL, 60 mL)

Cataflam® Oral see diclofenac sodium on page 141

Catapres® Oral see clonidine on page 108

Catapres-TTS® Transdermal see clonidine on page 108

cbdca see carboplatin on page 76

ccnu see lomustine on page 272

C-Crystals® [OTC] see ascorbic acid on page 34

2-cda see cladribine on page 103

cddp see cisplatin on page 103

Ceclor® see cefaclor on next page

Cecon® [OTC] see ascorbic acid on page 34

CeeNU® Oral see lomustine on page 272

Ceepryn® [OTC] see cetylpyridinium chloride on page 86

cefaclor (sef' a klor)

Brand Names Ceclor®

Therapeutic Category Antibiotic, Cephalosporin (Second Generation)

Use Infections caused by susceptible organisms involving the respiratory tract, otitis media, sinusitis, skin and skin structure, bone and joint, and urinary tract and gynecologic as well as septicemia

Usual Dosage Oral:

Children >1 month: 20-40 mg/kg/day divided every 8-12 hours; maximum dose: 2 g/day (twice daily option is for treatment of otitis media or pharyngitis)

Adults: 250-500 mg every 8 hours or daily dose can be given in 2 divided doses

Dosage Forms

Capsule: 250 mg, 500 mg

Powder for oral suspension (strawberry flavor): 125 mg/5 mL (75 mL, 150 mL); 187 mg/5 mL (50 mL, 100 mL); 250 mg/5 mL (75 mL, 150 mL); 375 mg/5 mL (50 mL, 100 mL)

cefadroxil monohydrate (sef a drox' ill)

Brand Names Duricef®; Ultracef®

Therapeutic Category Antibiotic, Cephalosporin (First Generation)

Use Treatment of susceptible bacterial infections, including those caused by group A beta-hemolytic *Streptococcus*

Usual Dosage Oral:

Children: 30 mg/kg/day divided twice daily up to a maximum of 2 g/day

Adults: 1-2 g/day in 2 divided doses

Dosage Forms

Capsule, as monohydrate: 500 mg

Powder for oral suspension: 125 mg/5 mL (50 mL, 100 mL); 250 mg/5 mL (50 mL, 100 mL); 500 mg/5 mL (50 mL, 100 mL)

Tablet, as monohydrate: 1 g

Cefadyl® *see* cephapirin sodium *on page 85*

cefamandole nafate (sef a man' dole)

Brand Names Mandol®

Therapeutic Category Antibiotic, Cephalosporin (Second Generation)

Use Treatment of susceptible bacterial infection; mainly respiratory tract, skin and skin structure, bone and joint, urinary tract and gynecologic as well as septicemia, perioperative prophylaxis

Usual Dosage I.M., I.V.:

Children: 100-150 mg/kg/day in divided doses every 4-6 hours

Adults: 4-12 g/24 hours divided every 4-6 hours 500-1000 mg every 4-8 hours

Dosage Forms Powder for injection: 1 g (10 mL, 100 mL); 2 g (20 mL, 100 mL); 10 g (100 mL)

Cefanex® *see* cephalexin monohydrate *on page 84*

cefazolin sodium (sef a' zoe lin)

Brand Names Ancef®; Kefzol®; Zolicef®

Therapeutic Category Antibiotic, Cephalosporin (First Generation)

Use Treatment of gram-positive bacilli and cocci (except enterococcus); some gram-negative bacilli including *E. coli, Proteus,* and *Klebsiella* may be susceptible

Usual Dosage I.M., I.V.:

Neonates:

Postnatal age <7 days: 40 mg/kg/day divided every 12 hours

Postnatal age >7 days:

<2000 g: 40 mg/kg/day in 2 divided doses

>2000 g: 60 mg/kg/day in 3 divided doses

(Continued)

79

cefazolin sodium *(Continued)*

Infants and Children: 50-100 mg/kg/day in 3 divided doses; maximum dose: 6 g/day

Adults: 1-2 g every 8 hours

Dosage Forms
Infusion, premixed, in D_5W (frozen) (Ancef®): 500 mg (50 mL); 1 g (50 mL)
Powder for injection: 250 mg, 500 mg, 1 g, 5 g, 10 g, 20 g

cefixime (sef ix' eem)

Brand Names Suprax®
Therapeutic Category Antibiotic, Cephalosporin (Third Generation)
Use Treatment of urinary tract infections, otitis media, respiratory infections due to suscepti-
ble organisms; documented poor compliance with other oral antimicrobials; outpatient
therapy of serious soft tissue or skeletal infections due to susceptible organisms.
Usual Dosage Oral:
Children: 8 mg/kg/day in 1-2 divided doses; maximum dose: 400 mg/day
Children >50 kg or >12 years and Adults: 400 mg/day in 1-2 divided doses
Dosage Forms
Powder for oral suspension (strawberry flavor): 100 mg/5 mL (50 mL, 100 mL)
Tablet, film coated: 200 mg, 400 mg

Cefizox® *see* ceftizoxime sodium *on page 82*

cefmetazole sodium (sef met' a zole)

Brand Names Zefazone®
Therapeutic Category Antibiotic, Cephalosporin (Second Generation)
Use Second generation cephalosporin with an antibacterial spectrum similar to cefoxitin, use-
ful on many aerobic and anaerobic gram-positive and gram-negative bacteria
Usual Dosage Adults: I.V.:
Infections: 2 g every 6-12 hours for 5-14 days
Prophylaxis: 2 g 30-90 minutes before surgery
Dosage Forms Powder for injection: 1 g, 2 g

Cefobid® *see* cefoperazone sodium *on this page*

cefonicid sodium (se fon' i sid)

Brand Names Monocid®
Therapeutic Category Antibiotic, Cephalosporin (Second Generation)
Use Treatment of susceptible bacterial infection; mainly respiratory tract, skin and skin struc-
ture, bone and joint, urinary tract and gynecologic as well as septicemia; second generation
cephalosporin
Usual Dosage Adults: I.M., I.V.: 1 g every 24 hours
Dosage Forms Powder for injection: 500 mg, 1 g, 10 g

cefoperazone sodium (sef oh per' a zone)

Brand Names Cefobid®
Therapeutic Category Antibiotic, Cephalosporin (Third Generation)
Use Treatment of susceptible bacterial infection; mainly respiratory tract, skin and skin struc-
ture, bone and joint, urinary tract and gynecologic as well as septicemia
Usual Dosage I.M., I.V.:
Neonates: 50 mg/kg/dose every 12 hours
Children: 100-150 mg/kg/day divided every 8-12 hours
Adults: 2-4 g/day in divided doses every 12 hours (up to 12 g/day)
Dosage Forms
Injection, premixed (frozen): 1 g (50 mL); 2 g (50 mL)
Powder for infection: 1 g, 2 g

Cefotan® *see* cefotetan disodium *on this page*

cefotaxime sodium (sef oh taks' eem)
Brand Names Claforan®
Therapeutic Category Antibiotic, Cephalosporin (Third Generation)
Use Treatment of a documented or suspected meningitis due to susceptible organisms; non-pseudomonal gram-negative rod infection in a patient at risk of developing aminoglycoside-induced nephrotoxicity and/or ototoxicity; infection due to an organism whose susceptibilities clearly favor cefotaxime over cefuroxime or an aminoglycoside
Usual Dosage I.M., I.V.:
Neonates:
Postnatal age <7 days: 100 mg/kg/day in 2 divided doses
Postnatal age >7 days:
<1200 g: 100 mg/kg/day divided every 12 hours
>1200 g: 150 mg/kg/day in 3 divided doses

Infants and Children 1 month to 12 years:
<50 kg: 100-200 mg/kg/day in 3-4 divided doses
Meningitis: 200 mg/kg/day in 4 divided doses
>50 kg: Moderate to severe infection: 1-2 g every 6-8 hours; life-threatening infection: 2 g/dose every 4 hours; maximum dose: 12 g/day

Children >12 years and Adults: 1-2 g every 6-8 hours (up to 12 g/day)
Dosage Forms
Infusion, premixed, in D_5W (frozen): 1 g (50 mL); 2 g (50 mL)
Powder for injection: 1 g, 2 g, 10 g

cefotetan disodium (sef' oh tee tan)
Brand Names Cefotan®
Therapeutic Category Antibiotic, Cephalosporin (Second Generation)
Use Treatment of susceptible bacterial infection; mainly respiratory tract, skin and skin structure, bone and joint, urinary tract and gynecologic as well as septicemia
Usual Dosage I.M., I.V.:
Children: 40-80 mg/kg/day divided every 12 hours

Adults: 1-6 g/day in divided doses every 12 hours, 1-2 g may be given every 24 hours for urinary tract infection
Dosage Forms Powder for injection: 1 g (10 mL, 100 mL); 2 g (20 mL, 100 mL); 10 g (100 mL)

cefoxitin sodium (se fox' i tin)
Brand Names Mefoxin®
Therapeutic Category Antibiotic, Cephalosporin (Second Generation)
Use Less active against staphylococci and streptococci than first generation cephalosporins, but active against anaerobes including *Bacteroides fragilis*; active against gram-negative enteric bacilli including *E. coli*, *Klebsiella*, and *Proteus*
Usual Dosage I.M., I.V.:
Infants >3 months and Children:
Mild-moderate infection: 80-100 mg/kg/day in divided doses every 4-6 hours
Severe infection: 100-160 mg/kg/day in divided doses every 4-6 hours
Maximum dose: 12 g/day

Adults: 1-2 g every 6-8 hours (I.M. injection is painful)
Dosage Forms
Infusion, premixed, in D_5W (frozen): 1 g (50 mL); 2 g (50 mL)
Powder for injection: 1 g, 2 g, 10 g

cefpodoxime proxetil (sef pode ox' eem)
Brand Names Vantin®
Therapeutic Category Antibiotic, Cephalosporin (Second Generation)
Use Infections caused by susceptible organisms involving the respiratory tract, otitis media, sinusitis, skin and skin structure, bone and joint, and urinary tract and gynecologic as well as septicemia
(Continued)

81

cefpodoxime proxetil *(Continued)*

Usual Dosage Oral:
Children >6 months to 12 years: 10 mg/kg/day, divided every 12 hours, for 10 days
Adults: 100-400 mg every 12 hours, for 7-14 days

Dosage Forms
Granules for oral suspension (lemon creme flavor): 50 mg/5 mL (100 mL); 100 mg/5 mL (100 mL)
Tablet, film coated: 100 mg, 200 mg

cefprozil (sef proe' zil)

Brand Names Cefzil™
Therapeutic Category Antibiotic, Cephalosporin (Second Generation)
Use Infections caused by susceptible organisms involving the respiratory tract, otitis media, sinusitis, skin and skin structure, bone and joint, and urinary tract and gynecologic as well as septicemia
Usual Dosage Oral:
Infants and Children >6 months to 12 years: 15 mg/kg every 12 hours for 10 days
Children >13 years and Adults: 250-500 mg every 12-24 hours for 10 days
Dosage Forms
Powder for oral suspension, as anhydrous: 125 mg/5 mL (50 mL, 75 mL, 100 mL); 250 mg/5 mL (50 mL, 75 mL, 100 mL)
Tablet, as anhydrous: 250 mg, 500 mg

ceftazidime (sef' tay zi deem)

Brand Names Ceptaz™; Fortaz®; Pentacef™; Tazicef®; Tazidime®
Therapeutic Category Antibiotic, Cephalosporin (Third Generation)
Use Treatment of documented susceptible *Pseudomonas aeruginosa* infection; *Pseudomonas* infection in patient at risk of developing aminoglycoside-induced nephrotoxicity and/or ototoxicity; empiric therapy of a febrile, granulocytopenic patient
Usual Dosage
Neonates:
Postnatal age <7 days: 30-50 mg/kg/dose every 12 hours
Postnatal age >7 days: 30-50 mg/kg/dose every 8 hours
Infants and Children 1 month to 12 years: 30-50 mg/kg/dose every 8 hours; maximum dose: 6 g/day
Adults: 1-2 g every 8-12 hours (250-500 mg every 12 hours for urinary tract infections)
Dosage Forms
Infusion, premixed (frozen) (Fortaz®): 1 g (50 mL); 2 g (50 mL)
Powder for injection: 500 mg, 1 g, 2 g, 6 g

Ceftin® Oral *see cefuroxime on next page*

ceftizoxime sodium (sef ti zox' eem)

Brand Names Cefizox®
Therapeutic Category Antibiotic, Cephalosporin (Third Generation)
Use Treatment of susceptible bacterial infection; mainly respiratory tract, skin and skin structure, bone and joint, urinary tract and gynecologic as well as septicemia
Usual Dosage I.M., I.V.:
Children ≥6 months: 50 mg/kg every 6-8 hours to 200 mg/kg/day to maximum of 12 g/24 hours
Adults: 1-2 g every 8-12 hours, up to 2 g every 4 hours or 4 g every 8 hours for life-threatening infections
Dosage Forms
Injection, in D_5W (frozen): 1 g (50 mL); 2 g (50 mL)
Powder for injection: 500 mg, 1 g, 2 g, 10 g

ceftriaxone sodium (sef try ax' one)
Brand Names Rocephin®
Therapeutic Category Antibiotic, Cephalosporin (Third Generation)
Use Treatment of documented infection due to susceptible organisms in patients without I.V. line access; documented or suspected infection due to susceptible organisms in home care patients; treatment of documented or suspected gonococcal infection or chancroid; emergency room management of patients at high risk for bacteremia, periorbital or buccal cellulitis, salmonellosis or shigellosis and pneumonia of unestablished etiology (<5 years of age)
Usual Dosage
Neonates: I.M., I.V.:
    Postnatal age <7 days: 50 mg/kg/day given every 24 hours
    Postnatal age >7 days:
        <2000 g: 50 mg/kg/day given every 24 hours
        >2000 g: 75 mg/kg/day given every 24 hours

Gonococcal prophylaxis:
    LBW neonates: 25-50 mg/kg as a single dose (dose not to exceed 125 mg)
    Neonates: 125 mg as a single dose

Neonatal gonococcal ophthalmia: 25-50 mg/kg/day given every 24 hours

Infants and Children: 50-100 mg/kg/day in 1-2 divided doses
    Meningitis: 100 mg/kg/day divided every 12 hours; loading dose of 75 mg/kg may be administered at the start of therapy
    Chancroid, uncomplicated gonorrhea: I.M.:
        <45 kg: 125 mg as a single dose
        >45 kg: 250 mg as a single dose

Adults: 1-2 g every 12-24 hours depending on the type and severity of the infection; maximum dose: 4 g/day
Dosage Forms
Infusion, premixed (frozen): 1 g in $D_{3.8}$W (50 mL); 2 g in $D_{2.4}$W (50 mL)
Powder for injection: 250 mg, 500 mg, 1 g, 2 g, 10 g

cefuroxime (se fyoor ox' eem)
Brand Names Ceftin® Oral; Kefurox® Injection; Zinacef® Injection
Therapeutic Category Antibiotic, Cephalosporin (Second Generation)
Use Treatment of infections caused by staphylococci, group B streptococci, *H. influenzae* (type A and B), *E. coli*, *Enterobacter*, *Salmonella*, and *Klebsiella*; treatment of susceptible infections of the lower respiratory tract, otitis media, urinary tract, skin and soft tissue, bone and joint, sepsis and gonorrhea
Usual Dosage
Neonates: 10-25 mg/kg/dose every 12 hours

Children:
    Oral:
        <12 years: 125 mg twice daily
        >12 years: 250 mg twice daily
    I.M., I.V.: 75-150 mg/kg/day divided every 8 hours; maximum dose: 9 g/day

Adults:
    Oral: 125-500 mg twice daily, depending on severity of infection
    I.M., I.V.: 100-150 mg/kg/day in divided doses every 6-8 hours; maximum: 6 g/24 hours
Dosage Forms
Infusion, premixed (frozen) (Zinacef®): 750 mg (50 mL); 1.5 g (50 mL)
Powder for injection, as sodium (generic): 750 mg, 1.5 g, 7.5 g
Powder for injection, as sodium (Kefurox®, Zinacef®): 750 mg, 1.5 g, 7.5 g
Tablet, as axetil (Ceftin®): 125 mg, 250 mg, 500 mg

Cefzil™ see cefprozil on previous page

Celestone® see betamethasone on page 52

Celestone® Soluspan® see betamethasone on page 52

cellulose, oxidized
Brand Names Oxycel®; Surgicel®
Synonyms absorbable cotton
Therapeutic Category Hemostatic Agent
Use Temporary packing for the control of capillary, venous, or small arterial hemorrhage
Usual Dosage Minimal amounts of an appropriate size are laid on the bleeding site
Dosage Forms
Pad (Oxycel™): 3" x 3", 8 ply
Pledget (Oxycel™): 2" x 1" x 1"
Strip:
Oxycel™: 18" x 2", 4 ply; 5" x ½", 4 ply; 36" x ½", 4 ply;
Surgicel™: 2" x 14"; 4" x 8"; 2" x 3"; ½" x 2"

cellulose sodium phosphate
Brand Names Calcibind®
Synonyms csp; sodium cellulose phosphate
Therapeutic Category Urinary Tract Product
Use Adjunct to dietary restriction to reduce renal calculi formation in absorptive hypercalciuria type I
Usual Dosage Adults: Oral: 5 g 3 times/day with meals; decrease dose to 5 g with main meal and 2.5 g with each of two other meals when urinary calcium declines to <150 mg/day
Dosage Forms Powder: 2.5 g packets (90s), 300 g bulk pack

Celluvisc® [OTC] see carboxymethylcellulose sodium on page 76

Celontin® see methsuximide on page 297

Cel-U-Jec® see betamethasone on page 52

Cenafed® [OTC] see pseudoephedrine on page 397

Cenafed® Plus [OTC] see triprolidine and pseudoephedrine on page 474

Cena-K® see potassium chloride on page 378

Cenolate® see sodium ascorbate on page 425

Centrax® see prazepam on page 382

cephalexin monohydrate (sef a lex' in)
Brand Names Biocef; Cefanex®; Keflex®; Keftab®; Zartan
Therapeutic Category Antibiotic, Cephalosporin (First Generation)
Use Treatment of susceptible bacterial infections, including those caused by group A beta-hemolytic *Streptococcus*, *Staphylococcus*, *Klebsiella pneumoniae*, *E. coli*, *Proteus mirabilis*, and *Shigella*
Usual Dosage Oral:
Children: 25-50 mg/kg/day every 6 hours; severe infections: 50-100 mg/kg/day in divided doses every 6 hours; maximum: 3 g/24 hours

Adults: 250-1000 mg every 6 hours
Dosage Forms
Capsule: 250 mg, 500 mg
Powder for oral suspension: 125 mg/5 mL (5 mL unit dose, 60 mL, 100 mL, 200 mL); 250 mg/5 mL (5 mL unit dose, 100 mL, 200 mL)
Suspension, oral, pediatric: 100 mg/mL [5 mg/drop] (10 mL)
Tablet: 500 mg, 1 g
Tablet, as hydrochloride: 500 mg

cephalothin sodium (sef a' loe thin)
Brand Names Keflin® Injection
Therapeutic Category Antibiotic, Cephalosporin (First Generation)
Use Treatment of susceptible bacterial infections, including those caused by group A beta-hemolytic *Streptococcus*

Usual Dosage I.M., I.V.:
Neonates:
  Postnatal age <7 days:
    <2000 g: 20 mg every 12 hours
    >2000 g: 20 mg every 8 hours
  Postnatal age >7 days:
    <2000 g: 20 mg every 8 hours
    >2000 g: 20 mg every 6 hours

Children: 75-125 mg/kg/day divided every 4-6 hours; maximum dose: 10 g in a 24-hour period

Adults: 500 mg to 2 g every 4-6 hours

Dosage Forms
Infusion, in D$_5$W (frozen): 1 g (50 mL); 2 g (50 mL)
Powder for injection: 1 g, 2 g

cephapirin sodium (sef a pye' rin)
Brand Names Cefadyl®
Therapeutic Category Antibiotic, Cephalosporin (First Generation)
Use Treatment of infections when caused by susceptible strains in serious respiratory, genitourinary, gastrointestinal, skin and soft-tissue, bone and joint infections; septicemia; endocarditis
Usual Dosage I.M., I.V.:
Children: 10-20 mg/kg every 6 hours up to 4 g/24 hours
Adults: 1 g every 6 hours up to 12 g/day
Dosage Forms Powder for injection: 500 mg, 1 g, 2 g, 4 g, 20 g

cephradine (sef' ra deen)
Brand Names Velosef®
Therapeutic Category Antibiotic, Cephalosporin (First Generation)
Use Treatment of susceptible bacterial infections, including those caused by group A beta-hemolytic *Streptococcus*
Usual Dosage Oral, I.M., I.V.:
Children ≥9 months: 25-100 mg/kg/day in equally divided doses every 6-12 hours up to 4 g/day
Adults: 2-4 g/day in 4 equally divided doses up to 8 g/day
Dosage Forms
Capsule: 250 mg, 500 mg
Powder for injection: 250 mg, 500 mg, 1 g, 2 g
Powder for oral suspension: 125 mg/5 mL (5 mL, 100 mL, 200 mL); 250 mg/5 mL (5 mL, 100 mL, 200 mL)

Cephulac® *see* lactulose *on page 261*

Ceptaz™ *see* ceftazidime *on page 82*

Ceredase® Injection *see* alglucerase *on page 12*

Cerespan® Oral *see* papaverine hydrochloride *on page 348*

Cerezyme® *see* imglucerase *on page 242*

Cerose-DM® [OTC] *see* chlorpheniramine, phenylephrine, and dextromethorphan *on page 95*

Cerubidine® *see* daunorubicin hydrochloride *on page 126*

Cerumenex® Otic *see* triethanolamine polypeptide oleate-condensate *on page 470*

ces *see* estrogens, conjugated *on page 174*

Cesamet® *see* nabilone *on page 315*

Cetacaine® *see* benzocaine, butyl aminobenzoate, tetracaine, and benzalkonium chloride *on page 49*

Cetamide® Ophthalmic *see* sodium sulfacetamide *on page 431*

Cetapred® *see* sodium sulfacetamide and prednisolone *on page 431*

cetylpyridinium chloride (see' til peer i di' nee um)
Brand Names Ceepryn® [OTC]; Cēpacol® [OTC]
Therapeutic Category Local Anesthetic, Topical
Use Temporary relief of sore throat
Dosage Forms
Lozenge: 1:1500 (24s)
Mouthwash: 0.05% and alcohol 14% (180 mL)

cetylpyridinium chloride and benzocaine (see' til peer i di' nee um)
Brand Names Cēpacol® Anesthetic Troches [OTC]
Synonyms benzocaine and cetylpyridinium chloride
Therapeutic Category Local Anesthetic, Oral
Use Symptomatic relief of sore throat
Usual Dosage Use as needed for sore throat
Dosage Forms Troche: Cetylpyridinium chloride 1:1500 and benzocaine 10 mg per troche (18s)

Cevalin® [OTC] *see* ascorbic acid *on page 34*

Ce-Vi-Sol® [OTC] *see* ascorbic acid *on page 34*

cg *see* chorionic gonadotropin *on page 101*

Charcoaid® [OTC] *see* charcoal *on this page*

charcoal
Brand Names Actidose-Aqua® [OTC]; Actidose® With Sorbitol [OTC]; Charcoaid® [OTC]; Charcocaps'' [OTC]; Liqui-Char® [OTC]
Synonyms activated carbon; activated charcoal; adsorbent charcoal; liquid antidote; medicinal carbon; medicinal charcoal
Therapeutic Category Antidiarrheal; Antidote, Adsorbent; Antiflatulent
Use Emergency treatment in poisoning by drugs and chemicals; repetitive doses for gastric dialysis in uremia to adsorb various waste products
Usual Dosage Oral:
Acute poisoning: Single dose: Charcoal with sorbitol:
Children 1-12 years: 1-2 g/kg/dose or 15-30 g or approximately 5-10 times the weight of the ingested poison; 1 g absorbs 100-1000 mg of poison; the use of repeat oral charcoal with sorbitol doses is not recommended. In young children sorbitol should be repeated no more than 1-2 times/day.
Adults: 30-100 g

Charcoal in water:
Single dose:
Infants <1 year: 1 g/kg
Children 1-12 years: 15-30 g or 1-2 g/kg
Adults: 30-100 g or 1-2 g/kg
Multiple dose:
Infants <1 year: 1 g/kg every 4-6 hours
Children 1-12 years: 20-60 g or 1-2 g/kg every 2-6 hours until clinical observations and serum drug concentration have returned to a subtherapeutic range
Adults: 20-60 g or 1-2 g/kg every 2-6 hours

Gastric dialysis: Adults: 20-50 g every 6 hours for 1-2 days
Dosage Forms
Capsule. (Charcocaps''): 260 mg
Liquid, activated:
Actidose-Aqua'': 12.5 g (60 mL); 25 g (120 mL)

Liqui-Char®: 12.5 g (60 mL); 15 g (75 mL); 25 g (120 mL); 30 g (120 mL); 50 g (240 mL)
Liquid, activated, with propylene glycol: 12.5 g (60 mL); 25 g (120 mL)
Liquid, activated, with sorbitol:
Actidose® With Sorbitol: 25 g (120 mL); 50 g (240 mL)
Charcoaid®: 30 g (150 mL)
Powder for suspension, activated:
15 g, 30 g, 40 g, 120 g, 240 g

Charcocaps® [OTC] *see* charcoal *on previous page*

Chealamide® *see* edetate disodium *on page 163*

Chemet® *see* succimer *on page 437*

Chemstrip® 7 [OTC] *see* diagnostic aids *(in vitro)*, urine *on page 137*

Chemstrip® 9 [OTC] *see* diagnostic aids *(in vitro)*, urine *on page 137*

Chemstrip® bG [OTC] *see* diagnostic aids *(in vitro)*, blood *on page 136*

Chemstrip® K [OTC] *see* diagnostic aids *(in vitro)*, urine *on page 137*

Chemstrip® uG [OTC] *see* diagnostic aids *(in vitro)*, urine *on page 137*

Chemstrip® uGK [OTC] *see* diagnostic aids *(in vitro)*, urine *on page 137*

chenodeoxycholic acid *see* chenodiol *on this page*

chenodiol (kee noe dye' ole)
Synonyms chenodeoxycholic acid
Therapeutic Category Bile Acid; Gallstone Dissolution Agent
Use Oral dissolution of cholesterol gallstones in selected patients
Usual Dosage Adults: Oral: 13-16 mg/kg/day in 2 divided doses, starting with 250 mg twice daily the first 2 weeks and increasing by 250 mg/day each week thereafter until the recommended or maximum tolerated dose is achieved
Dosage Forms Tablet, film coated: 250 mg

Cheracol® *see* guaifenesin and codeine *on page 214*

Cheracol® D [OTC] *see* guaifenesin and dextromethorphan *on page 214*

Chibroxin™ Ophthalmic *see* norfloxacin *on page 332*

Chiggertox® [OTC] *see* benzocaine *on page 48*

Children's Advil® *see* ibuprofen *on page 240*

Children's Hold® [OTC] *see* dextromethorphan hydrobromide *on page 135*

Children's Kaopectate® [OTC] *see* attapulgite *on page 39*

Children's Motrin® *see* ibuprofen *on page 240*

Children's Silfedrine® [OTC] *see* pseudoephedrine *on page 397*

children's vitamins *see* vitamin, multiple (pediatric) *on page 491*

Chlo-Amine® Oral [OTC] *see* chlorpheniramine maleate *on page 95*

Chlorafed® *see* chlorpheniramine and pseudoephedrine *on page 94*

chloral *see* chloral hydrate *on this page*

chloral hydrate (klor' al hye' drate)
Brand Names Aquachloral® Supprettes®
Synonyms chloral; hydrated chloral; trichloroacetaldehyde monohydrate
Therapeutic Category Hypnotic; Sedative
Use Short-term sedative and hypnotic (<2 weeks), sedative/hypnotic for dental and diagnostic procedures; sedative prior to EEG evaluations
Usual Dosage
Neonates: 25 mg/kg/dose for sedation prior to a procedure
(Continued)

chloral hydrate (Continued)

Children:
    Sedation, anxiety: Oral, rectal: 5-15 mg/kg/dose every 8 hours, maximum: 500 mg/dose
    Prior to EEG: Oral, rectal: 20-25 mg/kg/dose, 30-60 minutes prior to EEG; may repeat in
        30 minutes to maximum of 100 mg/kg or 2 g total
    Hypnotic: Oral, rectal: 20-40 mg/kg/dose up to a maximum of 50 mg/kg/24 hours or 1 g/
        dose or 2 g/24 hours
    Sedation, nonpainful procedure: Oral: 50-75 mg/kg/dose 30-60 minutes prior to proce-
        dure; may repeat 30 minutes after initial dose if needed, to a total maximum dose of
        120 mg/kg or 1 g total
Adults: Oral, rectal:
    Sedation, anxiety: 250 mg 3 times/day
    Hypnotic: 500-1000 mg at bedtime or 30 minutes prior to procedure, not to exceed 2 g/24
        hours

Dosage Forms
Capsule: 250 mg, 500 mg
Suppository, rectal: 324 mg, 500 mg, 648 mg
Syrup: 250 mg/5 mL (10 mL); 500 mg/5 mL (5 mL, 10 mL, 480 mL)

chlorambucil (klor am' byoo sil)

Brand Names Leukeran®
Therapeutic Category Antineoplastic Agent, Alkylating Agent (Nitrogen Mustard)
Use Management of chronic lymphocytic leukemia, Hodgkin's and non-Hodgkin's lymphoma;
macroglobulinemia, polycythemia vera, trophoblastic neoplasms, ovarian neoplasms; man-
agement of nephrotic syndrome unresponsive to conventional therapy
Usual Dosage Oral (refer to individual protocols):
Children and Adults: General short courses: 0.1-0.2 mg/kg/day or 4-8 mg/m^2/day for 2-3
    weeks for remission induction, then adjust dose on basis of blood counts; maintenance
    therapy: 0.03-0.1 mg/kg/day
    Nephrotic syndrome: 0.1-0.2 mg/kg/day every day for 5-15 weeks with low-dose predni-
        sone
    Chronic lymphocytic leukemia:
        Biweekly regimen: Initial: 0.4 mg/kg dose is increased by 0.1 mg/kg every 2 weeks until
            a response occurs and/or myelosuppression occurs
        Monthly regimen: Initial: 0.4 mg/kg, increase dose by 0.2 mg/kg every 4 weeks until a
            response occurs and/or myelosuppression occurs
    Malignant lymphomas:
        Non-Hodgkins lymphoma: 0.1 mg/kg/day
        Hodgkins: 0.2 mg/kg/day
Dosage Forms Tablet, sugar coated: 2 mg

Chloramine-T® see chlorazene on next page

chloramphenicol (klor am fen' i kole)

Brand Names AK-Chlor® Ophthalmic; Chloromycetin®; Chloroptic® Ophthalmic; Ophtho-
chlor® Ophthalmic
Therapeutic Category Antibiotic, Miscellaneous; Antibiotic, Ophthalmic; Antibiotic, Otic
Use Treatment of serious infections due to organisms resistant to other less toxic antibiotics
or when its penetrability into the site of infection is clinically superior to other antibiotics to
which the organism is sensitive; useful in infections caused by Bacteroides, H. influenzae,
Neisseria meningitidis, Salmonella, and Rickettsia
Usual Dosage
Neonates: Initial loading dose: Oral, I.V. (I.M. administration is not recommended): 20 mg/kg
    (the first maintenance dose should be given 12 hours after the loading dose)
    Maintenance dose:
        Postnatal age 0-4 weeks, <2000 g: 25 mg/kg/day once every 24 hours;
        Postnatal age 7-28 days, >2000 g: 50 mg/kg/day divided every 12 hours
Meningitis: Infants and Children: Maintenance dose: I.V.: 75-100 mg/kg/day divided every 6
    hours

Other infections: Oral, I.V.:
  Infants and Children: 50-75 mg/kg/day divided every 6 hours; maximum daily dose: 4 g/day
  Adults: 50 mg/kg/day in divided doses every 6 hours; maximum daily dose: 4 g/day
Children and Adults:
  Ophthalmic: Instill 1-2 drops or small amount of ointment every 3-6 hours; increase interval between applications after 48 hours
Dosage Forms
Capsule: 250 mg
Ointment, ophthalmic (AK-Chlor®, Chloromycetin®, Chloroptic®): 1% [10 mg/g] (3.5 g)
Powder for injection, as sodium succinate: 1 g
Powder for ophthalmic solution (Chloromycetin®): 25 mg/vial
Solution:
  Ophthalmic (AK-Chlor®, Chloroptic®, Ophthochlor®): 0.5% [5 mg/mL] (2.5 mL, 7.5 mL, 15 mL)
  Otic (Chloromycetin®): 0.5% (15 mL)

chloramphenicol and prednisolone
Brand Names Chloroptic-P® Ophthalmic
Therapeutic Category Antibiotic, Ophthalmic; Corticosteroid, Ophthalmic
Use Topical anti-infective and corticosteroid for treatment of ocular infections
Usual Dosage Ophthalmic: Instill 1-2 drops in eye(s) 2-4 times/day
Dosage Forms Ointment, ophthalmic: Chloramphenicol 1% and prednisolone 0.5% (3.5 g)

chloramphenicol, polymyxin b, and hydrocortisone
Brand Names Ophthocort® Ophthalmic
Therapeutic Category Antibiotic, Ophthalmic
Use Topical anti-infective and corticosteroid for treatment of ocular infections
Usual Dosage Apply ½" ribbon every 3-4 hours until improvement occurs
Dosage Forms Solution, ophthalmic: Chloramphenicol 1%, polymyxin b sulfate 10,000 units, and hydrocortisone acetate 0.5% per g (3.75 g)

Chloraseptic® Oral [OTC] see phenol on page 362
Chlorate® Oral [OTC] see chlorpheniramine maleate on page 95

chlorazene
Brand Names Chloramine-T®
Therapeutic Category Antibacterial, Topical
Use Topical antiseptic and deodorant

chlordiazepoxide (klor dye az e pox' ide)
Brand Names Libritabs®; Librium®; Mitran® Oral; Reposans-10® Oral
Synonyms methaminodiazepoxide hydrochloride
Therapeutic Category Benzodiazepine; Hypnotic; Sedative
Use Management of anxiety and as a preoperative sedative, symptoms of alcohol withdrawal
Usual Dosage
Children >6 years: Anxiety: Oral, I.M.: 0.5 mg/kg/24 hours divided every 6-8 hours
Adults:
  Anxiety: Oral: 15-100 mg divided 3-4 times/day
  Severe anxiety: 20-25 mg 3-4 times/day
  Preoperative sedation:
    Oral: 5-10 mg 3-4 times/day, 1-day preop
    I.M.: 50-100 mg 1-hour preop
  Alcohol withdrawal symptoms: Oral, I.V.: 50-100 mg to start, dose may be repeated in 2-4 hours as necessary to a maximum of 300 mg/24 hours
(Continued)

chlordiazepoxide *(Continued)*
Dosage Forms
Capsule, as hydrochloride: 5 mg, 10 mg, 25 mg
Powder for injection, as hydrochloride: 100 mg
Tablet: 5 mg, 10 mg, 25 mg

chlordiazepoxide and amitriptyline *see* amitriptyline and chlordiazepoxide *on page 21*

chlordiazepoxide and clidinium *see* clidinium and chlordiazepoxide *on page 105*

Chlordrine® S.R. *see* chlorpheniramine and pseudoephedrine *on page 94*

Chloresium® [OTC] *see* chlorophyll *on this page*

chlorhexidine gluconate *(klor hex' i deen)*
Brand Names BactoShield® Topical [OTC]; Dyna-Hex® Topical [OTC]; Exidine® Scrub [OTC]; Hibiclens™ Topical [OTC]; Hibistat® Topical [OTC]; Peridex® Oral Rinse
Therapeutic Category Antibiotic, Oral Rinse; Antibiotic, Topical
Use Skin cleanser for surgical scrub, cleanser skin wounds, germicidal hand rinse, and as antibacterial dental rinse
Usual Dosage Oral rinse (Peridex®)
Precede use of solution by flossing and brushing teeth, completely rinse toothpaste from mouth; swish 15 mL undiluted oral rinse around in mouth for 30 seconds, then expectorate. Caution patient not to swallow the medicine; avoid eating for 2-3 hours after treatment. (The cap on bottle of oral rinse is a measure for 15 mL.)
When used as a treatment of gingivitis, the regimen begins with oral prophylaxis. Patient treats mouth with 15 mL chlorhexidine; swish for 30 seconds, then expectorate. This is repeated twice daily (morning and evening). Patient should have a re-evaluation followed by a dental prophylaxis every 6 months.
Dosage Forms
Foam, topical, with isopropyl alcohol 4% (BactoShield®): 4% (180 mL)
Liquid, topical, with isopropyl alcohol 4%:
Dyna-Hex™ Skin Cleanser: 2% (120 mL, 240 mL, 480 mL, 960 mL, 4000 mL); 4% (120 mL, 240 mL, 480 mL, 4000 mL)
BactoShield™ 2: 2% (960 mL)
BactoShield™, Exidine® Skin Cleanser, Hibiclens® Skin Cleanser: 4% (15 mL, 120 mL, 240 mL, 480 mL, 960 mL, 4000 mL)
Rinse:
Oral (mint flavor) (Peridex™): 0.12% with alcohol 11.6% (480 mL)
Topical (Hibistat® Hand Rinse): 0.5% with isopropyl alcohol 70% (120 mL, 240 mL)
Sponge/Brush (Hibiclens™): 4% with isopropyl alcohol 4% (22 mL)
Wipes (Hibistat®): 0.5% (50s)

2-chlorodeoxyadenosine *see* cladribine *on page 103*

chloroethane *see* ethyl chloride *on page 181*

Chloromycetin® *see* chloramphenicol *on page 88*

chlorophylin *see* chlorophyll *on this page*

chlorophyll *(klor' oh fill)*
Brand Names Chloresium™ [OTC]; Derifil® [OTC]; Nullo® [OTC]; PALS® [OTC]
Synonyms chlorophylin
Therapeutic Category Gastrointestinal Agent, Miscellaneous; Topical Skin Product
Use Topically promotes normal healing, relieves pain and inflammation, and reduces malodors in wounds, burns, surface ulcers, abrasions and skin irritations; used orally to control fecal and urinary odors in colostomy, ileostomy, or incontinence

Usual Dosage
Oral: 1-2 tablets/day
Topical: Apply generously and cover with gauze, linen, or other appropriate dressing; do not change dressings more often than every 48-72 hours
Dosage Forms
Ointment, topical (Chloresium®): Chlorophyllin copper complex 0.5% (30 g, 120 g)
Solution, topical, in isotonic saline (Chloresium®): Chlorophyllin copper complex 0.2% (240 mL, 946 mL)
Tablet:
Chloresium®: Chlorophyllin copper complex 14 mg
Derifil®: Water soluble chlorophyll: 100 mg
Nullo®: Chlorophyllin copper complex 33.3 mg
PALS®: Chlorophyllin copper complex 100 mg
Sodium free, sugar free: 20 mg

chloroprocaine hydrochloride (klor oh proe' kane)
Brand Names Nesacaine®; Nesacaine®-MPF
Therapeutic Category Local Anesthetic, Injectable
Use For infiltration anesthesia and for peripheral and epidural anesthesia
Usual Dosage Dosage varies with anesthetic procedure, the area to be anesthetized, the vascularity of the tissues, depth of anesthesia required, degree of muscle relaxation required, and duration of anesthesia
Dosage Forms Injection:
Preservative free (Nesacaine®-MPF): 2% (30 mL); 3% (30 mL)
With preservative (Nesacaine®): 1% (30 mL); 2% (30 mL)

Chloroptic® Ophthalmic see chloramphenicol on page 88
Chloroptic-P® Ophthalmic see chloramphenicol and prednisolone on page 89

chloroquine and primaquine
Brand Names Aralen® Phosphate With Primaquine Phosphate
Synonyms primaquine and chloroquine
Therapeutic Category Antimalarial Agent
Use Prophylaxis of malaria, regardless of species, in all areas where the disease is endemic
Usual Dosage
Children: For suggested weekly dosage (based on body weight), see table.

Adults: Start at least 1 day before entering the endemic area; take 1 tablet/week on the same day each week; continue for 8 weeks after leaving the endemic area.
Dosage Forms Tablet: Chloroquine phosphate 500 mg [base 300 mg] and primaquine phosphate 79 mg [base 45 mg]

chloroquine phosphate (klor' oh kwin)
Brand Names Aralen® Phosphate
Therapeutic Category Amebicide; Antimalarial Agent
Use Suppression or chemoprophylaxis of malaria; treatment of uncomplicated or mild-moderate malaria; extraintestinal amebiasis; rheumatoid arthritis
Usual Dosage Oral:
Malaria (excluding resistant P. falciparum):
Suppression or prophylaxis in endemic areas (begin 1-2 weeks prior to, and continue for 6-8 weeks after the period of potential exposure):
Children: 5 mg base/kg/dose weekly, up to a maximum of 300 mg/dose
Adults: 300 mg/dose weekly
Treatment:
Children: 10 mg base/kg/dose, up to a maximum of 600 mg base/dose one time, followed by 5 mg base/kg/dose one time after 6 hours, and then daily for 2 days (total dose of 25 mg base/kg).
(Continued)

chloroquine phosphate *(Continued)*

Adults: 600 mg base/dose one time, followed by 300 mg base/dose one time after 6 hours, and then daily for 2 days

Extraintestinal amebiasis: Dosage expressed in mg base:
Children: 10 mg/kg once daily for 2-3 weeks (up to 300 mg base/day)
Adults: 600 mg base/day for 2 days followed by 300 mg base/day for at least 2-3 weeks

Rheumatoid arthritis: Adults: 150 mg base once daily

Melanoma treatment: Children: 10 mg/kg base/dose (maximum: 600 mg) as a single dose followed by 5 mg/kg base one time after 6 hours, then daily for 2 days

Dosage Forms Tablet: 250 mg [150 mg base]; 500 mg [300 mg base]

chlorothiazide (klor oh thye' a zide)
Brand Names Diurigen®; Diuril®
Therapeutic Category Diuretic, Thiazide
Use Management of mild to moderate hypertension, or edema associated with congestive heart failure, pregnancy, or nephrotic syndrome in patients unable to take oral hydrochlorothiazide, when a thiazide is the diuretic of choice
Usual Dosage I.V. has been limited in infants and children and is generally not recommended

Infants <6 months and patients with pulmonary interstitial edema:
Oral: 20-40 mg/kg/day in 2 divided doses
I.V.: 2-8 mg/kg/day in 2 divided doses

Infants >6 months and Children:
Oral: 20 mg/kg/day in 2 divided doses
I.V.: 4 mg/kg/day

Adults:
Oral: 500 mg to 2 g/day divided in 1-2 doses
I.V.: 100-500 mg/day

Dosage Forms
Powder for injection, lyophilized, as sodium: 500 mg
Suspension, oral: 250 mg/5 mL (237 mL)
Tablet: 250 mg, 500 mg

chlorothiazide and methyldopa
Brand Names Aldoclor®
Synonyms methyldopa and chlorothiazide
Therapeutic Category Antihypertensive, Combination
Use Treatment of hypertension
Usual Dosage Oral: 1 tablet 2-3 times/day for first 48 hours, then adjust
Dosage Forms Tablet:
150: Chlorothiazide 150 mg and methyldopa 250 mg
250: Chlorothiazide 250 mg and methyldopa 250 mg

chlorothiazide and reserpine
Brand Names Diupres-250®; Diupres-500®
Synonyms reserpine and chlorothiazide
Therapeutic Category Antihypertensive, Combination
Use Management of hypertension
Usual Dosage Oral: 1-2 tablets 1-2 times/day
Dosage Forms Tablet:
250: Chlorothiazide 250 mg and reserpine 0.125 mg
500: Chlorothiazide 500 mg and reserpine 0.125 mg

chlorotrianisene (klor oh trye an' i seen)
Brand Names TACE®
Therapeutic Category Estrogen Derivative; Estrogen Derivative, Oral
Use Treat inoperable prostatic cancer; management of atrophic vaginitis, female hypogonadism, vasomotor symptoms of menopause; prevention of postpartum breast engorgement (no longer recommended because increased risk of thrombophlebitis)

Usual Dosage Adults: Oral:
Prostatic cancer: 12-25 mg/day

Atrophic vaginitis: 12-25 mg/day in 28-day cycles (21 days on and 7 days off)

Female hypogonadism: 12-25 mg for 21 days followed by I.M. progesterone 100 mg or 5 days of oral progestin; next course may begin on days of induced uterine bleeding

Menopause: 12-25 mg for 30 days

Postpartum breast engorgement: 12 mg 4 times/day for 7 days or 72 mg twice daily for 2 days

Dosage Forms Capsule: 12 mg, 25 mg

chloroxine (klor ox' een)
Brand Names Capitrol®
Therapeutic Category Antiseborrheic Agent, Topical; Shampoos
Use Treatment of dandruff or seborrheic dermatitis of the scalp
Usual Dosage Use twice weekly, massage into wet scalp, avoid contact with eyes, lather should remain on the scalp for approximately 3 minutes, then rinsed; application should be repeated and the scalp rinsed thoroughly
Dosage Forms Shampoo: 2% (120 mL)

Chlorphed®-LA Nasal Solution [OTC] *see* oxymetazoline hydrochloride
on page 343
Chlorphed® [OTC] *see* brompheniramine maleate *on page 59*

chlorphenesin carbamate (klor fen' e sin car' baa mate)
Brand Names Maolate®
Therapeutic Category Skeletal Muscle Relaxant
Use Adjunctive treatment of discomfort in short-term, acute, painful musculoskeletal conditions
Usual Dosage Adults: Oral: 800 mg 3 times/day, then adjusted to lowest effective dosage, usually 400 mg 4 times/day for up to a maximum of 2 months
Dosage Forms Tablet: 400 mg

chlorpheniramine and acetaminophen
Brand Names Coricidin® [OTC]
Therapeutic Category Analgesic, Non-Narcotic; Antihistamine; Antipyretic
Use Symptomatic relief of congestion, headache, aches and pains of colds and flu
Usual Dosage Adults: Oral: 2 tablets every 4 hours, up to 20/day
Dosage Forms Tablet: Chlorpheniramine maleate 2 mg and acetaminophen 325 mg

chlorpheniramine and phenylephrine
Brand Names Dallergy-D®; Decohistine®; Dihistine®; Histor-D® Liquid; Novahistine® Elixir [OTC]; Prehist®; Ru-Tuss® Liquid
Synonyms phenylephrine and chlorpheniramine
Therapeutic Category Antihistamine/Decongestant Combination
Use Temporary relief of nasal congestion and eustachian tube congestion as well as runny nose, sneezing, itching of nose or throat, itchy and watery eyes
Usual Dosage Oral:
Children:
2-5 years: 2.5 mL every 4 hours
6-12 years: 5 mL every 4 hours

Adults: 10 mL every 4 hours
Dosage Forms
Capsule, sustained release: Chlorpheniramine maleate 8 mg and phenylephrine hydrochloride 20 mg
(Continued)

93

chlorpheniramine and phenylephrine *(Continued)*

Liquid: Chlorpheniramine maleate 5 mg and phenylephrine hydrochloride 2 mg per 5 mL (120 mL, 480 mL, 4000 mL)

chlorpheniramine and phenylpropanolamine

Brand Names Allerest™ 12 Hour Capsule [OTC]; Condrin-LA®; Contac® Maximum Strength [OTC]; CPA TR™; Demazin® [OTC]; Drize®; Genamin® Cold Syrup [OTC]; Myminic® Syrup [OTC]; Oragest SR™; Ornade® Spansule®; Parhist SR®; Resaid®; Rescon Liquid [OTC]; Rhinolar-EX™ 12; Ru-Tuss II®; Triaminic-12® [OTC]; Triaminic® Syrup [OTC]; Trind® Liquid [OTC]; Tripalgen™ Cold [OTC]; Triphenyl® Syrup [OTC]

Synonyms phenylpropanolamine and chlorpheniramine

Therapeutic Category Antihistamine/Decongestant Combination

Use Symptomatic relief of nasal congestion, runny nose, sneezing, itchy nose or throat, and itchy or watery eyes due to the common cold or allergic rhinitis

Usual Dosage

Children <12 years: 5 mL every 3-4 hours

Children >12 years and Adults: 1 capsule every 12 hours or 5-10 mL every 3-4 hours

Dosage Forms

Capsule, sustained release: Chlorpheniramine maleate 12 mg and phenylpropanolamine hydrochloride 75 mg

Liquid: Chlorpheniramine maleate 2 mg and phenylpropanolamine hydrochloride 12.5 mg per 5 mL

Syrup: Chlorpheniramine maleate 2 mg and phenylpropanolamine hydrochloride 12.5 mg per 5 mL

Tablet, sustained release: Chlorpheniramine maleate 12 mg and phenylpropanolamine hydrochloride 75 mg

chlorpheniramine and pseudoephedrine

Brand Names Anamine T.D.®; Brexin® L.A.; Chlorafed®; Chlordrine® S.R.; Codimal-L.A.®; Colfed-A™; Co-Pyronil® 2 [OTC]; Deconamine® SR; Deconamine® Tablet; Duralex®; Dura-Tap/PD™; Fedahist™ Timecaps®; Isoclor® Tablet; Isoclor® Timesules®; Klerist-D®; Kronofed-A-Jr™; N D Clear™; Novafed® A; Pseudo-Chlor® [OTC]; Pseudo-gest Plus® [OTC]; Rescon; Rescon-ED™; Rescon Jr; Sudafed Plus® Tablet

Synonyms pseudoephedrine and chlorpheniramine

Therapeutic Category Antihistamine/Decongestant Combination

Use Relief of nasal congestion associated with the common cold, hay fever, and other allergies, sinusitis, eustachian tube blockage, and vasomotor and allergic rhinitis

Usual Dosage Oral:

Capsule: One every 12 hours

Tablet: One 3-4 times/day

Dosage Forms

Capsule: Chlorpheniramine maleate 4 mg and pseudoephedrine hydrochloride 60 mg; chlorpheniramine maleate 12 mg and pseudoephedrine hydrochloride 120 mg

Capsule, sustained release: Chlorpheniramine maleate 4 mg and pseudoephedrine hydrochloride 60 mg; chlorpheniramine maleate 8 mg and pseudoephedrine hydrochloride 120 mg

Tablet: Chlorpheniramine maleate 4 mg and pseudoephedrine hydrochloride 60 mg

chlorpheniramine, ephedrine, phenylephrine, and carbetapentane

Brand Names Rentamine®; Rynatuss® Pediatric Suspension; Tri-Tannate Plus®

Therapeutic Category Antihistamine/Decongestant Combination

Use Symptomatic relief of cough

Usual Dosage Children:

<2 years: Titrate dose individually

2-6 years: 2.5-5 mL every 12 hours

>6 years: 5-10 mL every 12 hours

Dosage Forms Liquid: Carbetapentane tannate 30 mg, phenylephrine tannate 5 mg, ephedrine tannate 5 mg, and chlorpheniramine tannate 4 mg per 5 mL

chlorpheniramine maleate (klor fen ir' a meen mal' ee ate)

Brand Names Aller-Chlor® Oral [OTC]; Chlo-Amine® Oral [OTC]; Chlorate® Oral [OTC]; Chlor-Pro® Injection; Chlor-Trimeton® Injection; Chlor-Trimeton® Oral [OTC]; Phenetron® Oral; Telachlor® Oral; Teldrin® Oral [OTC]

Therapeutic Category Antihistamine

Use Perennial and seasonal allergic rhinitis and other allergic symptoms including urticaria

Usual Dosage Oral:

  Children: 0.35 mg/kg/day in divided doses every 4-6 hours

    2-6 years: 1 mg every 4-6 hours

    6-12 years: 2 mg every 4-6 hours, not to exceed 12 mg/day

  Adults: 4 mg every 4-6 hours, not to exceed 24 mg/day or sustained release 8-12 mg every 12 hours

Dosage Forms

  Capsule: 12 mg

  Capsule, timed release: 6 mg, 8 mg, 12 mg

  Injection: 10 mg/mL (1 mL, 30 mL); 100 mg/mL (10 mL)

  Liquid: 1 mg/5 mL (120 mL)

  Syrup: 2 mg/5 mL (120 mL, 480 mL, 4000 mL)

  Tablet: 4 mg, 8 mg, 12 mg

  Tablet:

    Chewable: 2 mg

    Timed release: 8 mg, 12 mg

chlorpheniramine, phenindamine, and phenylpropanolamine

Brand Names Nolamine®

Therapeutic Category Antihistamine/Decongestant Combination

Use Upper respiratory and nasal congestion

Usual Dosage Adults: Oral: 1 tablet every 8-12 hours

Dosage Forms Tablet, timed release: Chlorpheniramine maleate 4 mg, phenindamine tartrate 24 mg, and phenylpropanolamine hydrochloride 50 mg

chlorpheniramine, phenylephrine, and codeine

Brand Names Pediacof®; Pedituss®

Therapeutic Category Antihistamine/Decongestant Combination; Cough Preparation

Use Symptomatic relief of rhinitis, nasal congestion and cough due to colds or allergy

Usual Dosage Children 6 months to 12 years: 1.25-10 mL every 4-6 hours

Dosage Forms Liquid: Chlorpheniramine maleate 0.75 mg, phenylephrine hydrochloride 2.5 mg, and codeine phosphate 5 mg with potassium iodide 75 mg per 5 mL

chlorpheniramine, phenylephrine, and dextromethorphan

Brand Names Cerose-DM® [OTC]

Therapeutic Category Antihistamine/Decongestant Combination; Cough Preparation

Use Temporary relief of cough due to minor throat and bronchial irritation; relieves nasal congestion, runny nose and sneezing

Usual Dosage Adults: Oral: 5-10 mL 4 times/day

Dosage Forms Liquid: Chlorpheniramine maleate 4 mg, phenylephrine hydrochloride 10 mg, and dextromethorphan hydrobromide 15 mg per 5 mL

chlorpheniramine, phenylephrine and methscopolamine

Brand Names Alersule Forte®; Dallergy®; Extendryl® SR; Histor-D® Timecelles®

Therapeutic Category Antihistamine/Decongestant Combination

Use Relieves nasal congestion, runny nose and sneezing

Usual Dosage Adults: Oral: 1 capsule every 12 hours

Dosage Forms

  Caplet, sustained release: Chlorpheniramine maleate 8 mg, phenylephrine hydrochloride 20 mg, and methscopolamine nitrate 2.5 mg

(Continued)

95

chlorpheniramine, phenylephrine and methscopolamine
(Continued)
Capsule, sustained release: Chlorpheniramine maleate 8 mg, phenylephrine hydrochloride 10 mg, and methscopolamine nitrate 2.5 mg

Syrup: Chlorpheniramine maleate 2 mg, phenylephrine hydrochloride 10 mg, and methscopolamine nitrate 0.625 mg per 5 mL

chlorpheniramine, phenylephrine, and phenyltoloxamine
Brand Names Comhist®; Comhist® LA

Therapeutic Category Antihistamine/Decongestant Combination

Use Symptomatic relief of rhinitis and nasal congestion due to colds or allergy

Usual Dosage Oral: 1 capsule every 8-12 hours or 1-2 tablets 3 times/day

Dosage Forms
Capsule, sustained release (Comhist® LA): Chlorpheniramine maleate 4 mg, phenylephrine hydrochloride 20 mg, and phenyltoloxamine citrate 50 mg

Tablet (Comhist®): Chlorpheniramine maleate 2 mg, phenylephrine hydrochloride 10 mg, and phenyltoloxamine citrate 25 mg

chlorpheniramine, phenylpropanolamine, and acetaminophen
Brand Names BQ® Tablet [OTC]; Congestant D® [OTC]; Coricidin 'D'® [OTC]; Dapacin® Cold Capsule [OTC]; Duadacin® Capsule [OTC]; Tylenol® Cold Effervescent Medication Tablet [OTC]

Therapeutic Category Analgesic, Non-Narcotic; Antihistamine/Decongestant Combination; Antipyretic

Use Symptomatic relief of nasal congestion and headache from colds/sinus congestion

Usual Dosage Adults: Oral: 2 tablets every 4 hours, up to 12 tablets/day

Dosage Forms
Capsule: Chlorpheniramine maleate 2 mg, phenylpropanolamine hydrochloride 12.5 mg, and acetaminophen 325 mg

Tablet: Chlorpheniramine maleate 2 mg, phenylpropanolamine hydrochloride 12.5 mg, and acetaminophen 325 mg

chlorpheniramine, phenylpropanolamine, and dextromethorphan
Brand Names Triaminicol® Multi-Symptom Cold Syrup [OTC]

Therapeutic Category Antihistamine/Decongestant Combination; Cough Preparation

Use Provides relief of runny nose, sneezing, suppresses cough, promotes nasal and sinus drainage

Usual Dosage
Children 6-12 years: 5 mL every 4 hours
Adults: 10 mL every 4 hours

Dosage Forms Liquid: Chlorpheniramine maleate 2 mg, phenylpropanolamine hydrochloride 12.5 mg, and dextromethorphan hydrobromide 10 mg per 5 mL

chlorpheniramine, phenyltoloxamine, phenylpropanolamine and phenylephrine
Brand Names Naldecon®; Naldelate®; Nalgest®; Nalspan®; New Decongestant®; Par Decon'''; Quadra-Hist®; Tri-Phen-Chlor®; Uni-Decon®

Therapeutic Category Antihistamine/Decongestant Combination

Use Symptomatic treatment of nasal and eustachian tube congestion associated with sinusitis and acute upper respiratory infection; symptomatic relief of perennial and allergic rhinitis

Usual Dosage Oral:
Children:
3-6 months: 0.25 mL (pediatric drops) every 3-4 hours
6-12 months: 2.5 mL (pediatric syrup) or 0.5 mL (pediatric drops) every 3-4 hours
1-6 years: 5 mL (pediatric syrup) or 1 mL (pediatric drops) every 3-4 hours
6-12 years: 2.5 mL (syrup) or 10 mL (pediatric syrup) or $1/_2$ tablet every 3-4 hours

Children >12 years and 5 mL (syrup) or 1 tablet every 3-4 hours
Dosage Forms
Drops, pediatric: Chlorpheniramine maleate 0.5 mg, phenyltoloxamine citrate 2 mg, phenyl-propanolamine hydrochloride 5 mg, and phenylephrine hydrochloride 1.25 mg per mL
Syrup: Chlorpheniramine maleate 2.5 mg, phenyltoloxamine citrate 7.5 mg, phenylpropanol-amine hydrochloride 20 mg, and phenylephrine hydrochloride 5 mg per 5 mL
Syrup, pediatric: Chlorpheniramine maleate 0.5 mg, phenyltoloxamine citrate 2 mg, phenyl-propanolamine hydrochloride 5 mg, and phenylephrine hydrochloride 1.25 mg per 5 mL
Tablet, sustained release: Chlorpheniramine maleate 5 mg, phenyltoloxamine citrate 15 mg, phenylpropanolamine hydrochloride 40 mg, and phenylephrine hydrochloride 10 mg

chlorpheniramine, pseudoephedrine, and codeine
Brand Names Codehist® DH; Decohistine® DH; Dihistine® DH; Novahistine® DH; Phen DH® w/Codeine; Ryna-C® Liquid
Therapeutic Category Antihistamine/Decongestant Combination; Cough Preparation
Use Temporary relief of cough associated with minor throat or bronchial irritation or nasal congestion due to common cold, allergic rhinitis, or sinusitis
Usual Dosage Oral:
Children:
25-50 lb: 1.25-2.50 mL every 4-6 hours, up to 4 doses in 24-hour period
50-90 lb: 2.5-5 mL every 4-6 hours, up to 4 doses in 24-hour period

Adults: 10 mL every 4-6 hours, up to 4 doses in 24-hour period
Dosage Forms Liquid: Chlorpheniramine maleate 2 mg, pseudoephedrine hydrochloride 30 mg, and codeine phosphate 10 mg (120 mL, 480 mL)

chlorpheniramine, pyrilamine, and phenylephrine
Brand Names Rynatan® Pediatric Suspension; Tritan®; Tritann® Pediatric
Therapeutic Category Antihistamine/Decongestant Combination
Use Symptomatic relief of nasal congestion associated with upper respiratory tract condition
Usual Dosage Children:
<2 years: Titrate dose individually
2-6 years: 2.5-5 mL every 12 hours
>6 years: 5-10 mL every 12 hours
Dosage Forms
Liquid: Chlorpheniramine tannate 2 mg, pyrilamine tannate 12.5 mg, and phenylephrine tannate 5 mg per 5 mL
Tablet: Chlorpheniramine tannate 8 mg, pyrilamine maleate 12.5 mg, and phenylephrine tannate 25 mg

Chlor-Pro® Injection *see* chlorpheniramine maleate *on page 95*

chlorpromazine hydrochloride (klor proe' ma zeen)
Brand Names Ormazine; Thorazine®
Therapeutic Category Antiemetic; Antipsychotic Agent; Phenothiazine Derivative
Use Treatment of nausea and vomiting; psychoses; Tourette's syndrome; mania; intractable hiccups (adults); behavioral problems (children)
Usual Dosage
Children >6 months:
Psychosis:
Oral: 0.5-1 mg/kg/dose every 4-6 hours; older children may require 200 mg/day or higher
I.M., I.V.: 0.5-1 mg/kg/dose every 6-8 hours; maximum I.M./I.V. dose for <5 years (22.7 kg) = 40 mg/day; maximum I.M./I.V. for 5-12 years (22.7-45.5 kg) = 75 mg/day
Nausea and vomiting:
Oral: 0.5-1 mg/kg/dose every 4-6 hours as needed
I.M., I.V.: 0.5-1 mg/kg/dose every 6-8 hours; maximum dose: Same as psychosis
Rectal: 1 mg/kg/dose every 6-8 hours as needed
(Continued)

chlorpromazine hydrochloride *(Continued)*

Adults:
  Psychosis:
    Oral: Range: 30-800 mg/day in 1-4 divided doses, initiate at lower doses and titrate as needed; usual dose is 200 mg/day; some patients may require 1-2 g/day
    I.M., I.V.: 25 mg initially, may repeat (25-50 mg) in 1-4 hours, gradually increase to a maximum of 400 mg/dose every 4-6 hours until patient controlled; usual dose 300-800 mg/day
  Nausea and vomiting:
    Oral: 10-25 mg every 4-6 hours
    I.M., I.V.: 25-50 mg every 4-6 hours
    Rectal: 50-100 mg every 6-8 hours
  Intractable hiccups: Oral, I.M.: 25-50 mg 3-4 times/day

Dosage Forms
Capsule, sustained action: 30 mg, 75 mg, 150 mg, 200 mg, 300 mg
Concentrate, oral: 30 mg/mL (120 mL); 100 mg/mL (60 mL, 240 mL)
Injection: 25 mg/mL (1 mL, 2 mL, 10 mL)
Suppository, rectal, as base: 25 mg, 100 mg
Syrup: 10 mg/5 mL (120 mL)
Tablet: 10 mg, 25 mg, 50 mg, 100 mg, 200 mg

chlorpropamide (klor proe' pa mide)

Brand Names Diabinese"
Therapeutic Category Antidiabetic Agent; Hypoglycemic Agent, Oral; Sulfonylurea Agent
Use Control blood sugar in adult onset, noninsulin-dependent diabetes (type II). Unlabeled use includes: neurogenic diabetes insipidus
Usual Dosage The dosage of chlorpropamide is variable and should be individualized based upon the patient's response.

Adults: Oral: 250 mg once daily; initial dose in elderly patients: 100 mg once daily; subsequent dosages may be increased or decreased by 50-125 mg/day at 3- to 5-day intervals; maximum daily dose: 750 mg
Dosage Forms Tablet: 100 mg, 250 mg

chlorprothixene (klor proe thix' een)

Therapeutic Category Antipsychotic Agent; Thioxanthene Derivative
Use Management of psychotic disorders
Usual Dosage
Children >6 years: Oral: 10-25 mg 3-4 times/day

Adults:
  Oral: 25-50 mg 3-4 times/day, to be increased as needed; doses exceeding 600 mg/day are rarely required
  I.M.: 25-50 mg up to 3-4 times/day
Dosage Forms
Concentrate, oral, as lactate and hydrochloride (fruit flavor): 100 mg/5 mL (480 mL)
Injection, as hydrochloride: 12.5 mg/mL (2 mL)
Tablet: 10 mg, 25 mg, 50 mg, 100 mg

chlortetracyline hydrochloride (klor te tra sye' kleen)

Brand Names Aureomycin"
Therapeutic Category Antibiotic, Ophthalmic; Antibiotic, Tetracycline Derivative
Use Treatment of superficial infections of the skin due to susceptible organisms, also infection prophylaxis in minor skin abrasions
Usual Dosage Apply 1-5 times/day, cover with sterile bandage if needed
Dosage Forms Ointment:
Ophthalmic: 1% [10 mg/g] (3.5 g)
Topical: 3% (14.2 g, 30 g)

chlorthalidone (klor thal' i done)
Brand Names Hygroton®; Thalitone®
Therapeutic Category Diuretic, Miscellaneous
Use Management of mild to moderate hypertension, used alone or in combination with other agents; treatment of edema associated with congestive heart failure, nephrotic syndrome, or pregnancy
Usual Dosage Oral:
Children: 2 mg/kg 3 times/week
Adults: 25-100 mg/day or 100 mg 3 times/week
Dosage Forms Tablet:
Hygroton®: 25 mg, 50 mg, 100 mg
Thalitone®: 15 mg, 25 mg

Chlor-Trimeton® Injection *see* chlorpheniramine maleate *on page 95*
Chlor-Trimeton® Oral [OTC] *see* chlorpheniramine maleate *on page 95*

chlorzoxazone (klor zox' a zone)
Brand Names Flexaphen®; Lobac®; Mus-Lac®; Paraflex®; Parafon Forte™ DSC; Remular-S®
Therapeutic Category Centrally Acting Muscle Relaxant; Skeletal Muscle Relaxant
Use Symptomatic treatment of muscle spasm and pain associated with acute musculoskeletal conditions
Usual Dosage Oral:
Children: 20 mg/kg/day or 600 mg/m^2/day in 3-4 divided doses
Adults: 250-500 mg 3-4 times/day up to 750 mg 3-4 times/day
Dosage Forms
Caplet (Parafon Forte™ DSC): 500 mg
Capsule (Lobac®, Mus-Lac®): 250 mg with acetaminophen 300 mg
Tablet (Paraflex®): 250 mg

Cholac® *see* lactulose *on page 261*
Cholan-HMB® *see* dehydrocholic acid *on page 127*
Cholebrine® *see* radiological/contrast media (ionic) *on page 404*

cholecalciferol (kole e kal si' fer ole)
Brand Names Delta-D®
Synonyms d$_3$
Therapeutic Category Vitamin D Analog
Use Dietary supplement, treatment of vitamin D deficiency or prophylaxis of deficiency
Usual Dosage Adults: Oral: 400-1000 units/day
Dosage Forms Tablet: 400 units, 1000 units

Choledyl® *see* oxtriphylline *on page 341*

cholera vaccine (kol' er a)
Therapeutic Category Vaccine, Inactivated Bacteria
Use Primary immunization for cholera prophylaxis
Usual Dosage I.M., S.C.:
Children:
6 months to 4 years: 0.2 mL with same dosage schedule
5-10 years: 0.3 mL with same dosage schedule

Children >10 years and Adults: 0.5 mL in 2 doses 1 week to 1 month or more apart
Dosage Forms Injection: Suspension of killed *Vibrio cholerae* (Inaba and Ogawa types) 8 units of each serotype per mL (1.5 mL, 20 mL)

cholestyramine resin (koe less' tir a meen)
Brand Names Questran®; Questran® Light
Therapeutic Category Antilipemic Agent
Use Adjunct in the management of primary hypercholesterolemia; pruritus associated with elevated levels of bile acids; diarrhea associated with excess fecal bile acids; binding toxicologic agents; pseudomembraneous colitis
Usual Dosage Dosages are expressed in terms of anhydrous resin. Oral:
Children: 240 mg/kg/day in 3 divided doses; need to titrate dose depending on indication
Adults: 3-4 g 3-4 times/day to a maximum of 16-32 g/day in 2-4 divided doses
Dosage Forms
Powder: 4 g of resin/9 g of powder (9 g, 378 g)
Powder, for oral suspension, with aspartame: 4 g of resin/5 g of powder (5 g, 210 g)

choline magnesium trisalicylate
Brand Names Tricosal®; Trilisate®
Therapeutic Category Analgesic, Non-Narcotic; Anti-inflammatory Agent; Nonsteroidal Anti-Inflammatory Agent (NSAID), Oral; Salicylate
Use Management of osteoarthritis, rheumatoid arthritis, and other arthritides
Usual Dosage Oral (based on total salicylate content):
Children: 30-60 mg/kg/day given in 3-4 divided doses
Adults: 500 mg to 1.5 g 1-3 times/day
Dosage Forms
Liquid: 500 mg/5 mL [choline salicylate 293 mg and magnesium salicylate 362 mg per 5 mL] (237 mL)
Tablet:
500 mg: Choline salicylate 293 mg and magnesium salicylate 362 mg
750 mg: Choline salicylate 440 mg and magnesium salicylate 544 mg
1000 mg: Choline salicylate 587 mg and magnesium salicylate 725 mg

choline salicylate
Brand Names Arthropan® [OTC]
Therapeutic Category Analgesic, Non-Narcotic; Anti-inflammatory Agent; Nonsteroidal Anti-Inflammatory Agent (NSAID), Oral; Salicylate
Use Temporary relief of pain of rheumatoid arthritis, rheumatic fever, osteoarthritis, and other conditions for which oral salicylates are recommended; useful in patients in which there is difficulty in administering doses in a tablet or capsule dosage form, because of the liquid dosage form
Usual Dosage Adults: 5 mL every 3-4 hours, if necessary, but not more than 6 doses in 24 hours
Dosage Forms Liquid (mint flavor): 870 mg/5 mL (240 mL, 480 mL)

choline theophyllinate *see* oxtriphylline *on page 341*
Cholografin® Meglumine *see* radiological/contrast media (ionic) *on page 404*
Choloxin® *see* dextrothyroxine sodium *on page 135*

chondroitin sulfate-sodium hyaluronate
(kon droy' tin sul' fate-so' de um hi a lu ron' ate)
Brand Names Viscoat®
Synonyms sodium hyaluronate-chrondroitin sulfate
Therapeutic Category Ophthalmic Agent, Viscoeleastic
Use Surgical aid in anterior segment procedures, protects corneal endothelium and coats intraocular lens thus protecting it
Usual Dosage Carefully introduce into anterior chamber after thoroughly cleaning the chamber with a balanced salt solution
Dosage Forms Solution: Sodium chondroitin 40 mg and sodium hyaluronate 30 mg (0.25 mL, 0.5 mL)

Chooz® [OTC] *see* calcium carbonate *on page 66*

Chorex® *see* chorionic gonadotropin *on this page*

chorionic gonadotropin (kor re on' ik goe nad' oh troe pin)
Brand Names A.P.L.®; Chorex®; Choron®; Follutein®; Glukor®; Gonic®; Pregnyl®; Profasi® HP
Synonyms cg; hcg
Therapeutic Category Gonadotropin; Ovulation Stimulator
Use Induce ovulation and pregnancy; treatment of hypogonadotropic hypogonadism, prepubertal cryptorchidism
Usual Dosage Children: I.M.:
Prepubertal cryptorchidism: 1000-2000 units/m^2/dose 3 times/week for 3 weeks

Hypogonadotropic hypogonadism: 500-1000 USP units 3 times/week for 3 weeks, followed by the same dose twice weekly for 3 weeks
Dosage Forms Powder for injection: 200 units/mL (10 mL, 25 mL); 500 units/mL (10 mL); 1000 units/mL (10 mL); 2000 units/mL (10 mL)

Choron® *see* chorionic gonadotropin *on this page*

Chromagen® OB [OTC] *see* vitamin, multiple (prenatal) *on page 491*

Chroma-Pak® *see* trace metals *on page 465*

chromium *see* trace metals *on page 465*

Chronulac® *see* lactulose *on page 261*

Chymex® *see* bentiromide *on page 47*

Chymodiactin® *see* chymopapain *on this page*

chymopapain (kye' moe pa pane)
Brand Names Chymodiactin®; Discase®
Therapeutic Category Enzyme, Intradiscal; Enzyme, Proteolytic
Use Alternative to surgery in patients with herniated lumbar intervertebral disks
Usual Dosage 2000-4000 units/disk with a maximum cumulative dose not to exceed 8000 units for patients with multiple disk herniations
Dosage Forms Injection: 4000 units [4 nKat]; 10,000 units [10 nKat]

ciclopirox olamine (sye kloe peer' ox)
Brand Names Loprox®
Therapeutic Category Antifungal Agent, Topical
Use Treatment of tinea pedis, tinea cruris, tinea corporis, cutaneous candidiasis, tinea versicolor
Usual Dosage Children >10 years and Adults: Apply twice daily, gently massage into affected areas; safety and efficacy in children <10 years have not been established
Dosage Forms
Cream, topical: 1% (15 g, 30 g, 90 g)
Lotion: 1% (30 mL)

Ciloxan™ Ophthalmic *see* ciprofloxacin hydrochloride *on next page*

cimetidine (sye met' i deen)
Brand Names Tagamet®
Therapeutic Category Histamine-2 Antagonist
Use Short-term treatment of active duodenal ulcers and benign gastric ulcers; long-term prophylaxis of duodenal ulcer; gastric hypersecretory states; gastroesophageal reflux; prevention of upper gastrointestinal bleeding in critically ill patients
Usual Dosage Oral, I.M., I.V.:
Neonates: 5-10 mg/kg/day in divided doses every 8-12 hours
(Continued)
101

cimetidine *(Continued)*

Infants: 10-20 mg/kg/day divided every 6-12 hours
Children: 20-30 mg/kg/day in divided doses every 6 hours

Patients with an active bleed: Give cimetidine as a continuous infusion

Adults:
Short-term treatment of active ulcers:
Oral: 300 mg 4 times/day or 800 mg at bedtime or 400 mg twice daily for up to 8 weeks
I.M., I.V.: 300 mg every 6 hours or 37.5 mg/hour by continuous infusion; I.V. dosage should be adjusted to maintain an intragastric pH of 5 or greater
Duodenal ulcer prophylaxis: Oral: 400-800 mg at bedtime
Gastric hypersecretory conditions: Oral, I.M., I.V.: 300-600 mg every 6 hours; dosage not to exceed 2.4 g/day

Dosage Forms
Infusion, as hydrochloride, in NS: 300 mg (50 mL)
Injection, as hydrochloride: 150 mg/mL (2 mL, 8 mL)
Liquid, oral, as hydrochloride (mint-peach flavor): 300 mg/5 mL with alcohol 2.8% (5 mL, 240 mL)
Tablet: 200 mg, 300 mg, 400 mg, 800 mg

Cinobac® Pulvules® *see cinoxacin on this page*

cinoxacin (sin ox' a sin)

Brand Names Cinobac® Pulvules®
Therapeutic Category Antibiotic, Quinolone
Use Urinary tract infections
Usual Dosage Children >12 years and Adults: 1 g/day in 2-4 doses
Dosage Forms Capsule: 250 mg, 500 mg

ciprofloxacin hydrochloride (sip roe flox' a sin)

Brand Names Ciloxan™ Ophthalmic; Cipro™ Injection; Cipro™ Oral
Therapeutic Category Antibiotic, Ophthalmic; Antibiotic, Quinolone
Use Treatment of documented or suspected pseudomonal infection in home care patients; documented multi-drug resistant gram-negative organisms; documented infectious diarrhea due to *Campylobacter jejuni*, *Shigella*, or *Salmonella*; osteomyelitis caused by susceptible organisms in which parenteral therapy is not feasible; used ophthalmically for treatment of corneal ulcers and conjunctivitis due to strains of microorganisms susceptible to ciprofloxacin
Usual Dosage
Children: Oral: 20-30 mg/kg/day in 2 divided doses; maximum dose: 1.5 g/day

Adults:
Oral: 250-750 mg every 12 hours, depending on severity of infection and susceptibility
Ophthalmic: Instill 1-2 drops in eye(s) every 2 hours while awake for 2 days and 1-2 drops every 4 hours while awake for the next 5 days
I.V.: 200-400 mg every 12 hours depending on severity of infection

Dosage Forms
Infusion, in D₅W: 400 mg (200 mL)
Infusion, in NS or D₅W: 200 mg (100 mL)
Injection: 200 mg (20 mL); 400 mg (40 mL)
Solution, ophthalmic: 3.5 mg/mL (2.5 mL, 5 mL)
Tablet: 250 mg, 500 mg, 750 mg

Cipro™ Injection *see ciprofloxacin hydrochloride on this page*
Cipro™ Oral *see ciprofloxacin hydrochloride on this page*

cisapride (sis' a pride)

Brand Names Propulsid®
Therapeutic Category Antiemetic; Cholinergic Agent
Use Symptomatic treatment of patients with nocturnal heartburn due to gastrointestinal reflux disease

Usual Dosage Adults: Oral: 10 mg 4 times daily at least 15 minutes before meals and at bedtime; in some patients the dosage will need to be increased to 20 mg to obtain a satisfactory result

Dosage Forms Tablet: 10 mg, 20 mg

cisplatin (sis' pla tin)
Brand Names Platinol®; Platinol®-AQ
Synonyms cddp
Therapeutic Category Antineoplastic Agent, Alkylating Agent
Use Management of metastatic testicular or ovarian carcinoma, advanced bladder cancer, osteosarcoma, Hodgkin's and non-Hodgkin's lymphoma, head or neck cancer, cervical cancer, lung cancer, or other tumors; used alone or with other agents
Usual Dosage Children and Adults (refer to individual protocols):
I.V.: Intermittent dosing schedule: 37-75 mg/m^2 once every 2-3 weeks or 50-120 mg/m^2 once every 3-4 weeks
Daily dosing schedule: 15-20 mg/m^2/day for 5 days every 3-4 weeks
Dosage Forms
Injection, aqueous: 1 mg/mL (50 mL, 100 mL)
Powder for injection: 10 mg, 50 mg

13-*cis*-retinoic acid *see* isotretinoin *on page 254*

Citanest® Forte *see* prilocaine *on page 385*

Citanest® Plain *see* prilocaine *on page 385*

Citracal® [OTC] *see* calcium citrate *on page 67*

citrate of magnesia *see* magnesium citrate *on page 276*

citric acid and d-gluconic acid irrigant *see* citric acid bladder mixture *on this page*

citric acid bladder mixture
Brand Names Renacidin®
Synonyms citric acid and d-gluconic acid irrigant; hemiacidrin
Therapeutic Category Irrigating Solution
Use Preparing solutions for irrigating indwelling urethral catheters; to dissolve or prevent formation of calcifications
Usual Dosage 30-60 mL of 10% (sterile) solution 2-3 times/day by means of a rubber syringe
Dosage Forms
Powder for solution: Citric acid 156-171 g, magnesium hydroxycarbonate 75-87 g, d-gluconic acid 21-30 g, magnesium acid citrate 9-15 g, calcium carbonate 2-6 g (150 g, 300 g)
Solution, irrigation: Citric acid 6.602 g, magnesium hydroxycarbonate 3.177 g, glucono-delta-lactone 0.198 g and benzoic acid 0.023 g per 100 mL (500 mL)

citrovorum factor *see* leucovorin calcium *on page 263*

Citrucel® [OTC] *see* methylcellulose *on page 298*

cla *see* clarithromycin *on next page*

cladribine (kla' dri been)
Brand Names Leustatin™
Synonyms 2-cda; 2-chlorodeoxyadenosine
Therapeutic Category Antineoplastic Agent, Antimetabolite
Use Hairy cell and chronic lymphocytic leukemias
Usual Dosage Adults: I.V.: 0.09 mg/kg/day continuous infusion
Dosage Forms Injection, preservative free: 1 mg/mL (10 mL)

Claforan® *see* cefotaxime sodium *on page 81*

clarithromycin (kla rith' roe mye sin)
Brand Names Biaxin™ Filmtabs®
Synonyms cla
Therapeutic Category Antibiotic, Macrolide
Use Against most respiratory pathogens (eg, *S. pyogenes*, *S. pneumoniae*, *S. agalactiae*, *S. viridans*, *M. catarrhalis*, *C. trachomatis*, *Legionella* spp., *Mycoplasma pneumoniae*[, *S. aureus*). Clarithromycin is highly active (MICs ≤0.25 mcg/mL) against *H. influenzae*, the combination of clarithromycin and its metabolite demonstrate an additive effect. Additionally, clarithromycin has shown activity against *C. pneumoniae* (including strain TWAR) and *M. avium* infection.
Usual Dosage Usual dose: 250-500 mg every 12 hours for 7-14 days
Upper respiratory tract: 250-500 mg every 12 hours for 10-14 days
    Pharyngitis/tonsillitis: 250 mg every 12 hours for 10 days
    Acute maxillary sinusitis: 500 mg every 12 hours for 14 days

Lower respiratory tract: 250-500 mg every 12 hours for 7-14 days
    Acute exacerbation of chronic bronchitis due to:
      S. pneumoniae: 250 mg every 12 hours for 7-14 days
      M. catarrhalis: 250 mg every 12 hours for 7-14 days
      H. influenzae: 500 mg every 12 hours for 7-14 days
    Pneumonia due to:
      S. pneumoniae: 250 mg every 12 hours for 7-14 days
      M. pneumoniae: 250 mg every 12 hours for 7-14 days

Uncomplicated skin and skin structure: 250 mg every 12 hours for 7-14 days
Dosage Forms
Granules for oral suspension: 125 mg/5 mL (100 mL, 200 mL); 250 mg/5 mL (100 mL, 200 mL)
Tablet, film coated: 250 mg, 500 mg

Claritin® *see* loratadine *on page 273*
Clear Away® Disc [OTC] *see* salicylic acid *on page 416*
Clearblue® *see* diagnostic aids (*in vitro*), urine *on page 137*
Clear By Design® [OTC] *see* benzoyl peroxide *on page 50*
Clear Eyes® [OTC] *see* naphazoline hydrochloride *on page 319*
Clearplan® Easy *see* diagnostic aids (*in vitro*), urine *on page 137*
Clearsil® [OTC] *see* benzoyl peroxide *on page 50*

clemastine and phenylpropanolamine
Brand Names Tavist-D®
Therapeutic Category Antihistamine/Decongestant Combination
Use Symptomatic relief of allergic rhinitis; pruritus of the eyes, nose or throat, lacrimation and nasal congestion
Usual Dosage Children >12 years and Adults: Oral: 1 tablet every 12 hours
Dosage Forms Tablet: Clemastine fumarate 1.34 mg and phenylpropanolamine hydrochloride 75 mg

clemastine fumarate (klem' as teen fume' a rate)
Brand Names Antihist-1® [OTC]; Tavist®; Tavist®-1 [OTC]
Therapeutic Category Antihistamine
Use Perennial and seasonal allergic rhinitis and other allergic symptoms including urticaria
Usual Dosage Oral:
Children:
    <12 years: 0.67-1.34 mg every 8-12 hours as needed
    >12 years: 1.34 mg twice daily to 2.68 mg 3 times/day; do not exceed 8.04 mg/day

Adults: 1.34 mg twice daily to 2.68 mg 3 times/day; do not exceed 8.04 mg/day
Dosage Forms
Syrup (citrus flavor): 0.67 mg/5 mL with alcohol 5.5% (120 mL)
Tablet: 1.34 mg, 2.68 mg

Cleocin HCl® *see* clindamycin *on this page*
Cleocin Pediatric® *see* clindamycin *on this page*
Cleocin Phosphate® *see* clindamycin *on this page*
Cleocin T® *see* clindamycin *on this page*

clidinium and chlordiazepoxide
Brand Names Clindex®; Clinoxide®; Clipoxide®; Librax®; Lidox®; Zebrax®
Synonyms chlordiazepoxide and clidinium
Therapeutic Category Antispasmodic Agent, Gastrointestinal
Use Adjunct treatment of peptic ulcer, treatment of irritable bowel syndrome
Usual Dosage Oral: 1-2 capsules 3-4 times/day, before meals or food and at bedtime
Dosage Forms Capsule: Clidinium bromide 2.5 mg and chlordiazepoxide hydrochloride 5 mg

Clinda-Derm® Topical Solution *see* clindamycin *on this page*

clindamycin (klin da mye' sin)
Brand Names Cleocin HCl®; Cleocin Pediatric®; Cleocin Phosphate®; Cleocin T®; Clinda-Derm® Topical Solution
Therapeutic Category Acne Products; Antibiotic, Anaerobic; Antibiotic, Miscellaneous
Use Useful agent against aerobic and anaerobic streptococci (except enterococci), most staphylococci, *Bacteroides* sp. and *Actinomyces*; used topically in treatment of severe acne
Usual Dosage Avoid in neonates (contains benzyl alcohol)
 Neonates: I.M., I.V.:
  Postnatal age <7 days:
   ≤2000 g: 10 mg/kg/day in 2 equally divided doses
   >2000 g: 15 mg/kg/day in 3 divided doses
  Postnatal age >7 days:
   <1200 g: 10 mg/kg/day in 2 equally divided doses
   1200-2000 g: 15 mg/kg/day in 3 divided doses
   >2000 g: 20 mg/kg/day in 3-4 divided doses

 Infants and Children:
  Oral: 10-30 mg/kg/day in 3-4 divided doses
  I.M., I.V.: 25-40 mg/kg/day in 3-4 divided doses

 Children and Adults: Topical: Apply twice daily

 Adults:
  Oral: 150-450 mg/dose every 6-8 hours; maximum dose: 1.8 g/day
  I.M., I.V.: 1.2-1.8 g/day in 2-4 divided doses; maximum dose: 4.8 g/day
  Vaginal: One full applicator (100 mg) inserted intravaginally once daily before bedtime for
   seven consecutive days
Dosage Forms
 Capsule, as hydrochloride: 75 mg, 150 mg, 300 mg
 Cream, vaginal: 2% (40 g)
 Gel, topical, as phosphate: 1% [10 mg/g] (7.5 g, 30 g)
 Granules for oral solution, as palmitate: 75 mg/5 mL (100 mL)
 Infusion, as phosphate, in D_5W: 300 mg (50 mL); 600 mg (50 mL)
 Injection, as phosphate: 150 mg/mL (2 mL, 4 mL, 6 mL, 50 mL, 60 mL)
 Lotion: 1% [10 mg/mL] (60 mL)
 Solution, topical, as phosphate: 1% [10 mg/mL] (30 mL, 60 mL, 480 mL)

Clindex® *see* clidinium and chlordiazepoxide *on this page*
Clinistix® [OTC] *see* diagnostic aids (*in vitro*), urine *on page 137*
Clinitest® [OTC] *see* diagnostic aids (*in vitro*), urine *on page 137*

Clinoril® *see* sulindac *on page 443*

Clinoxide® *see* clidinium and chlordiazepoxide *on previous page*

clioquinol

Formerly Known As iodochlorhydroxyquin

Brand Names Vioform™ Topical [OTC]

Therapeutic Category Antifungal Agent, Topical

Use Used topically in the treatment of tinea pedis, tinea cruris, and skin infections caused by dermatophytic fungi (ring worm)

Usual Dosage Children and Adults: Topical: Apply 2-4 times/day; do not use for >7 days

Dosage Forms
  Cream: 3% (30 g)
  Ointment, topical: 3% (30 g)

clioquinol and hydrocortisone

Formerly Known As iodochlorhydroxyquin and hydrocortisone

Brand Names Ala-Quin® Topical; Corque® Topical; Cortin® Topical; Lanvisone® Topical; Pedi-Cort V™ Topical; Racet® Topical; UAD® Topical

Synonyms hydrocortisone and clioquinol

Therapeutic Category Antifungal Agent, Topical; Corticosteroid, Topical (Low Potency)

Use Contact or atopic dermatitis; eczema; neurodermatitis; anogenital pruritus; mycotic dermatoses; moniliasis

Usual Dosage Topical: Apply in a thin film 3-4 times/day

Dosage Forms
  Cream: Clioquinol 3% and hydrocortisone 0.5% (15 g, 30 g); clioquinol 3% and hydrocortisone 1% (15 g, 30 g)
  Lotion: Clioquinol 0.75% and hydrocortisone 0.25% (120 mL)
  Ointment, topical: Clioquinol 3% and hydrocortisone 1% (20 g, 480 g)

Clipoxide® *see* clidinium and chlordiazepoxide *on previous page*

clobetasol dipropionate (kloe bay' ta sol dye pro pee oh' nate)

Brand Names Temovate® Topical

Therapeutic Category Corticosteroid, Topical (Very High Potency)

Use Short-term relief of inflammation of moderate to severe corticosteroid-responsive dermatosis

Usual Dosage Apply twice daily for up to 2 weeks with no more than 50 g/week

Dosage Forms
  Cream: 0.05% (15 g, 30 g, 45 g)
  Gel: 0.05% (15 g, 30 g, 45 g)
  Ointment, topical: 0.05% (15 g, 30 g, 45 g)
  Scalp application: 0.05% (25 mL, 50 mL)

Clocort® Maximum Strength *see* hydrocortisone *on page 232*

clocortolone pivalate (kloe kor' toe lone)

Brand Names Cloderm™ Topical

Therapeutic Category Corticosteroid, Topical (Medium Potency)

Use Inflammation of corticosteroid-responsive dermatoses

Usual Dosage Topical: Apply sparingly and gently rub into affected area 1-4 times/day

Dosage Forms Cream: 0.1% (15 g, 45 g)

Cloderm® Topical *see* clocortolone pivalate *on this page*

clofazimine palmitate (kloe fa' zi meen)
Brand Names Lamprene®
Therapeutic Category Antibiotic, Miscellaneous
Use Treatment of dapsone-resistant leprosy; multibacillary dapsone-sensitive leprosy; erythema nodosum leprosum; *Mycobacterium avium* intracellular (MAI) infections
Usual Dosage Oral:
Children: Leprosy: 1 mg/kg/day every 24 hours in combination with dapsone and rifampin
Adults:
Dapsone-resistant leprosy: 50-100 mg/day in combination with one or more antileprosy drugs for 2 years; then alone 50-100 mg/day
Dapsone-sensitive multibacillary leprosy: 50-100 mg/day in combination with two or more antileprosy drugs for at least 2 years and continue until negative skin smears are obtained, then institute single drug therapy with appropriate agent
Erythema nodosum leprosum: 100-200 mg/day for up to 3 months or longer then taper dose to 100 mg/day when possible
MAI: Combination therapy using clofazimine 100 mg 1 or 3 times/day in combination with other antimycobacterial agents
Dosage Forms Capsule: 50 mg, 100 mg

clofibrate (kloe fye' brate)
Brand Names Atromid-S®
Therapeutic Category Antilipemic Agent
Use Adjunct to dietary therapy in the management of hyperlipidemias associated with high triglyceride levels
Usual Dosage Adults: Oral: 500 mg 4 times/day
Dosage Forms Capsule: 500 mg

Clomid® *see* clomiphene citrate *on this page*

clomiphene citrate (kloe' mi feen)
Brand Names Clomid®; Milophene®; Serophene®
Therapeutic Category Ovulation Stimulator
Use Treatment of ovulatory failure in patients desiring pregnancy
Usual Dosage Oral: 50 mg/day for 5 days (first course); start the regimen on or about the fifth day of cycle; if ovulation occurs do not increase dosage; if not, increase next course to 100 mg/day for 5 days
Dosage Forms Tablet: 50 mg

clomipramine hydrochloride (kloe mi' pra meen)
Brand Names Anafranil®
Therapeutic Category Antidepressant, Tricyclic
Use Treatment of obsessive-compulsive disorder (OCD)
Usual Dosage Oral:
Children: Initial: 25 mg/day and gradually increase, as tolerated to a maximum of 3 mg/kg or 100 mg, whichever is smaller
Adults: Initial: 25 mg/day and gradually increase, as tolerated to 100 mg/day the first 2 weeks, may then be increased to a total of 250 mg/day
Dosage Forms Capsule: 25 mg, 50 mg, 75 mg

clonazepam (kloe na' ze pam)
Brand Names Klonopin™
Therapeutic Category Anticonvulsant, Benzodiazepine
Use Prophylaxis of absence (petit mal), petit mal variant (Lennox-Gastaut), akinetic, and myoclonic seizures
Usual Dosage Oral:
Children <10 years or 30 kg:
Initial daily dose: 0.01-0.03 mg/kg/day (maximum: 0.05 mg/kg/day) given in 2-3 divided
(Continued)

clonazepam (Continued)

doses; increase by no more than 0.5 mg every third day until seizures are controlled or adverse effects are seen

Maintenance dose: 0.1-0.2 mg/kg/day divided 3 times/day; not to exceed 0.2 mg/kg/day

Adults:

Initial daily dose not to exceed 1.5 mg given in 3 divided doses; may increase by 0.5-1 mg every third day until seizures are controlled or adverse effects seen

Maintenance dose: 0.05-0.2 mg/kg; do not exceed 20 mg/day

Dosage Forms Tablet: 0.5 mg, 1 mg, 2 mg

clonidine (kloe' ni deen)

Brand Names Catapres® Oral; Catapres-TTS® Transdermal

Therapeutic Category Alpha-Adrenergic Agonist

Use Management of mild to moderate hypertension; either used alone or in combination with other antihypertensives; not recommended for first line therapy for hypertension; also used for heroin withdrawal and in smoking cessation therapy; other uses may include prophylaxis of migraines, glaucoma, paralytic ileus, and diabetes associated diarrhea

Usual Dosage Oral:

Children: Initial: 5-10 mcg/kg/day in divided doses every 8-12 hours; increase gradually to 5-25 mcg/kg/day in divided doses every 6 hours; maximum: 0.9 mg/day

Adults:

Initial dose: 0.1 mg twice daily

Maintenance dose: 0.2-1.2 mg/day in 2-4 divided doses; maximum recommended dose: 2.4 mg/day

Clonidine tolerance test (test of growth hormone release from the pituitary): 0.15 mg/m^2 or 4 mcg/kg as a single dose

Transdermal: Initial dose: 0.1 mg/day, increase every 1-2 weeks; maximum: doses exceeding 0.5 mg/day do not increase efficacy

Dosage Forms

Patch, transdermal: 1, 2, and 3 (0.1, 0.2, 0.3 mg/day to 7-day duration)

Tablet, as hydrochloride: 0.1 mg, 0.2 mg, 0.3 mg

clonidine and chlorthalidone

Brand Names Combipres®

Therapeutic Category Antihypertensive, Combination

Use Management of mild to moderate hypertension

Usual Dosage Oral: 1 tablet 1-2 times/day

Dosage Forms Tablet:

0.1: Clonidine 0.1 mg and chlorthalidone 15 mg

0.2: Clonidine 0.2 mg and chlorthalidone 15 mg

0.3: Clonidine 0.3 mg and chlorthalidone 15 mg

Clopra® see metoclopramide on page 302

clorazepate dipotassium (klor az' e pate)

Brand Names Gen-XENE®; Tranxene®

Therapeutic Category Anticonvulsant, Benzodiazepine; Benzodiazepine; Sedative

Use Treatment of generalized anxiety and panic disorders; management of alcohol withdrawal; adjunct anticonvulsant in management of partial seizures

Usual Dosage Oral:

Anticonvulsant:

Children:

<9 years: Dose not established

9-12 years: Anticonvulsant: Initial: 3.75-7.5 mg/dose twice daily; increase dose by 3.75 mg at weekly intervals, not to exceed 60 mg/day in 2-3 divided doses

Children >12 years and Adults: Initial: Up to 7.5 mg/dose 2-3 times/day; increase dose by 7.5 mg at weekly intervals; usual dose: 0.5-1 mg/kg/day; not to exceed 90 mg/day (up to 3 mg/kg/day has been used)

Anxiety: Adults: 7.5-15 mg 2-4 times/day, or given as single dose of 15-22.5 mg at bedtime

Alcohol withdrawal: Adults: Initial: 30 mg, then 15 mg 2-4 times/day on first day; maximum daily dose: 90 mg; gradually decrease dose over subsequent days

Dosage Forms
Capsule: 3.75 mg, 7.5 mg, 15 mg
Tablet: 3.75 mg, 7.5 mg, 15 mg
Tablet, single dose: 11.25 mg, 22.5 mg

Clorpactin® WCS-90 *see* oxychlorosene sodium *on page 342*

clotrimazole (kloe trim' a zole)
Brand Names Gyne-Lotrimin® [OTC]; Lotrimin®; Lotrimin AF® Cream [OTC]; Lotrimin AF® Lotion [OTC]; Lotrimin AF® Solution [OTC]; Mycelex®; Mycelex®-G
Therapeutic Category Antifungal Agent, Oral Nonabsorbed; Antifungal Agent, Topical; Antifungal Agent, Vaginal
Use Treatment of susceptible fungal infections, including oropharyngeal candidiasis, dermatophytoses, superficial mycoses, and cutaneous candidiasis, as well as vulvovaginal candidiasis; limited data suggests that the use of clotrimazole troches may be effective for prophylaxis against oropharyngeal candidiasis in neutropenic patients
Usual Dosage
Children >3 years and Adults:
Oral: 10 mg troche dissolved slowly 5 times/day
Topical: Apply twice daily

Adults: Vaginal: 100 mg/day for 7 days or 200 mg/day for 3 days or 500 mg single dose or 5 g (= 1 applicatorful) of 1% vaginal cream daily for 7-14 days
Dosage Forms
Cream:
Topical (Lotrimin®, Lotrimin® AF, Mycelex®, Mycelex® OTC) : 1% (15 g, 30 g, 45 g, 90 g)
Vaginal (Gyne-Lotrimin®, Mycelex®-G): 1% (45 g, 90 g)
Lotion (Lotrimin®): 1% (30 mL)
Solution, topical (Lotrimin®, Lotrimin® AF, Mycelex®, Mycelex® OTC): 1% (10 mL, 30 mL)
Tablet, vaginal (Gyne-Lotrimin®, Mycelex®-G): 100 mg (7s); 500 mg (1s)
Troche (Mycelex®): 10 mg
Twin pack (Mycelex®): Tablet 500 mg (1's) and vaginal cream 1% (7 g)

cloxacillin sodium (klox a sill' in)
Brand Names Cloxapen®; Tegopen®
Therapeutic Category Antibiotic, Penicillin
Use Treatment of susceptible bacterial infections, notably penicillinase-producing staphylococci causing respiratory tract, skin and skin structure, bone and joint, urinary tract infections, endocarditis, septicemia, and meningitis
Usual Dosage Oral:
Children >1 month: 50-100 mg/kg/day in divided doses every 6 hours; up to a maximum of 4 g/day

Adults: 250-500 mg every 6 hours
Dosage Forms
Capsule: 250 mg, 500 mg
Powder for oral suspension: 125 mg/5 mL (100 mL, 200 mL)

Cloxapen® *see* cloxacillin sodium *on this page*

clozapine (kloe' za peen)
Brand Names Clozaril®
Therapeutic Category Antipsychotic Agent
Use Management of schizophrenic patients
(Continued)

clozapine *(Continued)*

Usual Dosage Adults: Oral: 25 mg once or twice daily initially and increased, as tolerated to a target dose of 300-450 mg/day, but may require doses as high as 600-900 mg/day

Dosage Forms Tablet: 25 mg, 100 mg

Clozaril® *see clozapine on previous page*

Clysodrast® *see bisacodyl on page 54*

Cepacol® [OTC] *see cetylpyridinium chloride on page 86*

Cepacol® Anesthetic Troches [OTC] *see cetylpyridinium chloride and benzocaine on page 86*

Cepastat® [OTC] *see phenol on page 362*

cmv-igiv *see cytomegalovirus immune globulin intravenous, human on page 123*

coal tar

Brand Names AquaTar" [OTC]; Denorex® [OTC]; DHS® Tar [OTC]; Duplex® T [OTC]; Estar® [OTC]; Fototar® [OTC]; Neutrogena® T/Derm; Pentrax® [OTC]; Polytar® [OTC]; psoriGel® [OTC]; T/Gel" [OTC]; Zetar® [OTC]

Synonyms crude coal tar; lcd; pix carbonis

Therapeutic Category Antipsoriatic Agent, Topical; Antiseborrheic Agent, Topical

Use Topically for controlling dandruff, seborrheic dermatitis, or psoriasis

Usual Dosage

Bath: Add appropriate amount to bath water, for adults usually 60-90 mL of a 5% to 20% solution or 15-25 mL of 30% lotion; soak 5-20 minutes, then pat dry; use once daily to 3 days

Shampoo: Rub shampoo onto wet hair and scalp, rinse thoroughly; repeat; leave on 5 minutes; rinse thoroughly; apply twice weekly for the first 2 weeks then once weekly or more often if needed

Skin: Apply to the affected area 1-4 times/day; decrease frequency to 2-3 times/week once condition has been controlled

Scalp psoriasis: Tar oil bath or coal tar solution may be painted sparingly to the lesions 3-12 hours before each shampoo

Psoriasis of the body, arms, legs: Apply at bedtime; if thick scales are present, use product with salicylic acid and apply several times during the day

Dosage Forms

Cream: 1% to 5%

Gel: Coal tar 5%

Lotion: 2.5% to 30%

Lotion: Coal tar 2% to 5%

Shampoo: Coal tar extract 2% with salicylic acid 2% (60 mL)

Shampoo, topical: Coal tar: 0.5% to 5%

Solution:

Coal tar: 2.5%, 5%, 20%

Coal tar extract: 5%

Suspension, coal tar: 30% to 33.3%

coal tar and salicylic acid

Brand Names X-seb" T [OTC]

Therapeutic Category Antipsoriatic Agent, Topical; Antiseborrheic Agent, Topical

Use Seborrheal dermatitis; dandruff

Usual Dosage Shampoo twice weekly

Dosage Forms Shampoo: Coal tar solution 10% and salicylic acid 4% (120 mL)

coal tar, lanolin, and mineral oil

Brand Names Balnetar" [OTC]

Therapeutic Category Antipsoriatic Agent, Topical; Antiseborrheic Agent, Topical

Use Psoriasis; seborrheal dermatitis; atopic dermatitis; eczematoid dermatitis

Usual Dosage Add to bath water, soak for 5-20 minutes then pat dry
Dosage Forms Oil, bath: Water-dispersible emollient tar 2.5%, lanolin fraction, and mineral oil (240 mL)

Cobex® *see cyanocobalamin on page 119*

cocaine hydrochloride (koe kane')
Therapeutic Category Local Anesthetic, Topical
Use Topical anesthesia for mucous membranes
Usual Dosage Use lowest effective dose; do not exceed 1 mg/kg; patient tolerance, anesthetic technique, vascularity of tissue and area to be anesthetized will determine dose needed
Dosage Forms
Powder: 5 g, 25 g
Solution, topical: 4% [40 mg/mL] (2 mL, 4 mL, 10 mL); 10% [100 mg/mL] (4 mL, 10 mL)
Tablet, soluble, for topical solution: 135 mg

coccidioidin skin test (kox i dee oh' i din)
Brand Names Spherulin®
Therapeutic Category Diagnostic Agent, Fungus
Use Intradermal skin test in diagnosis of coccidioidomycosis; differential diagnosis of this disease from histoplasmosis, sarcoidosis and other mycotic and bacterial infections. The skin test may be negative in severe forms of disease (anergy) or when prolonged periods of time have passed since infection.
Usual Dosage Children and Adults: Intradermally: 0.1 mL of 1:100 or flexor surface of forearm
Positive reaction: Induration of 5 mm or more; erythema without induration is considered negative; read the test at 24 and 48 hours, since some reactions may not be noticeable after 36 hours. A positive reaction indicates present or past infection with *Coccidioides immitis*.
Negative reaction: A negative test means the individual has not been sensitized to coccidioidin or has lost sensitivity
Dosage Forms Injection: 1:10 (0.5 mL); 1:100 (1 mL)

Codafed® Expectorant *see guaifenesin, pseudoephedrine, and codeine on page 217*
Codamine® *see hydrocodone and phenylpropanolamine on page 231*
Codamine® Pediatric *see hydrocodone and phenylpropanolamine on page 231*
CodAphen® *see acetaminophen and codeine on page 3*
Codehist® DH *see chlorpheniramine, pseudoephedrine, and codeine on page 97*

codeine (koe' deen)
Synonyms methylmorphine
Therapeutic Category Analgesic, Narcotic; Antitussive
Use Treatment of mild to moderate pain; antitussive in lower doses
Usual Dosage Doses should be titrated to appropriate analgesic effect; when changing routes of administration, note that oral dose is $\frac{2}{3}$ as effective as parenteral dose

Analgesic: Oral, I.M., S.C.:
Children: 0.5-1 mg/kg/dose every 4-6 hours as needed; maximum: 60 mg/dose
Adults: 30 mg/dose; range: 15-60 mg every 4-6 hours as needed

Antitussive: Oral (for nonproductive cough):
Children: 1-1.5 mg/kg/day in divided doses every 4-6 hours as needed: Alternatively dose according to age:
2-6 years: 2.5-5 mg every 4-6 hours as needed; maximum: 30 mg/day
6-12 years: 5-10 mg every 4-6 hours as needed; maximum: 60 mg/day
Adults: 10-20 mg/dose every 4-6 hours as needed; maximum: 120 mg/day
Dosage Forms
Injection, as phosphate: 30 mg (1 mL, 2 mL); 60 mg (1 mL, 2 mL)
Solution, oral: 15 mg/5 mL
(Continued)

codeine *(Continued)*
Tablet, as sulfate: 15 mg, 30 mg, 60 mg
Tablet, as phosphate, soluble: 30 mg, 60 mg
Tablet, as sulfate, soluble: 15 mg, 30 mg, 60 mg

codeine and acetaminophen *see* acetaminophen and codeine *on page 3*

codeine and aspirin *see* aspirin and codeine *on page 36*

codeine and bromodiphenhydramine *see* bromodiphenhydramine and codeine *on page 58*

codeine and butalbital compound *see* butalbital compound and codeine *on page 63*

codeine and guaifenesin *see* guaifenesin and codeine *on page 214*

Codiclear® DH *see* hydrocodone and guaifenesin *on page 230*

Codimal-L.A.® *see* chlorpheniramine and pseudoephedrine *on page 94*

cod liver oil *see* vitamin a and vitamin d *on page 489*

Codoxy® *see* oxycodone and aspirin *on page 343*

Codroxomin® *see* hydroxocobalamin *on page 235*

Cogentin® *see* benztropine mesylate *on page 50*

Co-Gesic® *see* hydrocodone and acetaminophen *on page 230*

Cognex® Oral *see* tacrine hydrochloride *on page 444*

Colace® [OTC] *see* docusate *on page 153*

colaspase *see* asparaginase *on page 35*

Co-Lav® *see* polyethylene glycol-electrolyte solution *on page 375*

Colax® [OTC] *see* docusate and phenolphthalein *on page 154*

ColBENEMID® *see* colchicine and probenecid *on this page*

colchicine (kol' chi seen)
Therapeutic Category Anti-inflammatory Agent; Uricosuric Agent
Use Treat acute gouty arthritis attacks and to prevent recurrences of such attacks; management of familial Mediterranean fever
Usual Dosage
Treatment for acute gouty arthritis:
Oral: Initial: 0.5-1.2 mg, then 0.5-0.6 mg every 1-2 hours or 1-1.2 mg every 2 hours until relief or GI side effects occur to a maximum total dose of 8 mg, wait 3 days before initiating a second course
I.V.: Initial: 1-3 mg, then 0.5 mg every 6 hours until response, not to exceed 4 mg/day; following a full course of colchicine (4 mg), wait 7 days before initiating another course of colchicine (by any route)

Prophylaxis of recurrent attacks: Oral:
<1 attack/year: 0.5 or 0.6 mg/day/dose for 3-4 days/week
>1 attack/year: 0.5 or 0.6 mg/day/dose
Severe cases: 1-1.8 mg/day
Dosage Forms
Injection: 0.5 mg/mL (2 mL)
Tablet: 0.5 mg, 0.6 mg

colchicine and probenecid
Brand Names ColBENEMID®; Proben-C®
Synonyms probenecid and colchicine
Therapeutic Category Uricosuric Agent
Use Treatment of chronic gouty arthritis when complicated by frequent, recurrent acute attacks of gout

Usual Dosage Adults: Oral: 1 tablet daily for 1 week, then 1 tablet twice daily thereafter
Dosage Forms Tablet: Colchicine 0.5 mg and probenecid 0.5 g

Colestid® *see colestipol hydrochloride on this page*

colestipol hydrochloride (koe les' ti pole)
Brand Names Colestid®
Therapeutic Category Antilipemic Agent
Use Adjunct in the management of primary hypercholesterolemia; to relieve pruritus associated with elevated levels of bile acids, possibly used to decrease plasma half-life of digoxin as an adjunct in the treatment of toxicity
Usual Dosage 15-30 g/day in divided doses 2-4 times/day
Dosage Forms Granules: 5 g packet, 300 g, 500 g

Colfed-A® *see chlorpheniramine and pseudoephedrine on page 94*

colfosceril palmitate (kole fos' er il)
Brand Names Exosurf® Neonatal
Synonyms dipalmitoylphosphatidylcholine; dppc; synthetic lung surfactant
Therapeutic Category Lung Surfactant
Use Neonatal respiratory distress syndrome:
Prophylactic therapy: Body weight <1350 g in infants at risk for developing RDS; body weight >1350 g in infants with evidence of pulmonary immaturity
Rescue therapy: Treatment of infants with RDS based on respiratory distress not attributable to any other causes and chest radiographic findings consistent with RDS
Usual Dosage
Prophylactic treatment: Give 5 mL/kg as soon as possible; the second and third doses should be administered at 12 and 24 hours later to those infants remaining on ventilators
Rescue treatment: Give 5 mL/kg as soon as the diagnosis of RDS is made; the second 5 mL/kg dose should be administered 12 hours later
Dosage Forms Powder for injection, lyophilized: 108 mg (10 mL)

colistimethate sodium (koe lis ti meth' ate)
Brand Names Coly-Mycin® M Parenteral
Therapeutic Category Antibiotic, Miscellaneous
Use Treatment of infections due to sensitive strains of certain gram-negative bacilli
Usual Dosage Children and Adults: I.M., I.V.: 2.5-5 mg/kg/day in 2-4 divided doses
Dosage Forms Powder for injection, lyophilized: 150 mg

colistin, neomycin, and hydrocortisone
Brand Names Coly-Mycin® S Otic Drops
Therapeutic Category Antibiotic, Miscellaneous; Corticosteroid, Otic; Otic Agent, Anti-infective
Use Treatment of superficial and susceptible bacterial infections of the external auditory canal; for treatment of susceptible bacterial infections of mastoidectomy and fenestration cavities
Usual Dosage Otic:
Children: 3 drops in affected ear 3-4 times/day
Adults: 4 drops in affected ear 3-4 times/day
Dosage Forms Suspension, otic: Colistin sulfate 0.3%, neomycin sulfate 0.47%, and hydrocortisone acetate 1% (5 mL, 10 mL)

colistin sulfate (koe lis' tin)
Brand Names Coly-Mycin® S Oral
Synonyms polymyxin e
Therapeutic Category Antibiotic, Miscellaneous; Antidiarrheal
(Continued)

colistin sulfate *(Continued)*

Use Treat diarrhea in infants and children caused by susceptible organisms, especially *E. coli* and *Shigella*

Usual Dosage Children: 5-15 mg/kg/day in 3 divided doses given every 8 hours

Dosage Forms Powder for oral suspension: 25 mg/5 mL (60 mL)

collagenase (kol' la je nase)

Brand Names Biozyme-C®; Santyl®

Therapeutic Category Enzyme, Topical Debridement

Use Promote debridement of necrotic tissue in dermal ulcers and severe burns

Usual Dosage Topical: Apply daily or every other day

Dosage Forms Ointment, topical: 250 units/g (15 g, 30 g)

collagen implants

Therapeutic Category Ophthalmic Agent, Miscellaneous

Use For the relief of dry eyes; enhance the effect of ocular medications

Usual Dosage Implants inserted by physician

Dosage Forms Implant: 0.2 mm, 0.3 mm, 0.4 mm, 0.5 mm, 0.6 mm

Collyrium Fresh® Ophthalmic [OTC] *see* tetrahydrozoline hydrochloride *on page 452*

Colocare® [OTC] *see* diagnostic aids *(in vitro)*, feces *on page 137*

Color® Ovulation Test *see* diagnostic aids *(in vitro)*, urine *on page 137*

ColoScreen [OTC] *see* diagnostic aids *(in vitro)*, feces *on page 137*

Colovage® *see* polyethylene glycol-electrolyte solution *on page 375*

Coly-Mycin® M Parenteral *see* colistimethate sodium *on previous page*

Coly-Mycin® S Oral *see* colistin sulfate *on previous page*

Coly-Mycin® S Otic Drops *see* colistin, neomycin, and hydrocortisone *on previous page*

CoLyte® *see* polyethylene glycol-electrolyte solution *on page 375*

Combipres® *see* clonidine and chlorthalidone *on page 108*

Combistix® [OTC] *see* diagnostic aids *(in vitro)*, urine *on page 137*

Comfort® Ophthalmic [OTC] *see* naphazoline hydrochloride *on page 319*

Comhist® *see* chlorpheniramine, phenylephrine, and phenyltoloxamine *on page 96*

Comhist® LA *see* chlorpheniramine, phenylephrine, and phenyltoloxamine *on page 96*

Compazine® *see* prochlorperazine *on page 388*

compound e *see* cortisone acetate *on page 116*

compound f *see* hydrocortisone *on page 232*

compound s *see* zidovudine *on page 494*

Concentraid® Nasal *see* desmopressin acetate *on page 130*

Condrin-LA® *see* chlorpheniramine and phenylpropanolamine *on page 94*

Condylox® *see* podofilox *on page 373*

Conex® [OTC] *see* guaifenesin and phenylpropanolamine *on page 215*

Congess® Jr *see* guaifenesin and pseudoephedrine *on page 216*

Congess® Sr *see* guaifenesin and pseudoephedrine *on page 216*

Congestac® *see* guaifenesin and pseudoephedrine *on page 216*

Congestant D® [OTC] *see* chlorpheniramine, phenylpropanolamine, and acetaminophen *on page 96*

Conray® *see* radiological/contrast media (ionic) *on page 404*

Constilac® *see* lactulose *on page 261*

Constulose® *see* lactulose *on page 261*

Contac® Maximum Strength [OTC] *see* chlorpheniramine and phenylpropanolamine *on page 94*

Contac® Cough Formula Liquid [OTC] *see* guaifenesin and dextromethorphan *on page 214*

Control® [OTC] *see* phenylpropanolamine hydrochloride *on page 365*

Contuss® *see* guaifenesin, phenylpropanolamine, and phenylephrine *on page 217*

Contuss® XT *see* guaifenesin and phenylpropanolamine *on page 215*

Cophene-B® Injection *see* brompheniramine maleate *on page 59*

Cophene XP® *see* hydrocodone, pseudoephedrine, and guaifenesin *on page 231*

copper *see* trace metals *on page 465*

Co-Pyronil® 2 [OTC] *see* chlorpheniramine and pseudoephedrine *on page 94*

Cordarone® *see* amiodarone hydrochloride *on page 21*

Cordran® SP Topical *see* flurandrenolide *on page 199*

Cordran® Topical *see* flurandrenolide *on page 199*

Corgard® *see* nadolol *on page 316*

Coricidin 'D'® [OTC] *see* chlorpheniramine, phenylpropanolamine, and acetaminophen *on page 96*

Coricidin® [OTC] *see* chlorpheniramine and acetaminophen *on page 93*

Corque® Topical *see* clioquinol and hydrocortisone *on page 106*

Correctol® Extra Gentle [OTC] *see* docusate *on page 153*

Correctol® [OTC] *see* docusate and phenolphthalein *on page 154*

CortaGel® [OTC] *see* hydrocortisone *on page 232*

Cortaid® Maximum Strength [OTC] *see* hydrocortisone *on page 232*

Cortaid® with Aloe [OTC] *see* hydrocortisone *on page 232*

Cortatrigen® Otic *see* neomycin, polymyxin b, and hydrocortisone *on page 323*

Cort-Dome® *see* hydrocortisone *on page 232*

Cortef® *see* hydrocortisone *on page 232*

Cortef® Feminine Itch *see* hydrocortisone *on page 232*

Cortenema® *see* hydrocortisone *on page 232*

Corticaine® Topical *see* dibucaine and hydrocortisone *on page 140*

corticotropin (kor ti koe troe' pin)
Brand Names Acthar®; H.P. Acthar® Gel
Synonyms acth; adrenocorticotropic hormone
Therapeutic Category Adrenal Corticosteroid
Use Acute exacerbations of multiple sclerosis; diagnostic aid in adrenocortical insufficiency; severe muscle weakness in myasthenia gravis
Usual Dosage
Acute exacerbation of multiple sclerosis: I.M.: 80-120 units/day for 2-3 weeks

Diagnostic purposes:
I.M., S.C.: 20 units 4 times/day
I.V.: 10-25 units in 500 mL 5% dextrose in water over 8 hours
Dosage Forms
Injection, repository (H.P. Acthar® Gel): 40 units/mL (1 mL, 5 mL); 80 units/mL (1 mL, 5 mL)
(Continued)

corticotropin *(Continued)*
Powder for injection (Acthar®): 25 units, 40 units

Cortifoam® *see* hydrocortisone *on page 232*

Cortin® Topical *see* clioquinol and hydrocortisone *on page 106*

cortisol *see* hydrocortisone *on page 232*

cortisone acetate *(kor' ti sone)*
Brand Names Cortone® Acetate
Synonyms compound e
Therapeutic Category Adrenal Corticosteroid; Anti-inflammatory Agent; Corticosteroid, Systemic
Use Management of adrenocortical insufficiency
Usual Dosage Depends upon the condition being treated and the response of the patient
Children:
    Anti-inflammatory or immunosuppressive:
        Oral: 2.5-10 mg/kg/day or 20-300 mg/m^2/day in divided doses every 6-8 hours
        I.M.: 1-5 mg/kg/day or 14-375 mg/m^2/day in divided doses every 12-24 hours
    Physiologic replacement:
        Oral: 0.5-0.75 mg/kg/day in divided doses every 8 hours
        I.M.: 0.25-0.35 mg/kg/day once daily
   Stress coverage for surgery: I.M.: 1 and 2 days before preanesthesia, and 1-3 days after surgery: 50-62.5 mg/m^2/day; 4 days after surgery: 31-50 mg/m^2/day
   Adults: Oral, I.M.: 20-300 mg/day
Dosage Forms
   Injection: 50 mg/mL (10 mL)
   Tablet: 5 mg, 10 mg, 25 mg

Cortisporin® Ophthalmic Ointment *see* bacitracin, neomycin, polymyxin b, and hydrocortisone *on page 43*

Cortisporin® Ophthalmic Suspension *see* neomycin, polymyxin b, and hydrocortisone *on page 323*

Cortisporin® Otic *see* neomycin, polymyxin b, and hydrocortisone *on page 323*

Cortisporin® Topical Cream *see* neomycin, polymyxin b, and hydrocortisone *on page 323*

Cortisporin® Topical Ointment *see* bacitracin, neomycin, polymyxin b, and hydrocortisone *on page 43*

Cortizone®-5 [OTC] *see* hydrocortisone *on page 232*

Cortizone®-10 [OTC] *see* hydrocortisone *on page 232*

Cortone® Acetate *see* cortisone acetate *on this page*

Cortrosyn® Injection *see* cosyntropin *on this page*

Cosmegen® *see* dactinomycin *on page 124*

cosyntropin *(koe sin troe' pin)*
Brand Names Cortrosyn® Injection
Synonyms synacthen; tetracosactide
Therapeutic Category Adrenal Corticosteroid
Use Diagnostic test to differentiate primary adrenal from secondary (pituitary) adrenocortical insufficiency
Usual Dosage
   Adrenocortical insufficiency: I.M., I.V.:
      Neonates: 0.015 mg/kg/dose
      Children <2 years: 0.125 mg injected over 2 minutes

Children >2 years and Adults: 0.25 mg injected over 2 minutes

When greater cortisol stimulation is needed, an I.V. infusion may be used: I.V. infusion: 0.25 mg administered over 4-8 hours

Congenital adrenal hyperplasia evaluation: 1 mg/m^2/dose up to a maximum of 1 mg
Dosage Forms Powder for injection: 0.25 mg

Cotazym® *see* pancrelipase *on page 346*

Cotazym-S® *see* pancrelipase *on page 346*

Cotrim® *see* co-trimoxazole *on this page*

Cotrim® DS *see* co-trimoxazole *on this page*

co-trimoxazole (koe-trye mox' a zole)

Brand Names Bactrim™; Bactrim™ DS; Cotrim®; Cotrim® DS; Septra®; Septra® DS; Sulfamethoprim®; Sulfatrim®; Sulfatrim® DS; Uroplus® DS; Uroplus® SS

Synonyms sulfamethoxazole and trimethoprim; tmp-smx; trimethoprim and sulfamethoxazole smx-tmp

Therapeutic Category Antibiotic, Sulfonamide Derivative

Use Oral treatment of urinary tract infections; acute otitis media in children; acute exacerbations of chronic bronchitis in adults; prophylaxis of *Pneumocystis carinii* pneumonitis (PCP); I.V. treatment of documented PCP, empiric treatment of highly suspected PCP in immune compromised patients; treatment of documented or suspected shigellosis, typhoid fever, or *Nocardia asteroides* infection in patients who are NPO

Usual Dosage Oral, I.V. (dosage recommendations are based on the trimethoprim component):

Children >2 months:
  Mild to moderate infections: 6-12 mg TMP/kg/day in divided doses every 12 hours
  Serious infection/*Pneumocystis*: 15-20 mg TMP/kg/day in divided doses every 6 hours
  Urinary tract infection prophylaxis: 2 mg TMP/kg/dose daily
  Prophylaxis of *Pneumocystis*: 5-10 mg TMP/kg/day or 150 mg TMP/m^2/day in divided doses every 12 hours 3 days/week; dose should not exceed 320 mg trimethoprim and 1600 mg sulfamethoxazole 3 days/week; Mon, Tue, Wed

Adults: Urinary tract infection/chronic bronchitis: 1 double strength tablet every 12 hours for 10-14 days

Dosage Forms The 5:1 ratio (SMX to TMP) remains constant in all dosage forms:
Injection: Sulfamethoxazole 80 mg and trimethoprim 16 mg per mL (5 mL, 10 mL, 20 mL, 30 mL, 50 mL)
Suspension, oral: Sulfamethoxazole 200 mg and trimethoprim 40 mg per 5 mL (20 mL, 100 mL, 150 mL, 200 mL, 480 mL)
Tablet: Sulfamethoxazole 400 mg and trimethoprim 80 mg
Tablet, double strength: Sulfamethoxazole 800 mg and trimethoprim 160 mg

Coumadin® *see* warfarin sodium *on page 492*

Cozaar® *see* losartan potassium *on page 273*

CPA TR® *see* chlorpheniramine and phenylpropanolamine *on page 94*

cpm *see* cyclophosphamide *on page 121*

Creon® *see* pancreatin *on page 346*

Creon 10® *see* pancrelipase *on page 346*

Creon 20® *see* pancrelipase *on page 346*

Creo-Terpin® [OTC] *see* dextromethorphan hydrobromide *on page 135*

Cresylate® *see* m-cresyl acetate *on page 281*

cromoglicic acid *see* cromolyn sodium *on next page*

cromolyn sodium (kroe' moe lin)
Brand Names Gastrocrom® Oral; Intal® Inhalation Capsule; Intal® Nebulizer Solution; Intal® Oral Inhaler; Nasalcrom® Nasal Solution

Synonyms cromoglicic acid; disodium cromoglycate; dscg

Therapeutic Category Antihistamine, Inhalation; Inhalation, Miscellaneous

Use Adjunct in the prophylactic management of severe bronchial asthma, prevention of acute bronchospasm, prevention of exercise, induced bronchospasm, allergic rhinitis

Usual Dosage
Children:
    Inhalation: >2 years: 20 mg 4 times/day
    Nebulization solution: >5 years: 2 inhalations 4 times/day by metered spray, or 20 mg 4 times/day (Spinhaler®); taper frequency to the lowest effective level
    For prevention of exercise-induced bronchospasm: Single dose of 2 inhalations (aerosol) or 20 mg (powder inhalation) just prior to exercise
    Nasal: >6 years: 1 spray in each nostril 3-4 times/day

Adults:
    Inhalation: 20 mg 4 times/day (Spinhaler®), 2 inhalations 4 times/day by metered spray
    Nasal: 1 spray in each nostril 3-4 times/day

Systemic mastocytosis: Oral:
    Infants up to 2 years of age: 20 mg/kg/day in 4 divided doses, not to exceed 30 mg/kg/day
    Children 2-12 years: 100 mg 4 times/day; not to exceed 40 mg/kg/day
    Adults: 200 mg 4 times/day

Food allergy and inflammatory bowel disease: Oral:
    Children: 100 mg 4 times/day 15-20 minutes before meals, not to exceed 40 mg/kg/day
    Adults: 200 mg 4 times/day 15-20 minutes before meal, up to 400 mg 4 times/day

Dosage Forms
Capsule:
    Oral (Gastrocrom®): 100 mg
    Oral inhalation (Intal®): 20 mg [to be used with Spinhaler® turbo-inhaler]
Inhalation, oral (Intal®): 800 mcg/spray (8.1 g)
Solution, for nebulization (Intal®): 10 mg/mL (2 mL)
Solution: Nasal (Nasalcrom®): 40 mg/mL (13 mL)

crotaline antivenin, polyvalent *see* antivenin polyvalent (*Crotalidae*) *on page 31*

crotamiton (kroe tam' i tonn)
Brand Names Eurax® Topical

Therapeutic Category Antipruritic, Topical; Scabicidal Agent

Use Treatment of scabies and symptomatic treatment of pruritus

Usual Dosage Topical: Scabicide: Children and Adults: Wash thoroughly and scrub away loose scales, then towel dry; apply a thin layer and massage drug onto skin of the entire body from the neck to the toes (with special attention to skin folds, creases, and interdigital spaces). Repeat application in 24 hours. Take a cleansing bath 48 hours after the final application.

Dosage Forms
Cream: 10% (60 g)
Lotion: 10% (60 mL, 454 mL)

crude coal tar *see* coal tar *on page 110*

Cruex® Powder [OTC] *see* calcium undecylenate *on page 70*

Cruex® Topical [OTC] *see* undecylenic acid and derivatives *on page 479*

cryptenamine tannates and methyclothiazide *see* methyclothiazide and cryptenamine tannates *on page 297*

crystalline penicillin *see* penicillin g, parenteral *on page 353*

crystal violet *see* gentian violet *on page 207*
Crystamine® *see* cyanocobalamin *on this page*
Crysticillin® A.S. Injection *see* penicillin g procaine, aqueous *on page 354*
Crystodigin® *see* digitoxin *on page 144*
csp *see* cellulose sodium phosphate *on page 84*
ctx *see* cyclophosphamide *on page 121*
Culturette® 10 Minute Group A Strep ID *see* diagnostic aids (*in vitro*), other *on page 137*
Cuprimine® *see* penicillamine *on page 352*
Curretab® Oral *see* medroxyprogesterone acetate *on page 283*
Cutivate™ Topical *see* fluticasone propionate *on page 200*
cya *see* cyclosporine *on page 121*

cyanide antidote kit
Therapeutic Category Antidote, Cyanide
Use Treatment of cyanide poisoning
Usual Dosage For cyanide poisoning, a 0.3 mL ampul of amyl nitrite is crushed every minute and vapor is inhaled for 15-30 seconds until an I.V. sodium nitrite infusion is available. Following administration of 300 mg I.V. sodium nitrite, inject 12.5 g sodium thiosulfate I.V. (over ~10 minutes), if needed; injection of both may be repeated at $\frac{1}{2}$ the original dose.
Dosage Forms Kit: Sodium nitrite 300 mg/10 mL (#2); sodium thiosulfate 12.5 g/50 mL (#2); amyl nitrite 0.3 mL (#12); also disposable syringes, stomach tube, tourniquet and instructions

cyanocobalamin (sye an oh koe bal' a min)
Brand Names Berubigen®; Cobex®; Crystamine®; Cyanoject®; Cyomin®; Ener-B® [OTC]; Kaybovite-1000®; Redisol®; Rubramin-PC®; Sytobex®
Synonyms vitamin b_{12}
Therapeutic Category Vitamin, Water Soluble
Use Vitamin B_{12} deficiency; increased B_{12} requirements due to pregnancy, thyrotoxicosis, hemorrhage, malignancy, liver or kidney disease
Usual Dosage
Congenital pernicious anemia (if evidence of neurologic involvement): I.M.: 1000 mcg/day for at least 2 weeks; maintenance: 50 mcg/month

Vitamin B_{12} deficiency: I.M., S.C.: (oral is not recommended due to poor absorption)
    Children: 100 mcg/day for 10-15 days (total dose of 1-1.5 mg), then once or twice weekly for several months; may taper to 250-1000 mcg every month
    Adults: 100 mcg/day for 6-7 days
    Hematologic signs only:
        Children: 10-50 mcg/day for 5-10 days, then maintenance: 100-250 mcg/dose every 2-4 weeks
        Adults: 30 mcg/day for 5-10 days, followed by 100-200 mcg/month

Methylmalonic aciduria: I.M.: 1 mg/day
Dosage Forms
Gel, nasal (Ener-B®): 400 mcg/0.1 mL
Injection: 30 mcg/mL (30 mL); 100 mcg/mL (1 mL, 10 mL, 30 mL); 1000 mcg/mL (1 mL, 10 mL, 30 mL)
Tablet [OTC]: 25 mcg, 50 mcg, 100 mcg, 250 mcg, 500 mcg, 1000 mcg

Cyanoject® *see* cyanocobalamin *on this page*
Cyclan® *see* cyclandelate *on this page*

cyclandelate (sye klan' de late)
Brand Names Cyclan®; Cyclospasmol®
Therapeutic Category Vasodilator, Peripheral
Use Adjunctive therapy in peripheral vascular disease and possibly senility
(Continued)
119

cyclandelate *(Continued)*

Usual Dosage Oral: 400-800 mg/day in 2-4 divided doses
Dosage Forms
  Capsule: 200 mg, 400 mg
  Tablet: 200 mg, 400 mg

cyclizine (sye' kli zeen)

Brand Names Marezine® [OTC]
Therapeutic Category Antiemetic; Antihistamine
Use Prevention and treatment of nausea, vomiting and vertigo associated with motion sickness; control of postoperative nausea and vomiting
Usual Dosage Oral:
  Children 6-12 years: 25 mg up to 3 times/day
  Adults: 50 mg taken 30 minutes before departure, may repeat in 4-6 hours if needed, up to 200 mg/day
Dosage Forms Tablet, as hydrochloride: 50 mg

cyclobenzaprine hydrochloride (sye kloe ben' za preen)

Brand Names Flexeril®
Therapeutic Category Skeletal Muscle Relaxant
Use Treatment of muscle spasm associated with acute painful musculoskeletal conditions; supportive therapy in tetanus; ineffective in spasticity secondary to chronic neurologic disorders
Usual Dosage Oral:
  Children: Dosage has not been established
  Adults: 20-40 mg/day in 2-4 divided doses; maximum dose: 60 mg/day
Dosage Forms Tablet: 10 mg

Cyclocort® Topical *see amcinonide on page 18*

Cyclogyl® *see cyclopentolate hydrochloride on this page*

Cyclomydril® Ophthalmic *see cyclopentolate and phenylephrine on this page*

cyclopentolate and phenylephrine

Brand Names Cyclomydril® Ophthalmic
Synonyms phenylephrine and cyclopentolate
Therapeutic Category Ophthalmic Agent, Mydriatic
Use Induce mydriasis greater than that produced with cyclopentolate HCl alone
Usual Dosage Ophthalmic: Instill 1 drop every 5-10 minutes, not to exceed 3 instillations
Dosage Forms Solution, ophthalmic: Cyclopentolate hydrochloride 0.2% and phenylephrine hydrochloride 1% (2 mL, 5 mL)

cyclopentolate hydrochloride (sye kloe pen' toe late)

Brand Names AK-Pentolate®; Cyclogyl®; I-Pentolate®; Pentolair®
Therapeutic Category Anticholinergic Agent, Ophthalmic; Ophthalmic Agent, Mydriatic
Use Diagnostic procedures requiring mydriasis and cycloplegia
Usual Dosage Ophthalmic:
  Infants: Instill 1 drop of 0.5% into each eye 5-10 minutes before examination

  Children: Instill 1 drop of 0.5%, 1%, or 2% in eye followed by 1 drop of 0.5% or 1% in 5 minutes, if necessary

  Adults: Instill 1 drop of 1% followed by another drop in 5 minutes; 2% solution in heavily pigmented iris
Dosage Forms Solution, ophthalmic: 0.5% (2 mL, 5 mL, 15 mL); 1% (2 mL, 5 mL, 15 mL); 2% (2 mL, 5 mL, 15 mL)

cyclophosphamide (sye kloe foss' fa mide)

Brand Names Cytoxan® Injection; Cytoxan® Oral; Neosar® Injection

Synonyms cpm; ctx; cyt

Therapeutic Category Antineoplastic Agent, Alkylating Agent (Nitrogen Mustard)

Use Management of Hodgkin's disease, malignant lymphomas, multiple myeloma, leukemias, mycosis fungoides, neuroblastoma, ovarian carcinoma, breast carcinoma, a variety of other tumors; nephrotic syndrome, lupus erythematosus, severe rheumatoid arthritis, and rheumatoid vasculitis

Usual Dosage

Children with no hematologic problems:
  Induction:
    Oral: 2-8 mg/kg/day
    I.V.: 10-20 mg/kg/day divided once daily
  Maintenance: Oral: 2-5 mg/kg (50-150 mg/m^2) twice weekly
  Pediatric solid tumors: I.V.: 250-1800 mg/m^2 once daily for 1-5 days every 21-28 days

Adults with no hematologic problems:
  Induction:
    Oral: 1-5 mg/kg/day
    I.V.: 40-50 mg/kg (1.5-1.8 g/m^2) in divided doses over 2-5 days
  Maintenance:
    Oral: 1-5 mg/kg/day
    I.V.: 10-15 mg/kg (350-550 mg/m^2) every 7-10 days or 3-5 mg/kg (110-185 mg/m^2) twice weekly

Children and Adults: I.V.:
  SLE: 500-750 mg/m^2 every month; maximum: 1 g/m^2
  JRA/vasculitis: 10 mg/kg every 2 weeks

BMT conditioning regimen: I.V.: 50 mg/kg/day once daily for 3-4 days

Nephrotic syndrome: Oral: 2-3 mg/kg/day every day for up to 12 weeks when corticosteroids are unsuccessful

Dosage Forms

Powder for injection: 100 mg, 200 mg, 500 mg, 1 g, 2 g
Powder for injection, lyophilized: 100 mg, 200 mg, 500 mg, 1 g, 2 g
Tablet: 25 mg, 50 mg

cycloserine (sye kloe ser' een)

Brand Names Seromycin® Pulvules®

Therapeutic Category Antibiotic, Miscellaneous; Antitubercular Agent

Use Adjunctive treatment in pulmonary or extrapulmonary tuberculosis; treatment of acute urinary tract infections caused by *E. coli* or *Enterobacter* sp when less toxic therapy has failed or is contraindicated

Usual Dosage Oral:

Tuberculosis:
  Children: 10-20 mg/kg/day in 2 divided doses up to 1000 mg/day
  Adults: Initial: 250 mg every 12 hours for 14 days, then give 500 mg to 1 g/day in 2 divided doses

Urinary tract infection: Adults: 250 mg every 12 hours for 14 days

Dosage Forms Capsule: 250 mg

Cyclospasmol® see cyclandelate on page 119

cyclosporin a see cyclosporine on this page

cyclosporine (sye' kloe spor een)

Brand Names Sandimmune® Injection; Sandimmune® Oral

Synonyms cya; cyclosporin a

Therapeutic Category Immunosuppressant Agent

(Continued)

cyclosporine *(Continued)*

Use Immunosuppressant used with corticosteroids to prevent graft versus host disease in patients with kidney, liver, heart, and bone marrow transplants. Unlabeled use: Rheumatoid arthritis

Usual Dosage Children and Adults:

Oral: Initial: 14-18 mg/kg/dose daily, beginning 4-12 hours prior to organ transplantation; maintenance: 5-10 mg/kg/day

I.V.: Initial: 5-6 mg/kg/day in divided doses every 12-24 hours; patients should be switched to oral cyclosporine as soon as possible

Dosage Forms

Capsule: 25 mg, 100 mg

Injection: 50 mg/mL (5 mL)

Solution, oral: 100 mg/mL (50 mL)

Cycrin® Oral *see* medroxyprogesterone acetate *on page 283*

Cyklokapron® Injection *see* tranexamic acid *on page 465*

Cyklokapron® Oral *see* tranexamic acid *on page 465*

Cylert® *see* pemoline *on page 351*

Cyomin® *see* cyanocobalamin *on page 119*

cyproheptadine hydrochloride (si proe hep' ta deen)

Brand Names Periactin®

Therapeutic Category Antihistamine

Use Perennial and seasonal allergic rhinitis and other allergic symptoms including urticaria

Usual Dosage Oral:

Children: 0.25 mg/kg/day in 2-3 divided doses or

2-6 years: 2 mg every 8-12 hours (not to exceed 12 mg/day)

7-14 years: 4 mg every 8-12 hours (not to exceed 16 mg/day)

Adults: 12-16 mg/day every 8 hours (not to exceed 0.5 mg/kg/day)

Dosage Forms

Syrup: 2 mg/5 mL with alcohol 5% (473 mL)

Tablet: 4 mg

Cystagon® *see* cysteamine bitartrate *on this page*

cysteamine bitartrate (sis tee' a meen)

Brand Names Cystagon®

Therapeutic Category Urinary Tract Product

Use Nephropathic cystinosis in children and adults

Dosage Forms Capsule: 50 mg, 150 mg

cysteine hydrochloride (sis' te een)

Therapeutic Category Nutritional Supplement

Use Total parenteral nutrition of infants as an additive to meet the I.V. amino acid requirements

Usual Dosage Combine 500 mg of cysteine with 12.5 g of amino acid, then dilute with 50% dextrose

Dosage Forms Injection: 50 mg/mL (10 mL)

Cystografin® *see* radiological/contrast media (ionic) *on page 404*

Cystospaz® *see* hyoscyamine sulfate *on page 239*

Cystospaz-M® *see* hyoscyamine sulfate *on page 239*

cyt *see* cyclophosphamide *on previous page*

Cytadren® *see* aminoglutethimide *on page 19*

cytarabine hydrochloride (sye tare' a been)
Brand Names Cytosar-U®; Tarabine® PFS
Synonyms arabinosylcytosine; ara-c; cytosine arabinosine hydrochloride
Therapeutic Category Antineoplastic Agent, Antimetabolite
Use In combination regimens for the treatment of leukemias and non-Hodgkin's lymphomas
Usual Dosage Children and Adults (refer to individual protocols):
Induction remission:
I.T.: 5-75 mg/m^2 once daily for 4 days or 1 every 4 days until CNS
I.V.: 200 mg/m^2/day for 5 days at 2-week intervals; 100-200 mg/m^2/day for 5- to 10-day therapy course or every day until remission given I.V. continuous drip, or in 2-3 divided doses findings normalize

Maintenance remission:
I.M., S.C.: 1-1.5 mg/kg single dose for maintenance at 1- to 4-week intervals
I.V.: 70-200 mg/m^2/day for 2-5 days at monthly intervals

High-dose therapies: Doses as high as 1-3 g/m^2 have been used for refractory or secondary leukemias or refractory non-Hodgkins lymphoma; dosages of 3 g/m^2 every 12 hours for up to 12 doses have been used
Dosage Forms
Injection, preservative free (Tarabine® PFS): 20 mg/mL (5 mL, 50 mL)
Powder for injection: 100 mg, 500 mg, 1 g, 2 g
Powder for injection (Cytosar-U®): 100 mg, 500 mg, 1 g, 2 g

CytoGam™ *see* cytomegalovirus immune globulin intravenous, human *on this page*

cytomegalovirus immune globulin intravenous, human
(sye toe meg a low vi' rus)
Brand Names CytoGam™
Synonyms cmv-igiv
Therapeutic Category Immune Globulin
Use Attenuation of primary CMV disease associated with kidney transplantation
Usual Dosage I.V.: Initial: Administer at 15 mg/kg/hour, then increase to 30 mg/kg/hour after 30 minutes if no untoward reactions, then increase to 60 mg/kg/hour after another 30 minutes, volume not to exceed 75 mL/hour
Dosage Forms Powder for injection, lyophilized, detergent treated: 2500 mg ± 250 mg (50 mL)

Cytomel® Oral *see* liothyronine sodium *on page 269*

Cytosar-U® *see* cytarabine hydrochloride *on this page*

cytosine arabinosine hydrochloride *see* cytarabine hydrochloride *on this page*

Cytotec® *see* misoprostol *on page 308*

Cytovene® *see* ganciclovir *on page 204*

Cytoxan® Injection *see* cyclophosphamide *on page 121*

Cytoxan® Oral *see* cyclophosphamide *on page 121*

d$_3$ *see* cholecalciferol *on page 99*

25-d$_3$ *see* calcifediol *on page 65*

d-3-mercaptovaline *see* penicillamine *on page 352*

d4T *see* stavudine *on page 435*

dacarbazine (da kar' ba zeen)
Brand Names DTIC-Dome®
Synonyms dic; imidazole carboxamide
Therapeutic Category Antineoplastic Agent, Miscellaneous
(Continued)

dacarbazine *(Continued)*

Use Metastatic malignant melanoma; in combination with other agents, in Hodgkin's disease; has been used for soft tissue sarcomas and neuroblastomas

Usual Dosage I.V. (refer to individual protocols):

Children:

Solid tumors: 200-470 mg/m^2/day over 5 days every 21-28 days

Neuroblastoma: 800-900 mg/m^2 as a single dose every 3-4 weeks in combination therapy

Adults:

Malignant melanoma: 2-4.5 mg/kg/day for 10 days, repeat in 4 weeks or may use 250 mg/m^2/day for 5 days, repeat in 3 weeks

Hodgkin's disease: 150 mg/m^2/day for 5 days, repeat every 4 weeks or 375 mg/m^2 on day 1, repeat in 15 days of each 28-day cycle in combination with other agents

Dosage Forms Injection: 100 mg (10 mL, 20 mL); 200 mg (20 mL, 30 mL); 500 mg (50 mL)

dactinomycin (dak ti noe mye' sin)

Brand Names Cosmegen®

Synonyms act; actinomycin d

Therapeutic Category Antineoplastic Agent, Antibiotic

Use Management, either alone or with other treatment modalities of Wilms' tumor, rhabdomyosarcoma, neuroblastoma, retinoblastoma, Ewing's sarcoma, trophoblastic neoplasms, testicular carcinoma, and other malignancies

Usual Dosage Refer to individual protocols. Dosage should be based on body surface area in obese or edematous patients.

Children >6 months and Adults: I.V.: 15 mcg/kg/day or 400-600 mcg/m^2/day for 5 days, may repeat every 3-6 weeks; or 2.5 mg/m^2 given in divided doses over 1 week; 0.75-2 mg/m^2 as a single dose given at intervals of 1-4 weeks have been used

Dosage Forms Powder for injection, lyophilized: 0.5 mg

Dairy Ease® [OTC] *see* lactase enzyme *on page 260*

Daisy® 2 *see* diagnostic aids *(in vitro)*, urine *on page 137*

Dakin's solution *see* sodium hypochlorite solution *on page 428*

Dalalone® *see* dexamethasone *on page 131*

Dalalone D.P.® *see* dexamethasone *on page 131*

Dalalone L.A.® *see* dexamethasone *on page 131*

Dalgan® *see* dezocine *on page 136*

Dallergy® *see* chlorpheniramine, phenylephrine and methscopolamine *on page 95*

Dallergy-D® *see* chlorpheniramine and phenylephrine *on page 93*

Dallergy-JR® *see* brompheniramine and pseudoephedrine *on page 59*

Dalmane® *see* flurazepam hydrochloride *on page 200*

***d*-alpha tocopherol** *see* vitamin e *on page 490*

dalteparin

Brand Names Fragmin®

Therapeutic Category Anticoagulant

Use Prevent deep vein thrombosis following abdominal surgery

Dosage Forms Injection:

Damason-P® *see* hydrocodone and aspirin *on page 230*

danazol (da' na zole)

Brand Names Danocrine®

Therapeutic Category Androgen

Use Treatment of endometriosis, fibrocystic breast disease, and hereditary angioedema

Usual Dosage Adults: Oral:
Endometriosis: 100-400 mg twice daily
Fibrocystic breast disease: 50-200 mg twice daily for 2-6 months
Hereditary angioedema: 400-600 mg/day in 2-3 divided doses
Dosage Forms Capsule: 50 mg, 100 mg, 200 mg

Danocrine® *see* danazol *on previous page*
Dantrium® *see* dantrolene sodium *on this page*

dantrolene sodium (dan' troe leen)
Brand Names Dantrium®
Therapeutic Category Antidote, Malignant Hyperthermia; Hyperthermia, Treatment; Skeletal Muscle Relaxant
Use Treatment of spasticity associated with spinal cord injury, stroke, cerebral palsy, or multiple sclerosis; also used as treatment of malignant hyperthermia
Usual Dosage
Spasticity: Oral:
Children: Initial: 0.5 mg/kg/dose twice daily, increase frequency to 3-4 times/day at 4- to 7-day intervals, then increase dose by 0.5 mg/kg to a maximum of 3 mg/kg/dose 2-4 times/day up to 400 mg/day
Adults: 25 mg/day to start, increase frequency to 3-4 times/day, then increase dose by 25 mg every 4-7 days to a maximum of 100 mg 2-4 times/day or 400 mg/day

Hyperthermia: Children and Adults:
Oral: 4-8 mg/kg/day in 4 divided doses
I.V.: 1 mg/kg; may repeat dose up to cumulative dose of 10 mg/kg (mean effective dose: 2.5 mg/kg), then switch to oral dosage
Dosage Forms
Capsule: 25 mg, 50 mg, 100 mg
Powder for injection: 20 mg

Dapacin® Cold Capsule [OTC] *see* chlorpheniramine, phenylpropanolamine, and acetaminophen *on page 96*
Dapa® [OTC] *see* acetaminophen *on page 2*

dapiprazole hydrochloride (da' pi pray zole)
Brand Names Rēv-Eyes™
Therapeutic Category Alpha-Adrenergic Blocking Agent, Ophthalmic
Use Treatment of iatrogenically induced mydriasis produced by adrenergic or parasympatholytic agents
Usual Dosage Ophthalmic: Instill 2 drops followed 5 minutes later by an additional 2 drops applied to the conjunctiva
Dosage Forms Powder, lyophilized: 25 mg [0.5% solution when mixed with supplied diluent]

dapsone (dap' sone)
Synonyms dds; diaminodiphenylsulfone
Therapeutic Category Antibiotic, Sulfone
Use Treatment of leprosy and dermatitis herpetiformis
Usual Dosage Oral:
Children: Leprosy: 1-2 mg/kg/24 hours; maximum: 100 mg/day
Adults:
Leprosy: 50-100 mg/day
Dermatitis herpetiformis: Start at 50 mg/day, increase to 300 mg/day, or higher to achieve full control, reduce dosage to minimum level as soon as possible
Dosage Forms Tablet: 25 mg, 100 mg

Daranide® *see* dichlorphenamide *on page 141*

Daraprim® *see* pyrimethamine *on page 401*

Darbid® *see* isopropamide iodide *on page 253*

Daricon® *see* oxyphencyclimine hydrochloride *on page 344*

Darvocet-N® *see* propoxyphene and acetaminophen *on page 393*

Darvocet-N® 100 *see* propoxyphene and acetaminophen *on page 393*

Darvon® *see* propoxyphene *on page 393*

Darvon® Compound-65 Pulvules® *see* propoxyphene and aspirin *on page 394*

Darvon-N® *see* propoxyphene *on page 393*

daunomycin *see* daunorubicin hydrochloride *on this page*

daunorubicin hydrochloride (daw noe roo' bi sin)

Brand Names Cerubidine®
Synonyms daunomycin; dnr; rubidomycin hydrochloride
Therapeutic Category Antineoplastic Agent, Antibiotic
Use In combination with other agents in the treatment of leukemias
Usual Dosage I.V.:
Children:
Combination therapy: Remission induction for ALL: 25-45 mg/m^2 on day 1 every week for 4 cycles
<2 years or <0.5 m^2: The manufacturer recommends that the dose is based on body weight rather than body surface area

Adults: 30-60 mg/m^2/day for 3-5 days, repeat dose in 3-4 weeks; total cumulative dose should not exceed 400-600 mg/m^2
Single agent induction for AML: 60 mg/m^2/day for 3 days; repeat every 3-4 weeks
Combination therapy induction for AML: 45 mg/m^2/day for 3 days; Subsequent courses: Every day for 2 days
Combination therapy: Remission induction for ALL: 45 mg/m^2 on days 1, 2, and 3
Dosage Forms Powder for injection, lyophilized: 20 mg

Daypro™ *see* oxaprozin *on page 341*

Dayto Himbin® *see* yohimbine hydrochloride *on page 493*

Dazamide® *see* acetazolamide *on page 5*

DC 240® Softgel® [OTC] *see* docusate *on page 153*

dcf *see* pentostatin *on page 357*

DDAVP® Injection *see* desmopressin acetate *on page 130*

DDAVP® Nasal *see* desmopressin acetate *on page 130*

ddc *see* zalcitabine *on page 494*

ddi *see* didanosine *on page 142*

dds *see* dapsone *on previous page*

1-deamino-8-d-arginine vasopressin *see* desmopressin acetate *on page 130*

Debrisan® Topical [OTC] *see* dextranomer *on page 134*

Debrox® [OTC] *see* carbamide peroxide *on page 74*

Decadron® *see* dexamethasone *on page 131*

Decadron®-LA *see* dexamethasone *on page 131*

Decadron® Phosphate Cream *see* dexamethasone *on page 131*

Decadron® Phosphate Turbinaire® *see* dexamethasone *on page 131*

Deca-Durabolin® Injection see nandrolone on page 318

Decaject® see dexamethasone on page 131

Decaject-LA® see dexamethasone on page 131

Decaspray® see dexamethasone on page 131

Decholin® see dehydrocholic acid on this page

Declomycin® see demeclocycline hydrochloride on next page

Decofed® Syrup [OTC] see pseudoephedrine on page 397

Decohistine® see chlorpheniramine and phenylephrine on page 93

Decohistine® DH see chlorpheniramine, pseudoephedrine, and codeine on page 97

Decohistine® Expectorant see guaifenesin, pseudoephedrine, and codeine on page 217

Deconamine® SR see chlorpheniramine and pseudoephedrine on page 94

Deconamine® Tablet see chlorpheniramine and pseudoephedrine on page 94

Deconsal® II see guaifenesin and pseudoephedrine on page 216

Defen-LA® see guaifenesin and pseudoephedrine on page 216

deferoxamine mesylate (de fer ox' a meen)
Brand Names Desferal® Mesylate
Therapeutic Category Antidote, Aluminum Toxicity; Antidote, Iron Toxicity
Use Acute iron intoxication; chronic iron overload secondary to multiple transfusions; diagnostic test for iron overload; used investigationally in the treatment of aluminum accumulation in renal failure; iron overload secondary to congenital anemias; hemochromatosis; removal of corneal rust rings following surgical removal of foreign bodies
Usual Dosage
Children:
Acute iron intoxication:
I.M.: 90 mg/kg/dose every 8 hours; maximum: 6 g/day
I.V.: 15 mg/kg/hour; maximum: 6 g/day
Chronic iron overload:
I.V.: 15 mg/kg/hour
S.C.: 20-40 mg/kg/day over 8-12 hours
Aluminum induced bone disease: 20-40 mg/kg every hemodialysis treatment, frequency dependent on clinical status of the patient
Adults:
Acute iron intoxication:
I.M.: 1 g stat, then 0.5 g every 4 hours for two doses, then 0.5 g every 4-12 hours up to 6 g/day
I.V.: 15 mg/kg/hour; maximum: 6 g/day
Chronic iron overload:
I.M.: 0.5-1 g every day
S.C.: 1-2 g every day over 8-24 hours
Dosage Forms Powder for injection: 500 mg

Degest® 2 Ophthalmic [OTC] see naphazoline hydrochloride on page 319

Dehist® Injection see brompheniramine maleate on page 59

dehydrocholic acid (dee hye droe koe' lik)
Brand Names Cholan-HMB®; Decholin®
Therapeutic Category Bile Acid; Laxative, Hydrocholeretic
Use Relief of constipation; adjunct to various biliary tract conditions
Usual Dosage Children >12 years and Adults: 250-500 mg 2-3 times/day after meals up to 1.5 g/day
Dosage Forms Tablet: 250 mg

Deladumone® Injection *see* estradiol and testosterone *on page 174*

Delatest® Injection *see* testosterone *on page 449*

Delatestryl® Injection *see* testosterone *on page 449*

Delaxin® *see* methocarbamol *on page 295*

Delcort® *see* hydrocortisone *on page 232*

Delestrogen® Injection *see* estradiol *on page 173*

Delfen® [OTC] *see* nonoxynol 9 *on page 331*

Del-Mycin® *see* erythromycin, topical *on page 172*

Delsym® [OTC] *see* dextromethorphan hydrobromide *on page 135*

Delta-Cortef® Oral *see* prednisolone *on page 383*

deltacortisone *see* prednisone *on page 384*

Delta-D® *see* cholecalciferol *on page 99*

deltadehydrocortisone *see* prednisone *on page 384*

deltahydrocortisone *see* prednisolone *on page 383*

Deltasone® Oral *see* prednisone *on page 384*

Delta-Tritex® *see* triamcinolone *on page 467*

Demadex® Injection *see* torsemide *on page 465*

Demadex® Oral *see* torsemide *on page 465*

Demazin® [OTC] *see* chlorpheniramine and phenylpropanolamine *on page 94*

demecarium bromide (dem e kare' ee um)

Brand Names Humorsol® Ophthalmic
Therapeutic Category Cholinergic Agent, Ophthalmic; Ophthalmic Agent, Miotic
Use Management of chronic simple glaucoma, chronic and acute angle-closure glaucoma; counter effects of cycloplegics
Usual Dosage Ophthalmic:
  Children: Instill 1 drop into eyes twice weekly to a maximum dosage of 1 or 2 drops twice daily for up to 4 months

  Adults: Instill 1-2 drops into eyes twice weekly to a maximum dosage of 1 or 2 drops twice daily for up to 4 months
Dosage Forms Solution, ophthalmic: 0.125% (5 mL); 0.25% (5 mL)

demeclocycline hydrochloride (dem e kloe sye' kleen)

Brand Names Declomycin®
Synonyms demethylchlortetracycline
Therapeutic Category Antibiotic, Tetracycline Derivative
Use Treatment of susceptible bacterial infections (acne, gonorrhea, pertussis and urinary tract infections) caused by both gram-negative and gram-positive organisms; used when penicillin is contraindicated; the treatment of chronic syndrome of inappropriate secretion of antidiuretic hormone (SIADH)
Usual Dosage
  Children ≥8 years: 8-12 mg/kg/day divided every 6-12 hours

  Adults: 150 mg 4 times/day or 300 mg twice daily
    Uncomplicated gonorrhea: 600 mg stat, 300 mg every 12 hours for 4 days (3 g total)
    SIADH: 900-1200 mg/day or 13-15 mg/kg/day divided every 6-8 hours initially, then decrease to 0.6-0.9 g/day
Dosage Forms
  Capsule: 150 mg
  Tablet: 150 mg, 300 mg

Demerol® *see* meperidine hydrochloride *on page 286*

demethylchlortetracycline *see* demeclocycline hydrochloride *on previous page*

4-demothoxydaunorubicin *see* idarubicin hydrochloride *on page 241*

Demser® *see* metyrosine *on page 304*

Demulen® *see* ethinyl estradiol and ethynodiol diacetate *on page 177*

Denorex® [OTC] *see* coal tar *on page 110*

deodorized opium tincture *see* opium tincture *on page 338*

2'-deoxycoformycin *see* pentostatin *on page 357*

Depakene® *see* valproic acid and derivatives *on page 482*

Depakote® *see* valproic acid and derivatives *on page 482*

depAndrogyn® Injection *see* estradiol and testosterone *on page 174*

Depen® *see* penicillamine *on page 352*

depGynogen® Injection *see* estradiol *on page 173*

depMedalone® Injection *see* methylprednisolone *on page 300*

Depo®-Estradiol Injection *see* estradiol *on page 173*

Depogen® Injection *see* estradiol *on page 173*

Depoject® Injection *see* methylprednisolone *on page 300*

Depo-Medrol® Injection *see* methylprednisolone *on page 300*

Deponit® Patch *see* nitroglycerin *on page 329*

Depopred® Injection *see* methylprednisolone *on page 300*

Depo-Provera® Injection *see* medroxyprogesterone acetate *on page 283*

Depo-Testadiol® Injection *see* estradiol and testosterone *on page 174*

Depotest® Injection *see* testosterone *on page 449*

Depotestogen® Injection *see* estradiol and testosterone *on page 174*

Depo®-Testosterone Injection *see* testosterone *on page 449*

deprenyl *see* selegiline hydrochloride *on page 420*

Deproist® Expectorant with Codeine *see* guaifenesin, pseudoephedrine, and codeine *on page 217*

Derifil® [OTC] *see* chlorophyll *on page 90*

Dermacomb® Topical *see* nystatin and triamcinolone *on page 335*

Dermacort® *see* hydrocortisone *on page 232*

Dermaflex® Gel *see* lidocaine hydrochloride *on page 267*

Dermarest Dricort® *see* hydrocortisone *on page 232*

Derma-Smoothe/FS® Topical *see* fluocinolone acetonide *on page 195*

Dermatop® *see* prednicarbate *on page 383*

Dermatophytin® *see* *Trichophyton* skin test *on page 469*

Dermatophytin-O *see* *Candida albicans (Monilia)* *on page 71*

DermiCort® *see* hydrocortisone *on page 232*

Dermolate® *see* hydrocortisone *on page 232*

Dermoplast® [OTC] *see* benzocaine *on page 48*

Dermoxyl® [OTC] *see* benzoyl peroxide *on page 50*

des *see* diethylstilbestrol *on page 143*

Desenex® [OTC] *see* tolnaftate *on page 464*

Desferal® Mesylate *see* deferoxamine mesylate *on page 127*

desflurane (des floo' rane)
Brand Names Suprane®
Therapeutic Category General Anesthetic
Use Induction or maintenance of anesthesia for adults in outpatient and inpatient surgery
Dosage Forms Liquid: 240 mL

desiccated thyroid see thyroid on page 459

desipramine hydrochloride (dess ip' ra meen)
Brand Names Norpramin®; Pertofrane®
Synonyms desmethylimipramine hydrochloride
Therapeutic Category Antidepressant, Tricyclic
Use Treatment of various forms of depression, often in conjunction with psychotherapy
Usual Dosage Oral (not recommended for use in children <12 years):
Adolescents: Initial: 25-50 mg/day; gradually increase to 100 mg/day in single or divided doses; maximum: 150 mg/day

Adults: Initial: 75 mg/day in divided doses; increase gradually to 150-200 mg/day in divided or single dose; maximum: 300 mg/day
Dosage Forms
Capsule (Pertofrane®): 25 mg, 50 mg
Tablet (Norpramin®): 10 mg, 25 mg, 50 mg, 75 mg, 100 mg, 150 mg

Desitin® Topical [OTC] see zinc oxide, cod liver oil, and talc on page 496

desmethylimipramine hydrochloride see desipramine hydrochloride on this page

desmopressin acetate (des moe press' in)
Brand Names Concentraid® Nasal; DDAVP® Injection; DDAVP® Nasal
Synonyms 1-deamino-8-d-arginine vasopressin
Therapeutic Category Antihemophilic Agent; Hemostatic Agent; Vasopressin Analog, Synthetic
Use Treatment of diabetes insipidus and controlling bleeding in certain types of hemophilia
Usual Dosage
Children:
Diabetes insipidus: 3 months to 12 years: Intranasal: Initial: 5 mcg/day divided 1-2 times/day; range: 5-30 mcg/day divided 1-2 times/day
Hemophilia: >3 months: I.V.: 0.3 mcg/kg by slow infusion; may repeat dose if needed
Nocturnal enuresis: ≥6 years: Intranasal: Initial: 20 mcg at bedtime; range: 10-40 mcg
Adults:
Diabetes insipidus: I.V., S.C.: 2-4 mcg/day in 2 divided doses or $\frac{1}{10}$ of the maintenance intranasal dose; intranasal: 5-40 mcg/day 1-3 times/day
Hemophilia: I.V.: 0.3 mcg/kg by slow infusion
Dosage Forms
Injection (DDAVP®): 4 mcg/mL (1 mL)
Solution, nasal (Concentraid®, DDAVP®): 100 mcg/mL (2.5 mL, 5 mL)

Desogen® see ethinyl estradiol and desogestrel on page 177

desogestrel and ethinyl estradiol see ethinyl estradiol and desogestrel on page 177

desonide (dess' oh nide)
Brand Names DesOwen® Topical; Tridesilon® Topical
Therapeutic Category Corticosteroid, Topical (Low Potency)
Use Adjunctive therapy for inflammation in acute and chronic corticosteroid responsive dermatosis
Usual Dosage Topical: Apply 2-4 times/day
Dosage Forms
Cream, topical: 0.05% (15 g, 60 g)
Ointment, topical: 0.05% (15 g, 60 g)
Lotion: 0.05% (60 mL, 120 mL)

DesOwen® Topical *see* desonide *on previous page*

desoximetasone (des ox i met' a sone)
Brand Names Topicort®; Topicort®-LP
Therapeutic Category Corticosteroid, Topical (High Potency)
Use Relieve inflammation and pruritic symptoms of corticosteroid-responsive dermatosis
Usual Dosage Topical:
  Children: Apply sparingly in a very thin film to affected area 1-2 times/day
  Adults: Apply sparingly in a thin film twice daily
Dosage Forms
  Cream, topical:
    Topicort®: 0.25% (15 g, 60 g, 120 g)
    Topicort®-LP: 0.05% (15 g, 60 g)
  Gel, topical: 0.05% (15 g, 60 g)
  Ointment, topical (Topicort®): 0.25% (15 g, 60 g)

desoxyephedrine hydrochloride *see* methamphetamine hydrochloride *on page 292*

Desoxyn® *see* methamphetamine hydrochloride *on page 292*

desoxyphenobarbital *see* primidone *on page 386*

desoxyribonuclease and fibrinolysin *see* fibrinolysin and desoxyribonuclease *on page 191*

Despec® Liquid *see* guaifenesin, phenylpropanolamine, and phenylephrine *on page 217*

Desquam-X® *see* benzoyl peroxide *on page 50*

Desyrel® *see* trazodone hydrochloride *on page 466*

Detussin® Expectorant *see* hydrocodone, pseudoephedrine, and guaifenesin *on page 231*

Devrom® [OTC] *see* bismuth subgallate *on page 55*

Dexacidin® Ophthalmic *see* neomycin, polymyxin b, and dexamethasone *on page 322*

dexamethasone (dex a meth' a sone)
Brand Names Aeroseb-Dex®; AK-Dex®; Baldex®; Dalalone®; Dalalone D.P.®; Dalalone L.A.®; Decadron®; Decadron®-LA; Decadron® Phosphate Cream; Decadron® Phosphate Injection; Decadron® Phosphate Respihaler®; Decadron® Phosphate Turbinaire®; Decaject®; Decaject-LA®; Decaspray®; Dexasone®; Dexasone® L.A.; Dexone®; Dexone® LA; Dexotic®; Hexadrol®; Hexadrol® Phosphate; I-Methasone®; Maxidex®; Solurex®; Solurex L.A.®
Therapeutic Category Antiemetic; Anti-inflammatory Agent; Corticosteroid, Inhalant; Corticosteroid, Ophthalmic; Corticosteroid, Systemic; Corticosteroid, Topical (Low Potency)
Use Systemically and locally for chronic inflammation, allergic, hematologic, neoplastic, and autoimmune diseases; may be used in management of cerebral edema, septic shock, and as a diagnostic agent
Usual Dosage
Children:
  Antiemetic (prior to chemotherapy): 10 mg/m^2/dose for first dose then 5 mg/m^2/dose every 6 hours as needed
  Physiologic replacement: Oral, I.M., I.V.: 0.03-0.15 mg/kg/day or 0.6-0.75 mg/m^2/day in divided doses every 6-12 hours
  Extubation or airway edema: Oral, I.M., I.V.: 0.5-1 mg/kg/day in divided doses every 6 hours beginning 24 hours prior to extubation and continuing for 4-6 doses afterwards
  Ophthalmic: Instill 3-4 times/day
  Cerebral edema: Loading dose: 1-2 mg/kg/dose as a single dose; maintenance: 1 mg/kg/day (maximum: 16 mg/day) in divided doses every 4-6 hours
  Bacterial meningitis in infants and children >2 months: I.V.: 0.6 mg/kg/day in 4 divided doses for the first 4 days of antibiotic treatment; start dexamethasone at the time of the first dose of antibiotic

(Continued)

dexamethasone *(Continued)*

Adults:

Anti-inflammatory: Oral, I.M., I.V.: 0.75-9 mg/day in divided doses every 6-12 hours

Cerebral edema: I.V. 10 mg stat, 4 mg I.M./I.V. every 6 hours until response is maximized, then switch to oral regimen, then taper off if appropriate

Diagnosis for Cushing's syndrome: Oral: 1 mg at 11 PM, draw blood at 8 AM

ANLL protocol: I.V.: 2 mg/m^2/dose every 8 hours for 12 doses

Dosage Forms

Acetate: Injection:

Dalalone L.A.", Decadron"-LA, Decaject-LA®, Dexasone® L.A., Dexone® LA, Solurex L.A.": 8 mg/mL (1 mL, 5 mL)

Dalalone D.P.": 16 mg/mL (1 mL, 5 mL)

Base:

Aerosol, topical:

Aeroseb-Dex": 0.01% (58 g)

Decaspray": 0.04% (25 g)

Elixir (Decadron", Hexadrol®): 0.5 mg/5 mL (5 mL, 20 mL, 100 mL, 120 mL, 240 mL, 500 mL)

Solution, oral: 0.5 mg/5 mL (5 mL, 20 mL, 500 mL)

Solution, oral concentrate: 0.5 mg/0.5 mL (30 mL)

Suspension, ophthalmic (Maxidex"): 0.1% (5 mL, 15 mL)

Tablet (Decadron", Dexone", Hexadrol"): 0.25 mg, 0.5 mg, 0.75 mg, 1 mg, 1.5 mg, 2 mg, 4 mg, 6 mg

Therapeutic pack: Six 1.5 mg tablets and eight 0.75 mg tablets

Sodium phosphate:

Aerosol, nasal (Decadron" Phosphate Turbinaire®): 84 mcg/activation [170 metered doses] (12.6 g)

Aerosol, oral (Decadron" Phosphate Respihaler®): 84 mcg/activation [170 metered doses] (12.6 g)

Cream (Decadron" Phosphate): 0.1% (15 g, 30 g)

Injection:

Dalalone", Decadron" Phosphate, Decaject", Dexasone®, Hexadrol® Phosphate, Solurex": 4 mg/mL (1 mL, 2 mL, 2.5 mL, 5 mL, 10 mL, 30 mL)

Hexadrol" Phosphate: 10 mg/mL (1 mL, 10 mL); 20 mg/mL (5 mL)

Decadron" Phosphate: 24 mg/mL (5 mL, 10 mL)

Ointment, ophthalmic (AK-Dex", Baldex", Decadron® Phosphate, Maxidex®): 0.05% (3.5 g)

Solution, ophthalmic (AK-Dex", Baldex", Decadron® Phosphate, Dexotic®, I-Methasone"): 0.1% (5 mL)

dexamethasone and neomycin *see* neomycin and dexamethasone
on page 321

dexamethasone and tobramycin *see* tobramycin and dexamethasone
on page 462

Dexasone® *see* dexamethasone *on previous page*

Dexasone® L.A. *see* dexamethasone *on previous page*

Dexasporin® Ophthalmic *see* neomycin, polymyxin b, and dexamethasone
on page 322

Dexatrim® [OTC] *see* phenylpropanolamine hydrochloride *on page 365*

dexbrompheniramine and pseudoephedrine

Brand Names Disobrom" [OTC]; Disophrol® Chrontabs® [OTC]; Drixoral® [OTC]; Histrodrix® [OTC]; Resporal" [OTC]

Synonyms pseudoephedrine and dexbrompheniramine

Therapeutic Category Antihistamine/Decongestant Combination

Use Relief of symptoms of upper respiratory mucosal congestion in seasonal and perennial nasal allergies, acute rhinitis, rhinosinusitis and eustachian tube blockage

Usual Dosage Children >12 years and Adults: Oral: 1 tablet every 12 hours, may require 1 tablet every 8 hours

Dosage Forms Tablet, timed release: Dexbrompheniramine maleate 6 mg and pseudoephedrine sulfate 120 mg

Dexchlor® *see* dexchlorpheniramine maleate *on this page*

dexchlorpheniramine maleate (dex klor fen eer' a meen)

Brand Names Dexchlor®; Poladex®; Polaramine®; Polargen®
Therapeutic Category Antihistamine
Use Perennial and seasonal allergic rhinitis and other allergic symptoms including urticaria
Usual Dosage Oral:
Children:
2-5 years: 0.5 mg every 4-6 hours
6-11 years: 1 mg every 4-6 hours or 4 mg timed release at bedtime

Adults: 2 mg every 4-6 hours or 4-6 mg timed release at bedtime or 8-10 hours
Dosage Forms
Syrup (orange flavor): 2 mg/5 mL with alcohol 6% (480 mL)
Tablet: 2 mg
Tablet, sustained action: 4 mg, 6 mg

Dexedrine® *see* dextroamphetamine sulfate *on next page*

Dexone® *see* dexamethasone *on page 131*

Dexone® LA *see* dexamethasone *on page 131*

Dexotic® *see* dexamethasone *on page 131*

dexpanthenol (dex pan' the nole)

Brand Names Ilopan-Choline® Oral; Ilopan® Injection; Panthoderm® Cream [OTC]
Synonyms pantothenyl alcohol
Therapeutic Category Gastrointestinal Agent, Stimulant
Use Prophylactic use to minimize paralytic ileus, treatment of postoperative distention
Usual Dosage Adults: Oral: 2-3 tablets 3 times/day
Prevention of postoperative ileus: I.M.: 250-500 mg stat, repeat in 2 hours, followed by doses every 6 hours until danger passes

Paralyzed ileus: I.M.: 500 mg stat, repeat in 2 hours, followed by doses every 6 hours, if needed
Dosage Forms
Cream: 2% (30 g, 60 g)
Injection (Ilopan®): 250 mg/mL (2 mL, 10 mL, 30 mL)
Tablet (Ilopan-Choline®): 50 mg with choline bitartrate 25 mg

dexrazoxone (dex ray zoks' ane)

Brand Names Zinecard®
Therapeutic Category Cardiovascular Agent, Other
Use Prevention of cardiomyopathy associated with doxorubicin administration
Dosage Forms Injection

dextran

Brand Names Gentran®; LMD®; Macrodex®; Rheomacrodex®
Synonyms dextran 40; dextran 70; dextran 75; dextran, high molecular weight; dextran, low molecular weight
Therapeutic Category Plasma Volume Expander
Use Blood volume expander used in treatment of shock or impending shock when blood or blood products are not available
(Continued)
133

dextran *(Continued)*
Usual Dosage I.V.:
Children: Total dose should not be >20 mL/kg during first 24 hours
Adults: 500-1000 mL at rate of 20-40 mL/minute
Dosage Forms Injection:
High molecular weight:
6% dextran 75 in dextrose 5% (500 mL)
Gentran'": 6% dextran 75 in sodium chloride 0.9% (500 mL)
Gentran'", Macrodex'": 6% dextran 70 in sodium chloride 0.9% (500 mL)
Macrodex'": 6% dextran 70 in dextrose 5% (500 mL)

Low molecular weight: Gentran'", LMD®, Rheomacrodex®:
10% dextran 40 in dextrose 5% (500 mL)
10% dextran 40 in sodium chloride 0.9% (500 mL)

dextran 1
Brand Names Promit'"
Therapeutic Category Plasma Volume Expander
Use Prophylaxis of serious anaphylactic reactions to I.V. infusion of dextran
Usual Dosage I.V. (time between dextran 1 and dextran solution should not exceed 15 minutes):
Children: 0.3 mL/kg 1-2 minutes before I.V. infusion of dextran
Adults: 20 mL 1-2 minutes before I.V. infusion of dextran
Dosage Forms Injection: 150 mg/mL (20 mL)

dextran 40 *see dextran on previous page*

dextran 70 *see dextran on previous page*

dextran 75 *see dextran on previous page*

dextran, high molecular weight *see dextran on previous page*

dextran, low molecular weight *see dextran on previous page*

dextranomer (dex tran' oh mer)
Brand Names Debrisan'" Topical [OTC]
Therapeutic Category Topical Skin Product
Use Clean exudative wounds; no controlled studies have found dextranomer to be more effective than conventional therapy
Usual Dosage Topical: Apply to affected area once or twice daily
Dosage Forms
Beads: 4 g, 25 g, 60 g, 120 g
Paste: 10 g foil packets

dextroamphetamine sulfate (dex troe am fet' a meen)
Brand Names Dexedrine'"
Therapeutic Category Amphetamine; Anorexiant; Central Nervous System Stimulant, Amphetamine
Use Narcolepsy; abnormal behavioral syndrome in children; exogenous obesity
Usual Dosage Oral:
Children:
Narcolepsy: 6-12 years: Initial: 5 mg/day, may increase at 5 mg increments in weekly intervals until side effects appear; maximum dose: 60 mg/day
Attention deficit disorder:
3-5 years: Initial: 2.5 mg/day given every morning; increase by 2.5 mg/day in weekly intervals until optimal response is obtained, usual range is 0.1-0.5 mg/kg/dose every morning with maximum of 40 mg/day
≥6 years: 5 mg once or twice daily; increase in increments of 5 mg/day at weekly intervals until optimal response is reached, usual range is 0.1-0.5 mg/kg/dose every morning (5-20 mg/day) with maximum of 40 mg/day

Adults:
Narcolepsy: Initial: 10 mg/day, may increase at 10 mg increments in weekly intervals until
side effects appear; maximum: 60 mg/day
Exogenous obesity: 5-30 mg/day in divided doses of 5-10 mg 30-60 minutes before meals
Dosage Forms
Capsule, sustained release: 5 mg, 10 mg, 15 mg
Tablet: 5 mg, 10 mg

dextromethorphan and guaifenesin *see* guaifenesin and dextromethorphan
on page 214

dextromethorphan hydrobromide (dex troe meth or' fan)
Brand Names Benylin DM® [OTC]; Children's Hold® [OTC]; Creo-Terpin® [OTC]; Delsym®
[OTC]; Drixoral® Cough Liquid Caps [OTC]; Hold® DM [OTC]; Pertussin® CS [OTC]; Pertus-
sin® ES [OTC]; Robitussin® Cough Calmers [OTC]; Robitussin® Pediatric [OTC]; Scot-
Tussin DM® Cough Chasers [OTC]; Silphen DM® [OTC]; St. Joseph® Cough Suppressant
[OTC]; Sucrets® Cough Calmers [OTC]; Suppress® [OTC]; Trocal® [OTC]; Vicks® Formula
44® [OTC]; Vicks Formula 44® Pediatric Formula [OTC]
Therapeutic Category Antitussive
Use Symptomatic relief of coughs caused by minor viral upper respiratory tract infections or
inhaled irritants; most effective for a chronic nonproductive cough
Usual Dosage Oral:
Children:
2-5 years: 2.5-5 mg every 4 hours or 7.5 mg every 6-8 hours; extended release is 50 mg
twice daily
6-11 years: 5-10 mg every 4 hours or 15 mg every 6-8 hours; extended release is 30 mg
twice daily
Adults: 10-20 mg every 4 hours or 30 mg every 6-8 hours; extended release is 60 mg twice
daily
Dosage Forms
Capsule (Drixoral® Cough Liquid Caps): 30 mg
Liquid:
Pertussin® CS: 3.5 mg/5 mL (120 mL)
Robitussin® Pediatric, St. Joseph® Cough Suppressant: 7.5 mg/5 mL (60 mL, 120 mL,
240 mL)
Pertussin® ES, Vicks® Formula 44®: 15 mg/5 mL (120 mL, 240 mL)
Liquid, sustained release, as polistirex (Delsym®): 30 mg/5 mL (89 mL)
Lozenges:
Scot-Tussin DM® Cough Chasers: 2.5 mg
Children's Hold®, Hold® DM, Robitussin® Cough Calmers, Sucrets® Cough Calmers: 5
mg
Suppress®, Trocal®: 7.5 mg
Syrup:
Benylin DM®, Silphen DM®: 10 mg/5 mL (120 mL, 3780 mL)
Vicks® Formula 44® Pediatric Formula: 15 mg/15 mL (120 mL)

dextropropoxyphene *see* propoxyphene *on page 393*
Dextrostix® [OTC] *see* diagnostic aids (*in vitro*), blood *on next page*

dextrothyroxine sodium (dex troe thye rox' een)
Brand Names Choloxin®
Therapeutic Category Antilipemic Agent
Use Reduction of elevated serum cholesterol
Usual Dosage Oral:
Children: 0.1 mg/kg/day
Adults: 1-2 mg/day, up to 8 mg/day
Dosage Forms Tablet: 1 mg, 2 mg, 4 mg

Dey-Dose® Isoproterenol *see isoproterenol on page 253*

Dey-Dose® Metaproterenol *see metaproterenol sulfate on page 290*

Dey-Drop® Ophthalmic Solution *see silver nitrate on page 422*

Dey-Lute® Isoetharine *see isoetharine on page 251*

dezocine (dez' oh seen)
  Brand Names Dalgan'"
  Therapeutic Category Analgesic, Narcotic
  Use Relief of moderate to severe postoperative, acute renal and ureteral colic, and cancer pain
  Usual Dosage Adults:
    I.M.: Initial: 5-20 mg; may be repeated every 3-6 hours as needed; maximum: 120 mg/day
    I.V.: Initial: 2.5-10 mg; may be repeated every 2-4 hours as needed
  Dosage Forms Injection, single-dose vial: 5 mg/mL (2 mL); 10 mg/mL (2 mL); 15 mg/mL (2 mL)

dfmo *see eflornithine hydrochloride on page 164*

dfp *see isoflurophate on page 252*

dhad *see mitoxantrone hydrochloride on page 309*

DHC Plus® *see dihydrocodeine compound on page 145*

D.H.E. 45® Injection *see dihydroergotamine mesylate on page 145*

dhpg sodium *see ganciclovir on page 204*

DHS® Tar [OTC] *see coal tar on page 110*

DHS Zinc® [OTC] *see pyrithione zinc on page 401*

DHT™ *see dihydrotachysterol on page 146*

Diaβeta® *see glyburide on page 209*

Diabetic Tussin EX® [OTC] *see guaifenesin on page 213*

Diabinese® *see chlorpropamide on page 98*

diagnostic aids (*in vitro*), blood
  Brand Names Abbott HIVAB HIV-1 EIA; Abbott HIVAG-1; Abbott HTLV III Confirmatory EIA; Azostix" [OTC]; Chemstrip" bG [OTC]; Dextrostix® [OTC]; Diascan-S® [OTC]; Glucostix® [OTC]; MicroTrak" HSV 1/HSV 2 Culture Identification/Typing Test; Mono-Diff®; Monospot®; Monosticon" Dri-Dot"; Mono-Sure'"; Mono-Test"; Recombigen® HIV-1 LA; Rheumanosticon® Dri-Dot"; Rubacell" II; Rubazyme"; Sickledex™; TPM® Test; Tracer bG® [OTC]; Virogen® Rubella Microlatex"; Virogen'" Rubella Slide Test
  Therapeutic Category Diagnostic Agent
  Dosage Forms
    Diagnostic test for glucose in blood:
      Chemstrip bG"
      Dextrostix"
      Diascan-S"
      Tracer bG"
      Glucostix"
    Diagnostic test for blood urea nitrogen in blood: Azostix®
    Diagnostic test for infectious mononucleosis:
      Mono-Diff"
      Monospot"
      Monosticon" Dri-Dot"
      Mono-Sure"
      Mono-Test"
    Diagnostic test for sickle cell anemia: Sickledex™
    Diagnostic test for toxoplasmosis: TPM" Test
    Diagnostic test for virus:
      Abbott HIVAB HIV-1 EIA
      Abbott HIVAG-1

Abbott HTLV I EIA
Abbott HTLV III Confirmatory EIA
MicroTrak® HSV 1/HSV 2 Culture Identification/Typing Test
Recombigen® HIV-1 LA
Rubacell® II
Rubazyme®
Virogen® Rotatest®
Virogen® Rubella Microlatex®
Virogen® Rubella Slide Test

diagnostic aids (*in vitro*), feces
Brand Names Colocare® [OTC]; ColoScreen [OTC]; EZ-Detect® [OTC]; Hema-Chek® [OTC]; Hematest® [OTC]; Hemoccult® II [OTC]; Hemoccult® Slides; Rotalex®; Virogen® Rotatest®
Therapeutic Category Diagnostic Agent
Dosage Forms
Diagnostic tests for occult blood:
Colocare®
Early Detector®
EZ-Detect®
Hemocult® II
Diagnostic test for virus:
Rotalex®
Virogen® Rotatest®

diagnostic aids (*in vitro*), other
Brand Names Accusens T®; Biocult-GC®; Culturette® 10 Minute Group A Strep ID; Gastroccult®; Gonodecten®; Gonozyme®; Isocult® for *Neisseria gonorrhoeae*; Isocult® for *Staphylococcus aureus*; Isocult® for *Trichomonas vaginalis*; Isocult® Throat Streptococci; Lung Check®; *Neisseria gonorrhoeae*; RapidTest® Strep; Respiracult-Strep®; Respiralex®; Streptonase-B®; Strepto-Sac®; Virogen® Herpes Slide Test
Therapeutic Category Diagnostic Agent
Dosage Forms
Diagnostic test for gonorrhea:
Biocult-GC®
Gonodecten®
Gonozyme®
Isocult® for #*Neisseria gonorrhoeae*
MicroTrak® #*Neisseria gonorrhoeae*
Diagnostic test for precancerous lung cells: Lung Check®
Diagnostic test for occult blood (gastric contents): Gastrocult®
Diagnostic test for *Staphylococcus*: Isocult® for *Staphylococcus aureus*
Culturette® 10 Minute Group A Strep ID
Diagnostic test for *Streptococcus*:
Isocult® Throat Streptococci
RapidTest® Strep
Respiracult-Strep®
Respiralex®
Streptonase-B®
Strepto-Sac®
Taste function test: Accusens T®
Diagnostic test for *Trichomonas*: Isocult® for *Trichomonas vaginalis*
Diagnostic test for virus: Virogen® Herpes Slide Test

diagnostic aids (*in vitro*), urine
Brand Names Advance®; Answer®; Answer® Ovulation; Answer® Plus; Bili-Labstix® [OTC]; Chemstrip® 7 [OTC]; Chemstrip® 9 [OTC]; Chemstrip® K [OTC]; Chemstrip® uG [OTC]; Chemstrip® uGK [OTC]; Clearblue®; Clearplan® Easy; Clinistix® [OTC]; Clinitest® [OTC]; Color® Ovulation Test; Combistix® [OTC]; Daisy® 2; Diastix® [OTC]; e.p.t.® Stick; Fact Plus®;
(Continued)

diagnostic aids (*in vitro*), urine *(Continued)*

First Response™; Fortel® Home Ovulation; Hema-Combistix® [OTC]; Hemastix® [OTC]; Icto-test™ [OTC]; Isocult® for Bacteriuria; Isocult® for *Pseudomonas aeruginosa*; Keto-Diastix® [OTC]; Ketostix® [OTC]; Labstix® [OTC]; Microstix-3®; Multistix® [OTC]; Nimbus®; OvuKIT® Acetest™ [OTC]; OvuQUICK®; Pregnosis®; Pregnospia® II; Tes-Tape® [OTC]; UCG-Slide® Test; Uricult™; Uristix™

Therapeutic Category Diagnostic Agent

Dosage Forms

Diagnostic test for acetone, bilirubin, blood, glucose, pH and protein in urine: Bili-Labstix®
Diagnostic test for bilirubin in the urine: Ictotest®
Diagnostic test for acetone, blood, glucose, pH, and protein in urine: Labstix®
Diagnostic test for acetone in urine: Acetest®, Chemstrip® K, Ketostix®
Diagnostic test for bacteriuria:
   Microstix-3™
   Uricult™
   Isocult™ for bacteriuria
Diagnostic test for blood, glucose, pH, and protein in urine: Hema-Combistix [OTC]
Diagnostic test for blood in urine: Hemastix®
Diagnostic test for glucose and protein in urine: Uristix®
Diagnostic test for glucose and ketones in urine; Keto-Diastix®
Diagnostic test for glucose in urine:
   Chemstrip® uG
   Clinistix™
   Clinitest™
   Diastix™
   Tes-Tape™
Diagnostic test for glucose, pH, and protein in urine: Combistix®
Diagnostic test for multiple determinations in urine:
   Chemstrip™ 7
   Chemstrip™ 9
   Chemstrip™ uGK
   Hema-Combistix™
   Multistix™
Ovulation tests:
   Answer™ Ovulation
   Clearplan™ Easy
   Color™ Ovulation Test
   First Response®
   Fortel™ Home Ovulation
   OvuKIT™
   OvuQUICK™
Pregnancy tests:
   Advance™
   Answer™
   Answer™ Plus
   Clearblue™
   Daisy™ 2
   e.p.t.™ Stick
   Fact Plus™
   First Response™
   Pregnosis™
   UCG-Slide™ Test
   Nimbus™
   Pregnospia™ II
Diagnostic test for *Pseudomonas*: Isocult™ for *Pseudomonas aeruginosa*

Dialose® [OTC] *see* docusate *on page 153*

Dialose® Plus Capsule [OTC] *see* docusate and casanthranol *on page 154*

Dialose® Plus Tablet [OTC] *see* docusate and phenolphthalein *on page 154*

Dialume® [OTC] *see* aluminum hydroxide *on page 15*

Diamine T.D.® Oral [OTC] *see* brompheniramine maleate *on page 59*

diaminodiphenylsulfone *see* dapsone *on page 125*

Diamox® *see* acetazolamide *on page 5*

Diaparene® [OTC] *see* methylbenzethonium chloride *on page 298*

Diapid® Nasal Spray *see* lypressin *on page 275*

Diaqua® *see* hydrochlorothiazide *on page 229*

Diar-aid® [OTC] *see* loperamide hydrochloride *on page 272*

Diascan-S® [OTC] *see* diagnostic aids (*in vitro*), blood *on page 136*

Diasorb® [OTC] *see* attapulgite *on page 39*

Diastix® [OTC] *see* diagnostic aids (*in vitro*), urine *on page 137*

diatrizoate meglumine *see* radiological/contrast media (ionic) *on page 404*

diatrizoate meglumine and diatrizoate sodium *see* radiological/contrast media (ionic) *on page 404*

diatrizoate meglumine and iodipamide meglumine *see* radiological/contrast media (ionic) *on page 404*

diatrizoate sodium *see* radiological/contrast media (ionic) *on page 404*

diazepam (dye az' e pam)

Brand Names Valium®; Valrelease®; Zetran® Injection

Therapeutic Category Antianxiety Agent; Anticonvulsant, Benzodiazepine; Benzodiazepine; Sedative

Use Management of general anxiety disorders, panic disorders, and to provide preoperative sedation, light anesthesia, and amnesia; treatment of status epilepticus, alcohol withdrawal symptoms; used as a skeletal muscle relaxant

Usual Dosage

Neonates: I.V.: Status epilepticus: 0.5-1 mg/kg/dose every 15-30 minutes for 2-3 doses

Children:

Sedation or muscle relaxation or anxiety:

Oral: 0.12-0.8 mg/kg/day in divided doses every 6-8 hours

I.M., I.V.: 0.04-0.3 mg/kg/dose every 2-4 hours to a maximum of 0.6 mg/kg within an 8-hour period if needed

Status epilepticus: I.V.:

Infants 30 days to 5 years: 0.05-0.3 mg/kg/dose given over 2-3 minutes, every 15-30 minutes to a maximum total dose of 5 mg; repeat in 2-4 hours as needed or 0.2-0.5 mg/dose every 2-5 minutes to a maximum total dose of 5 mg

>5 years: 0.05-0.3 mg/kg/dose given over 2-3 minutes, every 15-30 minutes to a maximum total dose of 10 mg; repeat in 2-4 hours as needed or 1 mg/dose every 2-5 minutes to a maximum of 10 mg;

Adults:

Anxiety:

Oral: 2-10 mg 2-4 times/day

I.M., I.V.: 2-10 mg, may repeat in 3-4 hours if needed

Skeletal muscle relaxation:

Oral: 2-10 mg 2-4 times/day

I.M., I.V.: 5-10 mg, may repeat in 2-4 hours

Status epilepticus: I.V.: 0.2-0.5 mg/kg/dose every 15-30 minutes for 2-3 doses; maximum dose: 30 mg

Dosage Forms

Capsule, sustained release (Valrelease®): 15 mg

Injection: 5 mg/mL (1 mL, 2 mL, 5 mL, 10 mL)

Solution, oral (wintergreen-spice flavor): 5 mg/5 mL (5 mL, 10 mL, 500 mL)

Solution, oral concentrate: 5 mg/mL (30 mL)

Tablet: 2 mg, 5 mg, 10 mg

diazoxide (dye az ox' ide)
Brand Names Hyperstat® I.V.; Proglycem® Oral
Therapeutic Category Antihypertensive; Antihypoglycemic Agent
Use
  Oral: Hypoglycemia related to islet cell adenoma, carcinoma, hyperplasia, or adenomatosis, nesidioblastosis, leucine sensitivity, or extrapancreatic malignancy
  I.V.: Emergency lowering of blood pressure
Usual Dosage
  Hyperinsulinemic hypoglycemia: Oral:
    Newborns and Infants: 8-15 mg/kg/day in divided doses every 8-12 hours
    Children and Adults: 3-8 mg/kg/day in divided doses every 8-12 hours

  Hypertension: Children and Adults: I.V.: 1-3 mg/kg (maximum: 150 mg in a single injection); repeat dose in 5-15 minutes until blood pressure adequately reduced; repeat administration every 4-24 hours; monitor blood pressure closely
Dosage Forms
  Capsule (Proglycem®): 50 mg
  Injection (Hyperstat®): 15 mg/mL (1 mL, 20 mL)
  Suspension, oral (chocolate-mint flavor) (Proglycem®): 50 mg/mL (30 mL)

Dibent® Injection *see* dicyclomine hydrochloride *on page 142*

Dibenzyline® *see* phenoxybenzamine hydrochloride *on page 363*

dibucaine (dye' byoo kane)
Brand Names Nupercainal® Topical [OTC]
Therapeutic Category Local Anesthetic, Topical
Use Fast, temporary relief of pain and itching due to hemorrhoids, minor burns, other minor skin conditions
Usual Dosage Children and Adults:
  Rectal: Hemorrhoids: Insert ointment into rectum using a rectal applicator; administer each morning,evening, and after each bowel movement
  Topical: Apply gently to the affected areas; no more than 30 g for adults or 7.5 g for children should be used in any 24-hour period
Dosage Forms
  Cream: 0.5% (45 g)
  Ointment, topical: 1% (30 g, 60 g)

dibucaine and hydrocortisone
Brand Names Corticaine® Topical
Synonyms hydrocortisone and dibucaine
Therapeutic Category Corticosteroid, Topical (Low Potency); Local Anesthetic, Topical
Use Relief of the inflammatory and pruritic manifestations of corticosteroid-responsive dermatoses and for external anal itching
Usual Dosage Topical: Apply to affected areas 2-4 times/day
Dosage Forms Cream: Dibucaine 5% and hydrocortisone 5%

dic *see* dacarbazine *on page 123*

dicalcium phosphate *see* calcium phosphate, dibasic *on page 70*

Dicarbosil® [OTC] *see* calcium carbonate *on page 66*

dichlorodifluoromethane and trichloromonofluoromethane
Brand Names Fluori-Methane® Topical Spray
Therapeutic Category Analgesic, Topical
Use Management of myofascial pain, restricted motion, muscle pain; control of pain associated with injections

Usual Dosage Topical: Apply to area from approximately 12" away
Dosage Forms Spray, topical: Dichlorodifluoromethane 15% and trichloromonofluoromethane 85%

dichlorotetrafluoroethane and ethyl chloride *see* ethyl chloride and
dichlorotetrafluoroethane *on page 181*

dichlorphenamide (dye klor fen' a mide)
Brand Names Daranide®
Synonyms diclofenamide
Therapeutic Category Carbonic Anhydrase Inhibitor; Diuretic, Carbonic Anhydrase Inhibitor
Use Adjunct in treatment of open-angle glaucoma and perioperative treatment for angle-
closure glaucoma
Usual Dosage Adults: Oral: 100-200 mg to start followed by 100 mg every 12 hours until de-
sired response is obtained; maintenance dose: 25-50 mg 1-3 times/day
Dosage Forms Tablet: 50 mg

dichysterol *see* dihydrotachysterol *on page 146*

diclofenac sodium (dye kloe' fen ak)
Brand Names Cataflam® Oral; Voltaren® Ophthalmic; Voltaren® Oral
Therapeutic Category Analgesic, Non-Narcotic; Anti-inflammatory Agent; Nonsteroidal Anti-
Inflammatory Agent (NSAID), Ophthalmic; Nonsteroidal Anti-Inflammatory Agent (NSAID),
Oral
Use Acute and chronic treatment of rheumatoid arthritis, ankylosing spondylitis, and osteoar-
thritis; also used for juvenile rheumatoid arthritis, gout, dysmenorrhea, and pain relief; oph-
thalmic solution for postoperative inflammation after cataract extraction
Usual Dosage Adults:
Oral:
Rheumatoid arthritis: 150-200 mg/day in 2-4 divided doses
Osteoarthritis: 100-150 mg/day in 2-3 divided doses
Ankylosing spondylitis: 100-125 mg/day in 4-5 divided doses
Ophthalmic: Instill 1 drop into affected eye 4 times/day beginning 24 hours after cataract sur-
gery and continuing for 2 weeks
Dosage Forms
Solution, ophthalmic, as sodium (Voltaren®): 0.1% (2.5 mL, 5 mL)
Tablet, enteric coated, as sodium (Voltaren®): 25 mg, 50 mg, 75 mg
Tablet, as potassium (Cataflam®): 50 mg

diclofenamide *see* dichlorphenamide *on this page*

dicloxacillin sodium (dye klox a sill' in)
Brand Names Dycill®; Dynapen®; Pathocil®
Therapeutic Category Antibiotic, Penicillin
Use Treatment of systemic infections such as pneumonia, skin and soft tissue infections and
follow-up therapy for osteomyelitis caused by penicillinase-producing staphylococci
Usual Dosage Oral:
Children <40 kg: 12.5-50 mg/kg/day divided every 6 hours; doses of 50-100 mg/kg/day in di-
vided doses every 6 hours have been used for follow-up therapy of osteomyelitis

Children >40 kg and Adults: 125-500 mg every 6 hours
Dosage Forms
Capsule: 125 mg, 250 mg, 500 mg
Powder for oral suspension: 62.5 mg/5 mL (80 mL, 100 mL, 200 mL)

dicumarol (dye koo' ma role)
Synonyms bishydroxycoumarin
Therapeutic Category Anticoagulant
Use Prophylaxis and treatment of thromboembolic disorders
(Continued)

dicumarol *(Continued)*

Usual Dosage Adults: Oral: 25-200 mg/day based on prothrombin time (PT) determinations
Dosage Forms Tablet: 25 mg, 50 mg, 100 mg

dicyclomine hydrochloride (dye sye' kloe meen)

Brand Names Antispas® Injection; Bentyl® Hydrochloride Injection; Bentyl® Hydrochloride Oral; Byclomine® Injection; Dibent® Injection; Dilomine® Injection; Di-Spaz® Injection; Di-Spaz® Oral; Neoquess® Injection; Or-Tyl® Injection; Spasmoject® Injection
Synonyms dicycloverine hydrochloride
Therapeutic Category Antispasmodic Agent, Gastrointestinal
Use Treatment of functional disturbances of GI motility such as irritable bowel syndrome
Usual Dosage
Oral:
Infants >6 months: 5 mg/dose 3-4 times/day
Children: 10 mg/dose 3-4 times/day
Adults: Begin with 80 mg/day in 4 equally divided doses, then increase up to 160 mg/day
I.M. **(should not be used I.V.)**: 80 mg/day in 4 divided doses (20 mg/dose)
Dosage Forms
Capsule: 10 mg, 20 mg
Injection: 10 mg/mL (2 mL, 10 mL)
Syrup: 10 mg/5 mL (118 mL, 473 mL, 946 mL)
Tablet: 20 mg

dicycloverine hydrochloride *see* dicyclomine hydrochloride *on this page*

didanosine (dye dan' oh seen)

Brand Names Videx® Oral
Synonyms ddi
Therapeutic Category Antiviral Agent, Oral
Use Advanced HIV infection in patients who are intolerant of zidovudine therapy or who have demonstrated significant clinical or immunologic deterioration during zidovudine therapy
Usual Dosage Administer on an empty stomach
Children (dosing is based on body surface area (m^2)):
<0.4: 25 mg tablets twice daily or 31 mg powder twice daily
0.5-0.7: 50 mg tablets twice daily or 62 mg powder twice daily
0.8-1: 75 mg tablets twice daily or 94 mg powder twice daily
1.1-1.4: 100 mg tablets twice daily or 125 mg powder twice daily

Adults: Dosing is based on patient weight:
35-49 kg: 125 mg tablets twice daily or 167 mg buffered powder twice daily
50-74 kg: 200 mg tablets twice daily or 250 mg buffered powder twice daily
≥75 mg: 300 mg tablets twice daily or 375 mg buffered powder twice daily

Note: Children >1 year and Adults should receive 2 tablets per dose and children <1 year should receive 1 tablet per dose for adequate buffering and absorption; tablets should be chewed
Dosage Forms
Powder for oral solution:
Buffered (single dose packet): 100 mg, 167 mg, 250 mg, 375 mg
Pediatric: 2 g, 4 g
Tablet, buffered, chewable (mint flavor): 25 mg, 50 mg, 100 mg, 150 mg

dideoxycytidine *see* zalcitabine *on page 494*
Didrex® *see* benzphetamine hydrochloride *on page 50*
Didronel® I.V. *see* etidronate disodium *on page 182*
Didronel® Oral *see* etidronate disodium *on page 182*

dienestrol (dye en ess' trole)
Brand Names DV® Vaginal Cream; Ortho® Dienestrol Vaginal
Therapeutic Category Estrogen Derivative
Use Symptomatic management of atrophic vaginitis in postmenopausal women
Usual Dosage Adults: Vaginal: 1-2 applicatorfuls/day for 2 weeks and then $\frac{1}{2}$ of that dose for 2 weeks; maintenance dose: 1 applicatorful 1-3 times/week for 3 weeks each month
Dosage Forms Cream, vaginal: 0.01% (30 g, 78 g)

diethylpropion hydrochloride (dye eth il proe' pee on)
Brand Names Tenuate®; Tepanil®
Synonyms amfepramone
Therapeutic Category Anorexiant
Use Short-term adjunct in exogenous obesity
Usual Dosage Adults: Oral: 25 mg 3 times/day before meals or food or 75 mg controlled release tablet at midmorning
Dosage Forms
Tablet: 25 mg
Tablet, controlled release: 75 mg

diethylstilbestrol (dye eth il stil bess' trole)
Brand Names Stilphostrol®
Synonyms des; stilbestrol
Therapeutic Category Estrogen Derivative
Use Management of severe vasomotor symptoms of menopause, for estrogen replacement, and for palliative treatment of inoperable metastatic prostatic carcinoma
Usual Dosage Adults:
Hypogonadism and ovarian failure: Oral: 0.2-0.5 mg/day

Menopausal symptoms: Oral: 0.1-2 mg/day for 3 weeks and then off 1 week

Postmenopausal breast carcinoma: Oral: 15 mg/day

Prostate carcinoma: Oral: 1-3 mg/day

Prostatic cancer: I.V.: 0.5 g to start, then 1 g every 2-5 days followed by 0.25-0.5 g 1-2 times/week as maintenance

Diphosphate:
Oral: 50 mg 3 times/day; increase up to 200 mg or more 3 times/day
I.V.: Give 0.5 g, dissolved in 250 mL of saline or D_5W, administer slowly the first 10-15 minutes then adjust rate so that the entire amount is given in 1 hour
Dosage Forms
Injection, as diphosphate sodium (Stilphostrol®): 0.25 g (5 mL)
Tablet: 1 mg, 2.5 mg, 5 mg
Tablet (Stilphostrol®): 50 mg

difenoxin and atropine (dye fen ox' in)
Brand Names Motofen®
Therapeutic Category Antidiarrheal
Use Treatment of diarrhea
Usual Dosage Adults: Oral: Initial: 2 tablets, then 1 tablet after each loose stool; 1 tablet every 3-4 hours, up to 8 tablets in a 24-hour period; if no improvement after 48 hours, continued administration is not indicated
Dosage Forms Tablet: Difenoxin hydrochloride 1 mg and atropine sulfate 0.025 mg

diflorasone diacetate (dye flor' a sone)
Brand Names Florone® E Topical; Florone® Topical; Maxiflor® Topical; Psorcon™ Topical
Therapeutic Category Corticosteroid, Topical (High Potency)
Use Relieve inflammation and pruritic symptoms of corticosteroid-responsive dermatosis
(Continued)

diflorasone diacetate *(Continued)*
Usual Dosage Topical:
Cream: Apply 2-4 times/day
Ointment: Apply sparingly 1-3 times/day
Dosage Forms
Cream: 0.05% (15 g, 30 g, 60 g)
Ointment, topical: 0.05% (15 g, 30 g, 60 g)

Diflucan® Injection *see* fluconazole *on page 193*

Diflucan® Oral *see* fluconazole *on page 193*

diflunisal (dye floo' ni sal)
Brand Names Dolobid®
Therapeutic Category Analgesic, Non-Narcotic; Anti-inflammatory Agent; Nonsteroidal Anti-Inflammatory Agent (NSAID), Oral
Use Management of inflammatory disorders usually including rheumatoid arthritis and osteoarthritis; can be used as an analgesic for treatment of mild to moderate pain
Usual Dosage Adults: Oral:
Pain: Initial: 500-1000 mg followed by 250-500 mg every 8-12 hours
Inflammatory condition: 500-1000 mg/day in 2 divided doses
Dosage Forms Tablet: 250 mg, 500 mg

Di-Gel® [OTC] *see* aluminum hydroxide, magnesium hydroxide, and simethicone *on page 16*

Digibind® *see* digoxin immune fab (ovine) *on next page*

digitoxin (di ji tox' in)
Brand Names Crystodigin®
Therapeutic Category Antiarrhythmic Agent, Miscellaneous; Cardiac Glycoside
Use Congestive heart failure; atrial fibrillation; atrial flutter; paroxysmal atrial tachycardia; and cardiogenic shock
Usual Dosage
Children: The doses are very individualized; the maintenance range after neonatal period, the recommended digitalizing dose is as follows:
<1 year: 0.045 mg/kg
1-2 years: 0.04 mg/kg
2 years: 0.03 mg/kg which is equivalent to 0.75 mg/mm^2
Maintenance: Approximately $^1/_{10}$ of the digitalizing dose
Adults:
Rapid oral loading dose: Initial: 0.6 mg followed by 0.4 mg and then 0.2 mg at intervals of 4-6 hours
Slow oral loading dose: 0.2 mg twice daily for a period of 4 days followed by a maintenance dose
Maintenance: 0.05-0.3 mg/day
Most common dose: 0.15 mg/day
Dosage Forms Tablet: 0.1 mg

digoxin (di jox' in)
Brand Names Lanoxicaps®; Lanoxin®
Therapeutic Category Antiarrhythmic Agent, Miscellaneous; Cardiac Glycoside
Use Treatment of congestive heart failure; slows the ventricular rate in tachyarrhythmias such as atrial fibrillation, atrial flutter, supraventricular tachycardia, paroxysmal atrial tachycardia, cardiogenic shock
Usual Dosage Adults (based on lean body weight and normal renal function for age. Decrease dose in patients with decreased renal function)

Total digitalizing dose: Give $\frac{1}{2}$ as initial dose, then give $\frac{1}{4}$ of the total digitalizing dose (TDD) in each of 2 subsequent doses at 8- to 12-hour intervals. Obtain EKG 6 hours after each dose to assess potential toxicity.
    Oral: 0.75-1.5 mg
    I.M., I.V.: 0.5-1 mg

Daily maintenance dose:
    Oral: 0.125-0.5 mg
    I.M., I.V.: 0.1-0.4 mg
Dosage Forms
    Capsule: 50 mcg, 100 mcg, 200 mcg
    Elixir, pediatric (lime flavor): 50 mcg/mL with alcohol 10% (60 mL)
    Injection: 250 mcg/mL (1 mL, 2 mL)
    Injection, pediatric: 100 mcg/mL (1 mL)
    Tablet: 125 mcg, 250 mcg, 500 mcg

digoxin immune fab (ovine)
Brand Names Digibind®
Synonyms antidigoxin fab fragments
Therapeutic Category Antidote, Digoxin
Use Treatment of potentially life-threatening digoxin or digitoxin intoxication in carefully selected patients
Usual Dosage To determine the dose of digoxin immune Fab, first determine the total body load of digoxin (TBL) as follows (using either an approximation of the amount ingested or a postdistribution serum digoxin concentration):

TBL of digoxin (in mg) = C (in ng/mL) x 5.6 x body weight (in kg)/1000 or TBL = mg of digoxin ingested (as tablets or elixir) x 0.8; C = postdistribution digoxin concentration

Dose of digoxin immune Fab (in mg) I.V. = TBL x 66.7 or dose of digoxin immune Fab (in number of 40 mg vials) = [C of digoxin (in ng/mL) x body weight (in kg)]/100
Dosage Forms Powder for injection, lyophilized: 40 mg

Dihistine® *see* chlorpheniramine and phenylephrine *on page 93*
Dihistine® DH *see* chlorpheniramine, pseudoephedrine, and codeine *on page 97*
Dihistine® Expectorant *see* guaifenesin, pseudoephedrine, and codeine *on page 217*

dihydrocodeine compound (dye hye droe koe' deen)
Brand Names DHC Plus®; Synalgos®-DC
Therapeutic Category Analgesic, Narcotic
Use Management of mild to moderate pain that requires relaxation
Usual Dosage Adults: Oral: 1-2 capsules every 4-6 hours as needed for pain
Dosage Forms Capsule:
    DHC Plus®: Dihydrocodeine bitartrate 16 mg, acetaminophen 356.4 mg, and caffeine 30 mg
    Synalgos®-DC: Dihydrocodeine bitartrate 16 mg, aspirin 356.4 mg, and caffeine 30 mg

dihydroergotamine mesylate (dye hye droe er got' a meen)
Brand Names D.H.E. 45® Injection
Therapeutic Category Ergot Alkaloid
Use To abort or prevent vascular headaches
Usual Dosage
    I.M.: 1 mg at first sign of headache; 1 mg every 6 hours for 2 doses (not to exceed 6 mg in 24 hours)
    I.V.: Up to 2 mg for faster effects
Dosage Forms Injection: 1 mg/mL (1 mL)

dihydroergotoxine *see* ergoloid mesylates *on page 169*

dihydrohydroxycodeinone *see* oxycodone hydrochloride *on page 343*

dihydromorphinone *see* hydromorphone hydrochloride *on page 234*

dihydrotachysterol (dye hye droe tak iss' ter ole)
Brand Names DHT™; Hytakerol®
Synonyms dichysterol
Therapeutic Category Vitamin D Analog
Use Treatment of hypocalcemia associated with hypoparathyroidism; prophylaxis of hypocalcemic tetany following thyroid surgery
Usual Dosage Oral:
Hypoparathyroidism:
    Neonates: 0.05-0.1 mg/day
    Infants and young Children: 0.1-0.5 mg/day
    Older Children and Adults: 0.5-1 mg/day

Nutritional rickets: 0.5 mg as a single dose or 13-50 mcg/day until healing occurs

Renal osteodystrophy: 0.6-6 mg/24 hours; maintenance: 0.25-0.6 mg/24 hours adjusted as necessary to achieve normal serum calcium levels and promote bone healing
Dosage Forms
Capsule (Hytakerol®): 0.125 mg
Solution:
    Oral Concentrate (DHT™): 0.2 mg/mL (30 mL)
    Oral, in oil (Hytakerol®): 0.25 mg/mL (15 mL)
Tablet (DHT™): 0.125 mg, 0.2 mg, 0.4 mg

dihydroxyaluminum sodium carbonate (dye hye drox' i a loo' mi num)
Brand Names Rolaids® [OTC]
Therapeutic Category Antacid
Use Symptomatic relief of upset stomach associated with hyperacidity
Usual Dosage Oral: Chew 1-2 tablets as needed
Dosage Forms Tablet, chewable: 334 mg

1,25 dihydroxycholecalciferol *see* calcitriol *on page 65*

dihydroxypropyl theophylline *see* dyphylline *on page 161*

diiodohydroxyquin *see* iodoquinol *on page 249*

diisopropyl fluorophosphate *see* isoflurophate *on page 252*

Dilacor™ XR *see* diltiazem hydrochloride *on this page*

Dilantin® *see* phenytoin *on page 366*

Dilantin® With Phenobarbital *see* phenytoin with phenobarbital *on page 367*

Dilatrate®-SR *see* isosorbide dinitrate *on page 254*

Dilaudid-HP® Injection *see* hydromorphone hydrochloride *on page 234*

Dilaudid® Injection *see* hydromorphone hydrochloride *on page 234*

Dilaudid® Oral *see* hydromorphone hydrochloride *on page 234*

Dilaudid® Suppository *see* hydromorphone hydrochloride *on page 234*

Dilocaine® *see* lidocaine hydrochloride *on page 267*

Dilomine® Injection *see* dicyclomine hydrochloride *on page 142*

Dilor® *see* dyphylline *on page 161*

diltiazem hydrochloride (dil tye' a zem)
Brand Names Cardizem® CD; Cardizem® Injectable; Cardizem® SR; Cardizem® Tablet; Dilacor™ XR
Therapeutic Category Antianginal Agent; Calcium Channel Blocker

Use

Cardizem® CD capsule: Hypertension (alone or in combination); chronic stable angina or angina from coronary artery spasm

Cardizem® injection: Atrial fibrillation or atrial flutter; paroxysmal supraventricular tachycardias (PSVT)

Cardizem® SR capsule, Dilacor™ XR capsule: Hypertension (alone or in combination)

Cardizem® tablet: Chronic stable angina or angina from coronary artery spasm

Usual Dosage Adults:

Oral: 30-120 mg 3-4 times/day; dosage should be increased gradually, at 1- to 2-day intervals until optimum response is obtained; usual maintenance dose is usually 240-360 mg/day

Sustained-release capsules (SR): Initial dose of 60-120 mg twice daily

Sustained-release capsules (CD, XR): 180-300 mg once daily

I.V.: Initial 0.25 mg/kg as a bolus over 2 minutes, then continuous infusion of 5-15 mg/hour for up to 24 hours

Dosage Forms

Capsule, sustained release:
Cardizem® CD: 120 mg, 180 mg, 240 mg, 300 mg
Cardizem® SR: 60 mg, 90 mg, 120 mg
Dilacor™ XR: 180 mg, 240 mg
Injection (Cardizem®): 5 mg/mL (5 mL, 10 mL)
Tablet (Cardizem®): 30 mg, 60 mg, 90 mg, 120 mg

dimenhydrinate (dye men hye' dri nate)

Brand Names Calm-X® Oral [OTC]; Dimetabs® Oral; Dinate® Injection; Dramamine® Oral [OTC]; Dramilin® Injection; Dramoject® Injection; Dymenate® Injection; Hydrate® Injection; Marmine® Injection; Marmine® Oral [OTC]; Tega-Vert® Oral; TripTone® Caplets® [OTC]

Therapeutic Category Antiemetic; Antihistamine

Use Treatment and prevention of nausea, vertigo, and vomiting associated with motion sickness

Usual Dosage

Children: Oral, I.M.:
2-5 years: 12.5-25 mg every 6-8 hours, maximum: 75 mg/day
6-12 years: 25-50 mg every 6-8 hours, maximum: 75 mg/day
or
Alternately: 5 mg/kg/day in 4 divided doses, not to exceed 300 mg/day

Adults: Oral, I.M., I.V.: 50-100 mg every 4-6 hours, not to exceed 400 mg/day

Dosage Forms

Capsule: 50 mg
Injection: 50 mg/mL (1 mL, 5 mL, 10 mL)
Liquid: 12.5 mg/4 mL
Tablet: 50 mg
Tablet, chewable: 50 mg

dimercaprol (dye mer kap' role)

Brand Names BAL in Oil®

Synonyms bal; British anti-lewisite; dithioglycerol

Therapeutic Category Antidote, Arsenic Toxicity; Antidote, Gold Toxicity; Antidote, Lead Toxicity; Antidote, Mercury Toxicity

Use Antidote to gold, arsenic, and mercury poisoning; adjunct to edetate calcium disodium in lead poisoning

Usual Dosage Children and Adults: I.M.:

Mild arsenic and gold poisoning: 2.5 mg/kg/dose every 6 hours for 2 days, then every 12 hours on the third day, and once daily thereafter for 10 days

Severe arsenic and gold poisoning: 3 mg/kg/dose every 4 hours for 2 days then every 6 hours on the third day, then every 12 hours thereafter for 10 days

Mercury poisoning: Initial: 5 mg/kg followed by 2.5 mg/kg/dose 1-2 times/day for 10 days

Lead poisoning (use with edetate calcium disodium):
Mild: 3 mg/kg/dose every 4 hours for 5-7 days

(Continued)

dimercaprol *(Continued)*

    Severe: 4 mg/kg/dose every 4 hours for 5-7 days

    Acute encephalopathy: Initial: 4 mg/kg/dose, then every 4 hours

Dosage Forms Injection: 100 mg/mL (3 mL)

Dimetabs® Oral *see* dimenhydrinate *on previous page*

Dimetane®-DC *see* brompheniramine, phenylpropanolamine, and codeine *on page 60*

Dimetane® Oral [OTC] *see* brompheniramine maleate *on page 59*

Dimetapp® [OTC] *see* brompheniramine and phenylpropanolamine *on page 59*

Dimetapp® Extentabs® [OTC] *see* brompheniramine and phenylpropanolamine *on page 59*

dimethoxyphenyl penicillin sodium *see* methicillin sodium *on page 294*

β,β-**dimethylcysteine** *see* penicillamine *on page 352*

dimethyl sulfoxide (dye meth il sul fox' ide)

Brand Names Rimso®-50

Synonyms dmso

Therapeutic Category Urinary Tract Product

Use Symptomatic relief of interstitial cystitis

Usual Dosage Instill 50 mL directly into bladder and allow to remain for 15 minutes; repeat every 2 weeks until maximum symptomatic relief is obtained

Dosage Forms Solution: 50% [500 mg/mL] (50 mL)

dimethyl tubocurarine iodide *see* metocurine iodide *on page 302*

Dinate® Injection *see* dimenhydrinate *on previous page*

dinoprostone (dye noe prost' one)

Brand Names Prepidil® Vaginal Gel; Prostin E$_2$® Vaginal Suppository

Synonyms pge$_2$; prostaglandin e$_2$

Therapeutic Category Abortifacient; Prostaglandin

Use Terminate pregnancy from 12th through 28th week of gestation; evacuate uterus in cases of missed abortion or intrauterine fetal death; manage benign hydatidiform mole

Usual Dosage Insert 1 suppository high in vagina, repeat at 3- to 5-hour intervals until abortion occurs up to 240 mg (maximum dose)

Dosage Forms

Gel, vaginal: 0.5 mg in 3 g syringes [each package contains a 10-mm and 20-mm shielded catheter]

Suppository, vaginal: 20 mg

dinoprost tromethamine

Brand Names Prostin F$_2$ Alpha®

Synonyms pgf$_{2\alpha}$; prostaglandin f$_2$ alpha

Therapeutic Category Prostaglandin

Use Abort 2nd trimester pregnancy

Usual Dosage 40 mg (8 mL) via transabdominal tap, if abortion not completed in 24 hours, another 10-40 mg may be given

Dosage Forms Injection: 5 mg/mL (4 mL, 8 mL)

Diocto C® [OTC] *see* docusate and casanthranol *on page 154*

Diocto-K Plus® [OTC] *see* docusate and casanthranol *on page 154*

Diocto-K® [OTC] *see* docusate *on page 153*

Dioctolose Plus®　[OTC]　*see* docusate and casanthranol *on page 154*

Diocto®　[OTC]　*see* docusate *on page 153*

Dioeze®　[OTC]　*see* docusate *on page 153*

Dionosil Oily®　*see* radiological/contrast media (ionic) *on page 404*

Dioval®　Injection　*see* estradiol *on page 173*

dipalmitoylphosphatidylcholine　*see* colfosceril palmitate *on page 113*

Dipentum®　*see* olsalazine sodium *on page 336*

diphenhydramine hydrochloride (dye fen hye' dra meen)
Brand Names AllerMax® Oral [OTC]; Banophen® Oral [OTC]; Belix® Oral [OTC]; Bena-D® Injection; Benadryl® Injection; Benadryl® Oral [OTC]; Benadryl® Topical; Benahist® Injection; Benoject® Injection; Benylin® Cough Syrup [OTC]; Bydramine® Cough Syrup [OTC]; Diphen® Cough [OTC]; Dormin® Oral [OTC]; Genahist® Oral; Hydramyn® Syrup [OTC]; Maximum Strength Nytol® [OTC]; Nidryl® Oral [OTC]; Nordryl® Injection; Nordryl® Oral; Nytol® Oral [OTC]; Phendry® Oral [OTC]; Silphen® Cough [OTC]; Sleep-eze 3® Oral [OTC]; Sleepinal® [OTC]; Sominex® Oral [OTC]; Tusstat® Syrup; Twilite® Oral [OTC]; Uni-Bent® Cough Syrup; Wehdryl® Injection
Therapeutic Category Antidote, Hypersensitivity Reactions; Antihistamine; Sedative
Use Symptomatic relief of allergic symptoms caused by histamine release which include nasal allergies and allergic dermatosis; mild nighttime sedation, prevention of motion sickness, as an antitussive has antinauseant and topical anesthetic properties
Usual Dosage
Children: Oral, I.M., I.V.: 5 mg/kg/day or 150 mg/m²/day in divided doses every 6-8 hours, not to exceed 300 mg/day

Adults:
　　Oral: 25-50 mg every 4-6 hours
　　I.M., I.V.: 10-50 mg in a single dose every 2-4 hours, not to exceed 400 mg/day
Dosage Forms
Capsule: 25 mg, 50 mg
Cream: 1%, 2%
Elixir: 12.5 mg/5 mL (5 mL, 10 mL, 20 mL, 120 mL, 480 mL, 3780 mL)
Injection: 10 mg/mL (10 mL, 30 mL); 50 mg/mL (1 mL, 10 mL)
Lotion: 1% (75 mL)
Solution, topical spray: 1% (60 mL)
Syrup: 12.5 mg/5 mL (5 mL, 120 mL, 240 mL, 480 mL, 3780 mL)
Tablet: 25 mg, 50 mg

diphenidol hydrochloride (dye fen' i dole)
Brand Names Vontrol®
Therapeutic Category Antiemetic
Use Control of nausea and vomiting; peripheral vertigo and associated nausea and vomiting, Ménière's disease and middle and inner ear surgery
Dosage Forms Tablet: 25 mg

diphenoxylate and atropine (dye fen ox' i late)
Brand Names Lofene®; Logen®; Lomanate®; Lomodix®; Lomotil®; Lonox®; Low-Quel®
Synonyms atropine and diphenoxylate
Therapeutic Category Antidiarrheal
Use Treatment of diarrhea
Usual Dosage Oral (as diphenoxylate): Initial dose:
Children: 0.3-0.4 mg/kg/day in 2-4 divided doses
　　2-5 years: 2 mg 3 times/day
　　5-8 years: 2 mg 4 times/day
　　8-12 years: 2 mg 5 times/day
(Continued)

diphenoxylate and atropine *(Continued)*

Not recommended for children <2 years of age

Adults: 15-20 mg/day in 3-4 divided doses

Reduce dosage as soon as initial control of symptoms is achieved

Dosage Forms
Solution, oral: Diphenoxylate hydrochloride 2.5 mg and atropine sulfate 0.025 mg per 5 mL (4 mL, 10 mL, 60 mL)
Tablet: Diphenoxylate hydrochloride 2.5 mg and atropine sulfate 0.025 mg

Diphen® Cough [OTC] *see* diphenhydramine hydrochloride *on previous page*
Diphenylan Sodium® *see* phenytoin *on page 366*
diphenylhydantoin *see* phenytoin *on page 366*

diphtheria and tetanus toxoid (dif theer' ee a)

Synonyms dt; td; tetanus and diphtheria toxoid
Therapeutic Category Toxoid
Use Active immunity against diphtheria and tetanus
Usual Dosage I.M.:
Infants and Children:
6 weeks to 1 year: Three 0.5 mL doses at least 4 weeks apart; give a reinforcing dose 6-12 months after the third injection
1-6 years: Give two 0.5 mL doses at least 4 weeks apart; reinforcing dose 6-12 months after second injection; if final dose is given after seventh birthday, use adult preparation
4-6 years (booster immunization): 0.5 mL; not necessary if all 4 doses were given after fourth birthday – routinely give booster doses at 10-year intervals with the adult preparation

Adults >7 years: 2 primary doses of 0.5 mL each, given at an interval of 4-6 weeks; third (reinforcing) dose of 0.5 mL 6-12 months later; boosters every 10 years
Dosage Forms Injection:
Pediatric use:
Diphtheria 6.6 Lf units and tetanus 5 Lf units per 0.5 mL (5 mL)
Diphtheria 10 Lf units and tetanus 5 Lf units per 0.5 mL (0.5 mL, 5 mL)
Diphtheria 12.5 Lf units and tetanus 5 Lf units per 0.5 mL (5 mL)
Diphtheria 15 Lf units and tetanus 10 Lf units per 0.5 mL (5 mL)
Adult use:
Diphtheria 1.5 Lf units and tetanus 5 Lf units per 0.5 mL (0.5 mL, 5 mL)
Diphtheria 2 Lf units and tetanus 5 Lf units per 0.5 mL (5 mL)
Diphtheria 2 Lf units and tetanus 10 Lf units per 0.5 mL (5 mL)

diphtheria and tetanus toxoids and pertussis vaccine, adsorbed

Brand Names Tri-Immunol®
Synonyms dpt
Therapeutic Category Toxoid
Use Active immunization of infants and children through 6 years of age (between 2 months and the seventh birthday) against diphtheria, tetanus, and pertussis; recommended for both primary immunization and routine recall; start immunization at once if whooping cough or diphtheria is present in the community
Usual Dosage The primary immunization for children 2 months to 6 years of age, ideally beginning at the age of 2-3 months or at 6-week check-up. Administer 0.5 mL I.M. on 3 occasions at 4- to 8-week intervals with a re-enforcing dose administered 1 year after the third injection. The booster doses are given when the child is 4-6 years of age, 0.5 mL I.M.
Dosage Forms Injection:
Diphtheria 6.7 Lf units, tetanus 5 Lf units, and pertussis 4 protective units per 0.5 mL (7.5 mL)
Tri-Immunol®: Diphtheria 12.5 Lf units, tetanus 5 Lf units, and pertussis 4 protective units per 0.5 mL (7.5 mL)

diphtheria, tetanus toxoids, and whole-cell pertussis vaccine and hemophilus b conjugate vaccine

Brand Names Tetramune®
Therapeutic Category Toxoid
Use Active immunization of infants and children through 5 years of age (between 2 months and the sixth birthday) against diphtheria, tetanus, and pertussis and Hemophilus b disease when indications for immunization with DTP vaccine and HIB vaccine coincide
Usual Dosage The primary immunization for children 2 months to 5 years of age, ideally beginning at the age of 2-3 months or at 6-week check-up. Administer 0.5 mL I.M. on 3 occasions at ~2 month intervals, followed by a fourth 0.5 mL dose at ~15 months of age
Dosage Forms Injection: 5 mL

diphtheria antitoxin

Therapeutic Category Antitoxin
Use Passive prevention and treatment of diphtheria
Usual Dosage Administer I.M. or slow I.V. infusion: Dosage varies with a range from 20,000 units to 120,000 units
Dosage Forms Injection: 500 units/mL (20 mL, 40 mL)

diphtheria, tetanus toxoids, and acellular pertussis vaccine

Brand Names Acel-Immune®; Tripedia®
Synonyms dtap
Therapeutic Category Toxoid
Use Fourth or fifth immunization of children 15 months to 7 years of age (prior to seventh birthday) who have been previously immunized with 3 or 4 doses of whole-cell pertussis DTP vaccine
Dosage Forms Injection:
Acel-Immune®: Diphtheria 7.5 Lf units, tetanus 5 Lf units, and acellular pertussis vaccine 40 mcg per 0.5 mL (7.5 mL)
Tripedia®: Diphtheria 6.7 Lf units, tetanus 5 Lf units, and acellular pertussis vaccine 46.8 mcg per 0.5 mL (7.5 mL)

dipivalyl epinephrine *see* dipivefrin hydrochloride *on this page*

dipivefrin hydrochloride (dye pi' ve frin)

Brand Names Propine® Ophthalmic
Synonyms dipivalyl epinephrine; dpe
Therapeutic Category Adrenergic Agonist Agent, Ophthalmic; Ophthalmic Agent, Vasoconstrictor
Use Reduce elevated intraocular pressure in chronic open-angle glaucoma; also used to treat ocular hypertension, low tension, and secondary glaucomas
Usual Dosage Adults: Ophthalmic: Initial: 1 drop every 12 hours
Dosage Forms Solution, ophthalmic: 0.1% (5 mL, 10 mL, 15 mL)

Diprivan® Injection *see* propofol *on page 393*
Diprolene® *see* betamethasone *on page 52*
Diprolene® AF *see* betamethasone *on page 52*
dipropylacetic acid *see* valproic acid and derivatives *on page 482*
Diprosone® *see* betamethasone *on page 52*

dipyridamole (dye peer id' a mole)

Brand Names Persantine®
Therapeutic Category Antiplatelet Agent; Vasodilator, Coronary
Use Maintain patency after surgical grafting procedures including coronary artery bypass; with warfarin to decrease thrombosis in patients after artificial heart valve replacement; for
(Continued)

dipyridamole *(Continued)*

chronic management of angina pectoris; with aspirin to prevent coronary artery thrombosis; in combination with aspirin or warfarin to prevent other thromboembolic disorders

Usual Dosage
Children: Oral: 3-6 mg/kg/day in 3 divided doses
Dipyridamole stress test (for evaluation of myocardial perfusion): I.V.: 0.14 mg/kg/minute for a total of 4 minutes
Adults: Oral: 75-400 mg/day in 3-4 divided doses

Dosage Forms
Injection: 10 mg/2 mL
Tablet: 25 mg, 50 mg, 75 mg

Disalcid® *see* salsalate *on page 417*

disalicylic acid *see* salsalate *on page 417*

Disanthrol® [OTC] *see* docusate and casanthranol *on page 154*

Discase® *see* chymopapain *on page 101*

Disobrom® [OTC] *see* dexbrompheniramine and pseudoephedrine *on page 132*

disodium cromoglycate *see* cromolyn sodium *on page 118*

***d*-isoephedrine hydrochloride** *see* pseudoephedrine *on page 397*

Disolan® [OTC] *see* docusate and phenolphthalein *on page 154*

Disonate® [OTC] *see* docusate *on next page*

Disophrol® Chrontabs® [OTC] *see* dexbrompheniramine and pseudoephedrine *on page 132*

disopyramide phosphate (dye soe peer' a mide)

Brand Names Norpace®
Therapeutic Category Antiarrhythmic Agent, Class Ia
Use Suppression and prevention of unifocal and multifocal premature, ventricular premature complexes, coupled ventricular tachycardia; also effective in the conversion of atrial fibrillation, atrial flutter, and paroxysmal atrial tachycardia to normal sinus rhythm and prevention of the reoccurrence of these arrhythmias after conversion by other methods

Usual Dosage Oral:
Children:
<1 year: 10-30 mg/kg/24 hours in 4 divided doses
1-4 years: 10-20 mg/kg/24 hours in 4 divided doses
4-12 years: 10-15 mg/kg/24 hours in 4 divided doses
12-18 years: 6-15 mg/kg/24 hours in 4 divided doses

Adults:
<50 kg: 100 mg every 6 hours or 200 mg every 12 hours (controlled release)
>50 kg: 150 mg every 6 hours or 300 mg every 12 hours (controlled release); if no response, may increase to 200 mg every 6 hours; maximum dose required for patients with severe refractory ventricular tachycardia is 400 mg every 6 hours

Dosage Forms
Capsule: 100 mg, 150 mg
Capsule, sustained action: 100 mg, 150 mg

Disotate® *see* edetate disodium *on page 163*

Di-Spaz® Injection *see* dicyclomine hydrochloride *on page 142*

Di-Spaz® Oral *see* dicyclomine hydrochloride *on page 142*

Dispos-a-Med® Isoproterenol *see* isoproterenol *on page 253*

disulfiram (dye sul' fi ram)

Brand Names Antabuse®
Therapeutic Category Aldehyde Dehydrogenase Inhibitor Agent; Antialcoholic Agent
Use Management of chronic alcoholics

Usual Dosage Maximum daily dose: 500 mg/day in a single dose for 1-2 weeks; average maintenance dose: 250 mg/day; range: 125-500 mg; duration of therapy is to continue until the patient is fully recovered socially and a basis for permanent self control has been established; maintenance therapy may be required for months or even years
Dosage Forms Tablet: 250 mg, 500 mg

dithioglycerol see dimercaprol on page 147
dithranol see anthralin on page 29
Ditropan® see oxybutynin chloride on page 342
Diucardin® see hydroflumethiazide on page 234
Diupres-250® see chlorothiazide and reserpine on page 92
Diupres-500® see chlorothiazide and reserpine on page 92
Diurigen® see chlorothiazide on page 92
Diuril® see chlorothiazide on page 92
Diutensin® see methyclothiazide and cryptenamine tannates on page 297
divalproex sodium see valproic acid and derivatives on page 482
Dizmiss® [OTC] see meclizine hydrochloride on page 282
dl-alpha tocopherol see vitamin e on page 490
dl-norephedrine hydrochloride see phenylpropanolamine hydrochloride on page 365
d-mannitol see mannitol on page 279
4-dmdr see idarubicin hydrochloride on page 241
D-Med® Injection see methylprednisolone on page 300
dmso see dimethyl sulfoxide on page 148
dnase see dornase alfa on page 156
dnr see daunorubicin hydrochloride on page 126

dobutamine hydrochloride (doe byoo' ta meen)
Brand Names Dobutrex® Injection
Therapeutic Category Adrenergic Agonist Agent
Use Short-term management of patients with cardiac decompensation
Usual Dosage I.V. infusion:
Neonates: 2-15 mcg/kg/minute, titrate to desired response

Children: 2.5-15 mcg/kg/minute, titrate to desired response

Adults: 2.5-15 mcg/kg/minute; maximum: 40 mcg/kg/minute, titrate to desired response
Dosage Forms Injection: 12.5 mg/mL (20 mL)

Dobutrex® Injection see dobutamine hydrochloride on this page
Docucal-P® [OTC] see docusate and phenolphthalein on next page

docusate (dok' yoo sate)
Brand Names Colace® [OTC]; Correctol® Extra Gentle [OTC]; DC 240® Softgel® [OTC]; Dialose® [OTC]; Diocto® [OTC]; Diocto-K® [OTC]; Dioeze® [OTC]; Disonate® [OTC]; DOK® [OTC]; DOS® Softgel® [OTC]; D-S-S® [OTC]; Kasof® [OTC]; Modane® Soft [OTC]; Pro-Cal-Sof® [OTC]; Regulax SS® [OTC]; Regutol® [OTC]; Silace® [OTC]; Sulfalax® [OTC]; Surfak® [OTC]
Synonyms doss; dss
Therapeutic Category Laxative, Surfactant; Stool Softener
Use Stool softener in patients who should avoid straining during defecation and constipation associated with hard, dry stools
(Continued)

docusate *(Continued)*

Usual Dosage Docusate salts are interchangeable; the amount of sodium, calcium, or potassium per dosage unit is clinically insignificant

Infants and Children <3 years: Oral: 10-40 mg/day in 1-4 divided doses

Children: Oral:
3-6 years: 20-60 mg/day in 1-4 divided doses
6-12 years: 40-150 mg/day in 1-4 divided doses

Adolescents and Adults: Oral: 50-500 mg/day in 1-4 divided doses

Older Children and Adults: Rectal: Add 50-100 mg of docusate liquid to enema fluid (saline or water); give as retention or flushing enema

Dosage Forms
Capsule, as calcium:
DC 240" Softgel", Pro-Cal-Sof", Sulfalax": 240 mg
Surfak": 50 mg, 240 mg
Capsule, as potassium:
Diocto-K": 100 mg
Kasof": 240 mg
Capsule, as sodium:
Colace": 50 mg, 100 mg
Correctol" Extra Gentle: 100 mg
Dioeze": 250 mg
Disonate": 100 mg, 240 mg
DOK": 100 mg, 250 mg
DOS" Softgel®: 100 mg, 250 mg
D-S-S": 100 mg
Modane" Soft: 100 mg
Regulax SS": 100 mg, 250 mg
Liquid, as sodium (Diocto®, Colace®, Disonate®, DOK®): 150 mg/15 mL (30 mL, 60 mL, 480 mL)
Syrup, as sodium:
50 mg/15 mL (15 mL, 30 mL)
Colace", Diocto", Disonate®, DOK®, Silace®: 60 mg/15 mL (240 mL, 480 mL, 3780 mL)
Tablet, as sodium (Dialose®, Regutol®): 100 mg

docusate and casanthranol

Brand Names Dialose® Plus Capsule [OTC]; Diocto C® [OTC]; Diocto-K Plus® [OTC]; Dioctolose Plus" [OTC]; Disanthrol® [OTC]; DSMC Plus® [OTC]; D-S-S Plus® [OTC]; Genasoft® Plus [OTC]; Peri-Colace® [OTC]; Pro-Sof® Plus [OTC]; Regulace® [OTC]; Silace-C® [OTC]
Synonyms casanthranol and docusate; dss with casanthranol
Therapeutic Category Laxative, Surfactant; Stool Softener
Use Treatment of constipation generally associated with dry, hard stools and decreased intestinal motility
Usual Dosage Oral:
Children: 5-15 mL of syrup at bedtime or 1 capsule at bedtime

Adults: 1-2 capsules or 15-30 mL syrup at bedtime, may be increased to 2 capsules or 30 mL twice daily or 3 capsules at bedtime
Dosage Forms
Capsule (Dialose" Plus, Diocto-K Plus", Dioctolose Plus®, DSMC Plus®): Docusate potassium 100 mg and casanthranol 30 mg
Capsule (Disanthrol", D-S-S Plus®, Genasoft® Plus, Peri-Colace®, Pro-Sof® Plus, Regulace®): Docusate sodium 100 mg and casanthranol 30 mg
Syrup (Diocto C", Peri-Colace®, Silace-C"): Docusate sodium 60 mg and casanthranol 30 mg per 15 mL (240 mL, 480 mL, 4000 mL)

docusate and phenolphthalein

Brand Names Colax" [OTC]; Correctol® [OTC]; Dialose® Plus Tablet [OTC]; Disolan® [OTC]; Docucal-P" [OTC]; Doxidan® [OTC]; Ex-Lax", Extra Gentle Pills [OTC]; Feen-a-Mint® Pills [OTC]; Femilax" [OTC]; Modane® Plus [OTC]; Phillips'® LaxCaps® [OTC]; Unilax® [OTC]

Therapeutic Category Laxative, Stimulant; Laxative, Surfactant; Stool Softener
Use Management of chronic functional constipation
Usual Dosage Oral:
　Children 6-12 years: 1 capsule daily given at bedtime for 2-3 nights until bowel movements
　　are normal

　Children >12 years and Adults: 1-2 capsules daily given at bedtime for 2-3 nights until bowel
　　movements are normal
Dosage Forms
　Capsule:
　　　Disolan®: Docusate sodium 100 mg and phenolphthalein 65 mg
　　　Docucal-P®, Doxidan®: Docusate calcium 60 mg and phenolphthalein 65 mg
　　　Ex-Lax®, Extra Gentle Pills: Docusate sodium 60 mg and phenolphthalein 65 mg
　　　Phillips'® LaxCaps®: Docusate sodium 83 mg and phenolphthalein 90 mg
　　　Unilax®: Docusate sodium 230 mg and phenolphthalein 130 mg
　Tablet:
　　　Colax®, Correctol®, Dialose® Plus, Feen-A-Mint® Pills, Femilax®, Modane® Plus: Docu-
　　　　sate sodium 100 mg and phenolphthalein 65 mg

DOK® [OTC] *see docusate on page 153*

Doktors® Nasal Solution [OTC] *see phenylephrine hydrochloride on page 364*

Dolacet® *see hydrocodone and acetaminophen on page 230*

Dolene® *see propoxyphene on page 393*

Dolobid® *see diflunisal on page 144*

Dolophine® Oral *see methadone hydrochloride on page 292*

Domeboro® [OTC] *see aluminum acetate and calcium acetate on page 15*

Donnamar® *see hyoscyamine sulfate on page 239*

Donnapectolin-PG® *see hyoscyamine, atropine, scopolamine, kaolin, pectin, and
opium on page 239*

Donnapine® *see hyoscyamine, atropine, scopolamine, and phenobarbital
on page 238*

Donna-Sed® *see hyoscyamine, atropine, scopolamine, and phenobarbital
on page 238*

Donnatal® *see hyoscyamine, atropine, scopolamine, and phenobarbital
on page 238*

Donnazyme® *see pancreatin on page 346*

dopamine hydrochloride (doe' pa meen)
　Brand Names Intropin® Injection
　Therapeutic Category Adrenergic Agonist Agent
　Use Adjunct in the treatment of shock which persists after adequate fluid volume replace-
　　ment; dose-related inotropic and vasopressor effects; stimulates dopaminergic, beta and
　　alpha receptors; increased renal blood flow at low to moderate doses
　Usual Dosage I.V. infusion:
　Neonates: 1-20 mcg/kg/minute continuous infusion, titrate to desired response

　Children: 1-20 mcg/kg/minute, maximum: 50 mcg/kg/minute continuous infusion, titrate to
　　desired response

　Adults: 1 mcg/kg/minute up to 50 mcg/kg/minute, titrate to desired response

　If dosages >20-30 mcg/kg/minute are needed, a more direct acting pressor may be more
　　beneficial (ie, epinephrine, norepinephrine)

　The hemodynamic effects of dopamine are dose-dependent:
　　　Low-dose: 1-5 mcg/kg/minute, increased renal blood flow and urine output
　　　Intermediate-dose: 5-15 mcg/kg/minute, increased renal blood flow, heart rate, cardiac
　　　　contractility, and cardiac output
(Continued)

dopamine hydrochloride *(Continued)*
High-dose: >15 mcg/kg/minute, alpha-adrenergic effects begin to predominate, vaso-constriction, increased blood pressure
Dosage Forms
Infusion, in D_5W: 0.8 mg/mL (250 mL, 500 mL); 1.6 mg/mL (250 mL, 500 mL); 3.2 mg/mL (250 mL, 500 mL)
Injection: 40 mg/mL (5 mL, 10 mL, 20 mL); 80 mg/mL (5 mL, 20 mL); 160 mg/mL (5 mL)

Dopar® *see* levodopa *on page 265*
Dopram® Injection *see* doxapram hydrochloride *on this page*
Doral® *see* quazepam *on page 402*
Dorcol® [OTC] *see* acetaminophen *on page 2*
Dormin® Oral [OTC] *see* diphenhydramine hydrochloride *on page 149*

dornase alfa *(door' nace al' fa)*
Brand Names Pulmozyme®
Synonyms dnase; recombinant human deoxyribonuclease
Therapeutic Category Enzyme
Use Management of cystic fibrosis patients to reduce the frequency of respiratory infections that require parenteral antibiotics, and to improve pulmonary function
Usual Dosage Children >5 years and Adults: Inhalation: 2.5 mg once daily through selected nebulizers in conjunction with a Pulmo-Aide® or a Pari-Proneb® compressor
Dosage Forms Solution, inhalation: 1 mg/mL (2.5 mL)

Doryx® Oral *see* doxycycline *on page 158*

dorzolamide *(dor zole' a mide)*
Brand Names Trusopt®
Therapeutic Category Carbonic Anhydrase Inhibitor
Use Lowers intraocular pressure to treat glaucoma
Dosage Forms Solution, ophthalmic: 2%

DOS® Softgel® [OTC] *see* docusate *on page 153*
doss *see* docusate *on page 153*
Dovonex® *see* calcipotriene *on page 65*

doxacurium chloride *(dox a kyoo' rium)*
Brand Names Nuromax® Injection
Therapeutic Category Neuromuscular Blocker Agent, Nondepolarizing
Use Doxacurium is indicated for use as an adjunct to general anesthesia. It provides skeletal muscle relaxation during surgery.
Usual Dosage I.V. (in obese patients, use ideal body weight to calculate dosage):
Children >2 years: Initial: 0.03-0.05 mg/kg followed by maintenance doses of 0.005-0.01 mg/kg after 30-45 minutes
Adults: Surgery: 0.05 mg/kg with thiopental/narcotic or 0.025 mg/kg with succinylcholine; maintenance dose: 0.005-0.01 mg/kg after 60-100 minutes
Dosage Forms Injection: 1 mg/mL (5 mL)

doxapram hydrochloride *(dox' a pram)*
Brand Names Dopram® Injection
Therapeutic Category Central Nervous System Stimulant, Nonamphetamine; Respiratory Stimulant
Use Respiratory and CNS stimulant

Usual Dosage I.V.:
Neonatal apnea (apnea of prematurity):
Initial: 0.5 mg/kg/hour
Maintenance: 0.5-2.5 mg/kg/hour, titrated to the lowest rate at which apnea is controlled

Adults: Respiratory depression following anesthesia:
Initial: 0.5-1 mg/kg; may repeat at 5-minute intervals; maximum total dose: 2 mg/kg; single doses should not exceed 1.5 mg/kg
I.V. infusion: Initial: 5 mg/minute until adequate response or adverse effects seen; decrease to 1-3 mg/minute; usual total dose: 0.5-4 mg/kg; maximum: 300 mg
Dosage Forms Injection: 20 mg/mL (20 mL)

doxazosin mesylate (dox ay' zoe sin)
Brand Names Cardura®
Therapeutic Category Alpha-Adrenergic Blocking Agent, Oral
Use Alpha-adrenergic blocking agent for treatment of hypertension
Usual Dosage Adults: Oral: 1 mg once daily, may be increased to 2 mg once daily thereafter up to 16 mg if needed
Dosage Forms Tablet: 1 mg, 2 mg, 4 mg, 8 mg

doxepin hydrochloride (dox' e pin)
Brand Names Adapin® Oral; Sinequan® Oral; Zonalon® Topical Cream
Therapeutic Category Antianxiety Agent; Antidepressant, Tricyclic
Use Treatment of various forms of depression, usually in conjunction with psychotherapy; treatment of anxiety disorders; analgesic for certain chronic and neuropathic pain
Usual Dosage Oral:
Adolescents: Initial: 25-50 mg/day in single or divided doses; gradually increase to 100 mg/day
Adults: Initial: 30-150 mg/day at bedtime or in 2-3 divided doses; may increase up to 300 mg/day; single dose should not exceed 150 mg; select patients may respond to 25-50 mg/day
Dosage Forms
Capsule: 10 mg, 25 mg, 50 mg, 75 mg, 100 mg, 150 mg
Concentrate, oral: 10 mg/mL (120 mL)
Cream: 5% (30 g)

Doxidan® [OTC] *see* docusate and phenolphthalein *on page 154*

doxorubicin hydrochloride (dox oh roo' bi sin)
Brand Names Adriamycin PFS™; Adriamycin RDF™; Rubex®
Synonyms adr; hydroxydaunomycin hydrochloride
Therapeutic Category Antineoplastic Agent, Antibiotic
Use Treatment of various solid tumors including ovarian, breast and bladder, various lymphomas and leukemias, soft tissue sarcomas, neuroblastoma, osteosarcoma
Usual Dosage I.V. (refer to individual protocols. Patient's ideal weight should be used to calculate body surface area):
Children: 35-75 mg/m^2 as a single dose, repeat every 21 days; or 20 mg/m^2 once weekly
Adults: 60-75 mg/m^2 as a single dose, repeat every 21 days or other dosage regimens like 20-30 mg/m^2/day for 2-3 days, repeat in 4 weeks or 20 mg/m^2 once weekly
The lower dose regimen should be given to patients with decreased bone marrow reserve, prior therapy or marrow infiltration with malignant cells
Dosage Forms
Injection:
Aqueous, with NS: 2 mg/mL (5 mL, 10 mL, 25 mL)
Preservative free: 2 mg/mL (5 mL, 10 mL, 25 mL, 100 mL)
Powder for injection, lyophilized: 10 mg, 20 mg, 50 mg, 100 mg
Powder for injection, lyophilized, rapid dissolution formula: 10 mg, 20 mg, 50 mg, 150 mg

Doxychel® Injection *see* doxycycline *on this page*

Doxychel® Oral *see* doxycycline *on this page*

doxycycline (dox i sye' kleen)

Brand Names Bio-Tab™ Oral; Doryx™ Oral; Doxychel® Injection; Doxychel® Oral; Doxy® Oral; Monodox™ Oral; Vibramycin® Injection; Vibramycin® Oral; Vibra-Tabs®

Therapeutic Category Antibiotic, Tetracycline Derivative

Use Principally in the treatment of infections caused by susceptible *Rickettsia, Chlamydia,* and *Mycoplasma* along with uncommon susceptible gram-negative and gram-positive organisms

Usual Dosage Oral, I.V.:

Children ≥8 years: 2-4 mg/kg/day in 1-2 divided doses, not to exceed 200 mg/day

Adults: 100-200 mg/day in 1-2 divided doses

Dosage Forms

Capsule, as hyclate:

Doxychel™, Monodox™, Vibramycin®: 50 mg

Doxy™, Doxychel™, Monodox®, Vibramycin®: 100 mg

Capsule, coated pellets, as hyclate (Doryx®): 100 mg

Powder for injection, as hyclate (Doxy®, Doxychel®, Vibramycin® IV): 100 mg, 200 mg

Powder for oral suspension, as monohydrate (raspberry flavor) (Vibramycin®): 25 mg/5 mL (60 mL)

Syrup, as calcium (raspberry-apple flavor) (Vibramycin®): 50 mg/5 mL (30 mL, 473 mL)

Tablet, as hyclate

Doxychel™: 50 mg

Bio-Tab™, Doxychel™, Vibra-Tabs™: 100 mg

Doxy® Oral *see* doxycycline *on this page*

dpa *see* valproic acid and derivatives *on page 482*

dpe *see* dipivefrin hydrochloride *on page 151*

d-penicillamine *see* penicillamine *on page 352*

dph *see* phenytoin *on page 366*

dppc *see* colfosceril palmitate *on page 113*

dpt *see* diphtheria and tetanus toxoids and pertussis vaccine, adsorbed *on page 150*

Dramamine® Oral [OTC] *see* dimenhydrinate *on page 147*

Dramamine® II [OTC] *see* meclizine hydrochloride *on page 282*

Dramilin® Injection *see* dimenhydrinate *on page 147*

Dramoject® Injection *see* dimenhydrinate *on page 147*

Dri-Ear® Otic [OTC] *see* boric acid *on page 57*

Drisdol® Oral *see* ergocalciferol *on page 169*

Dristan® Allergy [OTC] *see* brompheniramine and pseudoephedrine *on page 59*

Dristan® Long Lasting Nasal Solution [OTC] *see* oxymetazoline hydrochloride *on page 343*

Drithocreme® *see* anthralin *on page 29*

Dritho-Scalp® *see* anthralin *on page 29*

Drixoral® Cough & Congestion Liquid Caps [OTC] *see* pseudoephedrine and dextromethorphan *on page 398*

Drixoral® Cough & Sore Throat Liquid Caps [OTC] *see* acetaminophen and dextromethorphan *on page 3*

Drixoral® Non-Drowsy [OTC] *see* pseudoephedrine *on page 397*

Drixoral® [OTC] *see* dexbrompheniramine and pseudoephedrine *on page 132*

Drixoral® Cough Liquid Caps [OTC] *see* dextromethorphan hydrobromide
on page 135

Drize® *see* chlorpheniramine and phenylpropanolamine *on page 94*

dronabinol (droe nab' i nol)
Brand Names Marinol®
Synonyms tetrahydrocannabinol; thc
Therapeutic Category Antiemetic
Use When conventional antiemetics fail to relieve the nausea and vomiting associated with cancer chemotherapy
Usual Dosage Oral:
Children: NCI protocol recommends 5 mg/m² starting 6-8 hours before chemotherapy and every 4-6 hours after to be continued for 12 hours after chemotherapy is discontinued

Adults: 5 mg/m² 1-3 hours before chemotherapy, then give 5 mg/m²/dose every 2-4 hours after chemotherapy for a total of 4-6 doses/day; dose may be increased up to a maximum of 15 mg/m²/dose if needed (dosage may be increased by 2.5 mg/m² increments)
Dosage Forms Capsule: 2.5 mg, 5 mg, 10 mg

droperidol (droe per' i dole)
Brand Names Inapsine®
Therapeutic Category Antiemetic; Antipsychotic Agent
Use Tranquilizer and antiemetic in surgical and diagnostic procedures; antiemetic for cancer chemotherapy; preoperative medication
Usual Dosage Titrate carefully to desired effect
Children 2-12 years:
Premedication: I.M.: 0.088-0.165 mg/kg; smaller doses may be sufficient for control of nausea or vomiting
Adjunct to general anesthesia: I.V. induction: 0.088-0.165 mg/kg
Nausea and vomiting: I.M., I.V.: 0.05-0.06 mg/kg/dose every 4-6 hours as needed
Adults:
Premedication: I.M., I.V.: 2.5-10 mg 30 minutes to 1 hour preoperatively
Adjunct to general anesthesia: I.V. induction: 0.22-0.275 mg/kg; maintenance: 1.25-2.5 mg/dose
Alone in diagnostic procedures: I.M.: Initial: 2.5-10 mg 30 minutes to 1 hour before; then 1.25-2.5 mg if needed
Nausea and vomiting: I.M., I.V.: 2.5-5 mg/dose every 3-4 hours as needed
Dosage Forms Injection: 2.5 mg/mL (1 mL, 2 mL, 5 mL, 10 mL)

droperidol and fentanyl
Brand Names Innovar®
Synonyms fentanyl and droperidol
Therapeutic Category Analgesic, Narcotic
Use Produce and maintain analgesia and sedation during diagnostic or surgical procedures (neuroleptanalgesia and neuroleptanesthesia); adjunct to general anesthesia
Usual Dosage
Children:
Premedication: I.M.: 0.03 mL/kg 30-60 minutes prior to surgery
Adjunct to general anesthesia: I.V.: Total dose: 0.05 mL/kg as slow infusion (1 mL/1-2 minutes) until sleep occurs
Adults:
Premedication: I.M.: 0.5-2 mL 30-60 minutes prior to surgery
Adjunct to general anesthesia: I.V.: 0.09-0.11 mL/kg as slow infusion (1 mL/1-2 minutes) until sleep occurs
Dosage Forms Injection: Droperidol 2.5 mg and fentanyl 50 mcg per mL (2 mL, 5 mL)

Drotic® Otic *see* neomycin, polymyxin b, and hydrocortisone *on page 323*

Dr Scholl's® Athlete's Foot [OTC] *see* tolnaftate *on page 464*

Dr Scholl's® Cracked Heel Relief Cream [OTC] *see* lidocaine hydrochloride *on page 267*

Dr Scholl's® Maximum Strength Tritin [OTC] *see* tolnaftate *on page 464*

Drysol™ *see* aluminum chloride hexahydrate *on page 15*

dscg *see* cromolyn sodium *on page 118*

DSMC Plus® [OTC] *see* docusate and casanthranol *on page 154*

dss *see* docusate *on page 153*

D-S-S Plus® [OTC] *see* docusate and casanthranol *on page 154*

D-S-S® [OTC] *see* docusate *on page 153*

dss with casanthranol *see* docusate and casanthranol *on page 154*

dt *see* diphtheria and tetanus toxoid *on page 150*

dtap *see* diphtheria, tetanus toxoids, and acellular pertussis vaccine *on page 151*

DTIC-Dome® *see* dacarbazine *on page 123*

dto *see* opium tincture *on page 338*

***d*-tubocurarine chloride** *see* tubocurarine chloride *on page 477*

Duadacin® Capsule [OTC] *see* chlorpheniramine, phenylpropanolamine, and acetaminophen *on page 96*

Dulcagen® [OTC] *see* bisacodyl *on page 54*

Dulcolax® [OTC] *see* bisacodyl *on page 54*

Dull-C® [OTC] *see* ascorbic acid *on page 34*

DuoCet™ *see* hydrocodone and acetaminophen *on page 230*

Duo-Cyp® Injection *see* estradiol and testosterone *on page 174*

Duofilm® Solution *see* salicylic acid and lactic acid *on page 416*

Duo-Medihaler® Aerosol *see* isoproterenol and phenylephrine *on page 253*

Duo-Trach® *see* lidocaine hydrochloride *on page 267*

Duotrate® *see* pentaerythritol tetranitrate *on page 355*

Duphalac® *see* lactulose *on page 261*

Duplex® T [OTC] *see* coal tar *on page 110*

Durabolin® Injection *see* nandrolone *on page 318*

Dura-Estrin® Injection *see* estradiol *on page 173*

Duragen® Injection *see* estradiol *on page 173*

Duragesic™ Transdermal *see* fentanyl citrate *on page 188*

Dura-Gest® *see* guaifenesin, phenylpropanolamine, and phenylephrine *on page 217*

Duralex® *see* chlorpheniramine and pseudoephedrine *on page 94*

Duralone® Injection *see* methylprednisolone *on page 300*

Duralutin® Injection *see* hydroxyprogesterone caproate *on page 236*

Duramorph® Injection *see* morphine sulfate *on page 311*

Duranest® Injection *see* etidocaine hydrochloride *on page 182*

Dura-Tap/PD® *see* chlorpheniramine and pseudoephedrine *on page 94*

Duratest® Injection *see* testosterone *on page 449*

Duratestrin® Injection *see* estradiol and testosterone *on page 174*

Durathate® Injection *see* testosterone *on page 449*

Duration® Nasal Solution [OTC] *see* oxymetazoline hydrochloride *on page 343*

Dura-Vent® *see* guaifenesin and phenylpropanolamine *on page 215*

Duricef® *see* cefadroxil monohydrate *on page 79*

Durrax® *see* hydroxyzine *on page 237*

Duvoid® *see* bethanechol chloride *on page 53*

DV® Vaginal Cream *see* dienestrol *on page 143*

d-xylose
Brand Names Xylo-Pfan® [OTC]
Synonyms wood sugar
Therapeutic Category Diagnostic Agent, Intestinal Absorption
Use Evaluating intestinal absorption and diagnosing malabsorptive states
Usual Dosage Oral:
Infants and young Children: 500 mg/kg as a 5% to 10% aqueous solution

Children: 5 g is dissolved in 250 mL water; additional fluids are permitted and are encouraged for children

Adults: 25 g dissolved in 200-300 mL water followed with an additional 200-400 mL water **or** 5 g dissolved in 200-300 mL water followed by an additional 200-400 mL water
Dosage Forms Powder for oral solution: 25 g

Dyazide® *see* hydrochlorothiazide and triamterene *on page 229*

Dycill® *see* dicloxacillin sodium *on page 141*

Dyclone® *see* dyclonine hydrochloride *on this page*

dyclonine hydrochloride (dye' kloe neen)
Brand Names Dyclone®; Sucrets® [OTC]
Therapeutic Category Local Anesthetic, Oral
Use Local anesthetic prior to laryngoscopy, bronchoscopy, or endotracheal intubation; use topically for temporary relief of pain associated with oral mucosa, skin, episiotomy, or anogenital lesions
Usual Dosage Children and Adults: Topical solution:
Mouth sores: 5-10 mL of 0.5% or 1% to oral mucosa (swab or swish and then spit) 3-4 times/day as needed; maximum single dose: 200 mg (40 mL of 0.5% solution or 20 mL of 1% solution)

Bronchoscopy: Use 2 mL of the 1% solution or 4 mL of the 0.5% solution sprayed onto the larynx and trachea every 5 minutes until the reflex has been abolished

Children >3 years and Adults: Lozenge: Dissolve 1 in mouth slowly every 2 hours
Dosage Forms
Lozenges: 1.2 mg, 3 mg
Solution, topical: 0.5% (30 mL); 1% (30 mL)

Dyflex® *see* dyphylline *on this page*

dyflos *see* isoflurophate *on page 252*

Dymelor® *see* acetohexamide *on page 6*

Dymenate® Injection *see* dimenhydrinate *on page 147*

Dynacin® Oral *see* minocycline hydrochloride *on page 307*

DynaCirc® *see* isradipine *on page 255*

Dyna-Hex® Topical [OTC] *see* chlorhexidine gluconate *on page 90*

Dynapen® *see* dicloxacillin sodium *on page 141*

dyphylline (dye' fi lin)
Brand Names Dilor®; Dyflex®; Lufyllin®; Neothylline®
Synonyms dihydroxypropyl theophylline
Therapeutic Category Bronchodilator; Theophylline Derivative
(Continued)
161

dyphylline *(Continued)*

Use Bronchodilator in reversible airway obstruction due to asthma or COPD
Usual Dosage
Children: I.M.: 4.4-6.6 mg/kg/day in divided doses

Adults:
Oral: Up to 15 mg/kg 4 times/day, individualize dosage
I.M.: 250-500 mg, do not exceed total dosage of 15 mg/kg every 6 hours
Dosage Forms
Elixir:
Lufyllin": 100 mg/15 mL with alcohol 20% (473 mL, 3780 mL)
Dilor": 160 mg/15 mL with alcohol 18% (473 mL)
Injection (Dilor", Lufyllin"): 250 mg/mL (2 mL)
Tablet: 200 mg, 400 mg
Dilor", Dyflex", Lufyllin", Neothylline®: 200 mg, 400 mg

Dyrenium® *see* triamterene *on page 468*

Easprin® *see* aspirin *on page 35*

echothiophate iodide (ek oh thye' oh fate)

Brand Names Phospholine Iodide" Ophthalmic
Synonyms ecostigmine iodide
Therapeutic Category Ophthalmic Agent, Miotic
Use Reverse toxic CNS effects caused by anticholinergic drugs; used as miotic in treatment of glaucoma
Usual Dosage Adults: Ophthalmic: Glaucoma: Instill 1 drop twice daily into eyes with one dose just prior to bedtime; some patients have been treated with 1 dose/day or every other day. Use lowest concentration and frequency which gives satisfactory response, with a maximum dose of 0.125% once daily, although more intensive therapy may be used for short periods of time
Dosage Forms Powder for reconstitution, ophthalmic: 1.5 mg [0.03%] (5 mL); 3 mg [0.06%] (5 mL); 6.25 mg [0.125%] (5 mL); 12.5 mg [0.25%] (5 mL)

econazole nitrate (e kone' a zole)

Brand Names Spectazole™ Topical
Therapeutic Category Antifungal Agent, Topical
Use Topical treatment of tinea pedis, tinea cruris, tinea corporis, tinea versicolor, and cutaneous candidiasis
Usual Dosage Children and Adults: Topical: Apply a sufficient amount to cover affected areas once daily; for cutaneous candidiasis: apply twice daily; candidal infections and tinea cruris, versicolor, and corporis should be treated for 2 weeks and tinea pedis for 1 month; occasionally, longer treatment periods may be required
Dosage Forms Cream: 1% (15 g, 30 g, 85 g)

Econopred® Ophthalmic *see* prednisolone *on page 383*

Econopred® Plus Ophthalmic *see* prednisolone *on page 383*

ecostigmine iodide *see* echothiophate iodide *on this page*

Ecotrin® [OTC] *see* aspirin *on page 35*

edathamil disodium *see* edetate disodium *on next page*

Edecrin® Oral *see* ethacrynic acid *on page 176*

Edecrin® Sodium Injection *see* ethacrynic acid *on page 176*

edetate calcium disodium (ed' e tate)

Brand Names Calcium Disodium Versenate"
Synonyms calcium edta
Therapeutic Category Antidote, Lead Toxicity

Use Treatment of acute and chronic lead poisoning; also used as an aid in the diagnosis of lead poisoning

Usual Dosage I.M., I.V.:

Children:

Diagnosis of lead poisoning: Mobilization test: (Asymptomatic patients or lead levels <55 mcg/dL): (**Note:** Urine is collected for 24 hours after first EDTA dose and analyzed for lead content; if the ratio of mcg of lead in urine to mg calcium EDTA given is >1, then test is considered positive): Children: 500 mg/m^2 (maximum: 1 g/dose) I.M. or I.V. over 1 hour **or** 2 doses of 500 mg/m^2 at 12-hour intervals

Asymptomatic lead poisoning: (Blood lead concentration >55 mcg/dL or blood lead concentrations of 25-55 mcg/dL with blood erythrocyte protoporphyrin concentrations of ≥35 mcg/dL and positive mobilization test) or symptomatic lead poisoning without encephalopathy with lead level <100 mcg/dL: 1 g/m^2/day I.M./I.V. in divided doses every 8-12 hours for 3-5 days (usually 5 days); maximum: 1 g/24 hours or 50 mg/kg/day

Symptomatic lead poisoning with encephalopathy with lead level >100 mcg/dL (treatment with calcium EDTA and dimercaprol is preferred): 250 mg/m^2 I.M. or intermittent I.V. infusion 4 hours after dimercaprol, then at 4-hour intervals thereafter for 5 days (1.5 g/m^2/day); dose (1.5 g/m^2/day) can also be given as a single I.V. continuous infusion over 12-24 hours/day for 5 days; maximum: 1 g/24 hours or 75 mg/kg/day

Note: Course of therapy may be repeated in 2-3 weeks until blood lead level is normal

Adults:

Diagnosis of lead poisoning: 500 mg/m^2 (maximum: 1 g/dose) over 1 hour

Treatment: 2 g/day or 1.5 g/m^2/day in divided doses every 12-24 hours for 5 days; may repeat course one time after at least 2 days (usually after 2 weeks)

Dosage Forms Injection: 200 mg/mL (5 mL)

edetate disodium (ed' e tate)

Brand Names Chealamide®; Disotate®; Endrate®

Synonyms edathamil disodium; edta; sodium edetate

Therapeutic Category Antidote, Hypercalcemia; Chelating Agent, Parenteral

Use Emergency treatment of hypercalcemia; control digitalis-induced cardiac dysrhythmias (ventricular arrhythmias)

Usual Dosage I.V.:

Hypercalcemia:

Children: 40-70 mg/kg slow infusion over 3-4 hours

Adults: 50 mg/kg/day over 3 or more hours

Dysrhythmias: Children and Adults: 15 mg/kg/hour up to 60 mg/kg/day

Dosage Forms Injection: 150 mg/mL (20 mL)

edrophonium chloride (ed roe foe' nee um)

Brand Names Enlon®; Reversol®; Tensilon®

Therapeutic Category Antidote, Neuromuscular Blocking Agent; Cholinergic Agent; Diagnostic Agent, Myasthenia Gravis

Use Diagnosis and differentiation of myasthenia gravis; to reverse nondepolarizing neuromuscular blockers; treatment of paroxysmal atrial tachycardia; a curare antagonist, also used for curare overdose to treat respiratory depression, reverses neuromuscular block produced by curare

Usual Dosage

Infants: I.V.: Initial: 0.1 mg, followed by 0.4 mg if no response; total dose: 0.5 mg

Children:

Diagnosis: Initial: 0.04 mg/kg followed by 0.16 mg/kg if no response, to a maximum total dose of 5 mg for children ≤34 kg, or 10 mg for children >34 kg

Titration of oral anticholinesterase therapy: 0.04 mg/kg once; if strength improves, an increase in neostigmine or pyridostigmine dose is indicated

Adults:

Diagnosis: I.V.: 2 mg test dose administered over 15-30 seconds; 8 mg given 45 seconds later if no response is seen. Test dose may be repeated after 30 minutes.

(Continued)

edrophonium chloride (Continued)

Titration of oral anticholinesterase therapy: 1-2 mg given 1 hour after oral dose of anticholinesterase; if strength improves, an increase in neostigmine or pyridostigmine dose is indicated

Differentiation of cholinergic from myasthenic crisis: I.V.: 1 mg, may repeat after 1 minute (**Note:** Intubation and controlled ventilation may be required if patient has cholinergic crises.)

Reversal of nondepolarizing neuromuscular blocking agents (neostigmine with atropine usually preferred): I.V.: 10 mg, may repeat every 5-10 minutes up to 40 mg

Termination of paroxysmal atrial tachycardia: I.V.: 5-10 mg

Dosage Forms Injection: 10 mg/mL (1 mL, 10 mL, 15 mL)

ED-SPAZ® see hyoscyamine sulfate on page 239

edta see edetate disodium on previous page

E.E.S.® Oral see erythromycin on page 170

Effer-K™ see potassium bicarbonate and potassium citrate, effervescent on page 377

Effer-Syllium® [OTC] see psyllium on page 398

Effexor® see venlafaxine on page 485

Efidac/24® [OTC] see pseudoephedrine on page 397

eflornithine hydrochloride (ee flor' ni theen)

Brand Names Ornidyl'' Injection

Synonyms dfmo

Therapeutic Category Antiprotozoal

Use Treatment of meningoencephalitic stage of *Trypanosoma brucei gambiense* infection (sleeping sickness)

Usual Dosage I.V. infusion: 100 mg/kg/dose given every 6 hours (over 45 minutes) for 14 days

Dosage Forms Injection, concentrate: 200 mg/mL (100 mL)

Efodine® [OTC] see povidone-iodine on page 380

Efudex® Topical see fluorouracil on page 198

ehdp see etidronate disodium on page 182

Elase-Chloromycetin® Topical see fibrinolysin and desoxyribonuclease on page 191

Elase® Topical see fibrinolysin and desoxyribonuclease on page 191

Elavil® see amitriptyline hydrochloride on page 22

Eldepryl® see selegiline hydrochloride on page 420

Eldopaque Forte® see hydroquinone on page 235

Eldopaque® [OTC] see hydroquinone on page 235

Eldoquin® Forte® see hydroquinone on page 235

Eldoquin® [OTC] see hydroquinone on page 235

electrolyte lavage solution see polyethylene glycol-electrolyte solution on page 375

Elimite™ Cream see permethrin on page 359

Elixicon® see theophylline on page 453

Elixophyllin® see theophylline on page 453

Elocon® Topical see mometasone furoate on page 310

E-Lor® see propoxyphene and acetaminophen on page 393

Elspar® see asparaginase on page 35

Eltroxin® *see* levothyroxine sodium *on page 266*

Emcyt® *see* estramustine phosphate sodium *on page 174*

Emecheck® [OTC] *see* phosphorated carbohydrate solution *on page 367*

Emetrol® [OTC] *see* phosphorated carbohydrate solution *on page 367*

Emgel™ *see* erythromycin, topical *on page 172*

Eminase® *see* anistreplase *on page 28*

Emko® [OTC] *see* nonoxynol 9 *on page 331*

EMLA® Topical *see* lidocaine and prilocaine *on page 267*

Empirin® [OTC] *see* aspirin *on page 35*

Empirin® With Codeine *see* aspirin and codeine *on page 36*

Emulsoil® [OTC] *see* castor oil *on page 78*

E-Mycin® Oral *see* erythromycin *on page 170*

enalapril (e nal' a pril)

Brand Names Vasotec® I.V.; Vasotec® Oral

Synonyms enalaprilat

Therapeutic Category Angiotensin-Converting Enzyme (ACE) Inhibitors

Use Management of mild to severe hypertension and congestive heart failure

Usual Dosage Use lower listed initial dose in patients with hyponatremia, hypovolemia, severe congestive heart failure, decreased renal function, or in those receiving diuretics

Children:

Investigational initial oral doses of enalapril of 0.1 mg/kg/day increasing over 2 weeks to 0.12-0.43 mg/kg/day have been used to treat severe congestive heart failure in infants (n=8)

Investigational I.V. doses of enalaprilat of 5-10 mcg/kg/dose administered every 8-24 hours (as determined by blood pressure readings) have been used for the treatment of neonatal hypertension (n=10); monitor patients carefully; select patients may require higher doses

Adults:

Oral: **Enalapril**: 2.5-5 mg/day then increase as required, usually 10-40 mg/day in 1-2 divided doses

I.V.: **Enalaprilat**: 0.625-1.25 mg/dose, given over 5 minutes every 6 hours

Dosage Forms

Injection, as enalaprilat: 1.25 mg/mL (1 mL, 2 mL)

Tablet, as maleate: 2.5 mg, 5 mg, 10 mg, 20 mg

enalapril and hydrochlorothiazide

Brand Names Vaseretic® 10-25

Therapeutic Category Antihypertensive, Combination

Use Treatment of hypertension

Dosage Forms Tablet: Enalapril maleate 10 mg and hydrochlorothiazide 25 mg

enalaprilat *see* enalapril *on this page*

encainide hydrochloride (en kay' nide)

Brand Names Enkaid®

Therapeutic Category Antiarrhythmic Agent, Class Ic

Use Ventricular arrhythmias; supraventricular arrhythmias

Usual Dosage Adults: Oral: 25 mg every 8 hours; may increase to 35 mg every 8 hours after 3-5 days if needed; increase to 50 mg every 8 hours in another 3-5 days if response is not achieved

Dosage Forms Capsule: 25 mg, 35 mg, 50 mg

Encare® **[OTC]** *see* nonoxynol 9 *on page 331*
Endep® *see* amitriptyline hydrochloride *on page 22*
End Lice® **[OTC]** *see* pyrethrins *on page 400*
Endolor® *see* butalbital compound *on page 63*
Endrate® *see* edetate disodium *on page 163*
Enduron® *see* methyclothiazide *on page 297*
Enduronyl® *see* methyclothiazide and deserpidine *on page 298*
Enduronyl® Forte *see* methyclothiazide and deserpidine *on page 298*
Enecat® *see* radiological/contrast media (ionic) *on page 404*
Ener-B® **[OTC]** *see* cyanocobalamin *on page 119*

enflurane (en' floo rane)
  Brand Names Ethrane®
  Therapeutic Category General Anesthetic
  Use General induction and maintenance of anesthesia (inhalation)
  Usual Dosage 0.5% to 3%
  Dosage Forms Liquid: 125 mL, 250 mL

Engerix-B® *see* hepatitis b vaccine *on page 224*
Enisyl® **[OTC]** *see* l-lysine hydrochloride *on page 271*
Enkaid® *see* encainide hydrochloride *on previous page*
Enlon® *see* edrophonium chloride *on page 163*
Enomine® *see* guaifenesin, phenylpropanolamine, and phenylephrine *on page 217*
Enovid® *see* mestranol and norethynodrel *on page 290*
Enovil® *see* amitriptyline hydrochloride *on page 22*

enoxacin (en ox' a sin)
  Brand Names Penetrex™ Oral
  Therapeutic Category Antibiotic, Quinolone
  Use Complicated and uncomplicated urinary tract infections caused by susceptible gram-negative and gram-positive bacteria
  Usual Dosage Adults: Oral: 400 mg twice daily
  Dosage Forms Tablet: 200 mg, 400 mg

enoxaparin sodium (e nox ah pair' in)
  Brand Names Lovenox® Injection
  Therapeutic Category Anticoagulant
  Use Prophylaxis and treatment of thromboembolic disorders (deep vein thrombosis)
  Usual Dosage Adults: S.C.: 30 mg twice daily
  Dosage Forms Injection, preservative free: 30 mg/0.3 mL

E.N.T.® *see* brompheniramine and phenylpropanolamine *on page 59*
Entex® *see* guaifenesin, phenylpropanolamine, and phenylephrine *on page 217*
Entex® LA *see* guaifenesin and phenylpropanolamine *on page 215*
Entex® PSE *see* guaifenesin and pseudoephedrine *on page 216*
Entrobar® *see* radiological/contrast media (ionic) *on page 404*
Enulose® *see* lactulose *on page 261*
Enzone® *see* pramoxine and hydrocortisone *on page 381*
epeg *see* etoposide *on page 183*

ephedrine sulfate (e fed' rin)
Brand Names Kondon's Nasal® [OTC]; Pretz-D® [OTC]
Therapeutic Category Adrenergic Agonist Agent
Use Bronchial asthma; nasal congestion; acute bronchospasm; acute hypotensive states
Usual Dosage
Children: Oral, I.V., S.C.: 3 mg/kg/day or 100 mg/m²/day divided into 4-6 doses

Adults:
Oral: 25-50 mg every 3-4 hours as needed
I.M., I.V., S.C.: 25-50 mg
Dosage Forms
Capsule: 25 mg, 50 mg
Injection: 25 mg/mL (1 mL); 50 mg/mL (1 mL, 10 mL)
Jelly (Kondon's Nasal®): 1% (20 g)
Spray (Pretz-D®): 0.25% (15 mL)

Epi-C® *see radiological/contrast media (ionic) on page 404*

Epifrin® *see epinephrine on this page*

E-Pilo-x® Ophthalmic *see pilocarpine and epinephrine on page 369*

Epinal® *see epinephrine on this page*

epinephrine (ep i nef' rin)
Brand Names Adrenalin®; AsthmaHaler®; AsthmaNefrin® [OTC]; Bronitin®; Bronkaid® Mist [OTC]; Epifrin®; Epinal®; EpiPen®; EpiPen® Jr; Eppy/N®; Glaucon®; Medihaler-Epi®; microNefrin®; Primatene® Mist [OTC]; Sus-Phrine®; Vaponefrin®
Synonyms adrenaline
Therapeutic Category Adrenergic Agonist Agent; Antidote, Hypersensitivity Reactions; Bronchodilator
Use Bronchospasms; anaphylactic reactions; cardiac arrest; management of open-angle (chronic simple) glaucoma
Usual Dosage
Neonates: Cardiac arrest: I.V. or intratracheal: 0.01-0.03 mg/kg (0.1-0.3 mL/kg 1:10,000 solution) every 3-5 minutes as needed

Children:
Bronchodilator: S.C.: 10 mcg/kg (single doses not to exceed 0.5 mg); injection suspension (1:200): 0.005 mL/kg/dose to a maximum of 0.15 mL every 8-12 hours
Cardiac arrest: I.V. or intratracheal: 0.01 mg/kg (0.1 mL/kg) of 1:10,000 solution (to maximum 5 mL) every 3-5 minutes as needed; infusion rate 0.1-4 mcg/kg/minute.
Refractory hypotension (refractory to dopamine/dobutamine): Start infusion 0.1 mcg/kg/minute, titrate to desired effect
Hypersensitivity reaction: S.C.: 0.01 mg/kg every 15 minutes for 2 doses then every 4 hours as needed (single doses not to exceed 0.5 mg)
Nebulization (racemic epinephrine):
<10 kg: 2 mL of 1:8 dilution over 15 minutes every 1-4 hours
10-15 kg: 2 mL of 1:6 dilution over 15 minutes every 1-4 hours
15-20 kg: 2 mL of 1:4 dilution over 15 minutes every 1-4 hours
>20 kg: 2 mL of 1:3 dilution over 15 minutes every 1-4 hours

Adults:
Bronchodilator:
I.M., S.C.: 0.1-0.5 mg every 10-15 minutes
I.V.: 0.1-0.25 mg (single dose maximum 1 mg)
Cardiac arrest: I.V., intracardiac: 0.1-1 mg every 5 minutes as needed; intratracheal: 1 mg
Hypersensitivity reaction: I.M., S.C.: 0.2-0.5 mg every 20 minutes to 4 hours (single dose maximum 1 mg)
Ophthalmic: Instill 1-2 drops in eye(s) once or twice daily
Dosage Forms
Aerosol, oral:
Bitartrate (AsthmaHaler®, Bronitin®, Medihaler-Epi®, Primatene® Suspension): 0.3 mg/spray [epinephrine base 0.16 mg/spray] (10 mL, 15 mL, 22.5 mL)
(Continued)

167

epinephrine *(Continued)*

      Bronkaid": 0.5% (10 mL, 15 mL, 22.5 mL)
      Primatene": 0.2 mg/spray (15 mL, 22.5 mL)
    Auto-injector:
      EpiPen": Delivers 0.3 mg I.M. of epinephrine 1:1000 (2 mL)
      EpiPen" Jr.: Delivers 0.15 mg I.M. of epinephrine 1:2000 (2 mL)
    Solution:
      Inhalation:
        Adrenalin": 1% [10 mg/mL, 1:100] (7.5 mL)
        AsthmaNefrin", microNefrin", Nephron®: Racepinephrine 2% [epinephrine base 1.125%] (7.5 mL, 15 mL, 30 mL)
        Vaponefrin'": Racepinephrine 2% [epinephrine base 1%] (15 mL, 30 mL)
      Injection:
        Adrenalin'": 0.01 mg/mL [1:100,000] (5 mL); 0.1 mg/mL [1:10,000] (3 mL, 10 mL); 1 mg/mL [1:1000] (1 mL, 2 mL, 30 mL)
        Suspension (Sus-Phrine'"): 5 mg/mL [1:200] (0.3 mL, 5 mL)
        Nasal (Adrenalin"): 0.1% [1 mg/mL, 1:1000] (30 mL)
        Ophthalmic, as borate (Epinal'", Eppy/N®): 0.5% (7.5 mL); 1% (7.5 mL); 2% (7.5 mL)
        Ophthalmic, as hydrochloride (Epifrin'", Glaucon®): 0.1% (1 mL, 30 mL); 0.25% (15 mL); 0.5% (15 mL); 1% (1 mL, 10 mL, 15 mL); 2% (10 mL, 15 mL)
        Topical (Adrenalin"): 0.1% [1 mg/mL, 1:1000] (30 mL, 10 mL)

EpiPen® *see epinephrine on previous page*

EpiPen® Jr *see epinephrine on previous page*

Epitol'® *see carbamazepine on page 73*

epo *see epoetin alfa on this page*

epoetin alfa (e poe' e tin al' fa)

Brand Names Epogen"; Procrit"
Synonyms epo; erythropoietin; rhuepo-α
Therapeutic Category Recombinant Human Erythropoietin
Use Treatment of anemia associated with chronic renal failure; anemia related to therapy with AZT-treated HIV-infected patients; anemia of prematurity
Usual Dosage

    In patients on dialysis epoetin alfa usually has been administered as an I.V. bolus 3 times/week. While the administration is independent of the dialysis procedure, it may be administered into the venous line at the end of the dialysis procedure to obviate the need for additional venous access; in patients with CRF not on dialysis, epoetin alfa may be given either as an I.V. or S.C. injection.

    AZT-treated HIV-infected patients: I.V., S.C.: Initial: 100 units/kg/dose 3 times/week for 8 weeks; after 8 weeks of therapy the dose can be adjusted by 50-100 units/kg increments 3 times/week to a maximum dose of 300 units/kg 3 times/week; if the hematocrit exceeds 40%, the dose should be discontinued until the hematocrit drops to 36%

    Anemia of prematurity: S.C.: 25-100 units/kg/dose 3 times/week
Dosage Forms Injection, preservative free: 2000 units (1 mL); 3000 units (1 mL); 4000 units (1 mL); 10,000 units (1 mL)

Epogen® *see epoetin alfa on this page*

Eppy/N® *see epinephrine on previous page*

epsom salts *see magnesium sulfate on page 278*

ept *see teniposide on page 446*

e.p.t.® Stick *see diagnostic aids (in vitro), urine on page 137*

Equagesic® *see aspirin and meprobamate on page 36*

Equalactin'® Chewablet Tablet [OTC] *see calcium polycarbophil on page 70*

Equanil® *see* meprobamate *on page 288*
Equilet® [OTC] *see* calcium carbonate *on page 66*
Ercaf® *see* ergotamine derivatives *on this page*
Ergamisol® *see* levamisole hydrochloride *on page 264*

ergocalciferol (er goe kal sif' e role)
Brand Names Calciferol™ Injection; Calciferol™ Oral; Drisdol® Oral
Synonyms activated ergosterol; viosterol; vitamin d_2
Therapeutic Category Vitamin D Analog
Use Refractory rickets; hypophosphatemia; hypoparathyroidism
Usual Dosage
Dietary supplementation: Oral:
Premature infants: 10-20 mcg/day (400-800 units), up to 750 mcg/day (30,000 units)
Infants and healthy Children: 10 mcg/day (400 units)

Renal failure: Oral:
Children: 0.1-1 mg/day (4000-40,000 units)
Adults: 0.5 mg/day (20,000 units)

Hypoparathyroidism: Oral:
Children: 1.25-5 mg/day (50,000-200,000 units) and calcium supplements
Adults: 625 mcg to 5 mg/day (25,000-200,000 units) and calcium supplements

Vitamin D-dependent rickets: Oral:
Children: 75-125 mcg/day (3000-5000 units)
Adults: 250 mcg to 1.5 mg/day (10,000-60,000 units)

Nutritional rickets and osteomalacia:
Oral:
Children and Adults (with normal absorption): 25 mcg/day (1000 units)
Children with malabsorption: 250-625 mcg/day (10,000-25,000 units)
I.M.: Adults: 250 mcg/day
Dosage Forms
Capsule (Drisdol®): 50,000 units [1.25 mg]
Injection (Calciferol™): 500,000 units/mL [12.5 mg/mL] (1 mL)
Liquid (Calciferol™, Drisdol®): 8000 units/mL [200 mcg/mL] (60 mL)
Tablet (Calciferol™): 50,000 units [1.25 mg]

ergoloid mesylates (er' goe loyd)
Brand Names Germinal®; Hydergine®; Hydergine® LC; Hydro-Ergoloid®
Synonyms dihydroergotoxine; hydrogenated ergot alkaloids
Therapeutic Category Ergot Alkaloid
Use Treatment of cerebrovascular insufficiency in primary progressive dementia, Alzheimer's dementia, and senile onset
Usual Dosage Adults: Oral: 1 mg 3 times/day up to 4.5-12 mg/day; up to 6 months of therapy may be necessary
Dosage Forms
Capsule, liquid (Hydergine® LC): 1 mg
Liquid (Hydergine®): 1 mg/mL (100 mL)
Tablet:
Oral: 0.5 mg
Gerimal®, Hydergine®: 1 mg
Sublingual: Gerimal®, Hydergine®: 0.5 mg, 1 mg

Ergomar® *see* ergotamine derivatives *on this page*
Ergostat® *see* ergotamine derivatives *on this page*

ergotamine derivatives (er got' a meen)
Brand Names Cafatine®; Cafergot®; Cafetrate®; Ercaf®; Ergomar®; Ergostat®; Medihaler Ergotamine™; Wigraine®
Therapeutic Category Adrenergic Blocking Agent; Ergot Alkaloid
(Continued)

ergotamine derivatives *(Continued)*

Use Vascular headache, such as migraine or cluster

Usual Dosage

Older Children and Adolescents: Oral: 1 tablet at onset of attack; then 1 tablet every 30 minutes as needed, up to a maximum of 3 tablets per attack

Adults:

Oral (Cafergot®): 2 tablets at onset of attack; then 1 tablet every 30 minutes as needed; maximum: 6 tablets per attack; do not exceed 10 tablets/week

Oral (Ergostat®): 1 tablet under tongue at first sign, then 1 tablet every 30 minutes, 3 tablets/24 hours, 5 tablets/week

Rectal (Cafergot® suppositories, Wigraine® suppositories, Cafatine-PB® suppositories): 1 at first sign of an attack; follow with second dose after 1 hour, if needed; maximum dose: 2 per attack; do not exceed 5/week

Dosage Forms

Suppository, rectal (Cafatine®, Cafergot®, Cafetrate®, Wigraine®): Ergotamine tartrate 2 mg and caffeine 100 mg (12s)

Tablet (Cafergot®, Ercaf®, Wigraine®): Ergotamine tartrate 1 mg and caffeine 100 mg

Tablet, sublingual (Ergostat®): Ergotamine tartrate 2 mg

Erycette® *see erythromycin, topical on page 172*

Eryc® Oral *see erythromycin on this page*

EryDerm® *see erythromycin, topical on page 172*

Erygel® *see erythromycin, topical on page 172*

Erymax® *see erythromycin, topical on page 172*

EryPed® Oral *see erythromycin on this page*

Ery-sol® *see erythromycin, topical on page 172*

Ery-Tab® Oral *see erythromycin on this page*

erythrityl tetranitrate (e ri' thri till te tra nye' trate)

Brand Names Cardilate®

Therapeutic Category Antianginal Agent; Nitrate; Vasodilator, Coronary

Use Prophylaxis and long-term treatment of frequent or recurrent anginal pain and reduced exercise tolerance associated with angina pectoris

Usual Dosage Adults: Oral: 5 mg under the tongue or in the buccal pouch 3 times/day or 10 mg before meals or food, chewed 3 times/day, increasing in 2-3 days if needed

Dosage Forms Tablet, oral or sublingual: 10 mg

Erythrocin® Oral *see erythromycin on this page*

erythromycin (er ith roe mye' sin)

Brand Names E.E.S.® Oral; E-Mycin® Oral; Eryc® Oral; EryPed® Oral; Ery-Tab® Oral; Erythrocin® Oral; Ilosone® Oral; PCE® Oral

Therapeutic Category Antibiotic, Macrolide

Use Treatment of susceptible bacterial infections including *M. pneumoniae*, *Legionella* pneumonia, Lyme disease, diphtheria, pertussis, chancroid, *Chlamydia*, and *Campylobacter* gastroenteritis; used in conjunction with neomycin for decontaminating the bowel

Usual Dosage

Neonates:

Oral:

Postnatal age <7 days: 20 mg/kg/day in divided doses every 12 hours

Postnatal age >7 days, <1200 g: 20 mg/kg/day in divided doses every 12 hours; ≥1200 g: 30 mg/kg/day in divided doses every 8 hours

Prophylaxis of neonatal gonococcal or chlamydial conjunctivitis: 0.5-1 cm ribbon of ointment should be instilled into each conjunctival sac

Infants and Children:
    Oral: Do not exceed 2 g/day
        Base and ethylsuccinate: 30-50 mg/kg/day divided every 6-8 hours
        Estolate: 30-50 mg/kg/day divided every 8-12 hours
        Stearate: 20-40 mg/kg/day divided every 6 hours
    Pre-op bowel preparation: 20 mg/kg erythromycin base at 1, 2, and 11 PM on the day before surgery combined with mechanical cleansing of the large intestine and oral neomycin
    I.V.: Lactobionate: 20-40 mg/kg/day divided every 6 hours, not to exceed 4 g/day

Adults:
    Oral:
        Base: 333 mg every 8 hours
        Estolate, stearate or base: 250-500 mg every 6-12 hours
        Ethylsuccinate: 400-800 mg every 6-12 hours
    Pre-op bowel preparation: 1 g erythromycin base at 1, 2, and 11 PM on the day before surgery combined with mechanical cleansing of the large intestine and oral neomycin
    I.V.: 15-20 mg/kg/day divided every 6 hours or given as a continuous infusion over 24 hours

Dosage Forms
Erythromycin base:
    Capsule, delayed release: 250 mg
    Capsule, delayed release, enteric coated pellets (Eryc®): 250 mg
    Tablet, delayed release: 333 mg
    Tablet, enteric coated (E-Mycin®, Ery-Tab®, E-Base®): 250 mg, 333 mg, 500 mg
    Tablet, film coated: 250 mg, 500 mg
    Tablet, polymer coated particles (PCE®): 333 mg, 500 mg

Erythromycin estolate:
    Capsule (Ilosone® Pulvules®): 250 mg
    Suspension, oral (Ilosone®): 125 mg/5 mL (480 mL); 250 mg/mL (480 mL)
    Tablet (Ilosone®): 500 mg

Erythromycin ethylsuccinate:
    Granules for oral suspension (EryPed®): 400 mg/5 mL (60 mL, 100 mL, 200 mL)
    Powder for oral suspension (E.E.S.®): 200 mg/5 mL (100 mL, 200 mL)
    Suspension, oral (E.E.S.®, EryPed®): 200 mg/5 mL (5 mL, 100 mL, 200 mL, 480 mL); 400 mg/5 mL (5 mL, 60 mL, 100 mL, 200 mL, 480 mL)
    Suspension, oral [drops] (EryPed®): 100 mg/2.5 mL (50 mL)
    Tablet (E.E.S.®): 400 mg
    Tablet, chewable (EryPed®): 200 mg

Erythromycin gluceptate: Injection: 1000 mg (30 mL)

Erythromycin lactobionate: Powder for injection: 500 mg, 1000 mg

Erythromycin stearate: Tablet, film coated (Eramycin®, Erythrocin®): 250 mg, 500 mg

erythromycin and benzoyl peroxide
Brand Names Benzamycin®
Therapeutic Category Acne Products
Use Topical control of acne vulgaris
Usual Dosage Apply twice daily, morning and evening
Dosage Forms Gel: Erythromycin 30 mg and benzoyl peroxide 50 mg per g

erythromycin and sulfisoxazole
Brand Names Eryzole®; Pediazole®
Synonyms sulfisoxazole and erythromycin
Therapeutic Category Antibiotic, Macrolide; Antibiotic, Sulfonamide Derivative
Use Treatment of susceptible bacterial infections of the upper and lower respiratory tract; otitis media in children caused by susceptible strains of *Haemophilus influenzae*; and other infections in patients allergic to penicillin
(Continued)

erythromycin and sulfisoxazole (Continued)

Usual Dosage Dosage recommendation is based on the product's erythromycin content

Oral:

Children ≥2 months: 40-50 mg/kg/day of erythromycin in divided doses every 6-8 hours; not to exceed 2 g erythromycin or 6 g sulfisoxazole/day or approximately 1.25 mL/kg/day divided every 6-8 hours

Adults: 400 mg erythromycin and 1200 mg sulfisoxazole every 6 hours

Dosage Forms Suspension, oral: Erythromycin ethylsuccinate 200 mg and sulfisoxazole acetyl 600 mg per 5 mL (100 mL, 150 mL, 200 mL)

erythromycin, topical

Brand Names AK-Mycin®; Akne-Mycin®; A/T/S®; Del-Mycin®; Emgel™; Erycette®; EryDerm®; Erygel"; Erymax®; Ery-sol®; ETS-2%®; Ilotycin®; Romycin®; Staticin®; Theramycin Z®; T-Stat"

Therapeutic Category Acne Products; Antibiotic, Ophthalmic; Antibiotic, Topical

Use Topical treatment of acne vulgaris

Usual Dosage Children and Adults:

Ophthalmic: Instill one or more times daily depending on the severity of the infection

Topical: Apply 2% solution over the affected area twice daily after the skin has been thoroughly washed and patted dry

Dosage Forms

Gel: 2% (30 g, 60 g)

Gel (A/T/S", Emgel™, Erygel®): 2% (27 g, 30 g, 60 g)

Ointment:

Ophthalmic (Ilotycin", AK-Mycin"): 0.5% (1 g, 3.5 g, 3.75 g)

Topical (Akne-mycin"): 2% (25 g)

Solution, topical:

Staticin": 1.5% (60 mL)

Akne-mycin", A/T/S", Del-Mycin®, Eryderm™, Ery-sol®, ETS-2%®, Romycin®, Theramycin Z", T-Stat": 2% (60 mL, 66 mL, 120 mL)

Pad (T-Stat"): 2% (60s)

Swab (Erycette®): 2% (60s)

erythropoietin see epoetin alfa on page 168

Eryzole® see erythromycin and sulfisoxazole on previous page

eserine salicylate see physostigmine on page 368

Esgic® see butalbital compound on page 63

Esgic-Plus® see butalbital compound on page 63

Esidrix® see hydrochlorothiazide on page 229

Eskalith® see lithium on page 270

esmolol hydrochloride (ess' moe lol)

Brand Names Brevibloc" Injection

Therapeutic Category Antiarrhythmic Agent, Class II; Beta-Adrenergic Blocker

Use Supraventricular tachycardia (primarily to control ventricular rate) and hypertension (especially perioperatively)

Usual Dosage Must be adjusted to individual response and tolerance

Children: An extremely limited amount of information regarding esmolol use in pediatric patients is currently available. Some centers have utilized doses of 100-500 mcg/kg given over 1 minute for control of supraventricular tachycardias. Loading doses of 500 mcg/kg/minute over 1 minute with maximal doses of 50-250 mcg/kg/minute (mean 173) have been used in addition to nitroprusside in a small number of patients (7 patients; 7-19 years of age; median 13 years) to treat postoperative hypertension after coarctation of aorta repair.

Adults: I.V.: Loading dose: 500 mcg/kg over 1 minute; follow with a 50 mcg/kg/minute infusion for 4 minutes; if response is inadequate, rebolus with another 500 mcg/kg loading dose over 1 minute, and increase the maintenance infusion to 100 mcg/kg/minute. Repeat

this process until a therapeutic effect has been achieved or to a maximum recommended maintenance dose of 200 mcg/kg/minute. Usual dosage range: 50-200 mcg/kg/minute with average dose = 100 mcg/kg/minute.
Dosage Forms Injection: 10 mg/mL (10 mL); 250 mg/mL (10 mL)

Esoterica® Facial [OTC] *see* hydroquinone *on page 235*
Esoterica® Regular [OTC] *see* hydroquinone *on page 235*
Esoterica® Sensitive Skin Formula [OTC] *see* hydroquinone *on page 235*
Esoterica® Sunscreen [OTC] *see* hydroquinone *on page 235*
Espotabs® [OTC] *see* phenolphthalein *on page 362*
Estar® [OTC] *see* coal tar *on page 110*

estazolam (ess ta' zoe lam)
Brand Names ProSom™
Therapeutic Category Benzodiazepine; Hypnotic; Sedative
Use Short-term management of insomnia
Usual Dosage Adults: Oral: 1 mg at bedtime, some patients may require 2 mg
Dosage Forms Tablet: 1 mg, 2 mg

Estinyl® *see* ethinyl estradiol *on page 177*
Estivin® II Ophthalmic [OTC] *see* naphazoline hydrochloride *on page 319*
Estrace® Oral *see* estradiol *on this page*
Estraderm® Transdermal *see* estradiol *on this page*
Estra-D® Injection *see* estradiol *on this page*

estradiol (ess tra dye' ole)
Brand Names Delestrogen® Injection; depGynogen® Injection; Depo®-Estradiol Injection; Depogen® Injection; Dioval® Injection; Dura-Estrin® Injection; Duragen® Injection; Estrace® Oral; Estraderm® Transdermal; Estra-D® Injection; Estra-L® Injection; Estro-Cyp® Injection; Estroject-L.A.® Injection; Gynogen L.A.® Injection; Valergen® Injection
Therapeutic Category Estrogen Derivative
Use Treatment of atrophic vaginitis, atrophic dystrophy of vulva, menopausal symptoms, female hypogonadism, ovariectomy, primary ovarian failure, inoperable breast cancer, inoperable prostatic cancer, mild to severe vasomotor symptoms associated with menopause; prevention of postmenopausal osteoporosis
Usual Dosage Adults (all dosage needs to be adjusted based upon the patient's response):

Male: Prostate cancer: Valerate:
    I.M.: ≥30 mg or more every 1-2 weeks
    Oral: 1-2 mg 3 times/day

Female:
    Hypogonadism:
        Oral: 1-2 mg/day in a cyclic regimen for 3 weeks on drug, then 1 week off drug
        I.M.: Cypionate: 1.5-2 mg/month; valerate: 10-20 mg/month
        Transdermal: 0.05 mg patch initially (titrate dosage to response) applied twice weekly in a cyclic regimen, for 3 weeks on drug and 1 week off drug
    Atrophic vaginitis, kraurosis vulvae: Vaginal: Insert 2-4 g/day for 2 weeks then gradually reduce to ½ the initial dose for 2 weeks followed by a maintenance dose of 1 g 1-3 times/week
    Moderate to severe vasomotor symptoms: I.M.:
        Cypionate: 1-5 mg every 3-4 months
        Valerate: 10-20 mg every 4 weeks
    Postpartum breast engorgement: I.M.: Valerate: 10-25 mg at end of first stage of labor
Dosage Forms
Cream, vaginal (Estrace®): 0.1 mg/g (42.5 g)
(Continued)

estradiol *(Continued)*

Injection, as cypionate (depGynogen™, Depo™-Estradiol, Depogen®, Dura-Estrin®, Estra-D®, Estro-Cyp™, Estroject-L.A.®): 5 mg/mL (5 mL, 10 mL)

Injection, as valerate:

Delestrogen™, Valergen™: 10 mg/mL (5 mL, 10 mL); 20 mg/mL (1 mL, 5 mL, 10 mL); 40 mg/mL (5 mL, 10 mL)

Dioval™, Duragen™, Estra-L™, Gynogen L.A.®: 20 mg/mL (10 mL); 40 mg/mL (10 mL)

Tablet, micronized (Estrace®): 1 mg, 2 mg

Transdermal system (Estraderm™):

0.05 mg/24 hours [10 cm^2], total estradiol 4 mg

0.1 mg/24 hours [20 cm^2], total estradiol 8 mg

estradiol and testosterone

Brand Names Andro/Fem® Injection; Deladumone® Injection; depAndrogyn® Injection; Depo-Testadiol™ Injection; Depotestogen™ Injection; Duo-Cyp® Injection; Duratestrin® Injection; Estra-Testrin™ Injection; Valertest No.1® Injection

Synonyms testosterone and estradiol

Therapeutic Category Estrogen and Androgen Combination

Use Vasomotor symptoms associated with menopause; postpartum breast engorgement

Dosage Forms Injection:

Andro/Fem™, depAndrogyn™, Depo-Testadiol®, Depotestogen®, Duo-Cyp®, Duratestrin®: Estradiol cypionate 2 mg and testosterone cypionate 50 mg per mL in cottonseed oil (1 mL, 10 mL)

Androgyn L.A.™, Deladumone™, Estra-Testrin™, Valertest No.1®: Estradiol valerate 4 mg and testosterone enanthate 90 mg per mL in sesame oil (5 mL, 10 mL)

Estra-L® Injection *see* estradiol *on previous page*

estramustine phosphate sodium (ess tra muss' teen)

Brand Names Emcyt™

Therapeutic Category Antineoplastic Agent, Hormone (Estrogen/Nitrogen Mustard)

Use Palliative treatment of prostatic carcinoma

Usual Dosage Oral: 1 capsule for each 22 lb/day, in 3-4 divided doses

Dosage Forms Capsule: 140 mg

Estratab® *see* estrogens, esterified *on next page*

Estratest H.S.® Oral *see* estrogens with methyltestosterone *on next page*

Estratest® Oral *see* estrogens with methyltestosterone *on next page*

Estra-Testrin® Injection *see* estradiol and testosterone *on this page*

Estro-Cyp® Injection *see* estradiol *on previous page*

estrogenic substance aqueous *see* estrone *on next page*

estrogens, conjugated (ess' troe jenz)

Brand Names Premarin®

Synonyms ces

Therapeutic Category Estrogen Derivative

Use Atrophic vaginitis; hypogonadism; primary ovarian failure; vasomotor symptoms of menopause; prostatic carcinoma; osteoporosis prophylactic

Usual Dosage Adults:

Male: Prostate cancer: Oral: 1.25-2.5 mg 3 times/day

Female:

Hypogonadism: Oral: 2.5-7.5 mg/day for 20 days, off 10 days and repeat until menses occur

Abnormal uterine bleeding:

Oral: 2.5-5 mg/day for 7-10 days; then decrease to 1.25 mg/day for 2 weeks

I.V.: 25 mg every 6-12 hours until bleeding stops
Moderate to severe vasomotor symptoms: Oral: 0.625-1.25 mg/day
Postpartum breast engorgement: Oral: 3.75 mg every 4 hours for 5 doses, then 1.25 mg every 4 hours for 5 days
Atrophic vaginitis, kraurosis vulvae: Vaginal: 2-4 g instilled/day 3 weeks on and 1 week off
Dosage Forms
Cream, vaginal: 0.625 mg/g (42.5 g)
Injection: 25 mg (5 mL)
Tablet: 0.3 mg, 0.625 mg, 0.9 mg, 1.25 mg, 2.5 mg

estrogens, esterified
Brand Names Estratab®; Menest®
Therapeutic Category Estrogen Derivative
Use Atrophic vaginitis; hypogonadism; primary ovarian failure; vasomotor symptoms of menopause; prostatic carcinoma; osteoporosis prophylactic
Usual Dosage Adults: Oral:
Male: Prostate cancer: 1.25-2.5 mg 3 times/day

Female:
Hypogonadism: 2.5-7.5 mg/day for 20 days, off 10 days and repeat until menses occur
Moderate to severe vasomotor symptoms: 0.3-1.25 mg/day
Dosage Forms Tablet: 0.3 mg, 0.625 mg, 1.25 mg, 2.5 mg

estrogens with methyltestosterone
Brand Names Estratest H.S.® Oral; Estratest® Oral; Premarin® With Methyltestosterone Oral
Therapeutic Category Estrogen and Androgen Combination
Use Atrophic vaginitis; hypogonadism; primary ovarian failure; vasomotor symptoms of menopause; prostatic carcinoma; osteoporosis prophylactic
Usual Dosage Lowest dose that will control symptoms should be chosen, normally given 3 weeks on and 1 week off
Dosage Forms Tablet:
Estratest®: Esterified estrogen 1.25 mg and methyltestosterone 2.5 mg
Estratest H.S.®: Esterified estrogen 0.625 mg and methyltestosterone 1.25 mg
Premarin® With Methyltestosterone: Conjugated estrogen 0.625 mg and methyltestosterone 5 mg; conjugated estrogen 1.25 mg and methyltestosterone 10 mg

Estroject-L.A.® Injection *see* estradiol *on page 173*

estrone (es' trone)
Brand Names Aquest®; Kestrone®; Theelin®
Synonyms estrogenic substance aqueous
Therapeutic Category Estrogen Derivative
Use Atrophic vaginitis; hypogonadism; primary ovarian failure; vasomotor symptoms of menopause; prostatic carcinoma; osteoporosis prophylactic
Usual Dosage Adults: I.M.:
Vasomotor symptoms, atrophic vaginitis: 0.1-0.5 mg 2-3 times/week
Primary ovarian failure, hypogonadism: 0.1-1 mg/week, up to 2 mg/week
Prostatic carcinoma: 2-4 mg 2-3 times/week
Dosage Forms Injection: 2 mg/mL (10 mL, 30 mL); 5 mg/mL (10 mL)

estropipate (ess' troe pih pate)
Brand Names Ogen®; Ortho-Est®
Synonyms piperazine estrone sulfate
Therapeutic Category Estrogen Derivative
Use Atrophic vaginitis; hypogonadism; primary ovarian failure; vasomotor symptoms of menopause; prostatic carcinoma; osteoporosis prophylactic
(Continued)

estropipate *(Continued)*

Usual Dosage Adults: Female:
Moderate to severe vasomotor symptoms: Oral: 0.625-5 mg/day
Hypogonadism: Oral: 1.25-7.5 mg/day for 3 weeks followed by an 8- to 10-day rest period
Atrophic vaginitis or kraurosis vulvae: Vaginal: Instill 2-4 g/day 3 weeks on and 1 week off

Dosage Forms
Cream, vaginal: 0.15% [estropipate 1.5 mg/g] (42.5 g tube)
Tablet: 0.625 mg [estropipate 0.75 mg]; 1.25 mg [estropipate 1.5 mg]; 2.5 mg [estropipate 3 mg]; 5 mg [estropipate 6 mg]

Estrovis® *see* quinestrol *on page 402*

ethacrynic acid (eth a krin' ik)

Brand Names Edecrin® Oral; Edecrin® Sodium Injection
Synonyms sodium ethacrynate
Therapeutic Category Diuretic, Loop
Use Management of edema secondary to congestive heart failure; hepatic or renal disease
Usual Dosage
Children:
Oral: 25 mg/day to start, increase by 25 mg/day at intervals of 2-3 days as needed, to a maximum of 3 mg/kg/day
I.V.: 1 mg/kg/dose, (maximum: 50 mg/dose); repeat doses not recommended

Adults:
Oral: 50-100 mg/day increased in increments of 25-50 mg at intervals of several days to a maximum of 400 mg/24 hours
I.V.: 0.5-1 mg/kg/dose (maximum: 50 mg/dose); repeat doses not recommended

Dosage Forms
Powder for injection, as ethacrynate sodium: 50 mg (50 mL)
Tablet: 25 mg, 50 mg

ethambutol hydrochloride (e tham' byoo tole)

Brand Names Myambutol®
Therapeutic Category Antitubercular Agent
Use Treatment of tuberculosis and other mycobacterial diseases in conjunction with other antituberculosis agents
Usual Dosage Oral (not recommended in children <12 years of age):
Children >12 years: 15 mg/kg/day once daily
Adolescents and Adults: 15-25 mg/kg/day once daily, not to exceed 2.5 g/day
Dosage Forms Tablet: 100 mg, 400 mg

Ethamolin® Injection *see* ethanolamine oleate *on this page*

eth and c *see* terpin hydrate and codeine *on page 448*

ethanoic acid *see* acetic acid *on page 5*

ethanol *see* alcohol, ethyl *on page 11*

ethanolamine oleate (eth' a nol a meen)

Brand Names Ethamolin® Injection
Therapeutic Category Sclerosing Agent
Use Mild sclerosing agent used for bleeding esophageal varices
Usual Dosage Adults: 1.5-5 mL per varix, up to 20 mL total or 0.4 mL/kg; patients with severe hepatic dysfunction should receive less than recommended maximum dose
Dosage Forms Injection: 5% [50 mg/mL] (2 mL)

Ethaquin® *see* ethaverine hydrochloride *on next page*

Ethatab® *see* ethaverine hydrochloride *on this page*

ethaverine hydrochloride
Brand Names Ethaquin®; Ethatab®; Ethavex-100®; Isovex®
Therapeutic Category Vasodilator
Use Peripheral and cerebral vascular insufficiency associated with arterial spasm
Usual Dosage Adults: Oral: 100 mg three times/daily
Dosage Forms
  Capsule (Isovex®): 100 mg
  Tablet (Ethaquin®, Ethatab®, Ethavex-100®): 100 mg

Ethavex-100® *see* ethaverine hydrochloride *on this page*

ethchlorvynol (eth klor vi' nole)
Brand Names Placidyl®
Therapeutic Category Hypnotic; Sedative
Use Short-term management of insomnia
Usual Dosage Oral: 500-1000 mg at bedtime
Dosage Forms Capsule: 200 mg, 500 mg, 750 mg

ethinyl estradiol (eth' in il ess tra dye' ole)
Brand Names Estinyl®
Therapeutic Category Estrogen Derivative
Use Atrophic vaginitis; hypogonadism; primary ovarian failure; vasomotor symptoms of menopause; prostatic carcinoma; osteoporosis prophylactic
Usual Dosage Adults: Oral:
  Hypogonadism: 0.05 mg 1-3 times/day for 2 weeks
  Prostatic carcinoma: 0.15-2 mg/day
  Vasomotor symptoms: 0.02-0.05 mg for 21 days, off 7 days and repeat
Dosage Forms Tablet: 0.02 mg, 0.05 mg, 0.5 mg

ethinyl estradiol and desogestrel (lee' voe nor jess trel)
Brand Names Desogen®; Ortho-Cept™
Synonyms desogestrel and ethinyl estradiol
Therapeutic Category Contraceptive, Oral
Use Prevention of pregnancy
Usual Dosage Contraception: Oral: 1 tablet daily, beginning on day 5 of menstrual cycle (first day of menstrual flow is day 1). With 21-tablet packages, new dosing cycle begins 7 days after last tablet taken. With 28-tablet packages, dosage is 1 tablet daily without interruption; extra tablets are placebos, If next menstrual period does not begin on schedule, rule out pregnancy before starting new dosing cycle. If menstrual period begins, start new dosing cycle 7 days after last tablet was taken. if all doses have been taken on schedule and 1 menstrual period is missed, continue dosing cycle. If 2 consecutive menstrual periods are missed, pregnancy test is required before new dosing cycle is started.
  One dose missed: Take as soon as remembered or take 2 tablets next day
  Two doses missed: Take 2 tablets as soon as remembered or 2 tablets next 2 days
  Three doses missed: Begin new compact of tablets starting on day 1 of next cycle
Dosage Forms Tablet: Ethinyl estradiol 0.03 mg and desogestrel 0.15 mg (21s, 28s)

ethinyl estradiol and ethynodiol diacetate
Brand Names Demulen®
Synonyms ethynodiol diacetate and ethinyl estradiol
Therapeutic Category Contraceptive, Oral
Use Prevention of pregnancy; treatment of hypermenorrhea, endometriosis, female hypogonadism
  (Continued)

177

ethinyl estradiol and ethynodiol diacetate *(Continued)*

Usual Dosage

For 21-tablet cycle packs, with 21 active tablets (28-day packs have 21 active tablets and 7 inert tablets): Take 1 tablet daily starting on the fifth day of menstrual cycle, with day 1 being the first day of menstruation; begin taking a new cycle pack on the eighth day after taking the last tablet from the previous pack

With 28-tablet packages, dosage is 1 tablet daily without interruption; extra tablets are placebos or contain iron. If next menstrual period does not begin on schedule, rule out pregnancy before starting new dosing cycle. If menstrual period begins, start new dosing cycle 7 days after last tablet was taken. if all doses have been taken on schedule and 1 menstrual period is missed, continue dosing cycle. If 2 consecutive menstrual periods are missed, pregnancy test is required before new dosing cycle is started.

One dose missed: Take as soon as remembered or take 2 tablets next day
Two doses missed: Take 2 tablets as soon as remembered or 2 tablets next 2 days
Three doses missed: Begin new compact of tablets starting on day 1 of next cycle

Dosage Forms Tablet:

1/35: Ethinyl estradiol 0.035 mg and ethynodiol diacetate 1 mg (21s, 28s)
1/50: Ethinyl estradiol 0.05 mg and ethynodiol diacetate 1 mg (21s, 28s)

ethinyl estradiol and fluoxymesterone

Synonyms fluoxymesterone and estradiol
Therapeutic Category Androgen; Estrogen Derivative
Use Moderate to severe vasomotor symptoms of menopause, postpartum breast engorgement
Usual Dosage Oral: 1-2 tablets at bedtime given cyclically, 3 weeks on and 1 week off
Dosage Forms Tablet: Ethinyl estradiol 0.02 mg and fluoxymesterone 1 mg

ethinyl estradiol and levonorgestrel

Brand Names Levlen®; Nordette®; Tri-Levlen®; Triphasil®
Synonyms levonorgestrel and ethinyl estradiol
Therapeutic Category Contraceptive, Oral
Use Prevention of pregnancy; treatment of hypermenorrhea, endometriosis, female hypogonadism
Usual Dosage

Contraception: Oral: 1 tablet daily, beginning on day 5 of menstrual cycle (first day of menstrual flow is day 1). With 20-tablet and 21-tablet packages, new dosing cycle begins 7 days after last tablet taken. With 28-tablet packages, dosage is 1 tablet daily without interruption; extra tablets are placebos or contain iron. If next menstrual period does not begin on schedule, rule out pregnancy before starting new dosing cycle. If menstrual period begins, start new dosing cycle 7 days after last tablet was taken. if all doses have been taken on schedule and 1 menstrual period is missed, continue dosing cycle. If 2 consecutive menstrual periods are missed, pregnancy test is required before new dosing cycle is started.

Triphasic oral contraceptive: 1 tablet/day in the sequence specified by the manufacturer

Dosage Forms Tablet:

Levlen®, Nordette®: Ethinyl estradiol 0.03 mg and levonorgestrel 0.15 mg (21s, 28s)
Tri-Levlen®, Triphasil®: Phase 1 (6 brown tablets): Ethinyl estradiol 0.03 mg and levonorgestrel 0.05 mg; Phase 2 (5 white tablets): Ethinyl estradiol 0.04 mg and levonorgestrel 0.075 mg; Phase 3 (10 yellow tablets): Ethinyl estradiol 0.03 mg and levonorgestrel 0.125 mg (21s, 28s)

ethinyl estradiol and norethindrone

Brand Names Brevicon®; Genora®; Loestrin®; Modicon™; N.E.E.® 1/35; Nelova™; Norcept-E® 1/35; Norethin™ 1/35E; Norinyl® 1+35; Norlestrin®; Ortho-Novum™ 1/35; Ortho-Novum™ 7/7/7; Ortho-Novum™ 10/11; Ovcon®; Tri-Norinyl®
Synonyms norethindrone acetate and ethinyl estradiol
Therapeutic Category Contraceptive, Oral

Use Prevention of pregnancy; treatment of hypermenorrhea, endometriosis, female hypogonadism

Usual Dosage

For 21-tablet cycle packs, with 21 active tablets (28-day packs have 21 active tablets and 7 inert tablets): Take 1 tablet daily starting on the fifth day of menstrual cycle, with day 1 being the first day of menstruation; begin taking a new cycle pack on the eighth day after taking the last tablet from the previous pack

With 28-tablet packages, dosage is 1 tablet daily without interruption; extra tablets are placebos or contain iron. If next menstrual period does not begin on schedule, rule out pregnancy before starting new dosing cycle. If menstrual period begins, start new dosing cycle 7 days after last tablet was taken. if all doses have been taken on schedule and 1 menstrual period is missed, continue dosing cycle. If 2 consecutive menstrual periods are missed, pregnancy test is required before new dosing cycle is started.

One dose missed: Take as soon as remembered or take 2 tablets next day

Two doses missed: Take 2 tablets as soon as remembered or 2 tablets next 2 days

Three doses missed: Begin new compact of tablets starting on day 1 of next cycle

Biphasic oral contraceptive (Ortho-Novum™ 10/11): 1 color tablet/day for 10 days, then next color tablet for 11 days

Triphasic oral contraceptive (Ortho-Novum™ 7/7/7, Tri-Norinyl®, Triphasil®): 1 tablet/day in the sequence specified by the manufacturer

Dosage Forms Tablet:

Brevicon®, Genora® 0.5/35, Modicon™, Nelova™ 0.5/35E: Ethinyl estradiol 0.035 mg and norethindrone 0.5 mg (21s, 28s)

Loestrin® 1.5/30: Ethinyl estradiol 0.03 mg and norethindrone acetate 1.5 mg (21s)

Loestrin® Fe 1.5/30: Ethinyl estradiol 0.03 mg and norethindrone acetate 1.5 mg with ferrous fumarate 75 mg in 7 inert tablets (28s)

Loestrin® 1/20: Ethinyl estradiol 0.02 mg and norethindrone acetate 1 mg (21s)

Loestrin® Fe 1/20: Ethinyl estradiol 0.02 mg and norethindrone acetate 1 mg with ferrous fumarate 75 mg in 7 inert tablets (28s)

Genora® 1/35, N.E.E.® 1/35, Nelova® 1/35E, Norcept-E® 1/35, Norethin™ 1/35E, Norinyl® 1+35, Ortho-Novum™ 1/35: Ethinyl estradiol 0.035 mg and norethindrone 1 mg (21s, 28s)

Norlestrin® 1/50: Ethinyl estradiol 0.05 mg and norethindrone acetate 1 mg (21s, 28s)

Norlestrin® Fe 1/50: Ethinyl estradiol 0.05 mg and norethindrone acetate 1 mg with ferrous fumarate 75 mg in 7 inert tablets (28s)

Norlestrin® 2.5/50: Ethinyl estradiol 0.05 mg and norethindrone acetate 2.5 mg (21s)

Norlestrin® Fe 2.5/50: Ethinyl estradiol 0.05 mg and norethindrone acetate 2.5 mg with ferrous fumarate 75 mg in 7 inert tablets (28s)

Ortho-Novum™ 7/7/7: Phase 1 (7 white tablets): Ethinyl estradiol 0.035 mg and norethindrone 0.5 mg; Phase 2 (7 light peach tablets): Ethinyl estradiol 0.035 mg and norethindrone 0.75 mg; Phase 3 (7 peach tablets): Ethinyl estradiol 0.035 mg and norethindrone 1 mg (21s, 28s)

Ortho-Novum™ 10/11: Phase 1 (10 white tablets): Ethinyl estradiol 0.035 mg and norethindrone 0.5 mg; Phase 2 (11 dark yellow tablets): Ethinyl estradiol 0.035 mg and norethindrone 1 mg (21s, 28s)

Ovcon® 35: Ethinyl estradiol 0.035 mg and norethindrone 0.4 mg (21s, 28s)

Ovcon® 50: Ethinyl estradiol 0.050 mg and norethindrone 1 mg (21s, 28s)

Tri-Norinyl®: Phase 1 (7 blue tablets): Ethinyl estradiol 0.035 mg and norethindrone 0.5 mg; Phase 2 (9 green tablets): Ethinyl estradiol 0.035 mg and norethindrone 1 mg; Phase 3 (5 blue tablets): Ethinyl estradiol 0.035 mg and norethindrone 0.5 mg (21s, 28s)

ethinyl estradiol and norgestimate

Brand Names Ortho-Cyclen®; Ortho™ Tri-Cyclen®

Synonyms norgestimate and ethinyl estradiol

Therapeutic Category Contraceptive, Oral

Use Prevention of pregnancy

Usual Dosage

Contraception: Oral: 1 tablet daily, beginning on day 5 of menstrual cycle (first day of menstrual flow is day 1). With 21-tablet packages, new dosing cycle begins 7 days after last

(Continued)

ethinyl estradiol and norgestimate *(Continued)*

tablet taken. With 28-tablet packages, dosage is 1 tablet daily without interruption; extra tablets are placebos or contain iron. If next menstrual period does not begin on schedule, rule out pregnancy before starting new dosing cycle. If menstrual period begins, start new dosing cycle 7 days after last tablet was taken. if all doses have been taken on schedule and 1 menstrual period is missed, continue dosing cycle. If 2 consecutive menstrual periods are missed, pregnancy test is required before new dosing cycle is started.

One dose missed: Take as soon as remembered or take 2 tablets next day

Two doses missed: Take 2 tablets as soon as remembered or 2 tablets next 2 days

Three doses missed: Begin new compact of tablets starting on day 1 of next cycle

Triphasic oral contraceptive: 1 tablet/day in the sequence specified by the manufacturer

Dosage Forms Tablet:

Ortho-Cyclen™: Ethinyl estradiol 0.035 mg and norgestimate 0.25 mg (21s, 28s)

Ortho™ Tri-Cyclen™: Phase 1 (7 white tablets): Ethinyl estradiol 0.035 mg and norgestimate 0.18 mg; Phase 2 (5 light blue tablets): Ethinyl estradiol 0.035 mg and norgestimate 0.215 mg; Phase 3 (10 blue tablets): Ethinyl estradiol 0.035 mg and norgestimate 0.25 mg (21s, 28s)

ethinyl estradiol and norgestrel

Brand Names Lo/Ovral™; Ovral®

Synonyms norgestrel and ethinyl estradiol

Therapeutic Category Contraceptive, Oral

Use Prevention of pregnancy; treatment of hypermenorrhea, endometriosis, female hypogonadism

Usual Dosage Contraception: Oral: 1 tablet daily, beginning on day 5 of menstrual cycle (first day of menstrual flow is day 1). With 20-tablet and 21-tablet packages, new dosing cycle begins 7 days after last tablet taken; with 28-tablet packages, dosage is 1 tablet daily without interruption; extra tablets are placebos or contain iron. If next menstrual period does not begin on schedule, rule out pregnancy before starting new dosing cycle; if menstrual period begins, start new dosing cycle 7 days after last tablet was taken; if all doses have been taken on schedule and 1 menstrual period is missed, continue dosing cycle; if two consecutive menstrual periods are missed, pregnancy test is required before new dosing cycle is started.

One dose missed: Take as soon as remembered or take 2 tablets next day

Two doses missed: Take 2 tablets as soon as remembered or 2 tablets next 2 days

Three doses missed: Begin new compact of tablets starting on day 1 of next cycle

Dosage Forms Tablet:

Lo/Ovral™: Ethinyl estradiol 0.03 mg and norgestrel 0.3 mg (21s and 28s)

Ovral™: Ethinyl estradiol 0.05 mg and norgestrel 0.5 mg (21s and 28s)

ethiodized oil *see* radiological/contrast media (ionic) *on page 404*

Ethiodol® *see* radiological/contrast media (ionic) *on page 404*

ethionamide (e thye on am' ide)

Brand Names Trecator™-SC

Therapeutic Category Antitubercular Agent

Use In conjunction with other antituberculosis agents in the treatment of tuberculosis and other mycobacterial diseases

Usual Dosage Oral:

Children: 15-20 mg/kg/day in 2 divided doses, not to exceed 1 g/day

Adults: 500-1000 mg/day in 1-3 divided doses

Dosage Forms Tablet, sugar coated: 250 mg

Ethmozine® *see* moricizine hydrochloride *on page 311*

ethopropazine hydrochloride (eth oh proe' pa zeen)
Brand Names Parsidol®
Therapeutic Category Anti-Parkinson's Agent
Use Treatment of Parkinsonism, drug induced extrapyramidal reactions, and congenital athetosis
Usual Dosage Adults: Oral: 50-600 mg/day
Dosage Forms Tablet: 10 mg, 50 mg

ethosuximide (eth oh sux' i mide)
Brand Names Zarontin®
Therapeutic Category Anticonvulsant, Succinimide
Use Management of absence (petit mal) seizures, myoclonic seizures, and akinetic epilepsy
Usual Dosage Oral:

Children 3-6 years: Initial: 250 mg; increment: 250 mg/day at 4- to 7-day intervals; maintenance: 20-40 mg/kg/day; maximum: 1500 mg/day in 2 divided doses

Children >6 years and Adults: Initial: 500 mg/day; maintenance: 20-40 mg/kg/day; increment: 250 mg/day at 4- to 7-day intervals; maximum: 1500 mg/day in 2 divided doses

Dosage Forms
Capsule: 250 mg
Syrup (raspberry flavor): 250 mg/5 mL (473 mL)

ethotoin (eth' o toin)
Brand Names Peganone®
Synonyms ethylphenylhydantoin
Therapeutic Category Anticonvulsant, Hydantoin
Use Generalized tonic-clonic or complex-partial seizures
Usual Dosage Oral:
Children: 250 mg twice daily, up to 250 mg 4 times/day

Adults: 250 mg 4 times/day after meals, may be increased up to 3 g/day in divided doses 4 times/day
Dosage Forms Tablet: 250 mg, 500 mg

ethoxynaphthamido penicillin sodium *see* nafcillin sodium *on page 316*

Ethrane® *see* enflurane *on page 166*

ethyl aminobenzoate *see* benzocaine *on page 48*

ethyl chloride
Synonyms chloroethane
Therapeutic Category Local Anesthetic, Topical
Use Local anesthetic in minor operative procedures and to relieve pain caused by insect stings and burns, and irritation caused by myofascial and visceral pain syndromes
Usual Dosage Dosage varies with use
Dosage Forms Spray: 100 mL, 120 mL

ethyl chloride and dichlorotetrafluoroethane
Brand Names Fluro-Ethyl® Aerosol
Synonyms dichlorotetrafluoroethane and ethyl chloride
Therapeutic Category Local Anesthetic, Topical
Use Topical refrigerant anesthetic to control pain associated with minor surgical procedures, dermabrasion, injections, contusions, and minor strains
Usual Dosage Press gently on side of spray valve allowing the liquid to emerge as a fine mist approximately 2" to 4" from site of application
Dosage Forms Aerosol: Ethyl chloride 25% and dichlorotetrafluoroethane 75% (225 g)

ethylnorepinephrine hydrochloride (eth il nor ep i nef' rin)
Brand Names Bronkephrine® Injection
Therapeutic Category Adrenergic Agonist Agent; Bronchodilator
Use Bronchial asthma and reversible bronchospasm
Usual Dosage I.M., S.C.:
  Children: Usually 0.1-0.5 mL
  Adults: 0.5-1 mL
Dosage Forms Injection: 2 mg/mL (1 mL)

ethylphenylhydantoin *see* ethotoin *on previous page*

ethynodiol diacetate and ethinyl estradiol *see* ethinyl estradiol and ethynodiol diacetate *on page 177*

etidocaine hydrochloride (e ti' doe kane)
Brand Names Duranest® Injection
Therapeutic Category Local Anesthetic, Injectable
Use Infiltration anesthesia; peripheral nerve blocks; central neural blocks
Usual Dosage Varies with procedure; use 1% for peripheral nerve block, central nerve block, lumbar peridural caudal; use 1.5% for maxillary infiltration or inferior alveolar nerve block; use 1% or 1.5% for intra-abdominal or pelvic surgery, lower limb surgery, or caesarean section
Dosage Forms
  Injection: 1% [10 mg/mL] (30 mL)
  Injection, with epinephrine 1:200,000: 1% [10 mg/mL] (30 mL); 1.5% [15 mg/mL] (20 mL)

etidronate disodium (e ti droe' nate)
Brand Names Didronel® I.V.; Didronel® Oral
Synonyms ehdp; sodium etidronate
Therapeutic Category Antidote, Hypercalcemia; Biphosphonate Derivative
Use Symptomatic treatment of Paget's disease and heterotopic ossification due to spinal cord injury or after total hip replacement, hypercalcemia associated with malignancy
Usual Dosage Adults: Oral:
  Paget's disease: 5 mg/kg/day given every day for no more than 6 months; may give 10 mg/kg/day for up to 3 months. Daily dose may be divided if adverse GI effects occur.

  Heterotopic ossification with spinal cord injury: 20 mg/kg/day for 2 weeks, then 10 mg/kg/day for 10 weeks (This dosage has been used in children, however, treatment greater than 1 year has been associated with a rachitic syndrome.)

  Hypercalcemia associated with malignancy: I.V.: 7.5 mg/kg/day for 3 days
Dosage Forms
  Injection: 50 mg/mL (6 mL)
  Tablet: 200 mg, 400 mg

etodolac (ee toe doe' lak)
Brand Names Lodine®
Therapeutic Category Analgesic, Non-Narcotic; Anti-inflammatory Agent; Nonsteroidal Anti-Inflammatory Agent (NSAID), Oral
Use Acute and long-term use in the management of signs and symptoms of osteoarthritis and management of pain
Usual Dosage Adults: Oral:
  Acute pain: 200-400 mg every 6-8 hours, as needed, not to exceed total daily doses of 1200 mg

  Osteoarthritis: Initial: 800-1200 mg/day given in divided doses: 400 mg 2 or 3 times/day; 300 mg 2, 3 or 4 times/day; 200 mg 3 or 4 times/day; total daily dose should not exceed 1200 mg; for patients weighing <60 kg, total daily dose should not exceed 20 mg/kg
Dosage Forms Capsule: 200 mg, 300 mg, 400 mg

etomidate (e tom' i date)
Brand Names Amidate® Injection
Therapeutic Category General Anesthetic
Use Induction of general anesthesia
Usual Dosage Children >10 years and Adults: I.V.: 0.2-0.6 mg/kg over period of 30-60 seconds
Dosage Forms Injection: 2 mg/mL (10 mL, 20 mL)

etoposide (e toe poe' side)
Brand Names VePesid® Injection; VePesid® Oral
Synonyms epeg; vp-16
Therapeutic Category Antineoplastic Agent, Miotic Inhibitor
Use Treatment of testicular and lung carcinomas, malignant lymphoma, Hodgkin's disease, leukemias, neuroblastoma; etoposide has also been used in the treatment of Ewing's sarcoma, rhabdomyosarcoma, Wilms' tumor and brain tumors
Usual Dosage Refer to individual protocols
Pediatric solid tumors: I.V.: 60-120 mg/m^2/day for 3-5 days every 3-6 weeks

Leukemia in children: I.V.: 100-200 mg/m^2/day for 5 days

Testicular cancer: I.V.: 50-100 mg/m^2/day on days 1-5 or 100 mg/m^2/day on days 1, 3 and 5 every 3-4 weeks for 3-4 courses

Small cell lung cancer:
  Oral: Twice the I.V. dose rounded to the nearest 50 mg given once daily if total dose ≤400 mg or in divided doses if >400 mg
  I.V.: 35 mg/m^2/day for 4 days or 50 mg/m^2/day for 5 days every 3-4 weeks
Dosage Forms
Capsule: 50 mg
Injection: 20 mg/mL (5 mL, 25 mL)

Etrafon® *see* amitriptyline and perphenazine *on page 21*

etretinate (e tret' i nate)
Brand Names Tegison®
Therapeutic Category Antipsoriatic Agent, Systemic
Use Treatment of severe recalcitrant psoriasis in patients intolerant of or unresponsive to standard therapies
Usual Dosage Adults: Oral: Individualized; Initial: 0.75-1 mg/kg/day in divided doses up to 1.5 mg/kg/day; maintenance dose established after 8-10 weeks of therapy 0.5-0.75 mg/kg/day
Dosage Forms Capsule: 10 mg, 25 mg

ETS-2%® *see* erythromycin, topical *on page 172*

Eudal-SR® *see* guaifenesin and pseudoephedrine *on page 216*

Eulexin® *see* flutamide *on page 200*

Eurax® Topical *see* crotamiton *on page 118*

Eutron® *see* methyclothiazide and pargyline *on page 298*

Evac-Q-Mag® [OTC] *see* magnesium citrate *on page 276*

Evac-U-Gen® [OTC] *see* phenolphthalein *on page 362*

Evac-U-Lax® [OTC] *see* phenolphthalein *on page 362*

Evalose® *see* lactulose *on page 261*

Everone® Injection *see* testosterone *on page 449*

E-Vista® *see* hydroxyzine *on page 237*

Exact® [OTC] *see* benzoyl peroxide *on page 50*

Excedrin®, Extra Strength [OTC] *see* acetaminophen and aspirin *on page 3*

Excedrin® P.M. [OTC] *see* acetaminophen and diphenhydramine *on page 4*

Excedrin® IB [OTC] *see* ibuprofen *on page 240*

Exelderm® Topical *see* sulconazole nitrate *on page 439*

Exidine® Scrub [OTC] *see* chlorhexidine gluconate *on page 90*

Ex-Lax®, Extra Gentle Pills [OTC] *see* docusate and phenolphthalein *on page 154*

Ex-Lax® [OTC] *see* phenolphthalein *on page 362*

Exna® *see* benzthiazide *on page 50*

Exosurf® Neonatal *see* colfosceril palmitate *on page 113*

Exsel® *see* selenium sulfide *on page 420*

Extendryl® SR *see* chlorpheniramine, phenylephrine and methscopolamine *on page 95*

Extra Action Cough Syrup [OTC] *see* guaifenesin and dextromethorphan *on page 214*

Extra Strength Bayer® Enteric 500 Aspirin [OTC] *see* aspirin *on page 35*

Eye-Sed® Ophthalmic [OTC] *see* zinc sulfate *on page 496*

Eyesine® Ophthalmic [OTC] *see* tetrahydrozoline hydrochloride *on page 452*

Eye-Zine® Ophthalmic [OTC] *see* tetrahydrozoline hydrochloride *on page 452*

EZ-Detect® [OTC] *see* diagnostic aids (*in vitro*), feces *on page 137*

Ezide® *see* hydrochlorothiazide *on page 229*

f₃t *see* trifluridine *on page 471*

factor viii:c (porcine)

Brand Names Hyate®:C
Therapeutic Category Hemophilic Agent
Use Treatment of congenital hemophiliacs with antibodies to human factor VIII:C and also for previously nonhemophiliac patients with spontaneously acquired inhibitors to human factor VIII:C; patients with inhibitors who are bleeding or who are to undergo surgery
Usual Dosage
Clinical response should be used to assess efficacy rather than relying upon a particular laboratory value for recovery of factor VIII:C.

Initial dose:
Antibody level to human factor VIII:C <50 BU/mL: Initial: 100-150 porcine units/kg (body weight) is recommended
Antibody level to human factor VIII:C >50 BU/mL: Activity of the antibody to porcine factor VIII:C should be determined; an antiporcine antibody level of >20 BU/mL indicates that the patient is unlikely to benefit from treatment; for lower titers, a dose of 100-150 porcine units/kg is recommended
If a patient has previously been treated with Hyate®:C, this may provide a guide a to his likely response and therefore assist in estimation of the preliminary dose

Subsequent doses: Following administration of the initial dose, if the recovery of factor VIII:C in the patient's plasma is not sufficient, a further higher dose should be administered. If recovery after the second dose is still insufficient a third and higher dose may prove effective
Dosage Forms Powder for injection, lyophilized: 400-700 porcine units to be reconstituted with 20 mL sterile water

factor ix complex (human)

Brand Names AlphaNine®; Konȳne® 80; Mononine®; Profilnine® Heat-Treated; Proplex® T
Therapeutic Category Antihemophilic Agent; Blood Product Derivative
Use Control bleeding in patients with factor IX deficiency (Hemophilia B or Christmas Disease); prevention/control of bleeding in hemophilia A patients with inhibitors to factor VIII
Usual Dosage Factor IX deficiency (1 unit/kg raises IX levels 1%): Children and Adults: I.V.: Hospitalized patients: 20-50 units/kg/dose; may be higher in special cases; may be given every 24 hours or more often in special cases

Inhibitor patients: 75-100 units/kg/dose; may be given every 6-12 hours
Dosage Forms Injection:
AlphaNine®: 500 units, 1000 units, 1500 units
Konÿne® 80: 10 mL, 20 mL
Mononine®: 250 units, 500 units, 1000 units
Profilnine® Heat-Treated: Single dose vial
Proplex® SX-T: Vial
Proplex® T: Vial

factor viii *see* antihemophilic factor (human) *on page 29*
Fact Plus® *see* diagnostic aids (*in vitro*), urine *on page 137*
Factrel® Injection *see* gonadorelin *on page 211*

famciclovir (fam sye' kloe veer)
Brand Names Famvir™
Therapeutic Category Antiviral Agent, Oral
Use Management of acute herpes zoster (shingles)
Usual Dosage Adult: Oral: 500 mg every 8 hours for 7 days
Dosing interval in renal impairment:
Cl_{cr} ≥60 mL/minute: Administer 500 mg every 8 hours
Cl_{cr} 40-59 mL/minute: Administer 500 mg every 12 hours
Cl_{cr} 20-39 mL/minute: Administer 500 mg every 24 hours
Dosage Forms Tablet: 500 mg

famotidine (fa moe' ti deen)
Brand Names Pepcid® I.V.; Pepcid® Oral
Therapeutic Category Histamine-2 Antagonist
Use Therapy and treatment of duodenal ulcer, gastric ulcer, control gastric pH in critically ill patients, symptomatic relief in gastritis, gastroesophageal reflux, active benign ulcer, and pathological hypersecretory conditions
Usual Dosage
Children: Oral, I.V.: Doses of 1-2 mg/kg/day have been used; maximum dose: 40 mg
Adults:
Oral:
Duodenal ulcer, gastric ulcer: 40 mg/day at bedtime for 4-8 weeks
Hypersecretory conditions: Initial: 20 mg every 6 hours, may increase up to 160 mg every 6 hours
GERD: 20 mg twice daily for 6 weeks
I.V.: 20 mg every 12 hours
Dosage Forms
Infusion, premixed in NS: 20 mg (50 mL)
Injection: 10 mg/mL (2 mL, 4 mL)
Powder for oral suspension (cherry-banana-mint flavor): 40 mg/5 mL (50 mL)
Tablet, film coated: 20 mg, 40 mg

Famvir™ *see* famciclovir *on this page*
Fansidar® *see* sulfadoxine and pyrimethamine *on page 440*
Fastin® *see* phentermine hydrochloride *on page 363*

fat emulsion
Brand Names Intralipid®; Liposyn®
Therapeutic Category Caloric Agent; Intravenous Nutritional Therapy
Use Source of calories and essential fatty acids for patients requiring parenteral nutrition of extended duration
(Continued)

fat emulsion *(Continued)*

Usual Dosage Fat emulsion should not exceed 60% of the total daily calories

Premature infants: Initial dose: 0.25-0.5 g/kg/day, increase by 0.25-0.5 g/kg/day to a maximum of 3-4 g/kg/day; maximum rate of infusion: 0.15 g/kg/hour (0.75 mL/kg/hour of 20% solution)

Infants and Children: Initial dose: 0.5-1 g/kg/day, increase by 0.5 g/kg/day to a maximum of 3-4 g/kg/day; maximum rate of infusion: 0.25 g/kg/hour (1.25 mL/kg/hour of 20% solution)

Children and Adults: Fatty acid deficiency: 8% to 10% of total caloric intake; infuse once or twice weekly

Adolescents and Adults: Initial dose: 1 g/kg/day, increase by 0.5-1 g/kg/day to a maximum of 2.5 g/kg/day; maximum rate of infusion: 0.25 g/kg/hour (1.25 mL/kg/hour of 20% solution); do not exceed 50 mL/hour (20%) or 100 mL/hour (10%)

Note: At the onset of therapy, the patient should be observed for any immediate allergic reactions such as dyspnea, cyanosis, and fever. Slower initial rates of infusion may be used for the first 10-15 minutes of the infusion, eg, 0.1 mL/minute of 10% of 0.05 mL/minute of 20% solution.

Dosage Forms Injection: 10% [100 mg/mL] (100 mL, 250 mL, 500 mL); 20% [200 mg/mL] (100 mL, 250 mL, 500 mL)

5-fc *see* flucytosine *on page 194*

Fedahist® Expectorant [OTC] *see* guaifenesin and pseudoephedrine *on page 216*

Fedahist® Expectorant Pediatric Drops [OTC] *see* guaifenesin and pseudoephedrine *on page 216*

Fedahist® Timecaps® *see* chlorpheniramine and pseudoephedrine *on page 94*

Feen-a-Mint® Pills [OTC] *see* docusate and phenolphthalein *on page 154*

Feen-a-Mint® [OTC] *see* phenolphthalein *on page 362*

Feiba VH Immuno® *see* anti-inhibitor coagulant complex *on page 30*

felbamate (fel' ba mate)

Brand Names Felbatol™

Therapeutic Category Anticonvulsant, Miscellaneous

Use Monotherapy and adjunctive therapy in patients 14 years of age and older with partial and secondarily generalized seizures; adjunctive therapy in children 2 years of age and older who have partial and generalized seizures associated with Lennox-Gastaut syndrome

Usual Dosage

Monotherapy: 1200 mg/day in divided doses 3 or 4 times/day; titrate previously untreated patients under close clinical supervision, increasing the dosage in 600 mg increments every 2 weeks to 2400 mg/day based on clinical response and thereafter to 3600 mg/day in clinically indicated

Conversion to monotherapy: Initiate at 1200 mg/day in divided doses 3 or 4 times/day, reduce the dosage of the concomitant anticonvulsant(s) by 33% at the initiation of felbamate therapy; at week 2, increase the felbamate dosage to 2400 mg/day while reducing the dosage of the other anticonvulsant(s) up to an additional 33% of their original dosage; at week 3, increase the felbamate dosage up to 3600 mg/day and continue to reduce the dosage of the other anticonvulsant(s) as clinically indicated

Adjunctive therapy:
  Week 1:
    Felbamate: 1200 mg/day initial dose
    Concomitant anticonvulsant(s): Reduce original dosage by 20% to 33%
  Week 2:
    Felbamate: 2400 mg/day (Therapeutic range)
    Concomitant anticonvulsant(s): Reduce original dosage by up to an additional 33%

Week 3:
Felbamate: 3600 mg/day (Therapeutic range)
Concomitant anticonvulsant(s): Reduce original dosage as clinically indicated
Dosage Forms
Suspension, oral: 600 mg/5 mL (240 mL, 960 mL)
Tablet: 400 mg, 600 mg

Felbatol™ *see* felbamate *on previous page*

Feldene® *see* piroxicam *on page 372*

felodipine (fe loe' di peen)
Brand Names Plendil®
Therapeutic Category Calcium Channel Blocker
Use Management of angina pectoris due to coronary insufficiency, hypertension
Usual Dosage Adults: Oral: 5-10 mg once daily
Dosage Forms Tablet, extended release: 2.5 mg, 5 mg, 10 mg

Femcet® *see* butalbital compound *on page 63*

Femilax® [OTC] *see* docusate and phenolphthalein *on page 154*

Femiron® [OTC] *see* ferrous fumarate *on page 189*

Femstat® *see* butoconazole nitrate *on page 63*

Fenesin DM® *see* guaifenesin and dextromethorphan *on page 214*

Fenesin™ [OTC] *see* guaifenesin *on page 213*

fenfluramine hydrochloride (fen flure' a meen)
Brand Names Pondimin®
Therapeutic Category Adrenergic Agonist Agent; Anorexiant
Use Short-term adjunct in exogenous obesity
Usual Dosage Adults: Oral: 20 mg 3 times/day before meals or food, up to 40 mg 3 times/day
Dosage Forms Tablet: 20 mg

fenofibrate (fen oh fye' brate)
Brand Names Lipidil®
Therapeutic Category Antilipemic Agent
Use Adjunct to dietary therapy for the treatment of adults with very high elevations of serum triglyceride levels (types IV and V hyperlipidemia) who are at risk of pancreatitis and who do not respond adequately to a determined dietary effort
Usual Dosage Adults: Oral: 100 mg/day

fenoprofen calcium (fen oh proe' fen)
Brand Names Nalfon®
Therapeutic Category Analgesic, Non-Narcotic; Anti-inflammatory Agent; Nonsteroidal Anti-Inflammatory Agent (NSAID), Oral
Use Symptomatic treatment of acute and chronic rheumatoid arthritis and osteoarthritis; relief of mild to moderate pain
Usual Dosage Oral:
Children: Juvenile arthritis: 900 mg/m^2/day, then increase over 4 weeks to 1.8 g/m^2/day
Adults:
Arthritis: 300-600 mg 3-4 times/day up to 3.2 g/day
Pain: 200 mg every 4-6 hours as needed
Dosage Forms
Capsule: 200 mg, 300 mg
Tablet: 600 mg

fentanyl and droperidol *see* droperidol and fentanyl *on page 159*

fentanyl citrate (fen' ta nil sit' rate)
Brand Names Duragesic™ Transdermal; Fentanyl Oralet®; Sublimaze® Injection
Therapeutic Category Analgesic, Narcotic; General Anesthetic
Use Sedation; relief of pain; preoperative medication; adjunct to general or regional anesthesia; management of chronic pain (transdermal product)
Usual Dosage Doses should be titrated to appropriate effects; wide range of doses, dependent upon desired degree of analgesia/anesthesia

Children:
> Sedation for minor procedures/analgesia: I.M., I.V.:
>> 1-3 years: 2-3 mcg/kg/dose; may repeat after 30-60 minutes as required
>> 3-12 years: 1-2 mcg/kg/dose; may repeat at 30- to 60-minute intervals as required.
>> **Note:** Children 18-36 months of age may require 2-3 mcg/kg/dose
>
> Continuous sedation/analgesia: Initial I.V. bolus: 1-2 mcg/kg then 1 mcg/kg/hour; titrate upward; usual: 1-3 mcg/kg/hour
> Transdermal: Not recommended

Children <12 years and Adults:
> Sedation for minor procedures/analgesia: 0.5-1 mcg/kg/dose; higher doses are used for major procedures
> Preoperative sedation, adjunct to regional anesthesia, postoperative pain: I.M., I.V.: 50-100 mcg/dose
> Adjunct to general anesthesia: I.M., I.V.: 2-50 mcg/kg
> General anesthesia without additional anesthetic agents: I.V. 50-100 mcg/kg with O_2 and skeletal muscle relaxant
> Transdermal: Initial: 25 mcg/hour system; if currently receiving opiates, convert to fentanyl equivalent and administer equianalgesic dosage (see package insert for further information)

Dosage Forms
Injection, as citrate: 0.05 mg/mL (2 mL, 5 mL, 10 mL, 20 mL, 50 mL)
Lozenge, oral transmucosal (raspberry flavored): 200 mcg, 300 mcg, 400 mcg
Transdermal system: 25 mcg/hour [10 cm^2]; 50 mcg/hour [20 cm^2]; 75 mcg/hour [30 cm^2]; 100 mcg/hour [40 cm^2] (all available in 5s)

Fentanyl Oralet® *see* fentanyl citrate *on this page*
Feosol® [OTC] *see* ferrous sulfate *on next page*
Feostat® [OTC] *see* ferrous fumarate *on next page*
Ferancee® [OTC] *see* ferrous salt and ascorbic acid *on page 190*
Feratab® [OTC] *see* ferrous sulfate *on next page*
Fergon® [OTC] *see* ferrous gluconate *on next page*
Fer-In-Sol® [OTC] *see* ferrous sulfate *on next page*
Fer-Iron® [OTC] *see* ferrous sulfate *on next page*
Fero-Grad 500® [OTC] *see* ferrous salt and ascorbic acid *on page 190*
Fero-Gradumet® [OTC] *see* ferrous sulfate *on next page*
Ferospace® [OTC] *see* ferrous sulfate *on next page*
Ferralet® [OTC] *see* ferrous gluconate *on next page*
Ferralyn® Lanacaps® [OTC] *see* ferrous sulfate *on next page*
Ferra-TD® [OTC] *see* ferrous sulfate *on next page*
Ferretts® [OTC] *see* ferrous fumarate *on next page*
Ferromar® [OTC] *see* ferrous salt and ascorbic acid *on page 190*
Ferro-Sequels® [OTC] *see* ferrous fumarate *on next page*

ferrous fumarate (fair' us fyoo' ma rate)
Brand Names Femiron® [OTC]; Feostat® [OTC]; Ferretts® [OTC]; Ferro-Sequels® [OTC]; Fumasorb® [OTC]; Fumerin® [OTC]; Hemocyte® [OTC]; Ircon® [OTC]; Nephro-Fer™ [OTC]; Span-FF® [OTC]

Therapeutic Category Iron Salt

Use Prevention and treatment of iron deficiency anemias

Usual Dosage
Children: 3 mg/kg 3 times/day
Adults: 200 mg 3-4 times/day

Dosage Forms Amount of elemental iron is listed in brackets
Capsule, controlled release (Span-FF®): 325 mg [106 mg]
Drops (Feostat®): 45 mg/0.6 mL [15 mg/0.6 mL] (60 mL)
Suspension, oral (Feostat®): 100 mg/5 mL [33 mg/5 mL] (240 mL)
Tablet:
325 mg [106 mg]
Ferretts®: 325 mg [106 mg]
Chewable (chocolate flavor) (Feostat®): 100 mg [33 mg]
Femiron®: 63 mg [20 mg]
Fumerin®: 195 mg [64 mg]
Fumasorb®, Ircon®: 200 mg [66 mg]
Hemocyte®: 324 mg [106 mg]
Nephro-Fer™: 350 mg [115 mg]
Timed release (Ferro-Sequels®): Ferrous fumarate 150 mg [50 mg] and docusate sodium 100 mg

ferrous gluconate (fair' us gloo' koe nate)
Brand Names Fergon® [OTC]; Ferralet® [OTC]; Simron® [OTC]

Therapeutic Category Iron Salt

Use Prevention and treatment of iron deficiency anemias

Usual Dosage Oral (dose expressed in terms of elemental iron):
Iron deficiency anemia: 3-6 Fe mg/kg/day in 3 divided doses

Maintenance:
Preterm infants:
Birthweight <1000 g: 4 Fe mg/kg/day
Birthweight 1000-1500 g: 3 Fe mg/kg/day
Birthweight 1500-2500 g: 2 Fe mg/kg/day
Term Infants and Children: 1-2 Fe mg/kg/day in 3 divided doses, up to a maximum of 18 Fe mg/day
Adults: 60-100 Fe mg/day in 3 divided doses

Dosage Forms Amount of elemental iron is listed in brackets
Capsule, soft gelatin (Simron®): 86 mg [10 mg]
Elixir (Fergon®): 300 mg/5 mL [34 mg/5 mL] with alcohol 7% (480 mL)
Tablet: 300 mg [34 mg]; 325 mg [38 mg]
Fergon®, Ferralet®: 320 mg [37 mg]
Sustained release (Ferralet® Slow Release): 320 mg [37 mg]

ferrous sulfate (fair' us sul fate)
Brand Names Feosol® [OTC]; Feratab® [OTC]; Fer-In-Sol® [OTC]; Fer-Iron® [OTC]; Fero-Gradumet® [OTC]; Ferospace® [OTC]; Ferralyn® Lanacaps® [OTC]; Ferra-TD® [OTC]; Mol-Iron® [OTC]; Slow FE® [OTC]

Synonyms $FeSO_4$

Therapeutic Category Iron Salt

Use Prevention and treatment of iron deficiency anemias

Usual Dosage Oral (dose expressed in terms of elemental iron):
Children:
Severe iron deficiency anemia: 4-6 mg Fe/kg/day in 3 divided doses
Mild to moderate iron deficiency anemia: 3 mg Fe/kg/day in 1-2 divided doses
Prophylaxis: 1-2 mg Fe/kg/day up to a maximum of 15 mg/day
(Continued)

ferrous sulfate *(Continued)*

Adults: Iron deficiency: 60-100 Fe/kg/day in divided doses

Dosage Forms Amount of elemental iron is listed in brackets

Capsule:

Exsiccated (Fer-In-Sol"): 190 mg [60 mg]

Exsiccated, timed release (Feosol"): 159 mg [50 mg]

Exsiccated, timed release (Ferralyn" Lanacaps®, Ferra-TD®): 250 mg [50 mg]

Ferospace": 250 mg [50 mg]

Drops, oral:

Fer-In-Sol": 75 mg/0.6 mL [15 mg/0.6 mL] (50 mL)

Fer-Iron": 75 mg/0.6 mL [15 mg/0.6 mL] (50 mL)

Elixir (Feosol"): 220 mg/5 mL [44 mg/5 mL] with alcohol 5% (473 mL, 4000 mL)

Syrup (Fer-In-Sol"): 90 mg/5 mL [18 mg/5 mL] with alcohol 5% (480 mL)

Tablet:

324 mg [65 mg]

Exsiccated (Feosol") 200 mg [65 mg]

Exsiccated, timed release (Slow FE®): 160 mg [50 mg]

Feratab": 300 mg [60 mg]

Mol-Iron": 195 mg [39 mg]

Timed release (Fero-Gradumet®): 525 mg [105 mg]

ferrous salt and ascorbic acid

Brand Names Ferancee® [OTC]; Fero-Grad 500® [OTC]; Ferromar® [OTC]

Synonyms ascorbic acid and ferrous sulfate

Therapeutic Category Iron Salt; Vitamin

Use Treatment of iron deficiency in nonpregnant adults; treatment and prevention of iron deficiency in pregnant adults

Usual Dosage Adults: Oral: 1 tablet daily

Dosage Forms Amount of elemental iron is listed in brackets

Caplet, sustained release (Ferromar"): Ferrous fumarate 201.5 mg [65 mg] and ascorbic acid 200 mg

Tablet (Fero-Grad 500"): Ferrous sulfate 525 mg [105 mg] and ascorbic acid 500 mg

Tablet, chewable (Ferancee"): Ferrous fumarate 205 mg [67 mg] and ascorbic acid 150 mg

ferrous sulfate, ascorbic acid, and vitamin b-complex

Brand Names Iberet®-Liquid [OTC]

Therapeutic Category Iron Salt; Vitamin

Use Conditions of iron deficiency with an increased needed for B-complex vitamins and vitamin C

Usual Dosage Oral:

Children 1-3 years: 5 mL twice daily after meals

Children >4 years and Adults: 10 mL 3 times/day after meals

Dosage Forms Liquid:

Ferrous sulfate: 78.75 mg

Ascorbic acid: 375 mg

B_1: 4.5 mg

B_2: 4.5 mg

B_3: 22.5 mg

B_5: 7.5 mg

B_6: 3.75 mg

B_{12}: 18.75 mg all per 15 mL

ferrous sulfate, ascorbic acid, vitamin b-complex, and folic acid

Brand Names Iberet-Folic-500"

Therapeutic Category Iron Salt; Vitamin

Use Treatment of iron deficiency and prevention of concomitant folic acid deficiency where there is an associated deficient intake or increased need for B-complex vitamins

Usual Dosage Adults: Oral: 1 tablet daily
Dosage Forms Tablet, controlled release:
  Ferrous sulfate: 105 mg
  Ascorbic acid: 500 mg
  B_1: 6 mg
  B_2: 6 mg
  B_3: 30 mg
  B_5: 10 mg
  B_6: 5 mg
  B_{12}: 25 mcg
  Folic acid: 800 mcg

FeSO₄ *see* ferrous sulfate *on page 189*

Feverall™ [OTC] *see* acetaminophen *on page 2*

Fiberall® Chewable Tablet [OTC] *see* calcium polycarbophil *on page 70*

Fiberall® Powder [OTC] *see* psyllium *on page 398*

Fiberall® Wafer [OTC] *see* psyllium *on page 398*

FiberCon® Tablet [OTC] *see* calcium polycarbophil *on page 70*

Fiber-Lax® Tablet [OTC] *see* calcium polycarbophil *on page 70*

FiberNorm® [OTC] *see* calcium polycarbophil *on page 70*

fibrinolysin and desoxyribonuclease
Brand Names Elase-Chloromycetin® Topical; Elase® Topical
Synonyms desoxyribonuclease and fibrinolysin
Therapeutic Category Enzyme, Topical Debridement
Use Debriding agent; cervicitis; and irrigating agent in infected wounds
Usual Dosage
  Ointment: 2-3 times/day
  Wet dressing: 3-4 times/day
Dosage Forms
  Ointment, topical:
    Elase®: Fibrinolysin 1 unit and desoxyribonuclease 666.6 units per g (10 g, 30 g)
    Elase-Chloromycetin®: Fibrinolysin 1 unit and desoxyribonuclease 666.6 units per g with chloramphenicol 10 mg per g (10 g, 30 g)
  Powder, dry: Fibrinolysin 25 units and desoxyribonuclease 15,000 units per 30 g

filgrastim (fil gra' stim)
Brand Names Neupogen® Injection
Synonyms granulocyte colony stimulating factor g-csf
Therapeutic Category Colony Stimulating Factor
Use Decrease the period of neutropenia and the associated risk of infection in patients with nonmyeloid malignancies receiving myelosuppressive chemotherapeutic regimens associated with a significant incidence of severe neutropenia with fever; it has also been used in AIDS patients on zidovudine and in patients with noncancer chemotherapy-induced neutropenia
Usual Dosage Children and Adults (refer to individual protocols): I.V., S.C.: 5-10 mcg/kg/day (approximately 150-300 mcg/m²/day) once daily for up to 14 days until ANC = 10,000/mm³; dose escalations at 5 mcg/kg/day may be required in some individuals when response at 5 mcg/kg/day is not adequate; dosages of 0.6-120 mcg/kg/day have been used in children ranging in age from 3 months to 18 years
Dosage Forms Injection, preservative free: 300 mcg/mL (1 mL, 1.6 mL)

Filibon® [OTC] *see* vitamin, multiple (prenatal) *on page 491*

finasteride (fi nas' teer ide)
Brand Names Proscar™ Oral
Therapeutic Category Antiandrogen; Antineoplastic Agent, Adjuvant
Use Early data indicate that finasteride is useful in the treatment of benign prostatic hyperplasia
Usual Dosage Adults: Benign prostatic hyperplasia: Oral: 5 mg/day as a single dose; clinical responses occur within 12 weeks to 6 months of initiation of therapy; long-term administration is recommended for maximal response
Dosage Forms Tablet, film coated: 5 mg

Fiorgen PF® *see* butalbital compound *on page 63*
Fioricet® *see* butalbital compound *on page 63*
Fiorinal® *see* butalbital compound *on page 63*
Fiorinal® With Codeine *see* butalbital compound and codeine *on page 63*
First Response® *see* diagnostic aids (*in vitro*), urine *on page 137*
fisalamine *see* mesalamine *on page 289*
Flagyl® Oral *see* metronidazole *on page 303*
Flarex® Ophthalmic *see* fluorometholone *on page 197*
Flatulex [OTC] *see* simethicone *on page 423*
Flavorcee® [OTC] *see* ascorbic acid *on page 34*

flavoxate hydrochloride (fla vox' ate)
Brand Names Urispas®
Therapeutic Category Antispasmodic Agent, Urinary
Use Antispasmodic to provide symptomatic relief of dysuria, nocturia, suprapubic pain, urgency, and incontinence
Usual Dosage Children >12 years and Adults: 100-200 mg 3-4 times/day
Dosage Forms Tablet, film coated: 100 mg

Flaxedil® *see* gallamine triethiodide *on page 204*

flecainide acetate (fle kay' nide)
Brand Names Tambocor®
Therapeutic Category Antiarrhythmic Agent, Class Ic
Use Prevention and suppression of documented life-threatening ventricular arrhythmias (ie, sustained ventricular tachycardia); controlling symptomatic, disabling supraventricular tachycardias in patients without structural heart disease
Usual Dosage Oral:
Children: Initial: 3 mg/kg/day in 3 divided doses; usual 3-6 mg/kg/day in 3 divided doses; up to 11 mg/kg/day for uncontrolled patients with subtherapeutic levels

Adults: Initial: 100 mg every 12 hours, increase by 100 mg/day (given in 2 doses/day) every 4 days to maximum of 400 mg/day; for patients receiving 400 mg/day who are not controlled and have trough concentrations <0.6 mcg/mL, dosage may be increased to 600 mg/day
Dosage Forms Tablet: 50 mg, 100 mg, 150 mg

Fleet® Phospho®-Soda [OTC] *see* sodium phosphate *on page 429*
Fleet® Laxative [OTC] *see* bisacodyl *on page 54*
Fleet® Flavored Castor Oil [OTC] *see* castor oil *on page 78*
Fleet® Babylax® Rectal [OTC] *see* glycerin *on page 210*
Fleet® Enema [OTC] *see* sodium phosphate *on page 429*
Flexaphen® *see* chlorzoxazone *on page 99*

Flexeril® *see* cyclobenzaprine hydrochloride *on page 120*

Flo-Coat® *see* radiological/contrast media (ionic) *on page 404*

Flonase® Nasal Spray *see* fluticasone propionate *on page 200*

Florical® [OTC] *see* calcium carbonate *on page 66*

Florinef® Acetate *see* fludrocortisone acetate *on next page*

Florone® E Topical *see* diflorasone diacetate *on page 143*

Florone® Topical *see* diflorasone diacetate *on page 143*

Floropryl® Ophthalmic *see* isoflurophate *on page 252*

Florvite® *see* vitamin, multiple (pediatric) *on page 491*

flosequinan (floe se' kwi nan)

Brand Names Manoplax®

Therapeutic Category Vasodilator, Peripheral

Use Management of congestive heart failure (CHF) in patients not responding to diuretics, with or without digitalis, who cannot tolerate an angiotensin-converting enzyme (ACE) inhibitor or who have not responded to a regimen including an ACE inhibitor

Usual Dosage Adults: Oral:

Patients not receiving ACE inhibitors: 100 mg administered daily as a single dose in the morning, if tolerated

Patients receiving concomitant ACE inhibitors: Initial: 50 mg once daily in the morning, titrating upward at weekly intervals up to 100 mg once daily up to 150 mg/day

Dosage Forms Tablet, film coated: 50 mg, 75 mg, 100 mg

Floxin® Injection *see* ofloxacin *on page 336*

Floxin® Oral *see* ofloxacin *on page 336*

floxuridine (flox yoor' i deen)

Brand Names FUDR®

Synonyms fluorodeoxyuridine

Therapeutic Category Antineoplastic Agent, Antimetabolite

Use Palliative management of carcinomas of head, neck, and brain as well as liver, gallbladder, and bile ducts

Usual Dosage Adults:

Intra-arterial infusion: 0.1-0.6 mg/kg/day for 14 days followed by heparinized saline for 14 days

Investigational: I.V.: 0.5-1 mg/kg/day for 6-15 days

Dosage Forms

Injection, preservative free: 100 mg/mL (5 mL)

Powder for injection: 500 mg (5 mL, 10 mL)

flubenisolone *see* betamethasone *on page 52*

fluconazole (floo koe' na zole)

Brand Names Diflucan® Injection; Diflucan® Oral

Therapeutic Category Antifungal Agent, Systemic

Use Treatment of susceptible fungal infections including oropharyngeal and esophageal candidiasis; treatment of systemic candidal infections including urinary tract infection, peritonitis, and pneumonia; treatment of cryptococcal meningitis

Usual Dosage The daily dose of fluconazole is the same for oral and I.V. administration

Efficacy of fluconazole has not been established in children; a small number of patients from ages 3-13 years have been treated with fluconazole using doses of 3-6 mg/kg/day once daily. Doses as high as 12 mg/kg/day once daily have been used to treat candidiasis in immunocompromised children.

(Continued)

fluconazole (Continued)

Indication	Day 1	Daily Therapy	Minimum Duration of Therapy
Oropharyngeal candidiasis	200 mg	100 mg	14 d
Esophageal candidiasis	200 mg	100 mg	21 d
Systemic candidiasis	400 mg	200 mg	28 d
Cryptococcal meningitis acute	400 mg	200 mg	10–12 wk after CSF culture becomes negative
relapse	200 mg	200 mg	

Adult doses of fluconazole: Oral, I.V.: For once daily dosing, see table.
Dosage Forms
Injection: 2 mg/mL (100 mL, 200 mL)
Tablet: 50 mg, 100 mg, 200 mg

flucytosine (floo sye' toe seen)
Brand Names Ancobon"
Synonyms 5-fc; 5-flurocytosine
Therapeutic Category Antifungal Agent, Systemic
Use Treatment of susceptible fungal infections, usually strains of *Candida* or *Cryptococcus*
Usual Dosage Children and Adults: Oral: 50-150 mg/kg/day in divided doses every 6 hours
Dosage Forms Capsule: 250 mg, 500 mg

Fludara® see fludarabine phosphate *on this page*

fludarabine phosphate (floo dare' a been)
Brand Names Fludara"
Therapeutic Category Antineoplastic Agent, Antimetabolite
Use Treatment of chronic lymphocytic leukemia (B-cell) in patients who have not responded to other alkylating agent regiment
Usual Dosage Adults: I.V.:
Chronic lymphocytic leukemia: 25 mg/m^2/day over a 30-minute period for 5 days
Non-Hodgkin's lymphoma: Loading dose: 20 mg/m^2 followed by 30 mg/m^2/day for 48 hours
Dosage Forms Powder for injection, lyophilized: 50 mg (6 mL)

fludrocortisone acetate (floo droe kor' ti sone)
Brand Names Florinef" Acetate
Synonyms fluohydrocortisone acetate; 9α-fluorohydrocortisone acetate
Therapeutic Category Mineralocorticoid
Use Addison's disease; partial replacement therapy for adrenal insufficiency and for treatment of salt-losing forms of congenital adrenogenital syndrome
Usual Dosage Oral:
Infants and Children: 0.05-0.1 mg/day
Adults: 0.05-0.2 mg/day
Dosage Forms Tablet: 0.1 mg

Flu-Imune® see influenza virus vaccine *on page 245*
Flumadine® **Oral** see rimantadine hydrochloride *on page 412*

flumazenil (floo' may ze nil)
Brand Names Romazicon™ Injection
Therapeutic Category Antidote, Benzodiazepine
Use Benzodiazepine antagonist – reverses sedative effects of benzodiazepines used in general anesthesia; for management of benzodiazepine overdose
Usual Dosage Reversal of conscious sedation or general anesthesia: 0.2 mg (2 mL) administered I.V. over 15 seconds; if desired effect is not achieved after 60 seconds, repeat in 0.2 mg (2 mL) increments every 60 seconds up to a total of 1 mg (10 mL); in event of resedation, repeat doses may be given at 20-minute intervals with no more than 1 mg (10 mL) given at any one time, with a maximum of 3 mg in any 1 hour
Dosage Forms Injection: 0.1 mg/mL (5 mL, 10 mL)

flunisolide (floo niss' oh lide)
Brand Names AeroBid®-M Oral Aerosol Inhaler; AeroBid® Oral Aerosol Inhaler; Nasalide® Nasal Aerosol
Therapeutic Category Anti-inflammatory Agent; Corticosteroid, Inhalant
Use Steroid-dependent asthma; nasal solution is used for seasonal or perennial rhinitis
Usual Dosage
Children:
Oral inhalation: >6 years: 2 inhalations twice daily up to 4 inhalations/day
Nasal: 6-14 years: 1 spray each nostril 2-3 times/day, not to exceed 4 sprays/day each nostril

Adults:
Oral inhalation: 2 inhalations twice daily up to 8 inhalations/day
Nasal: 2 sprays each nostril twice daily; maximum dose: 8 sprays/day in each nostril
Dosage Forms Inhalant:
Nasal (Nasalide®): 25 mcg/actuation [200 sprays] (25 mL)
Oral:
AeroBid®: 250 mcg/actuation [100 metered doses] (7 g)
AeroBid®-M (menthol flavor): 250 mcg/actuation [100 metered doses] (7 g)

fluocinolone acetonide (floo oh sin' oh lone)
Brand Names Derma-Smoothe/FS® Topical; Fluonid® Topical; Flurosyn® Topical; FS Shampoo® Topical; Synalar-HP® Topical; Synalar® Topical; Synemol® Topical
Therapeutic Category Corticosteroid, Topical (Medium Potency)
Use Relief of susceptible inflammatory dermatosis
Usual Dosage Children and Adults: Topical: Apply 2-4 times/day
Dosage Forms
Cream:
Flurosyn®, Synalar®: 0.01% (15 g, 30 g, 60 g, 425 g)
Flurosyn®, Synalar®, Synemol®: 0.025% (15 g, 60 g, 425 g)
Synalar-HP®: 0.2% (12 g)
Ointment, topical (Flurosyn®, Synalar®): 0.025% (15 g, 30 g, 60 g, 425 g)
Oil (Derma-Smoothe/FS®): 0.01% (120 mL)
Shampoo (FS Shampoo®): 0.01% (180 mL)
Solution, topical (Fluonid®, Synalar®): 0.01% (20 mL, 60 mL)

fluocinonide (floo oh sin' oh nide)
Brand Names Fluonex® Topical; Lidex-E® Topical; Lidex® Topical
Therapeutic Category Corticosteroid, Topical (High Potency)
Use Anti-inflammatory, antipruritic, relief of inflammatory and pruritic manifestations
Usual Dosage Children and Adults: Topical: Apply thin layer to affected area 2-4 times/day depending on the severity of the condition
Dosage Forms
Cream:
Anhydrous, emollient (Fluonex®, Lidex®): 0.05% (15 g, 30 g, 60 g, 120 g)
Aqueous, emollient (Lidex-E®): 0.05% (15 g, 30 g, 60 g, 120 g)
(Continued)
195

fluocinonide *(Continued)*

Gel, topical (Lidex"): 0.05% (15 g, 30 g, 60 g, 120 g)
Ointment, topical (Lidex"): 0.05% (15 g, 30 g, 60 g, 120 g)
Solution, topical (Lidex"): 0.05% (20 mL, 60 mL)

Fluogen® *see* influenza virus vaccine *on page 245*

fluohydrocortisone acetate *see* fludrocortisone acetate *on page 194*

Fluonex® Topical *see* fluocinonide *on previous page*

Fluonid® Topical *see* fluocinolone acetonide *on previous page*

Fluoracaine® Ophthalmic *see* proparacaine and fluorescein *on page 392*

fluorescein sodium (flure' e seen)

Brand Names AK-Fluor" Injection; Fluorescite® Injection; Fluorets® Ophthalmic Strips; Fluor-I-Strip"; Fluor-I-Strip-AT"; Fluress" Ophthalmic Solution; Ful-Glo® Ophthalmic Strips; Funduscein" Injection
Synonyms soluble fluorescein
Therapeutic Category Diagnostic Agent, Ophthalmic Dye
Use Demonstrates defects of corneal epithelium; diagnostic aid in ophthalmic angiography
Usual Dosage
Injection: Perform intradermal skin test before use to avoid possible allergic reaction
Children: 3.5 mg/lb (7.5 mg/kg) injected rapidly into antecubital vein
Adults: 500-750 mg injected rapidly into antecubital vein

Strips: Moisten with sterile water or irrigating solution, touch conjunctiva with moistened tip, blink several times after application

Topical solution: Instill 1-2 drops, allow a few seconds for staining, then wash out excess with sterile irrigation solution
Dosage Forms
Injection (AK-Fluor, Fluorescite", Funduscein", I-Rescein®): 10% [100 mg/mL] (5 mL, 10 mL); 25% [250 mg/mL] (2 mL, 3 mL)
Ophthalmic:
Solution:
2% [20 mg/mL] (1 mL, 2 mL, 15 mL)
Fluress": 0.25% [2.5 mg/mL] with benoxinate 0.4% (5 mL)
Strip:
Ful-Glo": 0.6 mg
Fluorets", Fluor-I-Strip-AT": 1 mg
Fluor-I-Strip": 9 mg

Fluorescite® Injection *see* fluorescein sodium *on this page*

Fluorets® Ophthalmic Strips *see* fluorescein sodium *on this page*

fluoride

Brand Names ACT" [OTC]; Fluorigard" [OTC]; Fluorinse®; Fluoritab®; Flura®; Flura-Drops®; Flura-Loz"; Gel Kam"; Gel-Tin" [OTC]; Karidium"; Karigel®; Karigel®-N; Listermint® with Fluoride [OTC]; Luride"; Luride" Lozi-Tab"; Luride"-SF Lozi-Tab"; Minute-Gel®; Pediaflor®; Pharmaflur"; Phos-Flur"; Point-Two"; Prevident"; Stop® [OTC]
Synonyms acidulated phosphate fluoride
Therapeutic Category Mineral, Oral; Mineral, Oral Topical
Use Prevention of dental caries
Usual Dosage Oral:
Recommended daily fluoride supplement (2.2 mg of sodium fluoride is equivalent to 1 mg of fluoride ion): See table.

Dental rinse or gel:
Children 6-12 years: 5-10 mL rinse or apply to teeth and spit daily after brushing
Adults: 10 mL rinse or apply to teeth and spit daily after brushing
Dosage Forms Fluoride ion content listed in brackets

Sodium Fluoride

Fluoride Content of Drinking Water	Daily Dose, Oral (mg)
<0.3 ppm Birth – 2 y	0.25–0.5
2–3 y	0.5
3–12 y	1
0.3–0.7 ppm Birth – 2 y	0.13
2–3 y	0.25
3–12 y	0.25–0.75

Drops, oral, as sodium:
  Fluoritab®, Flura-Drops®: 0.55 mg/drop [0.25 mg/drop] (22.8 mL, 24 mL)
  Karidium®, Luride®: 0.275 mg/drop [0.125 mg/drop] (30 mL, 60 mL)
  Pediaflor®: 1.1 mg/mL [0.5 mg/mL] (50 mL)
Gel, topical:
  Acidulated phosphate fluoride (Minute-Gel®): 1.23% (480 mL)
  Sodium fluoride (Karigel®, Karigel®-N, Prevident®): 1.1% [0.5%] (24 g, 30 g, 60 g, 120 g, 130 g, 250 g)
  Stannous fluoride (Gel Kam®, Gel-Tin®, Stop®): 0.4% [0.1%] (60 g, 65 g, 105 g, 120 g)
Lozenge, as sodium (Flura-Loz®)(raspberry flavor): 2.2 mg [1 mg]
Rinse, topical, as sodium:
  ACT®, Fluorigard®: 0.05% [0.02%] (90 mL, 180 mL, 300 mL, 360 mL, 480 mL)
  Fluorinse®, Point-Two®: 0.2% [0.09%] (240 mL, 480 mL, 3780 mL)
  Listermint® with Fluoride: 0.02% [0.01%] (180 mL, 300 mL, 360 mL, 480 mL, 540 mL, 720 mL, 960 mL, 1740 mL)
Solution, oral, as sodium (Phos-Flur®): 0.44 mg/mL [0.2 mg/mL] (250 mL, 500 mL, 3780 mL)
Tablet, as sodium:
  Chewable:
    Fluoritab®, Luride® Lozi-Tab®, Pharmaflur®: 1.1 mg [0.5 mg]
    Fluoritab®, Karidium®, Luride® Lozi-Tab®, Luride®-SF Lozi-Tab®, Pharmaflur®: 2.2 mg [1 mg]
  Flura®, Karidium®: 2.2 mg [1 mg]

Fluorigard® [OTC] *see* fluoride *on previous page*

Fluori-Methane® Topical Spray *see* dichlorodifluoromethane and trichloromonofluoromethane *on page 140*

Fluorinse® *see* fluoride *on previous page*

Fluor-I-Strip® *see* fluorescein sodium *on previous page*

Fluor-I-Strip-AT® *see* fluorescein sodium *on previous page*

Fluoritab® *see* fluoride *on previous page*

fluorodeoxyuridine *see* floxuridine *on page 193*

9α-fluorohydrocortisone acetate *see* fludrocortisone acetate *on page 194*

fluorometholone (flure oh meth' oh lone)
  Brand Names Flarex® Ophthalmic; Fluor-Op® Ophthalmic; FML® Forte Ophthalmic; FML® Ophthalmic
  Therapeutic Category Anti-inflammatory Agent; Corticosteroid, Ophthalmic
  Use Inflammatory conditions of the eye, including keratitis, iritis, cyclitis, and conjunctivitis
  Usual Dosage Children >2 years and Adults: Ophthalmic: 1-2 drops into conjunctival sac every hour during day, every 2 hours at night until favorable response is obtained, then use 1 drop every 4 hours; in mild or moderate inflammation: 1-2 drops into conjunctival sac 2-4 (Continued)
197

fluorometholone *(Continued)*

times/day. Ointment may be applied every 4 hours in severe cases or 1-3 times/day in mild to moderate cases.
Dosage Forms Ophthalmic:
Ointment (FML"): 0.1% (3.5 g)
Suspension:
Flarex", Fluor-Op", FML": 0.1% (5 mL, 10 mL, 15 mL)
FML" Forte: 0.25% (2 mL, 5 mL, 10 mL, 15 mL)

Fluoroplex® Topical *see* fluorouracil *on this page*

Fluor-Op® Ophthalmic *see* fluorometholone *on previous page*

fluorouracil (flure oh yoor' a sill)

Brand Names Adrucil" Injection; Efudex® Topical; Fluoroplex® Topical
Synonyms 5-fluorouracil; 5-fu
Therapeutic Category Antineoplastic Agent, Antimetabolite
Use Treatment of colon, breast, rectal, gastric, and pancreatic carcinomas; also used topically for management of multiple actinic or solar keratoses and superficial basal cell carcinomas
Usual Dosage Children and Adults (refer to individual protocol):
I.V.: Initial: 12 mg/kg/day (maximum: 800 mg/day) for 4-5 days; maintenance: 6 mg/kg every other day for 4 doses
Single weekly bolus dose of 15 mg/kg can be administered depending on the patient's reaction to the previous course of treatment; maintenance dose of 5-15 mg/kg/week as a single dose not to exceed 1 g/week
I.V. infusion: 15 mg/kg/day (maximum daily dose: 1 g) has been given by I.V. infusion over 4 hours for 5 days
Oral: 20 mg/kg/day for 5 days every 5 weeks for colorectal carcinoma; 15 mg/kg/week for hepatoma
Topical: 5% cream twice daily
Dosage Forms
Cream, topical:
Efudex": 5% (25 g)
Fluoroplex": 1% (30 g)
Injection (Adrucil"): 50 mg/mL (10 mL, 20 mL, 50 mL, 100 mL)
Solution, topical:
Efudex": 2% (10 mL); 5% (10 mL)
Fluoroplex": 1% (30 mL)

5-fluorouracil *see* fluorouracil *on this page*

Fluosol® *see* intravascular perfluorochemical emulsion *on page 248*

fluostigmin *see* isoflurophate *on page 252*

Fluothane® *see* halothane *on page 221*

fluoxetine hydrochloride (floo ox' e teen)

Brand Names Prozac"
Therapeutic Category Antidepressant; Serotonin Antagonist
Use Treatment of major depression
Usual Dosage Oral:
Children <18 years: Dose not established

Adults: 20 mg/day in the morning; may increase after several weeks by 20 mg/day increments; maximum: 80 mg/day; doses >20 mg should be divided into 2 daily doses
Note: Lower doses of 5 mg/day have been used for initial treatment
Dosage Forms
Capsule: 10 mg, 20 mg
Liquid (mint flavor): 20 mg/5 mL (120 mL)

fluoxymesterone (floo ox i mes' te rone)
Brand Names Halotestin®
Therapeutic Category Androgen
Use Replacement of endogenous testicular hormone; in female used as palliative treatment of breast cancer, postpartum breast engorgement
Usual Dosage Adults: Oral:
Male:
Hypogonadism: 5-20 mg/day
Delayed puberty: 2.5-20 mg/day for 4-6 months

Female:
Breast carcinoma: 10-40 mg/day in divided doses for 1-3 months
Breast engorgement: 2.5 mg after delivery, 5-10 mg/day in divided doses for 4-5 days
Dosage Forms Tablet: 2 mg, 5 mg, 10 mg

fluoxymesterone and estradiol see ethinyl estradiol and fluoxymesterone on page 178

fluphenazine (floo fen' a zeen)
Brand Names Permitil® Oral; Prolixin Decanoate® Injection; Prolixin Enanthate® Injection; Prolixin® Injection; Prolixin® Oral
Therapeutic Category Antipsychotic Agent; Phenothiazine Derivative
Use Management of manifestations of psychotic disorders
Usual Dosage Adults:
Oral: 0.5-10 mg/day in divided doses every 6-8 hours; usual maximum dose 20 mg/day
I.M.: 2.5-10 mg/day in divided doses every 6-8 hours; usual maximum dose 10 mg/day
I.M., S.C. (Decanoate®): Oral to I.M., S.C. conversion ratio = 12.5 mg, I.M., S.C. every 3 weeks for every 10 mg of oral fluphenazine
Dosage Forms
Concentrate, as hydrochloride:
Permitil®: 5 mg/mL with alcohol 1% (118 mL)
Prolixin®: 5 mg/mL with alcohol 14% (120 mL)
Elixir, as hydrochloride (Prolixin®): 2.5 mg/5 mL with alcohol 14% (60 mL, 473 mL)
Injection, as decanoate (Prolixin Decanoate®): 25 mg/mL (1 mL, 5 mL)
Injection, as enanthate (Prolixin Enanthate®): 25 mg/mL (5 mL)
Injection, as hydrochloride (Prolixin®): 2.5 mg/mL (10 mL)
Tablet, as hydrochloride
Permitil®: 2.5 mg, 5 mg, 10 mg
Prolixin®: 1 mg, 2.5 mg, 5 mg, 10 mg

Flura® see fluoride on page 196
Flura-Drops® see fluoride on page 196
Flura-Loz® see fluoride on page 196

flurandrenolide (flure an dren' oh lide)
Brand Names Cordran® SP Topical; Cordran® Topical
Synonyms flurandrenolone
Therapeutic Category Corticosteroid, Topical (Medium Potency)
Use Inflammation of corticosteroid-responsive dermatoses
Usual Dosage
Children:
Ointment or cream: Apply 1-2 times/day
Tape: Apply once daily

Adults: Cream, lotion, ointment: Apply 2-3 times/day
Dosage Forms
Cream, emulsified base (Cordran® SP): 0.025% (30 g, 60 g); 0.05% (15 g, 30 g, 60 g)
(Continued)
199

flurandrenolide (Continued)

Lotion (Cordran'''): 0.05% (15 mL, 60 mL)
Ointment, topical (Cordran'''): 0.025% (30 g, 60 g); 0.05% (15 g, 30 g, 60 g)
Tape, topical (Cordran'''): 4 mcg/cm^2 (7.5 cm x 60 cm, 7.5 cm x 200 cm rolls)

flurandrenolone *see flurandrenolide on previous page*

flurazepam hydrochloride (flure az' e pam)

Brand Names Dalmane'''
Therapeutic Category Benzodiazepine; Hypnotic; Sedative
Use Short-term treatment of insomnia
Usual Dosage Oral:
Children:
    <15 years: Dose not established
    >15 years: 15 mg at bedtime

Adults: 15-30 mg at bedtime
Dosage Forms Capsule: 15 mg, 30 mg

flurbiprofen sodium (flure bi' proe fen)

Brand Names Ansaid''' Oral; Ocufen''' Ophthalmic
Therapeutic Category Analgesic, Non-Narcotic; Anti-inflammatory Agent; Nonsteroidal Anti-Inflammatory Agent (NSAID), Ophthalmic
Use Inhibition of intraoperative miosis; acute or long-term treatment of signs of symptoms of rheumatoid arthritis and osteoarthritis; prevention and management of postoperative ocular inflammation and postoperative cystoid macular edema remains to be determined
Usual Dosage
Oral: Rheumatoid arthritis and osteoarthritis: 200-300 mg/day in 2, 3, or 4 divided doses

Ophthalmic: Instill 1 drop every 30 minutes, 2 hours prior to surgery (total of 4 drops to each affected eye)
Dosage Forms
Solution, ophthalmic (Ocufen''): 0.03% (2.5 mL, 5 mL, 10 mL)
Tablet (Ansaid''): 50 mg, 100 mg

Fluress'' Ophthalmic Solution *see fluorescein sodium on page 196*
5-flurocytosine *see flucytosine on page 194*
Fluro-Ethyl® Aerosol *see ethyl chloride and dichlorotetrafluoroethane on page 181*
Flurosyn® Topical *see fluocinolone acetonide on page 195*

flutamide (floo' ta mide)

Brand Names Eulexin''
Therapeutic Category Antiandrogen
Use In combination with LHRH agonistic analogs for the treatment of metastatic prostatic carcinoma
Usual Dosage Oral: 2 capsules every 8 hours
Dosage Forms Capsule: 125 mg

fluticasone propionate (floo tik' a sone)

Brand Names Cutivate™ Topical; Flonase'' Nasal Spray
Therapeutic Category Corticosteroid, Topical (Medium Potency)
Use
Nasal: Anti-inflammatory
Topical: Relief of inflammation and pruritus associated with corticosteroid-responsive dermatoses

Usual Dosage Apply sparingly in a thin film twice daily
Dosage Forms
Cream: 0.05% (15 g, 30 g, 60 g)
Ointment, topical: 0.005% (15 g, 60 g)
Spray, nasal:

fluvastatin (floo' va sta tin)
Brand Names Lescol®
Therapeutic Category Antilipemic Agent; HMG-CoA Reductase Inhibitor
Use Adjunct to dietary therapy to decrease elevated serum total and LDL cholesterol concentrations in primary hypercholesterolemia
Usual Dosage Adults: Oral: 20 mg at bedtime
Dosage Forms Capsule: 20 mg, 30 mg

fluvoxamine (floo vox' ah meen)
Brand Names Luvox®
Therapeutic Category Antidepressant; Serotonin Antagonist
Use Treatment of major depression and obsessive-compulsive disorder (OCD)
Dosage Forms Tablet: 50 mg, 100 mg

Fluzone® see influenza virus vaccine *on page 245*

FML® Forte Ophthalmic see fluorometholone *on page 197*

FML® Ophthalmic see fluorometholone *on page 197*

FML-S® see sodium sulfacetamide and fluoromethalone *on page 431*

Foille Plus® [OTC] see benzocaine *on page 48*

folacin see folic acid *on this page*

folate see folic acid *on this page*

Folbesyn® see vitamin b complex with vitamin c and folic acid *on page 490*

Folex® PFS see methotrexate *on page 295*

folic acid
Brand Names Folvite®
Synonyms folacin; folate; pteroylglutamic acid
Therapeutic Category Vitamin, Water Soluble
Use Treatment of megaloblastic and macrocytic anemias due to folate deficiency
Usual Dosage Folic acid deficiency:
Infants: 15 mcg/kg/dose daily or 50 mcg/day

Children: Oral, I.M., I.V., S.C.: 1 mg/day initial dosage; maintenance dose: 1-10 years: 0.1-0.3 mg/day

Children >11 years and Adults: Oral, I.M., I.V., S.C.: 1 mg/day initial dosage; maintenance dose: 0.5 mg/day
Dosage Forms
Injection, as sodium folate: 5 mg/mL (10 mL); 10 mg/mL (10 mL)
Folvite®: 5 mg/mL (10 mL)
Tablet: 0.1 mg, 0.4 mg, 0.8 mg, 1 mg
Folvite®: 1 mg

folinic acid see leucovorin calcium *on page 263*

Follutein® see chorionic gonadotropin *on page 101*

Folvite® see folic acid *on this page*

Forane® see isoflurane *on page 252*

5-formyl tetrahydrofolate see leucovorin calcium *on page 263*

Fortaz® *see* ceftazidime *on page 82*

Fortel® **Home Ovulation** *see* diagnostic aids (*in vitro*), urine *on page 137*

Fosamax® *see* alendronate *on page 12*

foscarnet (fos kar' net)
Brand Names Foscavir® Injection
Synonyms pfa; phosphonoformic acid
Therapeutic Category Antiviral Agent, Parenteral
Use Alternative to ganciclovir for treatment of CMV retinitis and other CMV infections; alternative to acyclovir for treatment of acyclovir-resistant HSV infections
Usual Dosage
Induction treatment: 60 mg/kg 3 times/day for 14-21 days
Maintenance therapy: 90-120 mg/kg/day
Dosage Forms Injection: 24 mg/mL (250 mL, 500 mL)

Foscavir® **Injection** *see* foscarnet *on this page*

fosinopril (foe sin' oh pril)
Brand Names Monopril®
Therapeutic Category Angiotensin-Converting Enzyme (ACE) Inhibitors
Use Treatment of hypertension, either alone or in combination with other antihypertensive agents
Usual Dosage Adults: Oral: 20-40 mg/day
Dosage Forms Tablet: 10 mg, 20 mg

Fostex® **[OTC]** *see* sulfur and salicylic acid *on page 442*

Fototar® **[OTC]** *see* coal tar *on page 110*

Fragmin® *see* dalteparin *on page 124*

Freezone® **Solution [OTC]** *see* salicylic acid *on page 416*

frusemide *see* furosemide *on next page*

FS Shampoo® **Topical** *see* fluocinolone acetonide *on page 195*

5-fu *see* fluorouracil *on page 198*

FUDR® *see* floxuridine *on page 193*

Ful-Glo® **Ophthalmic Strips** *see* fluorescein sodium *on page 196*

Fulvicin® **P/G** *see* griseofulvin *on page 213*

Fulvicin-U/F® *see* griseofulvin *on page 213*

Fumasorb® **[OTC]** *see* ferrous fumarate *on page 189*

Fumerin® **[OTC]** *see* ferrous fumarate *on page 189*

Funduscein® **Injection** *see* fluorescein sodium *on page 196*

Fungizone® *see* amphotericin B *on page 25*

Fungoid® *see* triacetin *on page 467*

Fungoid® **Creme** *see* miconazole *on page 305*

Fungoid® **HC Creme** *see* miconazole *on page 305*

Fungoid® **Tincture** *see* miconazole *on page 305*

Fungoid® **Topical Solution** *see* undecylenic acid and derivatives *on page 479*

Furacin® **Topical** *see* nitrofurazone *on page 329*

Furadantin® *see* nitrofurantoin *on page 329*

Furalan® *see* nitrofurantoin *on page 329*

Furan® *see* nitrofurantoin *on page 329*

Furanite® *see* nitrofurantoin *on page 329*

furazolidone (fur a zoe' li done)
Brand Names Furoxone®
Therapeutic Category Antibiotic, Miscellaneous; Antidiarrheal; Antiprotozoal
Use Treatment of bacterial or protozoal diarrhea and enteritis caused by susceptible organisms: *Giardia lamblia* and *Vibrio cholerae*
Usual Dosage Oral:
Children >1 month: 5-8.8 mg/kg/day in 3-4 divided doses for 7-10 days, not to exceed 400 mg/day
Adults: 100 mg 4 times/day for 7-10 days
Dosage Forms
Liquid: 50 mg/15 mL (60 mL, 473 mL)
Tablet: 100 mg

furazosin *see* prazosin hydrochloride *on page 383*

furosemide (fur oh' se mide)
Brand Names Lasix®
Synonyms frusemide
Therapeutic Category Diuretic, Loop
Use Management of edema associated with congestive heart failure and hepatic or renal disease; used alone or in combination with antihypertensives in treatment of hypertension
Usual Dosage
Neonates, premature:
Oral: Bioavailability is poor by this route. Doses of 1-4 mg/kg/dose 1-2 times/day have been used.
I.M., I.V.: 1-2 mg/kg/dose given every 12-24 hours
Children and Infants:
Oral: 2 mg/kg/dose increased in increments of 1 mg/kg/dose with each succeeding dose until a satisfactory effect is achieved to a maximum of 6 mg/kg/dose no more frequently than 6 hours
I.M., I.V.: 1 mg/kg/dose, increasing by each succeeding dose at 1 mg/kg/dose at intervals of 6-12 hours until a satisfactory response up to 6 mg/kg/dose
Adults:
Oral: 20-80 mg/dose initially increased in increments of 20-40 mg/dose at intervals of 6-8 hours; usual maintenance dose interval is twice daily or every day
I.M., I.V.: 20-40 mg/dose, may be repeated in 1-2 hours as needed and increased by 20 mg/dose with each succeeding dose up to 600 mg/day; usual dosing interval: 6-12 hours
Dosage Forms
Injection: 10 mg/mL (2 mL, 4 mL, 5 mL, 6 mL, 8 mL, 10 mL, 12 mL)
Solution, oral: 10 mg/mL (60 mL, 120 mL); 40 mg/5 mL (5 mL, 10 mL, 500 mL)
Tablet: 20 mg, 40 mg, 80 mg

Furoxone® *see* furazolidone *on this page*

gabapentin (ga' ba pen tin)
Brand Names Neurontin®
Therapeutic Category Anticonvulsant, Miscellaneous
Use Adjunct for treatment of drug-refractory partial and secondarily generalized seizures in adults with epilepsy
Usual Dosage Geriatrics and Adults: Oral: 900-1800 mg/day administered in 3 divided doses; therapy is initiated with a rapid titration, beginning with 300 mg on day 1, 300 mg twice daily on day 2, and 300 mg 3 times/day on day 3
(Continued)
203

gabapentin *(Continued)*

Dosing adjustment in renal impairment:
Cl_{cr} >60 mL/minute: Administer 1200 mg/day
Cl_{cr} 30-60 mL/minute: 600 mg/day
Cl_{cr} 15-30 mL/minute: 300 mg/day
Cl_{cr} <15 mL/minute: 150 mg/day
Hemodialysis: 200-300 mg after each 4-hour dialysis following a loading dose of 300-400 mg

Discontinuing therapy or replacing with an alternative agent should be done gradually over a minimum of 7 days
Dosage Forms Capsule: 100 mg, 300 mg, 400 mg

gadopentetate dimeglumine *see* radiological/contrast media (ionic) *on page 404*

gallamine triethiodide *(gal' a meen)*

Brand Names Flaxedil®
Therapeutic Category Neuromuscular Blocker Agent, Nondepolarizing; Skeletal Muscle Relaxant
Use Produce skeletal muscle relaxation during surgery after general anesthesia has been induced
Usual Dosage I.V.: 1 mg/kg then repeat dose of 0.5-1 mg/kg in 30-40 minutes for prolonged procedures
Dosage Forms Injection: 20 mg/mL (10 mL)

gallium nitrate *(gal' ee um)*

Brand Names Ganite™
Therapeutic Category Antidote, Hypercalcemia
Use Treatment of clearly symptomatic cancer-related hypercalcemia that has not responded to adequate hydration
Usual Dosage Adults: I.V. infusion: 200 mg/m^2 for 5 consecutive days
Dosage Forms Injection: 25 mg/mL (20 mL)

Gamastan® *see* immune globulin, intramuscular *on page 243*

Gamimune® N *see* immune globulin, intravenous *on page 243*

gamma benzene hexachloride *see* lindane *on page 269*

Gammagard® *see* immune globulin, intravenous *on page 243*

Gammagard® S/D *see* immune globulin, intravenous *on page 243*

gamma globulin *see* immune globulin, intramuscular *on page 243*

Gammar® *see* immune globulin, intramuscular *on page 243*

ganciclovir *(gan sye' kloe vir)*

Brand Names Cytovene®
Synonyms dhpg sodium; gcv sodium; nordeoxyguanosine
Therapeutic Category Antiviral Agent, Parenteral
Use CMV retinitis treatment of immunocompromised individuals, including patients with acquired immunodeficiency syndrome; investigational use in treatment of CMV pneumonia in marrow transplant recipients has not been rewarding, promising results have been achieved in AIDS patients and organ transplant recipients with CMV colitis, pneumonitis, and multiorgan involvement
Usual Dosage Slow I.V. infusion
Retinitis: Children >3 months and Adults: Induction therapy: 5 mg/kg/dose every 12 hours for 14-21 days followed by maintenance therapy; maintenance therapy: 5 mg/kg/day as a single daily dose for 7 days/week or 6 mg/kg/day for 5 days/week

Other CMV infections: 5 mg/kg/dose every 12 hours for 14-21 days or 2.5 mg/kg/dose every 8 hours; maintenance therapy: 5 mg/kg/day as a single daily dose for 7 days/week or 6 mg/kg/day for 5 days/week
Dosage Forms Powder for injection, lyophilized: 500 mg (10 mL)

Ganite™ *see* gallium nitrate *on previous page*

Gantanol® *see* sulfamethoxazole *on page 440*

Gantrisin® Ophthalmic *see* sulfisoxazole *on page 441*

Gantrisin® Oral *see* sulfisoxazole *on page 441*

Garamycin® Injection *see* gentamicin sulfate *on page 207*

Garamycin® Ophthalmic *see* gentamicin sulfate *on page 207*

Garamycin® Topical *see* gentamicin sulfate *on page 207*

Gastroccult® *see* diagnostic aids (*in vitro*), other *on page 137*

Gastrocrom® Oral *see* cromolyn sodium *on page 118*

Gastrografin® *see* radiological/contrast media (ionic) *on page 404*

Gastrosed™ *see* hyoscyamine sulfate *on page 239*

Gas-X® [OTC] *see* simethicone *on page 423*

Gaviscon®-2 Tablet [OTC] *see* aluminum hydroxide and magnesium trisilicate *on page 16*

Gaviscon® Liquid [OTC] *see* aluminum hydroxide and magnesium carbonate *on page 16*

Gaviscon® Tablet [OTC] *see* aluminum hydroxide and magnesium trisilicate *on page 16*

gcv sodium *see* ganciclovir *on previous page*

Gee Gee® [OTC] *see* guaifenesin *on page 213*

gelatin, absorbable
Brand Names Gelfilm® Ophthalmic; Gelfoam® Topical
Synonyms absorbable gelatin sponge
Therapeutic Category Hemostàtic Agent
Use Adjunct to provide hemostasis in surgery; also used in oral and dental surgery; in open prostatic surgery
Usual Dosage Hemostasis: Apply packs or sponges dry or saturated with sodium chloride. When applied dry, hold in place with moderate pressure. When applied wet, squeeze to remove air bubbles. Prostatectomy cones are designed for use with the Foley bag catheter. The powder is applied as a paste prepared by adding approximately 4 mL of sterile saline solution to the powder.
Dosage Forms

Gelfilm® (sterile)
    Film: 100 mm x 125 mm (1s)
    Ophthalmic: 25 mm x 50 mm (6s)

Gelfoam®
    Cones, prostatectomy:
        Size 13 cm (13 cm in diameter) (6s)
        Size 18 cm (18 cm in diameter) (6s)
    Packs:
        Size 2 cm (40 cm x 2 cm) (1s)
        Size 6 cm (40 cm x 6 cm) (6s)
    Packs, dental:
        Size 2 (10 mm x 20 mm x 7 mm) (15s)
        Size 4 (20 mm x 20 mm x 7 mm) (15s)
    Sponges:
        Size 12-3 mm (20 mm x 60 mm x 3 mm) (4s)
        Size 12-7 mm (20 mm x 60 mm x 7 mm) (4s)
        Size 50 (80 mm x 62.5 mm x 10 mm) (4s)
        Size 100 (80 mm x 125 mm x 10 mm) (6s)
        Size 100, compressed (80 mm x 125 mm) (6s)
        Size 200 (80 mm x 250 mm x 10 mm) (6s)

gelatin, pectin, and methylcellulose
Brand Names Orabase® Plain [OTC]
Therapeutic Category Protectant, Topical
Use Temporary relief from minor oral irritations
Usual Dosage Press small dabs into place until the involved area is coated with a thin film; do not try to spread onto area; may be used as often as needed
Dosage Forms Paste, oral: 5 g, 15 g

Gelfilm® Ophthalmic *see* gelatin, absorbable *on previous page*

Gelfoam® Topical *see* gelatin, absorbable *on previous page*

Gel Kam® *see* fluoride *on page 196*

Gelpirin® [OTC] *see* acetaminophen and aspirin *on page 3*

Gel-Tin® [OTC] *see* fluoride *on page 196*

Gelucast® *see* zinc gelatin *on page 495*

Gelusil® [OTC] *see* aluminum hydroxide, magnesium hydroxide, and simethicone *on page 16*

Gemcor® *see* gemfibrozil *on this page*

gemfibrozil (jem fi' broe zil)
Brand Names Gemcor®; Lopid®
Therapeutic Category Antilipemic Agent
Use Hypertriglyceridemia in types IV and V hyperlipidemia; increases HDL cholesterol
Usual Dosage Oral: 1200 mg/day in 2 divided doses, 30 minutes before breakfast and supper
Dosage Forms
  Capsule: 300 mg
  Tablet, film coated: 600 mg

Genabid® Oral *see* papaverine hydrochloride *on page 348*

Genac® [OTC] *see* triprolidine and pseudoephedrine *on page 474*

Genagesic® *see* propoxyphene and acetaminophen *on page 393*

Genahist® Oral *see* diphenhydramine hydrochloride *on page 149*

Genamin® Cold Syrup [OTC] *see* chlorpheniramine and phenylpropanolamine *on page 94*

Genamin® Expectorant [OTC] *see* guaifenesin and phenylpropanolamine *on page 215*

Genapap® [OTC] *see* acetaminophen *on page 2*

Genapax® Vaginal *see* gentian violet *on next page*

Genasoft® Plus [OTC] *see* docusate and casanthranol *on page 154*

Genaspor® [OTC] *see* tolnaftate *on page 464*

Genatuss DM® [OTC] *see* guaifenesin and dextromethorphan *on page 214*

Genatuss® [OTC] *see* guaifenesin *on page 213*

Gencalc® 600 [OTC] *see* calcium carbonate *on page 66*

Gen-K® *see* potassium chloride *on page 378*

Genoptic® Ophthalmic *see* gentamicin sulfate *on next page*

Genoptic® S.O.P. Ophthalmic *see* gentamicin sulfate *on next page*

Genora® *see* ethinyl estradiol and norethindrone *on page 178*

Genpril® [OTC] *see* ibuprofen *on page 240*

Gensan® [OTC] *see* aspirin *on page 35*

Gentab-LA® *see* guaifenesin and phenylpropanolamine *on page 215*

Gentacidin® Ophthalmic *see* gentamicin sulfate *on this page*

Gent-AK® Ophthalmic *see* gentamicin sulfate *on this page*

gentamicin and prednisolone *see* prednisolone and gentamicin *on page 384*

gentamicin sulfate (jen ta mye' sin)

Brand Names Garamycin® Injection; Garamycin® Ophthalmic; Garamycin® Topical; Genoptic® Ophthalmic; Genoptic® S.O.P. Ophthalmic; Gentacidin® Ophthalmic; Gent-AK® Ophthalmic; Gentrasul® Ophthalmic; G-myticin® Topical; Jenamicin® Injection

Therapeutic Category Antibiotic, Aminoglycoside; Antibiotic, Ophthalmic; Antibiotic, Topical

Use Treatment of susceptible bacterial infections, normally gram-negative organisms including *Pseudomonas*, *Proteus*, *Serratia*, and gram-positive *Staphylococcus*; treatment of bone infections, CNS infections, respiratory tract infections, skin and soft tissue infections, as well as abdominal and urinary tract infections, endocarditis, and septicemia

Usual Dosage Dosage should be based on an estimate of ideal body weight

Neonates: I.M., I.V.:
Postnatal age <7 days:
<1000 g and <28 weeks GA: 2.5 mg/kg/dose every 24 hours
<1500 g and <34 weeks GA: 2.5 mg/kg/dose every 18 hours
>1500 g and >34 weeks GA: 2.5 mg/kg/dose every 12 hours
Postnatal age >7 days:
<1200 g: 2.5 mg/kg/dose every 18-24 hours
>1200 g: 2.5 mg/kg/dose every 8 hours

Newborns: Intrathecal: 1 mg/day

Infants and Children >3 months: Intrathecal: 1-2 mg/day

Infants and Children <5 years: 2.5 mg/kg/dose every 8 hours

Children >5 years: 1.5-2.5 mg/kg/dose every 8 hours
Ophthalmic: Solution: 1-2 drops every 2-4 hours, up to 2 drops every hour for severe infections; ointment: 2-3 times/day
Topical: Apply 3-4 times/day

Adults:
Intrathecal: 4-8 mg/day
I.M., I.V.: 3-5 mg/kg/day in divided doses every 8 hours
Topical: Apply 3-4 times/day
Ophthalmic: Solution: 1-2 drops every 2-4 hours; ointment: 2-3 times/day

Dosage Forms
Cream, topical (Garamycin®, G-myticin®): 0.1% (15 g)
Infusion, in D₅W, as sulfate: 60 mg, 80 mg, 100 mg
Infusion, in NS, as sulfate: 40 mg, 60 mg, 80 mg, 90 mg, 100 mg, 120 mg
Injection, as sulfate: 40 mg/mL (1 mL, 1.5 mL, 2 mL)
Pediatric, as sulfate: 10 mg/mL (2 mL)
Intrathecal, preservative free, as sulfate (Garamycin®): 2 mg/mL (2 mL)
Ointment:
Ophthalmic:
Gent-AK®, Gentacidin®, Gentrasul®: 0.3% (3.5 g)
Sulfate (Garamycin®, Genoptic® S.O.P.): 0.3% (3.5 g)
Topical (Garamycin®, G-myticin®): 0.1% (15 g)
Solution, ophthalmic (Garamycin®, Genoptic®, Gentacidin®, Gent-AK®, Gentrasul®): 0.3% (1 mL, 5 mL, 15 mL)

gentian violet (jen' shun)
Brand Names Genapax® Vaginal
Synonyms crystal violet; methylrosaniline chloride
Therapeutic Category Antibacterial, Topical; Antifungal Agent, Topical
Use Treatment of cutaneous or mucocutaneous infections caused by *Candida albicans* and other superficial skin infections
(Continued)

gentian violet *(Continued)*
Usual Dosage
Infants: 3-4 drops of a 0.5% solution is applied under the tongue or on lesion after feedings

Children and Adults: Apply 0.5% to 2% with cotton to lesion 2-3 times/day for 3 days, do not swallow
Dosage Forms
Solution, topical: 1% (30 mL); 2% (30 mL)

Tampons: 5 mg (12s)

Gentran® *see dextran on page 133*

Gentrasul® Ophthalmic *see gentamicin sulfate on previous page*

Gen-XENE® *see clorazepate dipotassium on page 108*

Geocillin® *see carbenicillin on page 74*

Geref® Injection *see sermorelin acetate on page 421*

Geridium® *see phenazopyridine hydrochloride on page 360*

german measles vaccine *see rubella virus vaccine, live on page 415*

Germinal® *see ergoloid mesylates on page 169*

Gesterol® *see progesterone on page 389*

Gevrabon® [OTC] *see vitamin b complex on page 490*

gg *see guaifenesin on page 213*

GG-Cen® [OTC] *see guaifenesin on page 213*

Glaucon® *see epinephrine on page 167*

GlaucTabs® *see methazolamide on page 293*

glibenclamide *see glyburide on next page*

glipizide (glip' i zide)
Brand Names Glucotrol®; Glucotrol® XL

Synonyms glydiazinamide

Therapeutic Category Antidiabetic Agent; Hypoglycemic Agent, Oral; Sulfonylurea Agent

Use Management of noninsulin-dependent diabetes mellitus (type II)

Usual Dosage Adults: Oral: 2.5-40 mg/day; doses larger than 15-20 mg/day should be divided and given twice daily

Dosage Forms
Tablet: 5 mg, 10 mg

Tablet, extended release: 5 mg

glucagon (gloo' ka gon)
Therapeutic Category Antihypoglycemic Agent

Use Hypoglycemia; diagnostic aid in the radiologic examination of GI tract when a hypotonic state is needed; used with some success as a cardiac stimulant in management of severe cases of beta-adrenergic blocking agent overdosage

Usual Dosage
Hypoglycemia or insulin shock therapy: I.M., I.V., S.C.:

Neonates: 0.3 mg/kg/dose; maximum: 1 mg/dose

Children: 0.025-0.1 mg/kg/dose, not to exceed 1 mg/dose, repeated in 20 minutes as needed

Adults: 0.5-1 mg, may repeat in 20 minutes as needed

Diagnostic aid: Adults: I.M., I.V.: 0.25-2 mg 10 minutes prior to procedure

Dosage Forms Powder for injection, lyophilized: 1 mg [1 unit]; 10 mg [10 units]

glucocerebrosidase *see alglucerase on page 12*

glucose, instant
Brand Names B-D Glucose® [OTC]; Glutose® [OTC]; Insta-Glucose® [OTC]
Therapeutic Category Antihypoglycemic Agent
Use Management of hypoglycemia
Usual Dosage Oral: 10-20 g
Dosage Forms
Gel, oral (Glutose®, Insta-Glucose®): Dextrose 40% (25 g, 30.8 g, 80 g)
Tablet, chewable (B-D Glucose®): 5 g

glucose polymers (gloo' kose)
Brand Names Moducal® [OTC]; Polycose® [OTC]; Sumacal® [OTC]
Therapeutic Category Nutritional Supplement
Use Supplies calories for those persons not able to meet the caloric requirement with usual food intake
Dosage Forms
Liquid (Polycose®): 126 mL
Powder (Moducal®, Polycose®, Sumacal®): 350 g, 368 g, 400 g

Glucostix® [OTC] see diagnostic aids (in vitro), blood on page 136

Glucotrol® see glipizide on previous page

Glucotrol® XL see glipizide on previous page

Glukor® see chorionic gonadotropin on page 101

glutamic acid hydrochloride (gloo tam' ik)
Therapeutic Category Gastrointestinal Agent, Miscellaneous
Use Treatment of hypochlorhydria and achlorhydria
Usual Dosage Adults: Oral: 340 mg to 1.02 g 3 times/day before meals or food
Dosage Forms
Capsule, as hydrochloride: 340 mg
Powder: 100 g
Tablet: 500 mg

glutethimide (gloo teth' i mide)
Therapeutic Category Hypnotic; Sedative
Use Short-term treatment of insomnia
Usual Dosage Oral:
Adults: 250-500 mg at bedtime, dose may be repeated but not less than 4 hours before intended awakening; maximum: 1 g/day

Elderly/debilitated patients: Total daily dose should not exceed 500 mg
Dosage Forms Tablet: 250 mg

Glutose® [OTC] see glucose, instant on this page

Glyate® [OTC] see guaifenesin on page 213

glyburide (glye' byoor ide)
Brand Names Diaβeta®; Glynase™ Prestab™; Micronase®
Synonyms glibenclamide
Therapeutic Category Antidiabetic Agent; Hypoglycemic Agent, Oral; Sulfonylurea Agent
Use Management of noninsulin-dependent diabetes mellitus (type II)
Usual Dosage Adults: Oral: 1.25-5 mg to start then 1.25-20 mg maintenance dose/day divided in 1-2 doses
Prestab™: Initial: 0.75-3 mg/day, increase by 1.5 mg/day in weekly intervals; maximum: 12 mg/day
Dosage Forms
Tablet (Diaβeta®, Micronase®): 1.25 mg, 2.5 mg, 5 mg
Tablet, micronized (Glynase™ Prestab™): 1.5 mg, 3 mg

glycerin (glis' er in)

Brand Names Fleet™ Babylax® Rectal [OTC]; Ophthalgan® Ophthalmic; Osmoglyn® Ophthalmic; Sani-Supp™ Suppository [OTC]
Synonyms glycerol
Therapeutic Category Laxative, Hyperosmolar
Use Constipation; reduction of intraocular pressure; reduction of corneal edema; glycerin has been administered orally to reduce intracranial pressure
Usual Dosage
Constipation: Rectal:
Neonates: 0.5 mL/kg/dose
Children <6 years: 1 infant suppository 1-2 times/day as needed or 2-5 mL as an enema
Children >6 years and Adults: 1 adult suppository 1-2 times/day as needed or 5-15 mL as an enema

Children and Adults:
Reduction of intraocular pressure: Oral: 1-1.8 g/kg 1-1$\frac{1}{2}$ hours preoperatively; additional doses may be administered at 5-hour intervals
Reduction of corneal edema: Instill 1-2 drops in eye(s) every 3-4 hours
Reduction of intracranial pressure: Oral: 1.5 g/kg/day divided every 4 hours; dose of 1 g/kg/dose every 6 hours has also been used
Dosage Forms
Solution:
Ophthalmic, sterile (Ophthalgan®): Glycerin with chlorobutanol 0.55% (7.5 mL)
Oral (lime flavor)(Osmoglyn®): 50% (220 mL)
Rectal (Fleet® Babylax®): 4 mL/applicator (6's)
Suppository, rectal (Sani-Supp®): Glycerin with sodium stearate (infant and adult sizes)

glycerin, lanolin and peanut oil

Brand Names Massé® Breast Cream [OTC]
Therapeutic Category Topical Skin Product
Use Nipple care of pregnant and nursing women
Usual Dosage Topical: Apply as often as needed
Dosage Forms Cream: 2 oz

glycerol *see* glycerin *on this page*

glycerol guaiacolate *see* guaifenesin *on page 213*

Glycerol-T® *see* theophylline and guaifenesin *on page 454*

glycerol triacetate *see* triacetin *on page 467*

glyceryl trinitrate *see* nitroglycerin *on page 329*

Glycofed® *see* guaifenesin and pseudoephedrine *on page 216*

glycopyrrolate (glye koe pye' roe late)

Brand Names Robinul®; Robinul® Forte
Synonyms glycopyrronium bromide
Therapeutic Category Anticholinergic Agent; Antispasmodic Agent, Gastrointestinal
Use Adjunct in treatment of peptic ulcer disease; inhibit salivation and excessive secretions of the respiratory tract preoperatively; reversal of neuromuscular blockade; control of upper airway secretions
Usual Dosage
Children: Control of secretions:
Oral: 40-100 mcg/kg/dose 3-4 times/day
I.M., I.V.: 4-10 mcg/kg/dose every 3-4 hours; maximum: 0.2 mg/dose or 0.8 mg/24 hours
Children:
Intraoperative: I.V.: 4 mcg/kg not to exceed 0.1 mg; repeat at 2- to 3-minute intervals as needed
Preoperative: I.M.:
<2 years: 4.4-8.8 mcg/kg 30-60 minutes before procedure
>2 years: 4.4 mcg/kg 30-60 minutes before procedure

Children and Adults: Reverse neuromuscular blockade: I.V.: 0.2 mg for each 1 mg of neostigmine or 5 mg of pyridostigmine administered

Adults:
Intraoperative: I.V.: 0.1 mg repeated as needed at 2- to 3-minute intervals
Peptic ulcer:
Oral: 1-2 mg 2-3 times/day
I.M., I.V.: 0.1-0.2 mg 3-4 times/day
Preoperative: I.M.: 4.4 mcg/kg 30-60 minutes before procedure
Dosage Forms
Injection (Robinul®): 0.2 mg/mL (1 mL, 2 mL, 5 mL, 20 mL)
Tablet:
Robinul®: 1 mg
Robinul® Forte: 2 mg

glycopyrronium bromide see glycopyrrolate on previous page

Glycotuss-dM® [OTC] see guaifenesin and dextromethorphan on page 214

Glycotuss® [OTC] see guaifenesin on page 213

Glydeine® see guaifenesin and codeine on page 214

glydiazinamide see glipizide on page 208

Glynase™ Prestab™ see glyburide on page 209

Gly-Oxide® [OTC] see carbamide peroxide on page 74

Glytuss® [OTC] see guaifenesin on page 213

gm-csf see sargramostim on page 418

G-myticin® Topical see gentamicin sulfate on page 207

Go-Evac® see polyethylene glycol-electrolyte solution on page 375

gold sodium thiomalate
Brand Names Auralate®; Myochrysine®
Therapeutic Category Gold Compound
Use Treatment of progressive rheumatoid arthritis
Usual Dosage I.M.:
Children: Initial: Test dose of 10 mg I.M. is recommended, followed by 1 mg/kg I.M. weekly for 20 weeks; not to exceed 50 mg in a single injection; maintenance: 1 mg/kg/dose at 2- to 4-week intervals thereafter for as long as therapy is clinically beneficial and toxicity does not develop. Administration for 2-4 months is usually required before clinical improvement is observed

Adults: 10 mg first week; 25 mg second week; then 25-50 mg/week until 1 g cumulative dose has been given. If improvement occurs without adverse reactions, give 25-50 mg every 2-3 weeks, then every 3-4 weeks.
Dosage Forms Injection: 25 mg/mL (1 mL); 50 mg/mL (1 mL, 2 mL, 10 mL)

GoLYTELY® see polyethylene glycol-electrolyte solution on page 375

gonadorelin (goe nad oh rell' in)
Brand Names Factrel® Injection; Lutrepulse® Injection
Synonyms lrh
Therapeutic Category Diagnostic Agent, Gonadotrophic Hormone; Gonadotropin
Use Evaluation of the functional capacity and response of gonadotrophic hormones; used to evaluate abnormal gonadotropin regulation as in precocious puberty and delayed puberty
Usual Dosage Female:
Diagnostic test: Children >12 years and Adults: I.V., S.C. hydrochloride salt: 100 mcg administered in women during early phase of menstrual cycle (day 1-7)

Primary hypothalamic amenorrhea: Adults: Acetate: I.V.: 5 mcg every 90 minutes via Lutrepulse® pump kit at treatment intervals of 21 days (pump will pulsate every 90 minutes for 7 days)
(Continued)

211

gonadorelin *(Continued)*
Dosage Forms
Injection, as acetate (Lutrepulse®): 0.8 mg, 3.2 mg
Injection, as hydrochloride (Factrel®): 100 mcg, 500 mcg

Gonak™ [OTC] *see* hydroxypropyl methylcellulose *on page 236*

Gonic® *see* chorionic gonadotropin *on page 101*

gonioscopic ophthalmic solution *see* hydroxypropyl methylcellulose *on page 236*

Goniosol® [OTC] *see* hydroxypropyl methylcellulose *on page 236*

Gonodecten® *see* diagnostic aids (*in vitro*), other *on page 137*

Gonozyme® *see* diagnostic aids (*in vitro*), other *on page 137*

Goody's® Headache Powders *see* acetaminophen and aspirin *on page 3*

Gordofilm® Liquid *see* salicylic acid *on page 416*

Gormel® Creme [OTC] *see* urea *on page 480*

goserelin acetate *(goe' se rel in)*
Brand Names Zoladex® Implant
Therapeutic Category Gonadotropin Releasing Hormone Analog
Use Palliative treatment of advanced prostate cancer
Usual Dosage Adults: S.C.: 3.6 mg as a depot injection every 28 days into upper abdominal wall using sterile technique under the supervision of a physician. At the physician's option, local anesthesia may be used prior to injection. The injection should be repeated every 28 days as long as the patient can tolerate the side effects and there is satisfactory disease regression. While a delay of a few days is permissible, every effort should be made to adhere to the 28-day schedule.
Dosage Forms Injection, implant: 3.6 mg single-dose syringe

granisetron *(gra ni' se tron)*
Brand Names Kytril™ Injection; Kytril™ Tablet
Therapeutic Category Antiemetic
Use Prophylaxis and treatment of chemotherapy-related emesis; may be prescribed for patients who are refractory to or have severe adverse reactions to standard antiemetic therapy. Granisetron may be prescribed for young patients (ie, <45 years of age who are more likely to develop extrapyramidal reactions to high-dose metoclopramide) who are to receive highly emetogenic chemotherapeutic agents
Usual Dosage

Oral: One tablet (1 mg) twice daily
I.V.: 10-40 mcg/kg for 1-3 doses. Doses should be administered as a single IVPB over 5 minutes to 1 hour, given just prior to chemotherapy (15-60 minutes before)
  As intervention therapy for breakthrough nausea and vomiting, during the first 24 hours following chemotherapy, 2 or 3 repeat infusions (same dose) have been administered, separated by at least 10 minutes

Dosing interval in renal impairment: Creatinine clearance values have no relationship to granisetron clearance
Dosage Forms
Injection: 1 mg/mL
Tablet: 1 mg

Granulex *see* trypsin, balsam peru, and castor oil *on page 477*

granulocyte colony stimulating factor g-csf *see* filgrastim *on page 191*

granulocyte-macrophage colony stimulating factor *see* sargramostim *on page 418*

Grifulvin® V *see* griseofulvin *on this page*

Grisactin® *see* griseofulvin *on this page*

Grisactin® Ultra *see* griseofulvin *on this page*

griseofulvin (gri see oh ful' vin)

Brand Names Fulvicin® P/G; Fulvicin-U/F®; Grifulvin® V; Grisactin®; Grisactin® Ultra; Gris-PEG®

Therapeutic Category Antifungal Agent, Systemic

Use Treatment of susceptible tinea infections of the skin, hair, and nails

Usual Dosage Oral:

Children:

Microsize: 10-15 mg/kg/day in single or divided doses;

Ultramicrosize: >2 months: 5.5-7.3 mg/kg/day in single or divided doses

Adults:

Microsize: 500-1000 mg/day in single or divided doses

Ultramicrosize: 330-375 mg/day in single or divided doses; doses up to 750 mg/day have been used for infections more difficult to eradicate such as tinea unguium

Duration of therapy depends on the site of infection:

Tinea corporis: 2-4 weeks

Tinea capitis: 4-6 weeks or longer

Tinea pedis: 4-8 weeks

Tinea unguium: 3-6 months

Dosage Forms

Griseofulvin Microsize:

Capsule (Grisactin®): 125 mg, 250 mg

Suspension, oral (Grifulvin® V): 125 mg/5 mL with alcohol 0.2% (120 mL)

Tablet:

Fulvicin-U/F®, Grifulvin® V: 250 mg

Fulvicin-U/F®, Grifulvin® V, Grisactin®: 500 mg

Griseofulvin Ultramicrosize:

Tablet:

Fulvicin® P/G: 165 mg, 330 mg

Fulvicin® P/G, Grisactin® Ultra, Gris-PEG®: 125 mg, 250 mg

Grisactin® Ultra: 330 mg

Gris-PEG® *see* griseofulvin *on this page*

guaifenesin (gwye fen' e sin)

Brand Names Anti-Tuss® Expectorant [OTC]; Breonesin® [OTC]; Diabetic Tussin EX® [OTC]; Fenesin™ [OTC]; Gee Gee® [OTC]; Genatuss® [OTC]; GG-Cen® [OTC]; Glyate® [OTC]; Glycotuss® [OTC]; Glytuss® [OTC]; GuiaCough® Expectorant [OTC]; Guiatuss® [OTC]; Halotussin® [OTC]; Humibid® L.A. [OTC]; Humibid® Sprinkle [OTC]; Hytuss® [OTC]; Hytuss-2X® [OTC]; Liquibid®; Malotuss® [OTC]; Medi-Tuss® [OTC]; Mytussin® [OTC]; Naldecon® Senior EX [OTC]; Pneumomist®; Respa-GF®; Robitussin® [OTC]; Scot-Tussin® [OTC]; Siltussin® [OTC]; Sinumist®-SR Capsulets® [OTC]; Touro Ex®; Uni-Tussin® [OTC]

Synonyms gg; glycerol guaiacolate

Therapeutic Category Expectorant

Use Temporary control of cough due to minor throat and bronchial irritation

Usual Dosage Oral:

Children:

<2 years: 12 mg/kg/day in 6 divided doses

2-5 years: 50-100 mg (2.5-5 mL) every 4 hours, not to exceed 600 mg/day

6-11 years: 100-200 mg (5-10 mL) every 4 hours, not to exceed 1.2 g/day

Children >12 years and Adults: 200-400 mg (10-20 mL) every 4 hours to a maximum of 2.4 g/day (60 mL/day)

(Continued)

213

guaifenesin *(Continued)*
Dosage Forms
Caplet, sustained release (Touro Ex®): 600 mg
Capsule (Breonesin®, GG-Cen®, Hytuss-2X®): 200 mg
Capsule, sustained release (Humibid® Sprinkle): 300 mg
Liquid:
    Diabetic Tussin EX®: 100 mg/5 mL (118 mL)
    Naldecon® Senior EX: 200 mg/5 mL (118 mL, 480 mL)
Syrup (Anti-Tuss® Expectorant, Genatuss®, Glyate®, GuiaCough® Expectorant, Guiatuss®, Halotussin®, Malotuss®, Medi-Tuss®, Mytussin®, Robitussin®, Scot-tussin®, Siltussin®, Uni-Tussin®): 100 mg/5 mL (30 mL, 120 mL, 240 mL, 473 mL, 946 mL)
Tablet:
    Gee Gee®, Glytuss®: 200 mg
    Glycotuss®, Hytuss®: 100 mg
    Sustained release:
        Fenesin™, Humibid® L.A., Liquibid®, Pneumomist®, Respa-GF®, Sinumist®-SR Capsulets®: 600 mg

Guaifenesin AC® *see guaifenesin and codeine on this page*

guaifenesin and codeine
Brand Names Brontex® Liquid; Brontex® Tablet; Cheracol®; Glydeine®; Guaifenesin AC®; Guaituss AC®; Guiatussin® with Codeine; Halotussin® AC; Medi-Tuss® AC; Mytussin® AC; Robitussin® A-C
Synonyms codeine and guaifenesin
Therapeutic Category Antitussive; Cough Preparation; Expectorant
Use Temporary control of cough due to minor throat and bronchial irritation
Usual Dosage Oral:
Children:
    2-6 years: 1-1.5 mg/kg codeine/day divided into 4 doses administered every 4-6 hours
    6-12 years: 5 mL every 4 hours, not to exceed 30 mL/24 hours
    >12 years: 10 mL every 4 hours, up to 60 mL/24 hours

Adults: 10 mL or one tablet every 6-8 hours
Dosage Forms
Liquid (Brontex®): Guaifenesin 75 mg and codeine phosphate 2.5 mg per 5 mL
Syrup (Cheracol®, Glydeine®, Guaifenesin AC®, Guaituss AC®, Guiatussin® with Codeine, Halotussin® AC, Medi-Tuss® AC, Mytussin® AC, Robitussin® A-C): Guaifenesin 100 mg and codeine phosphate 10 mg per 5 mL (60 mL, 120 mL, 480 mL)
Tablet (Brontex®): Guaifenesin 300 mg and codeine phosphate 10 mg

guaifenesin and dextromethorphan
Brand Names Benylin® Expectorant [OTC]; Cheracol® D [OTC]; Contac® Cough Formula Liquid [OTC]; Extra Action Cough Syrup [OTC]; Fenesin DM®; Genatuss DM® [OTC]; Glycotuss-dM® [OTC]; GuiaCough® [OTC]; Guiatuss DM® [OTC]; Halotussin® DM [OTC]; Humibid® DM [OTC]; Kolephrin® GG/DM [OTC]; Mytussin® DM [OTC]; Naldecon® Senior DX [OTC]; Phanatuss® [OTC]; Queltuss® [OTC]; Respa-DM®; Rhinosyn-DMX® [OTC]; Robitussin®-DM [OTC]; Siltussin DM® [OTC]; Syracol-CF® [OTC]; Tolu-Sed® DM [OTC]; Tuss-DM® [OTC]; Uni-Tussin® DM [OTC]; Vicks® 44E
Synonyms dextromethorphan and guaifenesin
Therapeutic Category Antitussive; Cough Preparation; Expectorant
Use Temporary control of cough due to minor throat and bronchial irritation
Usual Dosage Oral:
Children:
    2-5 years: 2.5 mL every 6-8 hours; maximum: 10 mL/day
    6-12 years: 5 mL every 6-8 hours; maximum: 20 mL/24 hours
    >12 years: 10 mL every 6-8 hours; maximum: 40 mL/24 hours

Alternatively: 0.1-0.15 mL/kg/dose every 6-8 hours as needed

Adults: 10 mL every 6-8 hours

Dosage Forms

Syrup:

Benylin® Expectorant: Guaifenesin 100 mg and dextromethorphan hydrobromide 5 mg per 5 mL (118 mL, 236 mL)

Cheracol® D, Genatuss DM®, Mytussin® DM, Robitussin®-DM, Siltussin DM®, Tolu-Sed® DM: Guaifenesin 100 mg and dextromethorphan hydrobromide 10 mg per 5 mL (5 mL, 10 mL, 120 mL, 240 mL, 360 mL, 480 mL, 3780 mL)

Contac® Cough Formula Liquid: Guaifenesin 67 mg and dextromethorphan hydrobromide 10 mg per 5 mL (120 mL)

Extra Action Cough Syrup, GuiaCough®, Guiatuss DM®, Halotussin® DM, Rhinosyn-DMX®, Uni-tussin® DM: Guaifenesin 100 mg and dextromethorphan hydrobromide 15 mg per 5 mL (120 mL, 240 mL, 480 mL)

Kolephrin® GG/DM: Guaifenesin 150 mg and dextromethorphan hydrobromide 10 mg per 5 mL (120 mL)

Naldecon® Senior DX: Guaifenesin 200 mg and dextromethorphan hydrobromide 15 mg per 5 mL (118 mL, 480 mL)

Phanatuss®: Guaifenesin 85 mg and dextromethorphan hydrobromide 10 mg per 5 mL

Vicks® 44E: Guaifenesin 66.7 mg and dextromethorphan hydrobromide 6.7 mg per 5 mL

Tablet:

Extended release

Fenesin DM®, Humibid® DM, Respa-DM®: Guaifenesin 600 mg and dextromethorphan hydrobromide 30 mg

Glycotuss-dM®: Guaifenesin 100 mg and dextromethorphan hydrobromide 10 mg

Queltuss®: Guaifenesin 100 mg and dextromethorphan hydrobromide 15 mg

Syracol-CF®: Guaifenesin 200 mg and dextromethorphan hydrobromide 15 mg

Tuss-DM®: Guaifenesin 200 mg and dextromethorphan hydrobromide 10 mg

guaifenesin and hydrocodone see hydrocodone and guaifenesin on page 230

guaifenesin and phenylpropanolamine

Brand Names Ami-Tex LA®; Conex® [OTC]; Contuss® XT; Dura-Vent®; Entex® LA; Genamin® Expectorant [OTC]; Gentab-LA®; Guiapax®; Myminic® Expectorant [OTC]; Naldecon-EX® Children's Syrup [OTC]; Nolex® LA; Partuss® LA; Phenylfenesin® L.A.; Rymed-TR®; Silaminic® Expectorant [OTC]; Sildicon-E® [OTC]; Snaplets-EX® [OTC]; Theramin® Expectorant [OTC]; Triaminic® Expectorant [OTC]; Tri-Clear® Expectorant [OTC]; Triphenyl® Expectorant [OTC]; ULR-LA®; Vanex-LA®; Vicks® DayQuil® Sinus Pressure & Congestion Relief [OTC]

Synonyms phenylpropanolamine and guaifenesin

Therapeutic Category Decongestant; Expectorant

Use Symptomatic relief of those respiratory conditions where tenacious mucous plugs and congestion complicate the problem such as sinusitis, pharyngitis, bronchitis, asthma, and as an adjunctive therapy in serous otitis media

Usual Dosage Oral:

Children:

2-6 years: 2.5 mL every 4 hours

6-12 years: $\frac{1}{2}$ tablet every 12 hours or 5 mL every 4 hours

Children >12 years and Adults: 1 tablet every 12 hours or 10 mL every 4 hours

Dosage Forms

Caplet:

Vicks® DayQuil® Sinus Pressure & Congestion Relief: Guaifenesin 200 mg and phenylpropanolamine hydrochloride 25 mg

Gentab-LA®, Rymed-TR®: Guaifenesin 400 mg and phenylpropanolamine hydrochloride 75 mg

Drops (Sildicon-E®): Guaifenesin 30 mg and phenylpropanolamine hydrochloride 6.25 mg per mL (30 mL)

Granules (Snaplets-EX®): Guaifenesin 50 mg and phenylpropanolamine hydrochloride 6.25 mg (pack)

(Continued)

215

guaifenesin and phenylpropanolamine *(Continued)*
Liquid:
> Conex®, Genamin® Expectorant, Myminic® Expectorant, Silaminic® Expectorant, Theramine® Expectorant, Triaminic® Expectorant, Tri-Clear® Expectorant, Triphenyl® Expectorant: Guaifenesin 100 mg and phenylpropanolamine hydrochloride 12.5 mg per 5 mL (120 mL, 240 mL, 480 mL, 3780 mL)
> Naldecon-EX® Children's Syrup: Guaifenesin 100 mg and phenylpropanolamine hydrochloride 6.25 mg per 5 mL (120 mL)

Tablet, extended release:
> Ami-Tex LA®, Contuss® XT, Entex® LA, Guiapax®, Nolex® LA, Partuss® LA, Phenylfenesin® L.A., ULR-LA®, Vanex-LA®: Guaifenesin 400 mg and phenylpropanolamine hydrochloride 75 mg
> Dura-Vent®: Guaifenesin 600 mg and phenylpropanolamine hydrochloride 75 mg

guaifenesin and pseudoephedrine
Brand Names Congess® Jr; Congess® Sr; Congestac®; Deconsal® II; Defen-LA®; Entex® PSE; Eudal-SR®; Fedahist® Expectorant [OTC]; Fedahist® Expectorant Pediatric Drops [OTC]; Glycofed®; Guai-Vent/PSE®; Guiafed® [OTC]; Guiafed-PD®; GuiaMax-D®; Guiatab®; Guiatuss PE® [OTC]; Halotussin® PE [OTC]; Histalet X®; Nasabid®; Respa-1st®; Respaire®-60 SR; Respaire®-120 SR; Robitussin-PE® [OTC]; Robitussin® Severe Congestion Liqui-Gels [OTC]; Ru-Tuss® DE; Rymed®; Sinufed® Timecelles®; Sudex®; Touro LA®; Tuss-LA®; V-Dec-M®; Versacaps®; Zephrex®; Zephrex LA®

Synonyms pseudoephedrine and guaifenesin

Therapeutic Category Decongestant; Expectorant

Use Enhance the output of respiratory tract fluid and reduce mucosal congestion and edema in the nasal passage

Usual Dosage Oral:
Children:
> 2-6 years: 2.5 mL every 4 hours not to exceed 15 mL/24 hours
> 6-12 years: 5 mL every 4 hours not to exceed 30 mL/24 hours

> Children >12 years and Adults: 10 mL every 4 hours not to exceed 60 mL/24 hours

Dosage Forms
Capsule:
> Robitussin® Severe Congestion Liqui-Gels: Guaifenesin 200 mg and pseudoephedrine hydrochloride 30 mg
> Rymed®: Guaifenesin 250 mg and pseudoephedrine hydrochloride 30 mg

Capsule, extended release:
> Congess® Jr: Guaifenesin 125 mg and pseudoephedrine hydrochloride 60 mg
> Nasabid®: Guaifenesin 250 mg and pseudoephedrine hydrochloride 90 mg
> Congess® Sr, Guaifed®, Respaire®-120 SR,: Guaifenesin 250 mg and pseudoephedrine hydrochloride 120 mg
> Guiafed-PD®, Sinufed® Timecelles®, Versacaps®: Guaifenesin 300 mg and pseudoephedrine hydrochloride 60 mg
> Respaire®-60 SR: Guaifenesin 200 mg and pseudoephedrine hydrochloride 60 mg
> Tuss-LA® Capsule: Guaifenesin 500 mg and pseudoephedrine hydrochloride 120 mg

Drops, oral (Fedahist® Expectorant Pediatric): Guaifenesin 40 mg and pseudoephedrine hydrochloride 7.5 mg per mL (30 mL)

Syrup:
> Fedahist® Expectorant, Guiafed®: Guaifenesin 200 mg and pseudoephedrine hydrochloride 30 mg per 5 mL (120 mL, 240 mL)
> Guiatuss® PE, Halotussin® PE, Robitussin-PE®, Rymed®: Guaifenesin 100 mg and pseudoephedrine hydrochloride 30 mg per 5 mL (120 mL, 240 mL, 480 mL)
> Histalet X®: Guaifenesin 200 mg and pseudoephedrine hydrochloride 45 mg per 5 mL (473 mL)

Tablet:
> Congestac®, Guiatab®, Zephrex®: Guaifenesin 400 mg and pseudoephedrine hydrochloride 60 mg
> Glycofed®: Guaifenesin 100 mg and pseudoephedrine hydrochloride 30 mg

Tablet, extended release:

Deconsal® II, Defen-LA®, Respa-1st®: Guaifenesin 600 mg and pseudoephedrine hydrochloride 60 mg

Entex® PSE, GuiaMax-D®, Guai-Vent/PSE®, Ru-Tuss® DE, Sudex®, Zephrex LA®: Guaifenesin 600 mg and pseudoephedrine hydrochloride 120 mg

Eudal-SR®, Histalex® X, Touro LA®: Guaifenesin 400 mg and pseudoephedrine hydrochloride 120 mg

Tuss-LA® Tablet, V-Dec-M®: Guaifenesin 5mg and pseudoephedrine hydrochloride 120 mg

guaifenesin, phenylpropanolamine, and dextromethorphan

Brand Names Anatuss® [OTC]; Guiatuss CF® [OTC]; Naldecon® DX Adult Liquid [OTC]; Robafen® CF [OTC]; Robitussin-CF® [OTC]; Siltussin-CF® [OTC]

Therapeutic Category Cough Preparation; Decongestant; Expectorant

Use Temporarily relieves nasal congestion and controls cough due to minor throat and bronchial irritation; helps loosen phlegm and thin bronchial secretions to make coughs more productive

Usual Dosage Oral:

Children:

2-6 years: 2.5 mL every 4 hours not to exceed 15 mL/24 hours

6-12 years: 5 mL every 4 hours not to exceed 30 mL/24 hours

Children >12 years and Adults: 10 mL every 4 hours not to exceed 60 mL/24 hours

Dosage Forms

Syrup:

Anatuss®: Guaifenesin 100 mg, phenylpropanolamine hydrochloride 25 mg, and dextromethorphan hydrobromide 15 mg per 5 mL (120 mL, 473 mL)

Guiatuss® CF, Robafen® CF, Robitussin-CF®: Guaifenesin 100 mg, phenylpropanolamine hydrochloride 12.5 mg, and dextromethorphan hydrobromide 10 mg per 5 mL (120 mL, 240 mL, 360 mL, 480 mL)

Naldecon® DX Adult: Guaifenesin 200 mg, phenylpropanolamine hydrochloride 12.5 mg, and dextromethorphan hydrobromide 10 mg per 5 mL (120 mL, 473 mL)

Siltussin-CF®: Guaifenesin 100 mg, phenylpropanolamine hydrochloride 12.5 mg, and dextromethorphan hydrobromide 10 mg per 5 mL

Tablet: (Anatuss®): Guaifenesin 100 mg, phenylpropanolamine hydrochloride 25 mg, and dextromethorphan hydrobromide 15 mg

guaifenesin, phenylpropanolamine, and phenylephrine

Brand Names Contuss®; Despec® Liquid; Dura-Gest®; Enomine®; Entex®; Guiatex®; Respinol-G®; ULR®

Therapeutic Category Decongestant; Expectorant

Use Symptomatic relief of sinusitis, bronchitis, pharyngitis associated with nasal congestion and thick mucous secretions in lower respiratory tract

Usual Dosage Children >12 years and Adults: 1 capsule 4 times/day (every 6 hours) with food or fluid

Dosage Forms

Capsule (Contuss®, Dura-Gest®, Enomine®, Entex®, Guiatex®, ULR®): Guaifenesin 200 mg, phenylpropanolamine hydrochloride 45 mg, and phenylephrine hydrochloride 5 mg

Liquid (Contuss®, Despec®, Entex®): Guaifenesin 100 mg, phenylpropanolamine hydrochloride 20 mg, and phenylephrine hydrochloride 5 mg per 5 mL (118 mL, 480 mL)

Tablet (Respinol-G®): Guaifenesin 200 mg, phenylpropanolamine hydrochloride 45 mg, and phenylephrine hydrochloride 5 mg

guaifenesin, pseudoephedrine, and codeine

Brand Names Codafed® Expectorant; Decohistine® Expectorant; Deproist® Expectorant with Codeine; Dihistine® Expectorant; Guiatuss DAC®; Guiatussin® DAC; Halotussin® DAC; Isoclor® Expectorant; Mytussin® DAC; Novahistine® Expectorant; Nucofed®; Nucofed® Pediatric Expectorant; Nucotuss®; Phenhist® Expectorant; Robitussin®-DAC; Ryna-CX®

Therapeutic Category Cough Preparation; Decongestant; Expectorant

Use Temporarily relieves nasal congestion and controls cough due to minor throat and bron-
(Continued)

guaifenesin, pseudoephedrine, and codeine *(Continued)*

chial irritation; helps loosen phlegm and thin bronchial secretions to make coughs more productive

Usual Dosage Oral:

Children 6-12 years: 5 mL every 4 hours, not to exceed 40 mL/24 hours

Children >12 years and Adults: 10 mL every 4 hours, not to exceed 40 mL/24 hours

Dosage Forms Liquid:

Codafed™ Expectorant, Decohistine™ Expectorant, Deproist® Expectorant with Codeine, Dihistine™ Expectorant, Guiatuss DAC®, Guiatussin® DAC, Halotussin® DAC, Isoclor® Expectorant, Mytussin™ DAC, Novahistine® Expectorant, Nucofed® Pediatric Expectorant, Phenhist™ Expectorant, Robitussin®-DAC, Ryna-CX®: Guaifenesin 100 mg, pseudoephedrine hydrochloride 30 mg, and codeine phosphate 10 mg per 5 mL (120 mL, 480 mL, 4000 mL)

Nucofed™, Nucotuss™: Guaifenesin 200 mg, pseudoephedrine hydrochloride 60 mg, and codeine phosphate 20 mg per 5 mL (480 mL)

Guaituss AC® *see* guaifenesin and codeine *on page 214*

Guai-Vent/PSE® *see* guaifenesin and pseudoephedrine *on page 216*

guanabenz acetate *(gwahn' a benz)*

Brand Names Wytensin™

Therapeutic Category Alpha-Adrenergic Agonist

Use Management of hypertension

Usual Dosage Adults: Oral: Initial: 4 mg twice daily, increase in increments of 4-8 mg/day every 1-2 weeks to a maximum of 32 mg twice daily

Dosage Forms Tablet: 4 mg, 8 mg

guanadrel sulfate *(gwahn' a drel)*

Brand Names Hylorel™

Therapeutic Category Alpha-Adrenergic Agonist

Use Step 2 agent in stepped-care treatment of hypertension, usually with a diuretic

Usual Dosage Initial: 10 mg/day (5 mg twice daily); adjust dosage until blood pressure is controlled, usual dosage: 20-75 mg/day, given twice daily

Dosage Forms Tablet: 10 mg, 25 mg

guanethidine monosulfate *(gwahn eth' i deen)*

Brand Names Ismelin™

Therapeutic Category Alpha-Adrenergic Agonist

Use Treatment of moderate to severe hypertension

Usual Dosage

Children: Initial dose: 0.2 mg/kg/day, given daily; maximum dose: up to 3 mg/kg/24 hours

Adults: Initial dose: 10-12.5 mg/day, then 25-50 mg/day in 3 divided doses

Dosage Forms Tablet: 10 mg, 25 mg

guanfacine hydrochloride *(gwahn' fa seen)*

Brand Names Tenex™

Therapeutic Category Alpha-Adrenergic Agonist

Use Management of hypertension

Usual Dosage Adults: Oral: 1 mg usually at bedtime, may increase if needed at 3- to 4-week intervals to a maximum of 3 mg/day; 1 mg/day is most common dose

Dosage Forms Tablet: 1 mg

guanidine hydrochloride *(gwahn' i deen)*

Therapeutic Category Cholinergic Agent

Use Reduction of the symptoms of muscle weakness associated with the myasthenic syndrome of Eaton-Lambert, not for myasthenia gravis

Usual Dosage Adults: Oral: Initial: 10-15 mg/kg/day in 3-4 divided doses, gradually increase to 35 mg/kg/day
Dosage Forms Tablet: 125 mg

GuiaCough® Expectorant [OTC] *see* guaifenesin *on page 213*
GuiaCough® [OTC] *see* guaifenesin and dextromethorphan *on page 214*
Guiafed-PD® *see* guaifenesin and pseudoephedrine *on page 216*
Guiafed® [OTC] *see* guaifenesin and pseudoephedrine *on page 216*
GuiaMax-D® *see* guaifenesin and pseudoephedrine *on page 216*
Guiapax® *see* guaifenesin and phenylpropanolamine *on page 215*
Guiatab® *see* guaifenesin and pseudoephedrine *on page 216*
Guiatex® *see* guaifenesin, phenylpropanolamine, and phenylephrine *on page 217*
Guiatuss CF® [OTC] *see* guaifenesin, phenylpropanolamine, and dextromethorphan *on page 217*
Guiatuss DAC® *see* guaifenesin, pseudoephedrine, and codeine *on page 217*
Guiatuss DM® [OTC] *see* guaifenesin and dextromethorphan *on page 214*
Guiatussin® DAC *see* guaifenesin, pseudoephedrine, and codeine *on page 217*
Guiatussin® with Codeine *see* guaifenesin and codeine *on page 214*
Guiatuss PE® [OTC] *see* guaifenesin and pseudoephedrine *on page 216*
Guiatuss® [OTC] *see* guaifenesin *on page 213*
gum benjamin *see* benzoin *on page 49*
G-well® Lotion *see* lindane *on page 269*
G-well® Shampoo *see* lindane *on page 269*
Gynecort® [OTC] *see* hydrocortisone *on page 232*
Gyne-Lotrimin® [OTC] *see* clotrimazole *on page 109*
Gyne-Sulf® *see* sulfabenzamide, sulfacetamide, and sulfathiazole *on page 439*
Gynogen L.A.® Injection *see* estradiol *on page 173*
Gynol II® [OTC] *see* nonoxynol 9 *on page 331*
Habitrol™ Patch *see* nicotine *on page 327*

halazepam (hal az' e pam)
Brand Names Paxipam®
Therapeutic Category Antianxiety Agent; Benzodiazepine
Use Management of anxiety disorders; short-term relief of the symptoms of anxiety
Usual Dosage Adults: Oral: 20-40 mg 3 or 4 times daily
Dosage Forms Tablet: 20 mg, 40 mg

halcinonide (hal sin' oh nide)
Brand Names Halog-E® Topical; Halog® Topical
Therapeutic Category Corticosteroid, Topical (High Potency)
Use Inflammation of corticosteroid-responsive dermatoses
Usual Dosage Children and Adults: Topical: Apply sparingly 1-3 times/day, occlusive dressing may be used for severe or resistant dermatoses
Dosage Forms
Cream (Halog®): 0.025% (15 g, 60 g, 240 g); 0.1% (15 g, 30 g, 60 g, 240 g)
Cream, emollient base (Halog®-E) : 0.1% (15 g, 30 g, 60 g)
Ointment, topical (Halog®): 0.1% (15 g, 30 g, 60 g, 240 g)
Solution (Halog®): 0.1% (20 mL, 60 mL)

Halcion® *see* triazolam *on page 469*

Haldol® Decanoate Injection *see* haloperidol *on this page*

Haldol® Injection *see* haloperidol *on this page*

Haldol® Oral *see* haloperidol *on this page*

Haley's M-O® [OTC] *see* magnesium hydroxide and mineral oil emulsion *on page 277*

Halfan® *see* halofantrine *on this page*

Halfprin® 81 [OTC] *see* aspirin *on page 35*

halobetasol propionate (hal oh bay' ta sol)
Brand Names Ultravate™ Topical
Therapeutic Category Corticosteroid, Topical (Very High Potency)
Use Relief of inflammatory and pruritic manifestations of corticosteroid-response dermatoses
Usual Dosage Children and Adults: Topical: Apply sparingly to skin twice daily, rub in gently and completely
Dosage Forms
Cream: 0.05% (15 g, 45 g)
Ointment, topical: 0.05% (15 g, 45 g)

halofantrine (ha loe fan' trin)
Brand Names Halfan®
Therapeutic Category Antimalarial Agent
Use Treatment of mild to moderate acute malaria caused by susceptible strains of *Plasmodium falciparum* and *Plasmodium vivax*
Dosage Forms
Suspension: 100 mg/5 mL
Tablet: 250 mg

Halog-E® Topical *see* halcinonide *on previous page*

Halog® Topical *see* halcinonide *on previous page*

haloperidol (ha loe per' i dole)
Brand Names Haldol® Decanoate Injection; Haldol® Injection; Haldol® Oral
Therapeutic Category Antipsychotic Agent
Use Treatment of psychoses, Tourette's disorder, and severe behavioral problems in children; may be used for the emergency sedation of severely agitated or delirious patients
Usual Dosage
Children:
<3 years: Not recommended
3-6 years: Dose and indications are not well established
Control of agitation or hyperkinesia in disturbed children: Oral: 0.01-0.03 mg/kg/day once daily
Infantile autism: Oral: Daily doses of 0.5-4 mg have been reported to be helpful in this disorder
6-12 years: Dose not well established
I.M.: 1-3 mg/dose every 4-8 hours, up to a maximum of 0.1 mg/kg/day
Acute psychosis: Oral: Begin with 0.5-1.5 mg/day and increase gradually in increments of 0.5 mg/day, to a maintenance dose of 2-4 mg/day (0.05-0.1 mg/kg/day).
Tourette's syndrome and mental retardation with hyperkinesia: Oral: Begin with 0.5 mg/day and increase by 0.5 mg/day each day until symptoms are controlled or a maximum dose of 15 mg is reached
Children >12 years and Adults:
I.M.:
Acute psychosis: 2-5 mg/dose every 1-8 hours PRN up to a total of 10-30 mg, until control of symptoms is achieved

Mental retardation with hyperkinesia: Begin with 20 mg/day in divided doses, then increase slowly, up to a maximum of 60 mg/day; change to oral administration as soon as symptoms are controlled

Oral:

Acute psychosis: Begin with 1-15 mg/day in divided doses, then gradually increase until symptoms are controlled, up to a maximum of 100 mg/day; after control of symptoms is achieved, reduce dose to the minimal effective dose

Tourette's syndrome: Begin with 6-15 mg/day in divided doses, increase in increments of 2-10 mg/day until symptoms are controlled or adverse reactions become disabling; when symptoms are controlled, reduce to approximately 9 mg/day for maintenance

Dosage Forms
Concentrate, oral, as lactate: 2 mg/mL (5 mL, 10 mL, 15 mL, 120 mL, 240 mL)
Injection, as decanoate: 50 mg/mL (1 mL, 5 mL); 100 mg/mL (1 mL, 5 mL)
Injection, as lactate: 5 mg/mL (1 mL, 2 mL, 2.5 mL, 10 mL)
Tablet: 0.5 mg, 1 mg, 2 mg, 5 mg, 10 mg, 20 mg

haloprogin (ha loe proe' jin)
Brand Names Halotex® Topical
Therapeutic Category Antifungal Agent, Topical
Use Topical treatment of tinea pedis, tinea cruris, tinea corporis, tinea manuum caused by *Trichophyton rubrum*, *Trichophyton tonsurans*, *Trichophyton mentagrophytes*, *Microsporum canis*, or *Epidermophyton floccosum*
Usual Dosage Children and Adults: Topical: Twice daily for 2-3 weeks; intertriginous areas may require up to 4 weeks of treatment
Dosage Forms
Cream: 1% (15 g, 30 g)
Solution, topical: 1% with alcohol 75% (10 mL, 30 mL)

Halotestin® *see* fluoxymesterone *on page 199*
Halotex® Topical *see* haloprogin *on this page*

halothane (ha' loe thane)
Brand Names Fluothane®
Therapeutic Category General Anesthetic
Use General induction and maintenance of anesthesia (inhalation)
Usual Dosage Maintenance concentration varies from 0.5% to 1.5%
Dosage Forms Liquid: 125 mL, 250 mL

Halotussin® AC *see* guaifenesin and codeine *on page 214*
Halotussin® DAC *see* guaifenesin, pseudoephedrine, and codeine *on page 217*
Halotussin® [OTC] *see* guaifenesin *on page 213*
Halotussin® DM [OTC] *see* guaifenesin and dextromethorphan *on page 214*
Halotussin® PE [OTC] *see* guaifenesin and pseudoephedrine *on page 216*
Haltran® [OTC] *see* ibuprofen *on page 240*
hamamelis water *see* witch hazel *on page 492*
Havrix® *see* hepatitis a vaccine *on page 223*
hbig *see* hepatitis b immune globulin *on page 223*
H-BIG® *see* hepatitis b immune globulin *on page 223*
hcg *see* chorionic gonadotropin *on page 101*
hctz *see* hydrochlorothiazide *on page 229*
HD 85® *see* radiological/contrast media (ionic) *on page 404*
HD 200 Plus® *see* radiological/contrast media (ionic) *on page 404*

hdcv *see* rabies virus vaccine, human diploid *on page 404*

hdrs *see* rabies virus vaccine, human diploid *on page 404*

Head & Shoulders® [OTC] *see* pyrithione zinc *on page 401*

Healon® *see* sodium hyaluronate *on page 428*

Healon® GV *see* sodium hyaluronate *on page 428*

Healon® Yellow *see* sodium hyaluronate *on page 428*

Helistat® *see* microfibrillar collagen hemostat *on page 306*

Hemabate™ *see* carboprost tromethamine *on page 76*

Hema-Chek® [OTC] *see* diagnostic aids (*in vitro*), feces *on page 137*

Hema-Combistix® [OTC] *see* diagnostic aids (*in vitro*), urine *on page 137*

Hemastix® [OTC] *see* diagnostic aids (*in vitro*), urine *on page 137*

Hematest® [OTC] *see* diagnostic aids (*in vitro*), feces *on page 137*

hemiacidrin *see* citric acid bladder mixture *on page 103*

hemin
Brand Names Panhematin®
Therapeutic Category Blood Modifiers
Use Treatment of recurrent attacks of acute intermittent porphyria (AIP) only after an appropriate period of alternate therapy has been tried
Usual Dosage I.V.: 1-4 mg/kg/day administered over 10-15 minutes for 3-14 days; may be repeated no earlier than every 12 hours; not to exceed 6 mg/kg in any 24-hour period
Dosage Forms Powder for injection, preservative free: 313 mg/vial [hematin 7 mg/mL] (43 mL)

Hemoccult® II [OTC] *see* diagnostic aids (*in vitro*), feces *on page 137*

Hemoccult® Slides *see* diagnostic aids (*in vitro*), feces *on page 137*

Hemocyte® [OTC] *see* ferrous fumarate *on page 189*

Hemofil® M *see* antihemophilic factor (human) *on page 29*

hemophilus b conjugate vaccine (hem off' fil us)
Brand Names HibTITER®; OmniHIB®; PedvaxHIB™; ProHIBiT®
Synonyms Hib polysaccharide conjugate; prp-d
Therapeutic Category Vaccine, Inactivated Bacteria
Use Immunization of children 24 months to 6 years of age against diseases caused by *H. influenzae* type b
Dosage Forms Injection:
  HibTITER®, OmniHIB®: Capsular oligosaccharide 10 mcg and diphtheria CRM_{197} protein ~25 mcg per 0.5 mL (0.5 mL, 2.5 mL, 5 mL)
  PedvaxHIB™: Purified capsular polysaccharide 15 mcg and *Neisseria meningitidis* OMPC 250 mcg per dose (0.5 mL)
  ProHIBiT®: Purified capsular polysaccharide 25 mcg and conjugated diphtheria toxoid protein 18 mcg per dose (0.5 mL, 2.5 mL, 5 mL)

Hemotene® *see* microfibrillar collagen hemostat *on page 306*

Hemril-HC® Uniserts® *see* hydrocortisone *on page 232*

Hepalac® *see* lactulose *on page 261*

heparin (hep' a rin)
Brand Names Calciparine®; Hep-Lock®; Liquaemin®
Therapeutic Category Anticoagulant
Use Prophylaxis and treatment of thromboembolic disorders

Usual Dosage Note: For full-dose heparin (ie, nonlow-dose), the dose should be titrated according to PTT results. For anticoagulation, an APTT 1.5-2.5 times normal is usually desired. APTT is usually measured prior to heparin therapy, 6-8 hours after initiation of a continuous infusion (following a loading dose), and 6-8 hours after changes in the infusion rate; increase or decrease infusion by 2-4 units/kg/hour dependent on PTT. Continuous I.V. infusion is preferred vs I.V. intermittent injections. For intermittent I.V. injections, PTT is measured 3.5-4 hours after I.V. injection.

Children:
    Intermittent I.V.: Initial: 50-100 units/kg, then 50-100 units/kg every 4 hours
    I.V. infusion: Initial: 50 units/kg, then 15-25 units/kg/hour; increase dose by 2-4 units/kg/hour every 6-8 hours as required

Adults:
    Prophylaxis (low-dose heparin): S.C.: 5000 units every 8-12 hours
    Intermittent I.V.: Initial: 10,000 units, then 50-70 units/kg (5000-10,000 units) every 4-6 hours
    I.V. infusion: Initial: 75-100 units/kg, then 15 units/kg/hour with dose adjusted according to PTT results; usual range: 10-30 units/kg/hour

Dosage Forms
Heparin sodium:
    Lock flush injection:
        Beef lung source: 10 units/mL (1 mL, 2 mL, 2.5 mL, 3 mL, 5 mL, 10 mL, 30 mL); 100 units/mL (1 mL, 2 mL, 2.5 mL, 3 mL, 5 mL, 10 mL, 30 mL)
        Porcine intestinal mucosa source: 10 units/mL (1 mL, 2 mL, 10 mL, 30 mL); 100 units/mL (1 mL, 2 mL, 10 mL, 30 mL)
        Porcine intestinal mucosa source, preservative free: 10 units/mL (1 mL); 100 units/mL (1 mL)
    Multiple-dose vial injection:
        Beef lung source, with preservative: 1000 units/mL (5 mL, 10 mL, 30 mL); 5000 units/mL (10 mL); 10,000 units/mL (4 mL, 5 mL, 10 mL); 20,000 units/mL (2 mL, 5 mL, 10 mL); 40,000 units/mL (5 mL)
        Porcine intestinal mucosa source, with preservative: 1000 units/mL (10 mL, 30 mL); 5000 units/mL (10 mL); 10,000 units/mL (4 mL); 20,000 units/mL (2 mL, 5 mL)
    Single-dose vial injection:
        Beef lung source: 1000 units/mL (1 mL); 5000 units/mL (1 mL); 10,000 units/mL (1 mL); 20,000 units/mL (1 mL); 40,000 units/mL (1 mL)
        Porcine intestinal mucosa: 1000 units/mL (1 mL); 5000 units/mL (1 mL); 10,000 units/mL (1 mL); 20,000 units/mL (1 mL); 40,000 units/mL (1 mL)
    Unit dose injection:
        Porcine intestinal mucosa source, with preservative: 1000 units/dose (1 mL, 2 mL); 2500 units/dose (1 mL); 5000 units/dose (0.5 mL, 1 mL); 7500 units/dose (1 mL); 10,000 units/dose (1 mL); 15,000 units/dose (1 mL); 20,000 units/dose (1 mL)

Heparin sodium infusion, porcine intestinal mucosa source:
    D_5W: 40 units/mL (500 mL); 50 units/mL (250 mL, 500 mL); 100 units/mL (100 mL, 250 mL)
    NaCl 0.45%: 2 units/mL (500 mL, 1000 mL); 50 units/mL (250 mL); 100 units/mL (250 mL)
    NaCl 0.9%: 2 units/mL (500 mL, 1000 mL); 5 units/mL (1000 mL); 50 units/mL (250 mL, 500 mL, 1000 mL)

Heparin calcium:
    Unit dose injection, porcine intestinal mucosa, preservative free (Calciparine®): 5000 units/dose (0.2 mL); 12,500 units/dose (0.5 mL); 20,000 units/dose (0.8 mL)

hepatitis a vaccine
Brand Names Havrix®
Therapeutic Category Vaccine, Inactivated Virus
Dosage Forms Injection:

hepatitis b immune globulin
Brand Names H-BIG®; Hep-B-Gammagee®; HyperHep®
Synonyms hbig
Therapeutic Category Immune Globulin
(Continued)

hepatitis b immune globulin *(Continued)*

Use Provide prophylactic passive immunity to hepatitis B infection to those individuals exposed. Hepatitis B immune globulin is not indicated for treatment of active hepatitis B infections and is ineffective in the treatment of chronic active hepatitis B infection.

Usual Dosage I.M.:

Newborns: Hepatitis B: 0.5 mL as soon after birth as possible (within 12 hours)

Adults: Postexposure prophylaxis: 0.06 mL/kg; usual dose: 3-5 mL; maximum dose: 5 mL as soon as possible after exposure (within 7 days); repeat at 28-30 days after exposure

Dosage Forms Injection:
H-BIG™: 4 mL, 5 mL
Hep-B-Gammagee™: 5 mL
HyperHep™: 0.5 mL, 1 mL, 5 mL

hepatitis b vaccine

Brand Names Engerix-B®; Recombivax HB®

Therapeutic Category Vaccine, Inactivated Virus

Use Immunization against infection caused by all known subtypes of hepatitis B virus in individuals considered at high risk of potential exposure to hepatitis B virus or HB$_s$Ag-positive materials

Usual Dosage I.M.:

Neonates born to HB$_s$Ag-positive mothers: 5 mcg

Children:
≤11 years: 2.5 mcg doses
11-19 years: 5 mcg doses

Adults >20 years: 10 mcg doses

Dosage Forms Injection:
Recombinant DNA (Engerix-B™): Hepatitis B surface antigen 20 mcg/mL (1 mL)
Pediatric, recombinant DNA (Engerix-B®): Hepatitis B surface antigen 10 mcg/0.5 mL (0.5 mL)
Recombinant DNA (Recombivax HB™): Hepatitis B surface antigen 10 mcg/mL (1 mL, 3 mL)
Dialysis formulation, recombinant DNA (Recombivax HB®): Hepatitis B surface antigen 40 mcg/mL (1 mL)

Hep-B-Gammagee® *see* hepatitis b immune globulin *on previous page*

Hep-Lock® *see* heparin *on page 222*

Herplex® Ophthalmic *see* idoxuridine *on page 241*

hes *see* hetastarch *on this page*

Hespan® *see* hetastarch *on this page*

hetastarch (het' a starch)

Brand Names Hespan™

Synonyms hes; hydroxyethyl starch

Therapeutic Category Plasma Volume Expander

Use Blood volume expander used in treatment of shock or impending shock when blood or blood products are not available

Usual Dosage Up to 1500 mL/day

Dosage Forms Infusion, in sodium chloride 0.9%: 6% (500 mL)

Hexabrix™ *see* radiological/contrast media (ionic) *on page 404*

hexachlorocyclohexane *see* lindane *on page 269*

hexachlorophene (hex a klor' oh feen)

Brand Names pHisoHex™; Septisol®

Therapeutic Category Antibacterial, Topical; Soap

Use Surgical scrub and as a bacteriostatic skin cleanser; to control an outbreak of gram-positive infection when other procedures have been unsuccessful

Usual Dosage Children and Adults: Topical: Apply 5 mL cleanser and water to area to be cleansed; lather and rinse thoroughly under running water
Dosage Forms
Foam (Septisol®): 0.23% with alcohol 56% (180 mL, 600 mL)
Liquid, topical (pHisoHex®): 3% (8 mL, 150 mL, 500 mL, 3840 mL)

Hexadrol® *see* dexamethasone *on page 131*

Hexadrol® Phosphate *see* dexamethasone *on page 131*

Hexalen® *see* altretamine *on page 15*

hexamethylenetetramine *see* methenamine *on page 293*

hexamethylmelamine *see* altretamine *on page 15*

Hexlixate® *see* antihemophilic factor (recombinant) *on page 29*

H.H.R.® *see* hydralazine, hydrochlorothiazide, and reserpine *on page 228*

Hibiclens® Topical [OTC] *see* chlorhexidine gluconate *on page 90*

Hibistat® Topical [OTC] *see* chlorhexidine gluconate *on page 90*

Hib polysaccharide conjugate *see* hemophilus b conjugate vaccine *on page 222*

HibTITER® *see* hemophilus b conjugate vaccine *on page 222*

Hi-Cor-1.0® *see* hydrocortisone *on page 232*

Hi-Cor-2.5® *see* hydrocortisone *on page 232*

Hiprex® *see* methenamine *on page 293*

Hismanal® *see* astemizole *on page 36*

Histaject® Injection *see* brompheniramine maleate *on page 59*

Histalet X® *see* guaifenesin and pseudoephedrine *on page 216*

Histerone® Injection *see* testosterone *on page 449*

Histolyn-CYL® Injection *see* histoplasmin *on this page*

histoplasmin (hiss toe plaz' min)
Brand Names Histolyn-CYL® Injection
Synonyms histoplasmosis skin test antigen
Therapeutic Category Diagnostic Agent, Skin Test
Use Diagnosing histoplasmosis; to assess cell-mediated immunity
Usual Dosage Adults: Intradermally: 0.1 mL of 1:100 dilution 5-10 cm apart into volar surface of forearm; induration of ≥5 mm in diameter indicates a positive reaction
Dosage Forms Injection: 1:100 (0.1 mL, 1.3 mL)

histoplasmosis skin test antigen *see* histoplasmin *on this page*

Histor-D® Liquid *see* chlorpheniramine and phenylephrine *on page 93*

Histor-D® Timecelles® *see* chlorpheniramine, phenylephrine and methscopolamine *on page 95*

histrelin (his trel' in)
Brand Names Supprelin™ Injection
Therapeutic Category Gonadotropin Releasing Hormone Analog
Use Control central precocious puberty
Usual Dosage
Central idiopathic precocious puberty: S.C.: Usual dose is 10 mcg/kg/day given as a single daily dose at the same time each day

Acute intermittent porphyria in women:
S.C.: 5 mcg/day
(Continued)
225

histrelin *(Continued)*

Intranasal: 400-800 mcg/day

Endometriosis: S.C.: 100 mcg/day

Leiomyomata uteri: S.C.: 20-50 mcg/day or 4 mcg/kg/day

Dosage Forms Injection: 7-day kits of single use: 120 mcg/0.6 mL; 300 mcg/0.6 mL; 600 mcg/0.6 mL

Histrodrix® [OTC] *see* dexbrompheniramine and pseudoephedrine *on page 132*

Hi-Vegi-Lip® *see* pancreatin *on page 346*

Hivid® *see* zalcitabine *on page 494*

HMS Liquifilm® Ophthalmic *see* medrysone *on page 284*

HN₂ *see* mechlorethamine hydrochloride *on page 282*

Hold® DM [OTC] *see* dextromethorphan hydrobromide *on page 135*

homatropine and hydrocodone *see* hydrocodone and homatropine *on page 231*

homatropine hydrobromide (hoe ma' troe peen)

Brand Names AK-Homatropine" Ophthalmic; Isopto® Homatropine Ophthalmic
Therapeutic Category Anticholinergic Agent, Ophthalmic; Ophthalmic Agent, Mydriatic
Use Producing cycloplegia and mydriasis for refraction; treatment of acute inflammatory conditions of the uveal tract
Usual Dosage
Children:
Mydriasis and cycloplegia for refraction: 1 drop of 2% solution immediately before the procedure; repeat at 10-minute intervals as needed
Uveitis: 1 drop of 2% solution 2-3 times/day

Adults:
Mydriasis and cycloplegia for refraction: 1-2 drops of 2% solution or 1 drop of 5% solution before the procedure; repeat at 5- to 10-minute intervals as needed
Uveitis: 1-2 drops 2-3 times/day up to every 3-4 hours as needed
Dosage Forms Solution, ophthalmic:
2% (1 mL, 5 mL); 5% (1 mL, 2 mL, 5 mL)
AK-Homatropine": 5% (15 mL)
Isopto Homatropine 2% (5 mL, 15 mL); 5% (5 mL, 15 mL)

horse anti-human thymocyte gamma globulin *see* lymphocyte immune globulin, antithymocyte globulin (equine) *on page 275*

H.P. Acthar® Gel *see* corticotropin *on page 115*

human growth hormone

Brand Names Humatrope" Injection; Nutropin" Injection; Protropin® Injection
Synonyms somatrem; somatropin
Therapeutic Category Growth Hormone
Use Long-term treatment of growth failure from lack of adequate endogenous growth hormone secretion
Usual Dosage Children: I.M., S.C.:
Somatrem: Up to 0.1 mg (0.26 units)/kg/dose 3 times/week
Somatropin: Up to 0.06 mg (0.16 units)/kg/dose 3 times/week
Therapy should be discontinued when patient has reached satisfactory adult height, when epiphyses have fused, or when the patient ceases to respond
Dosage Forms Powder for injection (lyophilized):
Somatropin:
Humatrope": 5 mg ~13 units (5 mL)
Nutropin": 5 mg ~13 units (5 mL); 10 mg ~26 units (10 mL)
Somatrem, Protropin": 5 mg ~13 units (10 mL)

Humate-P® *see* antihemophilic factor (human) *on page 29*

Humatin® *see* paromomycin sulfate *on page 350*

Humatrope® Injection *see* human growth hormone *on previous page*

Humibid® L.A. [OTC] *see* guaifenesin *on page 213*

Humibid® Sprinkle [OTC] *see* guaifenesin *on page 213*

Humibid® DM [OTC] *see* guaifenesin and dextromethorphan *on page 214*

Humorsol® Ophthalmic *see* demecarium bromide *on page 128*

Humulin® 50/50 *see* insulin preparations *on page 245*

Humulin® 70/30 *see* insulin preparations *on page 245*

Humulin® L *see* insulin preparations *on page 245*

Humulin® N *see* insulin preparations *on page 245*

Humulin® R *see* insulin preparations *on page 245*

Humulin® U Utralente *see* insulin preparations *on page 245*

Hurricaine® *see* benzocaine *on page 48*

hyaluronic acid *see* sodium hyaluronate *on page 428*

hyaluronidase (hye al yoor on' i dase)
Brand Names Wydase® Injection
Therapeutic Category Antidote, Extravasation
Use Increase the dispersion and absorption of other drugs; increase rate of absorption of parenteral fluids given by hypodermoclysis; enhance diffusion of locally irritating or toxic drugs in the management of I.V. extravasation
Usual Dosage
Infants and Children:
Management of I.V. extravasation: Reconstitute the 150 unit vial of lyophilized powder with 1 mL normal saline; take 0.1 mL of this solution and dilute with 0.9 mL normal saline to yield 15 units/mL; using a 25- or 26-gauge needle, five 0.2 mL injections are made subcutaneously or intradermally into the extravasation site at the leading edge, changing the needle after each injection
Hypodermoclysis: S.C.: 15 units is added to each 100 mL of I.V. fluid to be administered
Adults: Absorption and dispersion of drugs: 150 units is added to the vehicle containing the drug
Dosage Forms
Injection, stabilized solution: 150 units/mL (1 mL, 10 mL)
Powder for injection, lyophilized: 150 units, 1500 units

Hyate®:C *see* factor viii:c (porcine) *on page 184*

Hybalamin® *see* hydroxocobalamin *on page 235*

Hybolin™ Decanoate Injection *see* nandrolone *on page 318*

Hybolin™ Improved Injection *see* nandrolone *on page 318*

HycoClear Tuss® *see* hydrocodone and guaifenesin *on page 230*

Hycodan® *see* hydrocodone and homatropine *on page 231*

Hycomine® *see* hydrocodone and phenylpropanolamine *on page 231*

Hycomine® Pediatric *see* hydrocodone and phenylpropanolamine *on page 231*

Hycort® *see* hydrocortisone *on page 232*

Hycotuss® Expectorant Liquid *see* hydrocodone and guaifenesin *on page 230*

Hydeltrasol® Injection *see* prednisolone *on page 383*

Hydeltra-T.B.A.® Injection *see* prednisolone *on page 383*

Hydergine® *see* ergoloid mesylates *on page 169*
Hydergine® LC *see* ergoloid mesylates *on page 169*

hydralazine and hydrochlorothiazide
Brand Names Apresazide®; Hydrazide®; Hy-Zide®
Synonyms hydrochlorothiazide and hydralazine
Therapeutic Category Antihypertensive, Combination
Use Management of moderate to severe hypertension and treatment of congestive heart failure
Usual Dosage Adults: Oral: 1 capsule twice daily
Dosage Forms Capsule:
   25/25: Hydralazine hydrochloride 25 mg and hydrochlorothiazide 25 mg
   50/50: Hydralazine hydrochloride 50 mg and hydrochlorothiazide 50 mg
   100/50: Hydralazine hydrochloride 100 mg and hydrochlorothiazide 50 mg

hydralazine hydrochloride (hye dral' a zeen)
Brand Names Alazine® Oral; Apresoline® Injection; Apresoline® Oral
Therapeutic Category Vasodilator
Use Management of moderate to severe hypertension, congestive heart failure, hypertension secondary to pre-eclampsia/eclampsia
Usual Dosage
   Children:
      Oral: Initial: 0.75-1 mg/kg/day in 2-4 divided doses, not to exceed 25 mg/dose; increase over 3-4 weeks to maximum of 7.5 mg/kg/day in 2-4 divided doses; maximum daily dose: 200 mg/day
      I.M., I.V.: 0.1-0.5 mg/kg/dose (initial dose not to exceed 20 mg) every 4-6 hours as needed
   Adults:
      Oral: Initial: 10 mg 4 times/day, increase by 10-25 mg/dose every 2-5 days to maximum of 300 mg/day
      I.M., I.V.:
         Hypertensive initial: 10-20 mg/dose every 4-6 hours as needed, may increase to 40 mg/dose
         Pre-eclampsia/eclampsia: 5 mg/dose then 5-10 mg every 20-30 minutes as needed
Dosage Forms
   Injection (Apresoline®): 20 mg/mL (1 mL)
   Tablet (Alazine®, Apresoline®): 10 mg, 25 mg, 50 mg, 100 mg

hydralazine, hydrochlorothiazide, and reserpine
Brand Names Cam-ap-es®; H.H.R.®; Hydrap-ES®; Marpres®; Ser-A-Gen®; Ser-Ap-Es®; Serathide®; Tri-Hydroserpine®; Unipres®
Therapeutic Category Antihypertensive, Combination
Use Hypertensive disorders
Usual Dosage Adults: Oral: 1-2 tablets 3 times/day
Dosage Forms Tablet: Hydralazine 25 mg, hydrochlorothiazide 15 mg, and reserpine 0.1 mg

Hydramyn® Syrup [OTC] *see* diphenhydramine hydrochloride *on page 149*
Hydrap-ES® *see* hydralazine, hydrochlorothiazide, and reserpine *on this page*
hydrated chloral *see* chloral hydrate *on page 87*
Hydrate® Injection *see* dimenhydrinate *on page 147*
Hydrazide® *see* hydralazine and hydrochlorothiazide *on this page*
Hydrea® *see* hydroxyurea *on page 237*
Hydrex® *see* benzthiazide *on page 50*
Hydrobexan® *see* hydroxocobalamin *on page 235*
Hydrocet® *see* hydrocodone and acetaminophen *on page 230*

hydrochlorothiazide (hye droe klor oh thye' a zide)
Brand Names Aquazide-H®; Diaqua®; Esidrix®; Ezide®; HydroDIURIL®; Hydro-Par®; Hydro-T®; Mictrin®; Oretic®
Synonyms hctz
Therapeutic Category Diuretic, Thiazide
Use Management of mild to moderate hypertension; treatment of edema in congestive heart failure and nephrotic syndrome
Usual Dosage Oral:
Children (daily dosages should be decreased if used with other antihypertensives):
<6 months: 2-3 mg/kg/day in 2 divided doses
>6 months: 2 mg/kg/day in 2 divided doses

Adults: 25-50 mg/day in 1-2 doses; maximum: 200 mg/day
Dosage Forms
Solution, oral (mint flavor): 50 mg/5 mL (50 mL)
Tablet: 25 mg, 50 mg, 100 mg

hydrochlorothiazide and amiloride *see* amiloride and hydrochlorothiazide
on page 19

hydrochlorothiazide and hydralazine *see* hydralazine and hydrochlorothiazide
on previous page

hydrochlorothiazide and methyldopa *see* methyldopa and hydrochlorothiazide
on page 299

hydrochlorothiazide and reserpine
Brand Names Hydropres®; Hydro-Serp®; Hydroserpine®
Synonyms reserpine and hydrochlorothiazide
Therapeutic Category Antihypertensive, Combination
Use Management of mild to moderate hypertension; treatment of edema in congestive heart failure and nephrotic syndrome
Usual Dosage Adults: Oral: 1-2 tablets once or twice daily
Dosage Forms Tablet:
25 Hydrochlorothiazide 25 mg and reserpine 0.125 mg
50 Hydrochlorothiazide 50 mg and reserpine 0.125 mg

hydrochlorothiazide and spironolactone
Brand Names Alazide®; Aldactazide®; Spironazide®; Spirozide®
Synonyms spironolactone and hydrochlorothiazide
Therapeutic Category Antihypertensive, Combination; Diuretic, Combination
Use Management of mild to moderate hypertension; treatment of edema in congestive heart failure and nephrotic syndrome
Usual Dosage Oral:
Children: 1.66-3.3 mg/kg/day (of spironolactone) in 2-4 divided doses
Adults: 1-8 tablets in 1-2 divided doses
Dosage Forms Tablet:
25/25: Hydrochlorothiazide 25 mg and spironolactone 25 mg
50/50: Hydrochlorothiazide 50 mg and spironolactone 50 mg

hydrochlorothiazide and triamterene
Brand Names Dyazide®; Maxzide®
Synonyms triamterene and hydrochlorothiazide
Therapeutic Category Diuretic, Combination
Use Management of mild to moderate hypertension; treatment of edema in congestive heart failure and nephrotic syndrome
Usual Dosage Adults: 1-2 capsules twice daily after meals
Dosage Forms
Capsule (Dyazide®): Hydrochlorothiazide 25 mg and triamterene 50 mg
(Continued)
229

hydrochlorothiazide and triamterene *(Continued)*
Tablet:
Maxzide"'-25: Hydrochlorothiazide 25 mg and triamterene 37.5 mg
Maxzide": Hydrochlorothiazide 50 mg and triamterene 75 mg

Hydrocil® [OTC] *see* psyllium *on page 398*
Hydro-Cobex® *see* hydroxocobalamin *on page 235*

hydrocodone and acetaminophen
Brand Names Anexsia"'; Bancap HC®; Co-Gesic®; Dolacet®; DuoCet™; Hydrocet®; Hydrogesic"'; Hy-Phen®; Lorcet®; Lorcet® 10/650; Lorcet®-HD; Lorcet® Plus; Margesic® H; Norcet"; Panacet® 5/500; Stagesic®; T-Gesic"; Vicodin®; Vicodin® ES; Zydone®
Synonyms acetaminophen and hydrocodone
Therapeutic Category Analgesic, Narcotic; Antipyretic
Use Relief of moderate to severe pain; antitussive (hydrocodone)
Usual Dosage Doses should be titrated to appropriate analgesic effect
Adults: 1-2 tablets or capsules every 4-6 hours
Dosage Forms
Capsule:
Bancap HC", Dolacet"', Hydrocet®, Hydrogesic®, Lorcet®-HD, Margesic® H, Norcet®, Stagesic", T-Gesic", Zydone": Hydrocodone bitartrate 5 mg and acetaminophen 500 mg
Solution, oral (tropical fruit punch flavor) (Lortab"): Hydrocodone bitartrate 2.5 mg and acetaminophen 120 mg per 5 mL with alcohol 7% (480 mL)
Tablet:
Lortab" 2.5/500: Hydrocodone bitartrate 2.5 mg and acetaminophen 500 mg
Anexsia" 5/500, Co-Gesic", DuoCet™, Hy-Phen®, Lorcet®, Lortab®® 5/500, Panacet® 5/500, Vicodin": Hydrocodone bitartrate 5 mg and acetaminophen 500 mg
Lorcet" 7.5/500: Hydrocodone bitartrate 7.5 mg and acetaminophen 500 mg
Anexsia" 7.5/650, Lorcet" Plus: Hydrocodone bitartrate 7.5 mg and acetaminophen 650 mg
Vicodin" ES: Hydrocodone bitartrate 7.5 mg and acetaminophen 750 mg
Lorcet" 10/650: Hydrocodone bitartrate 10 mg and acetaminophen 650 mg

hydrocodone and aspirin *(hye droe koe' done)*
Brand Names Azdone"'; Damason-P"; Lortab® ASA; Panasal® 5/500
Therapeutic Category Analgesic, Narcotic; Antipyretic
Use Relief of moderate to moderately severe pain
Usual Dosage Adults: Oral: 1-2 tablets every 4-6 hours as needed for pain
Dosage Forms Tablet: Hydrocodone bitartrate 5 mg and aspirin 500 mg

hydrocodone and chlorpheniramine
Brand Names Tussionex"'
Therapeutic Category Antitussive; Cough Preparation
Use Symptomatic relief of cough
Usual Dosage Oral:
Children 6-12 years: 2.5 mL every 12 hours; do not exceed 5 mL/24 hours
Adults: 5 mL every 12 hours; do not exceed 10 mL/24 hours
Dosage Forms Syrup, alcohol free: Hydrocodone polistirex 10 mg and chlorpheniramine polistirex 8 mg per 5 mL (480 mL, 900 mL)

hydrocodone and guaifenesin
Brand Names Codiclear" DH; HycoClear Tuss"; Hycotuss® Expectorant Liquid; Kwelcof®
Synonyms guaifenesin and hydrocodone
Therapeutic Category Antitussive; Cough Preparation
Use Symptomatic relief of nonproductive coughs associated with upper and lower respiratory tract congestion

Usual Dosage Oral:
Children:
<2 years: 0.3 mg/kg/day (hydrocodone) in 4 divided doses
2-12 years: 2.5 mL every 4 hours, after meals and at bedtime
>12 years: 5 mL every 4 hours, after meals and at bedtime

Adults: 5 mL every 4 hours, after meals and at bedtime, up to 30 mL/24 hours
Dosage Forms Liquid: Hydrocodone bitartrate 5 mg and guaifenesin 100 mg per 5 mL (120 mL, 480 mL)

hydrocodone and homatropine
Brand Names Hycodan®; Hydromet®; Hydropane®; Hydrotropine®; Tussigon®
Synonyms homatropine and hydrocodone
Therapeutic Category Antitussive; Cough Preparation
Use Symptomatic relief of cough
Usual Dosage Oral (based on hydrocodone component):
Children: 0.6 mg/kg/day in 3-4 divided doses; do not administer more frequently than every 4 hours

A single dose should not exceed 10 mg in children >12 years, 5 mg in children 2-12 years, and 1.25 mg in children <2 years of age

Adults: 5-10 mg every 4-6 hours, a single dose should not exceed 15 mg; do not administer more frequently than every 4 hours
Dosage Forms
Syrup (Hycodan®, Hydromet®, Hydropane®, Hydrotropine®): Hydrocodone bitartrate 5 mg and homatropine methylbromide 1.5 mg per 5 mL (120 mL, 480 mL, 4000 mL)
Tablet (Hycodan®, Tussigon®): Hydrocodone bitartrate 5 mg and homatropine methylbromide 1.5 mg

hydrocodone and phenylpropanolamine
Brand Names Codamine®; Codamine® Pediatric; Hycomine®; Hycomine® Pediatric
Synonyms phenylpropanolamine and hydrocodone
Therapeutic Category Cough Preparation; Decongestant
Use Symptomatic relief of cough and nasal congestion
Usual Dosage Oral:
Children 6-12 years: 2.5 mL every 4 hours, up to 6 doses/24 hours
Adults: 5 mL every 4 hours, up to 6 doses/24 hours
Dosage Forms Syrup:
Codamine®, Hycomine®: Hydrocodone bitartrate 5 mg and phenylpropanolamine hydrochloride 25 mg per 5 mL (480 mL, 3780 mL)
Codamine® Pediatric, Hycomine® Pediatric: Hydrocodone bitartrate 2.5 mg and phenylpropanolamine hydrochloride 12.5 mg per 5 mL (480 mL, 3780 mL)

hydrocodone, phenylephrine, pyrilamine, phenindamine, chlorpheniramine, and ammonium chloride
Brand Names P-V-Tussin®
Therapeutic Category Antihistamine/Decongestant Combination; Cough Preparation
Use Symptomatic relief of cough and nasal congestion
Usual Dosage Adults: Oral: 10 mL every 4-6 hours, up to 40 mL/day
Dosage Forms Syrup: Hydrocodone bitartrate 2.5 mg, phenylephrine hydrochloride 5 mg, pyrilamine maleate 6 mg, phenindamine tartrate 5 mg, chlorpheniramine maleate 2 mg, and ammonium chloride 50 mg per 5 mL with alcohol 5% (480 mL, 3780 mL)

hydrocodone, pseudoephedrine, and guaifenesin
Brand Names Cophene XP®; Detussin® Expectorant; SRC® Expectorant; Tussafin® Expectorant
Therapeutic Category Cough Preparation; Decongestant; Expectorant
(Continued)

hydrocodone, pseudoephedrine, and guaifenesin *(Continued)*

Use Symptomatic relief of irritating, nonproductive cough associated with respiratory conditions such as bronchitis, bronchial asthma, tracheobronchitis, and the common cold

Usual Dosage Adults: Oral: 5 mL every 4-6 hours

Dosage Forms Liquid: Hydrocodone bitartrate 5 mg, pseudoephedrine hydrochloride 60 mg, and guaifenesin 200 mg per 5 mL with alcohol 12.5% (480 mL)

Hydrocort® *see* hydrocortisone *on this page*

hydrocortisone (hye droe kor' ti sone)

Brand Names A-hydroCort™; Ala-Cort®; Ala-Scalp®; Anucort-HC® Suppository; Anuprep HC® Suppository; Anusol™ HC-1 [OTC]; Anusol® HC-2.5% [OTC]; Anusol-HC® Suppository; Caldecort™; Caldecort™ Anti-Itch Spray; Clocort® Maximum Strength; CortaGel® [OTC]; Cortaid™ Maximum Strength [OTC]; Cortaid™ with Aloe [OTC]; Cort-Dome®; Cortef®; Cortef® Feminine Itch; Cortenema®; Cortifoam®; Cortizone®-5 [OTC]; Cortizone®-10 [OTC]; Delcort™; Dermacort™; Dermarest Dricort®; DermiCort®; Dermolate®; Gynecort® [OTC]; Hemril-HC™ Uniserts®; Hi-Cor-1.0®; Hi-Cor-2.5®; Hycort®; Hydrocort®; Hydrocortone® Acetate; Hydrocortone™ Phosphate; HydroSKIN®; Hydro-Tex® [OTC]; Hytone®; LactiCare-HC®; Lanacort™ [OTC]; Locoid®; Nutracort®; Orabase® HCA; Penecort®; Proctocort™; Scalpicin®; Solu-Cortef™; S-T Cort™; Synacort®; Tegrin®-HC [OTC]; U-Cort™; Westcort®

Synonyms compound f; cortisol

Therapeutic Category Adrenal Corticosteroid; Anti-inflammatory Agent; Corticosteroid, Rectal; Corticosteroid, Systemic; Corticosteroid, Topical (Low Potency)

Use Management of adrenocortical insufficiency; relief of inflammation of corticosteroid-responsive dermatoses; adjunctive treatment of ulcerative colitis

Usual Dosage

Acute adrenal insufficiency: I.M., I.V.:
    Infants and young Children: 1-2 mg/kg/dose bolus, then 25-150 mg/day in divided doses
    Older Children: 1-2 mg/kg bolus then 150-250 mg/day in divided doses
    Adults: I.M., I.V., S.C.: 15-240 mg every 12 hours

Physiologic replacement: Children:
    Oral: 0.5-0.75 mg/kg/day or 20-25 mg/m^2/day every 8 hours
    I.M.: 0.25-0.35 mg/kg/day or 12-15 mg/m^2/day once daily

Anti-inflammatory or immunosuppressive:
    Infants and Children:
        Oral: 2.5-10 mg/kg/day or 75-300 mg/m^2/day every 6-8 hours
        I.M., I.V.: 1-5 mg/kg/day or 30-150 mg/m^2/day divided every 6-12 hours
    Adults: I.M., I.V., S.C.: 15-240 mg every 12 hours

Congenital adrenal hyperplasia: Oral: Initial: 30-36 mg/m^2/day with $^1/_3$ of dose every morning and $^1/_3$ every evening or $^1/_4$ every morning and midday and $^1/_2$ every evening; maintenance: 20-25 mg/m^2/day in divided doses

Status asthmaticus: Children: Loading: 1-2 mg/kg/dose every 6 hours for 24 hours then maintenance 0.5-1 mg/kg/dose every 6 hours

Shock: I.M., I.V.:
    Children: Initial: 50 mg/kg (succinate) and repeated in 4 hours and/or every 24 hours if needed
    Adults: 500 mg to 2 g every 2-6 hours (succinate)

Children and Adults:
    Rectal: Apply 1 application 1-2 times/day for 2-3 weeks
    Topical: Apply 3-4 times/day

Dosage Forms

Acetate:
    Aerosol, rectal (Cortifoam™): 10% [90 mg/applicatorful] 20 g
    Cream:
        Caldecort™, Gynecort™, Cortaid™ with Aloe, Cortef® Feminine Itch, Lanacort®: 0.5% (15 g, 22.5 g, 30 g)
        Anusol-HC-1™, Caldecort™, Clocort™ Maximum Strength, Cortaid® Maximum Strength, Dermarest Dricort™, U-cort™: 1% (15 g, 21 g, 30 g, 120 g)

Ointment, topical:
   Cortaid® with Aloe, Lanacort® 5: 0.5% (15 g, 30 g)
   Gynecort® 10, Lanacort® 10: 1% (15 g, 30 g)
Injection, suspension (Hydrocortone® Acetate): 25 mg/mL (5 mL, 10 mL); 50 mg/mL (5 mL, 10 mL)
Paste (Orabase® HCA): 0.5% (5 g)
Solution, topical (Scalpicin®): 1%
Suppository, rectal (Anucort-HC®, Anuprep HC®, Anusol-HC®, Hemril-HC® Uniserts®): 25 mg

Base:
   Aerosol, topical:
      Aeroseb-HC®, CaldeCORT® Anti-Itch Spray, Cortaid®: 0.5% (45 g, 58 g)
      Cortaid® Maximum Strength: 1% (45 mL)
   Cream:
      Cort-Dome®, Cortizone®-5, DermiCort®, Dermolate®, Dermtex® HC with Aloe, Hy-droSKIN®, Hydro-Tex®: 0.5% (15 g, 30 g, 120 g, 454 g)
      Ala-Cort®, Cort-Dome®, Delcort®, Dermacort®, DermiCort®, Eldecort®, Hi-Cor 1.0®, Hy-cort®, Hytone®, Nutracort®, Penecort®, Synacort®: 1% (15 g, 20 g, 30 g, 60 g, 120 g, 240 g, 454 g)
      Anusol-HC-2.5%®, Eldecort®, Hi-Cor-2.5®, Hydrocort®, Hytone®, Synacort®: 2.5% (15 g, 20 g, 30 g, 60 g, 120 g, 240 g, 454 g)
      Rectal (Proctocort™): 1% (30 g)
   Gel:
      CortaGel®: 0.5% (15 g, 30 g)
      CortaGel® Extra Strength: 1% (15 g, 30 g)
   Lotion:
      Cetacort®, DermiCort®, HydroSKIN®, S-T Cort®: 0.5% (60 mL, 120 mL)
      Acticort 100®, Cetacort®, Cortizone-10®, Dermacort®, HydroSKIN® Maximum Strength, Hytone®, LactiCare-HC®, Nutracort®: 1% (60 mL, 120 mL)
      Ala-Scalp®: 2% (30 mL)
      Hytone®, LactiCare-HC®, Nutracort®: 2.5% (60 mL, 120 mL)
   Ointment, topical:
      Cortizone®-5, HydroSKIN®: 0.5% (30 g)
      Cortizone®-10, Hycort®, HydroSKIN®, Hydro-Tex®, Hytone®, Tegrin®-HC: 1% (15 g, 20 g, 30 g, 60 g, 120 g, 240 g, 454 g)
      Hytone®: 2.5% (20 g, 30 g)
   Suspension, rectal (Cortenema®): 100 mg/60 mL (7s)
   Tablet:
      Cortef®: 5 mg, 10 mg, 20 mg
      Hydrocortone®: 10 mg, 20 mg
Butyrate (Locoid®):
   Cream: 0.1%
   Ointment, topical: 0.1%
   Solution, topical: 0.1% (20 mL, 60 mL)
Cypionate:
   Suspension, oral (Cortef®): 10 mg/5 mL (120 mL)
Sodium phosphate:
   Injection (Hydrocortone® Phosphate): 50 mg/mL (2 mL, 10 mL)
Sodium succinate (A-hydroCort®, Solu-Cortef®): 100 mg, 250 mg, 500 mg, 1000 mg
Valerate (Westcort®):
   Cream: 0.2% (15 g, 45 g, 60 g)
   Ointment, topical: 0.2% (15 g, 45 g, 60 g, 120 g)

hydrocortisone and clioquinol *see* clioquinol and hydrocortisone *on page 106*

hydrocortisone and dibucaine *see* dibucaine and hydrocortisone *on page 140*

hydrocortisone and pramoxine *see* pramoxine and hydrocortisone *on page 381*

hydrocortisone and urea *see* urea and hydrocortisone *on page 480*

Hydrocortone® Acetate *see* hydrocortisone *on previous page*

Hydrocortone® Phosphate *see* hydrocortisone *on page 232*
Hydro-Crysti-12® *see* hydroxocobalamin *on next page*
HydroDIURIL® *see* hydrochlorothiazide *on page 229*
Hydro-Ergoloid® *see* ergoloid mesylates *on page 169*

hydroflumethiazide (hye droe floo meth eye' a zide)
Brand Names Diucardin®; Saluron®
Therapeutic Category Diuretic, Thiazide
Use Management of mild to moderate hypertension; treatment of edema in congestive heart failure and nephrotic syndrome
Usual Dosage Oral: 1 tablet 1-2 times/day
Dosage Forms Tablet: 50 mg

hydroflumethiazide and reserpine
Brand Names Hydro-Fluserpine®; Salutensin®; Salutensin-Demi®
Therapeutic Category Antihypertensive, Combination
Use Management of hypertension
Usual Dosage Determined by individual titration, usually 1 tablet once or twice daily
Dosage Forms
Tablet (Salutensin™): Hydroflumethiazide 50 mg and reserpine 0.125 mg
Tablet (Hydro-Fluserpine™, Salutensin-Demi®): Hydroflumethiazide 25 mg and reserpine 0.125 mg

Hydro-Fluserpine® *see* hydroflumethiazide and reserpine *on this page*
hydrogenated ergot alkaloids *see* ergoloid mesylates *on page 169*
Hydrogesic® *see* hydrocodone and acetaminophen *on page 230*
hydromagnesium aluminate *see* magaldrate *on page 276*
Hydromet® *see* hydrocodone and homatropine *on page 231*

hydromorphone hydrochloride (hye droe mor' fone)
Brand Names Dilaudid-HP® Injection; Dilaudid® Injection; Dilaudid® Oral; Dilaudid® Suppository
Synonyms dihydromorphinone
Therapeutic Category Analgesic, Narcotic; Antitussive
Use Management of moderate to severe pain; antitussive at lower doses
Usual Dosage Doses should be titrated to appropriate analgesic effects; when changing routes of administration, note that oral doses are less than half as effective as parenteral doses (may be only $1/_5$ as effective)

Pain: Older children and Adults: Oral, I.M., I.V., S.C.: 1-4 mg/dose every 4-6 hours as needed; usual adult dose: 2 mg/dose

Antitussive: Oral:
Children 6-12 years: 0.5 mg every 3-4 hours as needed
Children >12 years and Adults: 1 mg every 3-4 hours as needed
Dosage Forms
Injection:
Dilaudid™: 1 mg/mL (1 mL); 2 mg/mL (1 mL, 20 mL); 3 mg/mL (1 mL); 4 mg/mL (1 mL)
Dilaudid-HP™: 10 mg/mL (1 mL, 2 mL, 5 mL)
Suppository, rectal: 3 mg (6s)
Tablet: 2 mg, 4 mg

Hydromox® *see* quinethazone *on page 403*
Hydropane® *see* hydrocodone and homatropine *on page 231*
Hydro-Par® *see* hydrochlorothiazide *on page 229*

Hydrophen® *see theophylline, ephedrine, and hydroxyzine on page 454*

Hydropres® *see hydrochlorothiazide and reserpine on page 229*

hydroquinone (hye' droe kwin one)

Brand Names Eldopaque® [OTC]; Eldopaque Forte®; Eldoquin® [OTC]; Eldoquin® Forte®; Esoterica® Facial [OTC]; Esoterica® Regular [OTC]; Esoterica® Sensitive Skin Formula [OTC]; Esoterica® Sunscreen [OTC]; Melanex®; Melpaque HP®; Melquin HP®; Nuquin HP®; Porcelana® [OTC]; Solaquin® [OTC]; Solaquin Forte®

Therapeutic Category Depigmenting Agent

Use Gradual bleaching of hyperpigmented skin conditions

Usual Dosage Topical: Apply thin layer and rub in twice daily

Dosage Forms

Cream, topical:

Esoterica® Sensitive Skin Formula: 1.5% (85 g)

Eldopaque®, Eldoquin®, Esoterica® Facial, Esoterica® Regular, Porcelana®: 2% (14.2 g, 28.4 g, 60 g, 85 g, 120 g)

Eldopaque Forte®, Eldoquin® Forte®, Melquin HP®: 4% (14.2 g, 28.4 g)

Cream, topical, with sunscreen:

Esoterica® Sunscreen, Porcelana®, Solaquin®: 2% (28.4 g, 120 g)

Melpaque HP®, Nuquin HP®, Solaquin Forte®: 4% (14.2 g, 28.4 g)

Gel, topical, with sunscreen (Solaquin Forte®): 4% (14.2 g, 28.4 g)

Solution, topical (Melanex®): 3% (30 mL)

Hydro-Serp® *see hydrochlorothiazide and reserpine on page 229*

Hydroserpine® *see hydrochlorothiazide and reserpine on page 229*

HydroSKIN® *see hydrocortisone on page 232*

Hydro-T® *see hydrochlorothiazide on page 229*

Hydro-Tex® [OTC] *see hydrocortisone on page 232*

Hydrotropine® *see hydrocodone and homatropine on page 231*

hydroxocobalamin (hye drox oh koe bal' a min)

Brand Names Alphamin®; Codroxomin®; Hybalamin®; Hydrobexan®; Hydro-Cobex®; Hydro-Crysti-12®; LA-12®

Synonyms vitamin b_{12a}

Therapeutic Category Vitamin, Water Soluble

Use Pernicious anemia, vitamin B_{12} deficiency, increased B_{12} requirements due to pregnancy, thyrotoxicosis, hemorrhage, malignancy, liver or kidney disease

Usual Dosage

Children:

Congenital pernicious anemia (if evidence of neurologic involvement): I.M.: 1000 mcg/day for at least 2 weeks; maintenance: 50 mcg/month

Vitamin B_{12} deficiency: I.M., S.C.: 1-5 mg given in single or S.C. doses of 100 mcg over 2 or more weeks

Adults:

Pernicious anemia: I.M., S.C.: 100 mcg/day for 6-7 days

Vitamin B_{12} deficiency:

Oral: Usually not recommended, maximum absorbed from a single oral dose is 2-3 mcg

I.M., S.C.: 30 mcg/day for 5-10 days, followed by 100-200 mcg/month

Dosage Forms Injection: 1000 mcg/mL (10 mL, 30 mL)

hydroxyamphetamine and tropicamide

Brand Names Paremyd® Ophthalmic

Therapeutic Category Ophthalmic Agent, Mydriatic

Use Mydriasis with cycloplegia

(Continued)

hydroxyamphetamine and tropicamide *(Continued)*
Usual Dosage Ophthalmic: Adults: Instill 1-2 drops into conjunctival sac(s)
Dosage Forms Solution, ophthalmic: Hydroxyamphetamine hydrobromide 1% and tropicamide 0.25% (5 mL, 15 mL)

hydroxychloroquine sulfate (hye drox ee klor' oh kwin)
Brand Names Plaquenil[®]
Therapeutic Category Antimalarial Agent
Use Suppress and treat acute attacks of malaria; treatment of systemic lupus erythematosus (SLE) and rheumatoid arthritis
Usual Dosage Oral:
Children:
  Chemoprophylaxis of malaria: 5 mg/kg (base) once weekly; should not exceed the recommended adult dose; begin 2 weeks before exposure; continue for 8 weeks after leaving endemic area
  Acute attack: 10 mg/kg (base) initial dose; followed by 5 mg/kg in 6 hours on day 1; 5 mg/kg in 1 dose on day 2 and on day 3
  Juvenile rheumatoid arthritis or SLE: 3-5 mg/kg/day divided 1-2 times/day to a maximum of 400 mg/day; not to exceed 7 mg/kg/day

Adults:
  Chemoprophylaxis of malaria: 2 tablets weekly on same day each week; begin 2 weeks before exposure; continue for 6-8 weeks after leaving epidemic area
  Acute attack: 4 tablets first dose day 1; 2 tablets in 6 hours day 1; 2 tablets in 1 dose day 2; and 2 tablets in 1 dose on day 3
  Rheumatoid arthritis: 2-3 tablets/day to start taken with food or milk; increase dose until optimum response level is reached; usually after 4-12 weeks dose should be reduced by $1/_2$ and a maintenance dose of 1-2 tablets/day given
  Lupus erythematosus: 2 tablets every day or twice daily for several weeks depending on response; 1-2 tablets/day for prolonged maintenance therapy
Dosage Forms Tablet: 200 mg [base 155 mg]

25-hydroxycholecalciferol *see* calcifediol *on page 65*

hydroxydaunomycin hydrochloride *see* doxorubicin hydrochloride *on page 157*

hydroxyethyl starch *see* hetastarch *on page 224*

hydroxyprogesterone caproate (hye drox ee proe jess' te rone)
Brand Names Duralutin[®] Injection; Hy-Gestrone[®] Injection; Hylutin[®] Injection; Hyprogest[®] Injection; Pro-Depo[®] Injection; Prodrox[®] Injection
Therapeutic Category Progestin
Use Treatment of amenorrhea, abnormal uterine bleeding, submucous fibroids, endometriosis, uterine carcinoma, and testing of estrogen production
Usual Dosage Adults: I.M.:
Amenorrhea: 375 mg; if no bleeding begin cyclic treatment with estradiol valerate

Endometriosis: Start cyclic therapy with estradiol valerate

Uterine carcinoma: 1 g one or more times/day (1-7 g/week) for up to 12 weeks

Test for endogenous estrogen production: 250 mg anytime; bleeding 7-14 days after injection indicate positive test
Dosage Forms Injection:
Pro-Depo[®]: 125 mg/mL (10 mL)
Duralutin[®], Gesterol[®] L.A., Hy-Gestrone[®], Hylutin[®], Hyprogest[®], Pro-Depo[®], Prodrox[®]: 250 mg/mL (5 mL)

hydroxypropyl methylcellulose (hye drox ee proe' pil meth e sell' yoo lose)
Brand Names Gonak™ [OTC]; Goniosol[®] [OTC]; Occucoat™
Synonyms gonioscopic ophthalmic solution
Therapeutic Category Ophthalmic Agent, Miscellaneous

Use Ophthalmic surgical aid in cataract extraction and intraocular implantation; gonioscopic examinations

Usual Dosage Introduced into anterior chamber of eye with 20-gauge or larger cannula

Dosage Forms Solution:
Occucoat™: 2% (1 mL syringe with cannula)
Gonak™, Goniosol®: 2.5% (15 mL)

hydroxyurea (hye drox ee yoor ee' a)
Brand Names Hydrea®
Therapeutic Category Antineoplastic Agent, Miscellaneous
Use Treatment of malignant neoplasms including melanoma, granulocytic leukemia, and ovarian carcinomas; also used with radiation in treatment of squamous cell carcinoma of the head and neck
Usual Dosage Oral (refer to individual protocols):
Children: No dosage regimens have been established. Dosages of 1500-3000 mg/m^2 as a single dose in combination with other agents every 4-6 weeks have been used in the treatment of pediatric astrocytoma, medulloblastoma and primitive neuroectodermal tumors

Adults:
Solid tumors: Intermittent therapy: 80 mg/kg as a single dose every third day; continuous therapy: 20-30 mg/kg/day given as a single dose/day
Concomitant therapy with irradiation: 80 mg/kg as a single dose every third day starting at least 7 days before initiation of irradiation
Resistant chronic myelocytic leukemia: 20-30 mg/kg/day divided daily
Dosage Forms Capsule: 500 mg

25-hydroxyvitamin d$_3$ see calcifediol on page 65

hydroxyzine (hye drox' i zeen)
Brand Names Anxanil®; Atarax®; Atozine®; Durrax®; E-Vista®; Hy-Pam®; Hyzine-50®; Neucalm®; Quiess®; Rezine®; Vamate®; Vistacon-50®; Vistaject-25®; Vistaject-50®; Vistaquel®; Vistaril®; Vistazine®
Therapeutic Category Antianxiety Agent; Antiemetic; Antihistamine; Sedative
Use Treatment of anxiety, as a preoperative sedative, an antipruritic, an antiemetic, and in alcohol withdrawal symptoms
Usual Dosage
Children:
Oral: 2 mg/kg/day divided every 6-8 hours
I.M.: 0.5-1 mg/kg/dose every 4-6 hours as needed

Adults:
Antiemetic: I.M.: 25-100 mg/dose every 4-6 hours as needed
Anxiety: Oral: 25-100 mg 4 times/day; maximum dose: 600 mg/day
Preoperative sedation:
Oral: 50-100 mg
I.M.: 25-100 mg
Management of pruritus: Oral: 25 mg 3-4 times/day
Dosage Forms
Hydrochloride:
Injection:
Vistaject-25®, Vistaril®: 25 mg/mL (1 mL, 2 mL, 10 mL)
E-Vista®, Hyzine-50®, Neucalm®, Quiess®, Vistacon-50®, Vistaject-50®, Vistaquel®, Vistaril®, Vistazine®: 50 mg/mL (1 mL, 2 mL, 10 mL)
Syrup (Atarax®): 10 mg/5 mL (120 mL, 480 mL, 4000 mL)
Tablet:
Anxanil®: 25 mg
Atarax®: 10 mg, 25 mg, 50 mg, 100 mg
Atozine®: 10 mg, 25 mg, 50 mg
Durrax®: 10 mg, 25 mg
(Continued)

hydroxyzine *(Continued)*

Rezine": 10 mg, 25 mg
Pamoate:
  Capsule:
    Hy-Pam": 25 mg, 50 mg
    Vamate": 25 mg, 50 mg, 100 mg
    Vistaril": 25 mg, 50 mg, 100 mg
  Suspension, oral (Vistaril":) 25 mg/5 mL (120 mL, 480 mL)

Hy-Gestrone® Injection see hydroxyprogesterone caproate *on page 236*

Hygroton® *see* chlorthalidone *on page 99*

Hylorel® *see* guanadrel sulfate *on page 218*

Hylutin® Injection see hydroxyprogesterone caproate *on page 236*

hyoscine *see* scopolamine *on page 418*

hyoscyamine, atropine, scopolamine, and phenobarbital

Brand Names Barbidonna®; Barophen®; Donnapine®; Donna-Sed®; Donnatal®; Hyosophen®; Kinesed"; Malatal®; Relaxadon®; Spasmolin®; Spasmophen®; Spasquid®; Susano®

Therapeutic Category Anticholinergic Agent; Antispasmodic Agent, Gastrointestinal

Use Adjunct in treatment of peptic ulcer disease, irritable bowel, spastic colitis, spastic bladder, and renal colic

Usual Dosage Oral:
Children 2-12 years:
  Kinesed" dose: $\frac{1}{2}$ to 1 tablet 3-4 times/day
  Donnatal": 0.1 mL/kg/dose every 4 hours; maximum dose: 5 mL

Adults: 0.125-0.25 mg (1-2 capsules or tablets) 3-4 times/day; or 0.375-0.75 mg (1 Donnatal® Extentab") in sustained release form every 12 hours; or 5-10 mL elixir 3-4 times/day or every 8 hours

Dosage Forms
Capsule (Donnatal", Spasmolin"): Hyoscyamine sulfate 0.1037 mg, atropine sulfate 0.0194 mg, scopolamine hydrobromide 0.0065 mg, and phenobarbital 16.2 mg
Elixir (Barophen", Donna-Sed", Donnatal®, Hyosophen®, Spasmophen®, Spasquid®, Susano"): Hyoscyamine sulfate 0.1037 mg, atropine sulfate 0.0194 mg, scopolamine hydrobromide 0.0065 mg, and phenobarbital 16.2 mg per 5 mL (120 mL, 480 mL, 4000 mL)
Tablet:
  Barbidonna": Hyoscyamine hydrobromide 0.1286 mg, atropine sulfate 0.025 mg, scopolamine hydrobromide 0.0074 mg, and phenobarbital 16 mg
  Barbidonna" No. 2: Hyoscyamine hydrobromide 0.1286 mg, atropine sulfate 0.025 mg, scopolamine hydrobromide 0.0074 mg, and phenobarbital 32 mg
  Chewable (Kinesed"): Hyoscyamine hydrobromide 0.12 mg, atropine sulfate 0.12 mg, scopolamine hydrobromide 0.007 mg, and phenobarbital 16 mg
  Donnapine", Donnatal", Hyosophen®, Malatal®, Relaxadon®, Susano®: Hyoscyamine sulfate 0.1037 mg, atropine sulfate 0.0194 mg, scopolamine hydrobromide 0.0065 mg, and phenobarbital 16.2 mg
  Donnatal" No. 2: Hyoscyamine sulfate 0.1037 mg, atropine sulfate 0.0194 mg, scopolamine hydrobromide 0.0065 mg, and phenobarbital 32.4 mg
  Long acting (Donnatal"): Hyoscyamine sulfate 0.3111 mg, atropine sulfate 0.0582 mg, scopolamine hydrobromide 0.0195 mg, and phenobarbital 48.6 mg
  Spasmophen": Hyoscyamine sulfate 0.1037 mg, atropine sulfate 0.0194 mg, scopolamine hydrobromide 0.0065 mg, and phenobarbital 15 mg

hyoscyamine, atropine, scopolamine, kaolin, and pectin

Therapeutic Category Antidiarrheal

Use Antidiarrheal; also used in gastritis, enteritis, colitis, and acute gastrointestinal upsets, and nausea which may accompany any of these conditions

Usual Dosage Oral:
Children:
  10-20 lb: 2.5 mL

20-30 lb: 5 mL
>30 lb: 5-10 mL
Adults:
Diarrhea: 30 mL at once and 15-30 mL with each loose stool
Other conditions: 15 mL every 3 hours as needed
Dosage Forms Suspension, oral: Hyoscyamine sulfate 0.1037 mg, atropine sulfate 0.0194 mg, scopolamine hydrobromide 0.0065 mg, kaolin 6 g, and pectin 142.8 mg per 30 mL

hyoscyamine, atropine, scopolamine, kaolin, pectin, and opium
Brand Names Donnapectolin-PG®; Kapectolin PG®
Therapeutic Category Antidiarrheal
Use Treatment of diarrhea
Usual Dosage
Children 6-12 years: Initial: 10 mL and 5-10 mL every 3 hours thereafter
Dosage recommendations (body weight/dosage): 10 lb/2.5 mL; 20 lb/5 mL; 30 lb and over/5-10 mL. Do not administer more than 4 doses in any 24-hour period

Children >12 years and Adults: Initial: 30 mL (1 fluid oz) followed by 15 mL every 3 hours
Dosage Forms Suspension, oral: Hyoscyamine sulfate 0.1037 mg, atropine sulfate 0.0194 mg, scopolamine hydrobromide 0.0065 mg, kaolin 6 g, pectin 142.8 mg, and powdered opium 24 mg per 30 mL with alcohol 5%

hyoscyamine sulfate (hye oh sye' a meen)
Brand Names Anaspaz®; Cystospaz®; Cystospaz-M®; Donnamar®; ED-SPAZ®; Gastrosed™; Levsin®; Levsinex®; Levsin/SL®
Synonyms l-hyoscyamine sulfate
Therapeutic Category Anticholinergic Agent; Antispasmodic Agent, Gastrointestinal
Use GI tract disorders caused by spasm, adjunctive therapy for peptic ulcers
Usual Dosage
Children:
<2 years: ¼ adult dosage
2-10 years: ½ adult dosage
Adults:
Oral, S.L.: 0.125-0.25 mg 3-4 times/day before meals or food and at bedtime; 0.375-0.75 mg (timed release) every 12 hours
I.M., I.V., S.C.: 0.25-0.5 mg every 6 hours
Dosage Forms
Capsule, timed release (Cystospaz-M®, Levsinex®): 0.375 mg
Elixir (Levsin®): 0.125 mg/5 mL with alcohol 20% (480 mL)
Injection (Levsin®): 0.5 mg/mL (1 mL, 10 mL)
Solution, oral (Gastrosed™, Levsin®): 0.125 mg/mL (15 mL)
Tablet:
Anaspaz®, Donnamar®, ED-SPAZ®, Gastrosed™, Levsin®: 0.125 mg
Cystospaz®: 0.15 mg
Sublingual (Levsin/SL®): 0.125 mg

Hyosophen® see hyoscyamine, atropine, scopolamine, and phenobarbital on previous page

Hy-Pam® see hydroxyzine on page 237

Hypaque-Cysto® see radiological/contrast media (ionic) on page 404

Hypaque® Meglumine see radiological/contrast media (ionic) on page 404

Hypaque® Sodium see radiological/contrast media (ionic) on page 404

Hyperab® see rabies immune globulin, human on page 404

HyperHep® see hepatitis b immune globulin on page 223

Hyperstat® I.V. see diazoxide on page 140

Hyper-Tet® *see* tetanus immune globulin, human *on page 450*

Hypertussis® *see* pertussis immune globulin, human *on page 360*

Hy-Phen® *see* hydrocodone and acetaminophen *on page 230*

HypRho®-D *see* Rh₀(D) immune globulin *on page 409*

HypRho®-D Mini-Dose *see* Rh₀(D) immune globulin *on page 409*

Hyprogest® Injection *see* hydroxyprogesterone caproate *on page 236*

Hytakerol® *see* dihydrotachysterol *on page 146*

Hytinic® [OTC] *see* polysaccharide-iron complex *on page 376*

Hytone® *see* hydrocortisone *on page 232*

Hytrin® *see* terazosin *on page 446*

Hytuss-2X® [OTC] *see* guaifenesin *on page 213*

Hytuss® [OTC] *see* guaifenesin *on page 213*

Hy-Zide® *see* hydralazine and hydrochlorothiazide *on page 228*

Hyzine-50® *see* hydroxyzine *on page 237*

ibenzmethyzin *see* procarbazine hydrochloride *on page 388*

Iberet-Folic-500® *see* ferrous sulfate, ascorbic acid, vitamin b-complex, and folic acid
on page 190

Iberet®-Liquid [OTC] *see* ferrous sulfate, ascorbic acid, and vitamin b-complex
on page 190

ibidomide hydrochloride *see* labetalol hydrochloride *on page 260*

Ibuprin® [OTC] *see* ibuprofen *on this page*

ibuprofen (eye byoo proe' fen)
    Brand Names Aches-N-Pain™ [OTC]; Advil® [OTC]; Arthritis Foundation® Ibuprofen [OTC];
    Bayer™ Select™ Pain Relief Formula [OTC]; Children's Advil®; Children's Motrin®; Excedrin®
    IB [OTC]; Genpril™ [OTC]; Haltran® [OTC]; Ibuprin® [OTC]; Ibuprohm® [OTC]; Ibu-Tab®;
    Medipren™ [OTC]; Menadol® [OTC]; Midol® IB [OTC]; Motrin®; Motrin® IB [OTC]; Nuprin®
    [OTC]; Rufen™; Saleto-200® [OTC]; Saleto-400®; Trendar® [OTC]; Uni-Pro® [OTC]
    Synonyms p-isobutylhydratropic acid
    Therapeutic Category Analgesic, Non-Narcotic; Anti-inflammatory Agent; Nonsteroidal Anti-
    Inflammatory Agent (NSAID), Oral
    Use Inflammatory diseases and rheumatoid disorders including juvenile rheumatoid arthritis;
    mild to moderate pain; fever; dysmenorrhea; gout
    Usual Dosage Oral:
        Children:
            Antipyretic: 6 months to 12 years: Temperature <102.5°F (39°C): 5 mg/kg/dose; tempera-
                ture >102.5°F: 10 mg/kg/dose given every 6-8 hours; maximum daily dose: 40 mg/kg/
                day
            Juvenile rheumatoid arthritis: 30-50 mg/kg/day in 4 divided doses; start at lower end of
                dosing range and titrate upward; maximum: 2.4 g/day
            Analgesic: 4-10 mg/kg/dose every 6-8 hours

        Adults:
            Inflammatory disease: 400-800 mg/dose 3-4 times/day; maximum dose: 3.2 g/day
            Pain/fever/dysmenorrhea: 200-400 mg/dose every 4-6 hours; maximum daily dose: 1.2 g
    Dosage Forms
        Suspension, oral: 100 mg/5 mL (120 mL, 480 mL)
        Tablet: 200 mg [OTC], 300 mg, 400 mg, 600 mg, 800 mg

Ibuprohm® [OTC] *see* ibuprofen *on this page*

Ibu-Tab® *see* ibuprofen *on this page*

Ictotest® [OTC] *see* diagnostic aids (*in vitro*), urine *on page 137*

Idamycin® *see* idarubicin hydrochloride *on this page*

idarubicin hydrochloride (eye da rue' bi sin)
Brand Names Idamycin®
Synonyms 4-demothoxydaunorubicin; 4-dmdr
Therapeutic Category Antineoplastic Agent, Antibiotic
Use In combination treatment of acute myeloid leukemia (AML), this includes classifications M1 through M7 of the French-American-British (FAB) classification system
Usual Dosage Adults: Slow I.V. infusion: 12 mg/m^2/day for 3 days in combination with Ara-C
Dosage Forms Powder for injection, lyophilized: 5 mg, 10 mg

idoxuridine (eye dox yoor' i deen)
Brand Names Herplex® Ophthalmic
Synonyms idu; iudr
Therapeutic Category Antiviral Agent, Ophthalmic
Use Treatment of herpes simplex keratitis
Usual Dosage Adults: Ophthalmic:
Ointment: Instill 5 times/day (every 4 hours) in the conjunctival sac with last dose at bedtime; continue therapy for 5-7 days after healing appears complete
Solution: Instill 1 drop in eye(s) every hour during day and every 2 hours at night, continue until definite improvement is noted, then reduce daytime dose to 1 drop every 2 hours and every 4 hours at night; continue for 5-7 days after healing appears complete
Dosage Forms Ointment, ophthalmic: 0.5% (4 g)

idu *see* idoxuridine *on this page*

Ifex® Injection *see* ifosfamide *on this page*

iflra *see* interferon alfa-2a *on page 247*

ifn *see* interferon alfa-2a *on page 247*

ifn-alpha 2 *see* interferon alfa-2b *on page 247*

ifosfamide (eye foss' fa mide)
Brand Names Ifex® Injection
Therapeutic Category Antineoplastic Agent, Alkylating Agent
Use In combination with certain other antineoplastics in treatment of lung cancer, Hodgkin's and non-Hodgkin's lymphoma, breast cancer, acute and chronic lymphocytic leukemia, ovarian cancer, testicular cancer, and sarcomas
Usual Dosage I.V. (refer to individual protocols):
Children: 1800 mg/m^2/day for 3-5 days every 21-28 days or 5000 mg/m^2 as a single 24-hour infusion or 3 g/m^2/day for 2 days

Adults: 700-2000 mg/m^2/day for 5 days or 2400 mg/m^2/day for 3 days every 21-28 days; 5000 mg/m^2 as a single dose over 24 hours
Dosage Forms Powder for injection: 1 g, 3 g

ig *see* immune globulin, intramuscular *on page 243*

igim *see* immune globulin, intramuscular *on page 243*

igiv *see* immune globulin, intravenous *on page 243*

Ilopan-Choline® Oral *see* dexpanthenol *on page 133*

Ilopan® Injection *see* dexpanthenol *on page 133*

Ilosone® Oral *see* erythromycin *on page 170*

Ilotycin® *see* erythromycin, topical *on page 172*

Ilozyme® *see* pancrelipase *on page 346*

Imdur™ *see* isosorbide mononitrate *on page 254*

I-Methasone® *see* dexamethasone *on page 131*

imglucerase (im glu' sir ase)
Brand Names Cerezyme®
Therapeutic Category Enzyme, Glucocerebrosidase
Use Long-term enzyme replacement therapy for patients with Type 1 Gaucher's disease
Usual Dosage I.V.: 2.5 units/kg 3 times a week up to as much as 60 units/kg administered as frequently as once a week or as infrequently as every 4 weeks; 60 units/kg administered every 2 weeks is the most common dose
Dosage Forms Powder for injection, preservative free (lyophilized): 212 units [equivalent to a withdrawal dose of 200 units]

imidazole carboxamide *see* dacarbazine *on page 123*

imipenem/cilastatin (i mi pen' em/sye la stat' in)
Brand Names Primaxin®
Therapeutic Category Antibiotic, Miscellaneous
Use Treatment of documented multidrug resistant gram-negative infection due to organisms proven or suspected to be susceptible to imipenem/cilastatin; treatment of multiple organism infection in which other agents have an insufficient spectrum of activity or are contraindicated due to toxic potential
Usual Dosage I.V. infusion (dosage recommendation based on imipenem component):
Children: 60-100 mg/kg/day in 4 divided doses

Adults:
Serious infection: 2-4 g/day in 3-4 divided doses
Mild to moderate infection: 1-2 g/day in 3-4 divided doses
Dosage Forms Powder for injection:
I.M.:
Imipenem 500 mg and cilastatin 500 mg
Imipenem 750 mg and cilastatin 750 mg
I.V.:
Imipenem 250 mg and cilastatin 250 mg
Imipenem 500 mg and cilastatin 500 mg

imipramine (im ip' ra meen)
Brand Names Janimine® Oral; Tofranil® Injection; Tofranil® Oral; Tofranil-PM® Oral
Therapeutic Category Antidepressant, Tricyclic
Use Treatment of various forms of depression, often in conjunction with psychotherapy; enuresis in children; analgesic for certain chronic and neuropathic pain
Usual Dosage
Children: Oral (safety and efficacy of imipramine therapy for treatment of depression in children <12 years have not been established):
Enuresis: ≥6 years: Initial: 10-25 mg at bedtime, if inadequate response still seen after 1 week of therapy, increase by 25 mg/day; dose should not exceed 2.5 mg/kg/day or 50 mg at bedtime if 6-12 years of age or 75 mg at bedtime if ≥12 years of age
Adjunct in the treatment of cancer pain: Initial: 0.2-0.4 mg/kg at bedtime; dose may be increased by 50% every 2-3 days up to 1-3 mg/kg/dose at bedtime

Adolescents: Oral: Initial: 25-50 mg/day; increase gradually; maximum: 100 mg/day in single or divided doses

Adults:
Oral: Initial: 25 mg 3-4 times/day, increase dose gradually, total dose may be given at bedtime; maximum: 300 mg/day
I.M.: Initial: Up to 100 mg/day in divided doses; change to oral as soon as possible
Dosage Forms
Capsule, as pamoate (Tofranil-PM®): 75 mg, 100 mg, 125 mg, 150 mg
Injection, as hydrochloride (Tofranil®): 12.5 mg/mL (2 mL)
Tablet, as hydrochloride (Janimine®, Tofranil®): 10 mg, 25 mg, 50 mg

Imitrex® Injection *see* sumatriptan succinate *on page 443*

Imitrex® Oral *see* sumatriptan succinate *on page 443*

immune globulin, intramuscular

Brand Names Gamastan®; Gammar®

Synonyms gamma globulin; ig; igim; immune serum globulin; isg

Therapeutic Category Immune Globulin

Use Prophylaxis against hepatitis A, measles, varicella, and possibly rubella and immunoglobulin deficiency, idiopathic thrombocytopenia purpura, Kawasaki syndrome, lymphocytic leukemia

Usual Dosage I.M.:

Hepatitis A: 0.02 mL/kg

IgG: 1.3 mL/kg then 0.66 mL/kg in 3-4 weeks

Measles: 0.25 mL/kg

Rubella: 0.55 mL/kg

Varicella: 0.6-1.2 mL/kg

Dosage Forms Injection: I.M.: 165 ± 15 mg (of protein)/mL (2 mL, 10 mL)

immune globulin, intravenous

Brand Names Gamimune® N; Gammagard®; Gammagard® S/D; Polygam®; Polygam® S/D; Sandoglobulin®; Venoglobulin®-I; Venoglobulin®-S

Synonyms igiv; ivig

Therapeutic Category Immune Globulin

Use Immunodeficiency syndrome, idiopathic thrombocytopenic purpura; used in conjunction with appropriate anti-infective therapy to prevent or modify acute bacterial or viral infections in patients with iatrogenically-induced or disease-associated immunodepression; autoimmune neutropenia, bone marrow transplantation patients, Kawasaki disease, Guillain-Barré syndrome, demyelinating polyneuropathies. Therapy should be guided by clinical observation and serial determination of serum IgG levels.

Usual Dosage Children and Adults: I.V. infusion:

Immunodeficiency syndrome: 100-200 mg/kg/dose every month; may increase to 400 mg/kg/dose as needed

Idiopathic thrombocytopenic purpura: 400-1000 mg/kg/dose for 2-5 consecutive days; maintenance dose: 400-1000 mg/kg/dose every 3-6 weeks based on clinical response and platelet count

Kawasaki disease: 400 mg/kg/day for 4 days or 2 g/kg as a single dose

Congenital and acquired antibody deficiency syndrome: 100-400 mg/kg/dose every 3-4 weeks

Bone marrow transplant: 500 mg/kg/week

Severe systemic viral and bacterial infections:

Neonates: 500 mg/kg/day for 2-6 days then once weekly

Children: 500-1000 mg/kg/week

Dosing comments in renal impairment: Cl_{cr} <10 mL/minute: Avoid use

Dosage Forms

Injection: Gamimune® N: 5% [50 mg/mL] (10 mL, 50 mL, 100 mL); 10% [100 mg/mL] (50 mL, 100 mL, 200 mL)

Powder for injection, lyophilized:

Gammagard®, Polygam®: 0.5 g, 2.5 g, 5 g, 10 g

Gammar®-IV: 1 g, 2.5 g, 5 g

Polygam®: 0.5 g, 2.5 g, 5 g, 10 g

Sandoglobulin®: 1 g, 3 g, 6 g

Venoglobulin®-I: 2.5 g, 5 g

Detergent treated:

Gammagard® S/D: 2.5 g, 5 g, 10 g

Polygam® S/D: 2.5 g, 5 g, 10 g

Venoglobulin®-S: 2.5 g, 5 g, 10 g

immune serum globulin see immune globulin, intramuscular *on previous page*

Imodium® see loperamide hydrochloride *on page 272*

Imodium® A-D [OTC] see loperamide hydrochloride *on page 272*

Imogam® see rabies immune globulin, human *on page 404*

Imovax® Rabies I.D. Vaccine see rabies virus vaccine, human diploid *on page 404*

Imovax® Rabies Vaccine see rabies virus vaccine, human diploid *on page 404*

Imuran® see azathioprine *on page 41*

I-Naphline® Ophthalmic see naphazoline hydrochloride *on page 319*

Inapsine® see droperidol *on page 159*

indapamide (in dap' a mide)
Brand Names Lozol®
Therapeutic Category Diuretic, Miscellaneous
Use Management of mild to moderate hypertension; treatment of edema in congestive heart failure and nephrotic syndrome
Usual Dosage Adults: Oral: 2.5-5 mg/day
Dosage Forms Tablet: 1.25 mg, 2.5 mg

Inderal® see propranolol hydrochloride *on page 394*

Inderal® LA see propranolol hydrochloride *on page 394*

Inderide® see propranolol and hydrochlorothiazide *on page 394*

Indocin® I.V. Injection see indomethacin *on this page*

Indocin® Oral see indomethacin *on this page*

Indocin® SR Oral see indomethacin *on this page*

indocyanine green (in doe sye' a neen)
Brand Names Cardio-Green®
Therapeutic Category Diagnostic Agent, Cardiac Function
Use Determining hepatic function, cardiac output and liver blood flow and for ophthalmic angiography
Usual Dosage Dilute dose in sterile water for injection or 0.9% NaCl to final volume of 1 mL if necessary doses may be repeated periodically; total dose should not exceed 2 mg/kg

Infants: 1.25 mg
Children: 2.5 mg
Adults: 5 mg
Dosage Forms Injection: 25 mg, 50 mg

indomethacin (in doe meth' a sin)
Brand Names Indocin® I.V. Injection; Indocin® Oral; Indocin® SR Oral
Therapeutic Category Analgesic, Non-Narcotic; Anti-inflammatory Agent; Nonsteroidal Anti-Inflammatory Agent (NSAID), Oral; Nonsteroidal Anti-Inflammatory Agent (NSAID), Parenteral
Use Management of inflammatory diseases and rheumatoid disorders; moderate pain; acute gouty arthritis; I.V. form used as alternative to surgery for closure of patent ductus arteriosus in neonates
Usual Dosage
Patent ductus arteriosus: Neonates: I.V.: Initial: 0.2 mg/kg; followed with: 2 doses of 0.1 mg/kg at 12- to 24-hour intervals if age <48 hours at time of first dose; 0.2 mg/kg 2 times if 2-7 days old at time of first dose; or 0.25 mg/kg 2 times if over 7 days at time of first dose; discontinue if significant adverse effects occur. Dose should be withheld if patient has anuria or oliguria.

Analgesia:
Children: Oral: Initial: 1-2 mg/kg/day in 2-4 divided doses; maximum: 4 mg/kg/day; not to exceed 150-200 mg/day

Adults: Oral, rectal: 25-50 mg/dose 2-3 times/day; maximum dose: 200 mg/day; extended release capsule should be given on a 1-2 times/day schedule

Dosage Forms
Capsule (Indocin®): 25 mg, 50 mg
Capsule, sustained release (Indocin® SR): 75 mg
Powder for injection, as sodium trihydrate (Indocin® I.V.): 1 mg
Suppository, rectal (Indocin®): 50 mg
Suspension, oral (Indocin®): 25 mg/5 mL (5 mL, 10 mL, 237 mL, 500 mL)

Infectrol® Ophthalmic see neomycin, polymyxin b, and dexamethasone on page 322

InFed™ Injection see iron dextran complex on page 251

Inflamase® Forte Ophthalmic see prednisolone on page 383

Inflamase® Mild Ophthalmic see prednisolone on page 383

influenza virus vaccine
Brand Names Flu-Imune®; Fluogen®; Fluzone®
Therapeutic Category Vaccine, Inactivated Virus
Use Provide active immunity to influenza virus strains contained in the vaccine
Usual Dosage Annual vaccination with current vaccine. Either whole- or split-virus vaccine may be used.
Dosage Forms Injection:
Purified surface antigen (Flu-Imune®): 5 mL
Split-virus (Fluogen®, Fluzone®): 0.5 mL, 5 mL
Whole-virus (Fluzone®): 5 mL

inh see isoniazid on page 252

INH™ see isoniazid on page 252

Innovar® see droperidol and fentanyl on page 159

Inocor® see amrinone lactate on page 27

insect sting kit
Brand Names Ana-Kit®
Therapeutic Category Antidote, Insect Sting
Use Anaphylaxis emergency treatment of insect bites or stings by the sensitive patient that may occur within minutes of insect sting or exposure to an allergic substance
Usual Dosage Children and Adults:
Epinephrine:
<2 years: 0.05-0.1 mL
2-6 years: 0.15 mL
6-12 years: 0.2 mL
>12 years : 0.3 mL

Chlorpheniramine:
<6 years: 1 tablet
6-12 years: 2 tablets
>12 years: 4 tablets
Dosage Forms Kit: Epinephrine hydrochloride 1:1000 (1 mL syringe), chlorpheniramine maleate chewable tablet 2 mg (4), sterile alcohol pads (2), tourniquet

Insta-Glucose® [OTC] see glucose, instant on page 209

insulin preparations
Brand Names Humulin® 50/50; Humulin® 70/30; Humulin® L; Humulin® N; Humulin® R; Humulin® U Utralente; Lente® Iletin® I; Lente® Iletin® II; Lente® Insulin; Lente® L; Novolin® 70/30; Novolin® 70/30 PenFil®; Novolin® L; Novolin® N; Novolin® N PenFil®; Novolin® R; Novolin® R
(Continued)

insulin preparations *(Continued)*

PenFil®; NPH Iletin® I; NPH Insulin; NPH-N; Pork NPH Iletin® II; Pork Regular Iletin® II; Regular (Concentrated) Iletin® II U-500; Regular Iletin® I; Regular Insulin; Regular Purified Pork Insulin; Ultralente® U; Velosulin® Human

Therapeutic Category Antidiabetic Agent

Use Treatment of insulin-dependent diabetes mellitus, also noninsulin-dependent diabetes mellitus unresponsive to treatment with diet and/or oral hypoglycemics

Usual Dosage Dose requires continuous medical supervision; only regular insulin may be given I.V. The daily dose should be divided up depending upon the product used and the patient's response, eg, regular insulin every 4-6 hours; NPH insulin every 8-12 hours.

Children and Adults: S.C.: 0.5-1 unit/kg/day

Adolescents (during growth spurt) S.C.: 0.8-1.2 units/kg/day

Diabetic ketoacidosis: Children: I.V. loading dose: 0.1 unit/kg, then maintenance continuous infusion: 0.1 unit/kg/hour (range: 0.05-0.2 units/kg/hour depending upon the rate of decrease of serum glucose – too rapid decrease of serum glucose may lead to cerebral edema).

Optimum rate of decrease (serum glucose): 80-100 mg/dL/hour

Note: Newly diagnosed patients with JODM presenting in DKA and patients with blood sugars <800 mg/dL may be relatively "sensitive" to insulin and should receive loading and initial maintenance doses approximately $1/2$ of those indicated above.

Note: The term "purified" refers to insulin preparations containing no more than 10 ppm proinsulin (purified and human insulins are less immunogenic)

Dosage Forms All insulins are 100 units/mL (10 mL) except where indicated:

Insulin injection (Regular Insulin)

Beef and pork: Regular Iletin® I [*Lilly*]

Human:

rDNA: Humulin® R [*Lilly*], Novolin® R [*Novo Nordisk*], Novolin® R PenFil® (1.5 mL) [*Novo Nordisk*]

Semisynthetic: Velosulin® Human [*Novo Nordisk*]

Pork: Regular Insulin [*Novo Nordisk*]

Purified pork:

Pork Regular Iletin® II [*Lilly*], Regular Purified Pork Insulin [*Novo Nordisk*]

Regular (Concentrated) Iletin® II U-500 (*Lilly*): 500 units/mL

Insulin zinc suspension (Lente)

Beef: Lente® Insulin [*Novo Nordisk*]

Beef and pork: Lente® Iletin® I [*Lilly*]

Human, rDNA: Humulin® L [*Lilly*], Novolin® L [*Novo Nordisk*]

Purified pork: Lente® Iletin® II [*Lilly*], Lente® L [*Novo Nordisk*]

Insulin zinc suspension, extended (Ultralente)

Beef: Ultralente® U [*Novo Nordisk*]

Human, rDNA: Humulin® U Utralente [*Lilly*]

Isophane insulin suspension (NPH)

Beef: NPH Insulin [*Novo Nordisk*]

Beef and pork: NPH Iletin® I [*Lilly*]

Human, rDNA: Humulin® N [*Lilly*], Novolin® N [*Novo Nordisk*], Novolin® N PenFil® (1.5 mL) [*Novo Nordisk*]

Purified pork: Pork NPH Iletin® II [*Lilly*], NPH-N [*Novo Nordisk*]

Isophane insulin suspension and insulin injection

Isophane insulin suspension (50%) and insulin injection (50%) human (rDNA): Humulin® 50/50 [*Lilly*]

Isophane insulin suspension (70%) and insulin injection (30%) human (rDNA): Humulin® 70/30 [*Lilly*], Novolin® 70/30 [*Novo Nordisk*], Novolin® 70/30 PenFil® (1.5 mL) [*Novo Nordisk*]

Intal® Inhalation Capsule *see* cromolyn sodium *on page 118*

Intal® Nebulizer Solution *see* cromolyn sodium *on page 118*

Intal® Oral Inhaler *see* cromolyn sodium *on page 118*
Intercept™ [OTC] *see* nonoxynol 9 *on page 331*
α-2-interferon *see* interferon alfa-2b *on this page*

interferon alfa-2a (in ter feer' on)
Brand Names Roferon-A®
Synonyms iflra; ifn; rifn-a
Therapeutic Category Antineoplastic Agent, Miscellaneous; Interferon
Use Hairy cell leukemia, AIDS related Kaposi's sarcoma in patients > 18 years of age, condyloma acuminata, multiple unlabeled uses. Indications and dosage regimens are specific for a particular brand of interferon.
Usual Dosage
Children: S.C.: Pulmonary hemangiomatosis: 1-3 million units/m²/day once daily

Adults > 18 years:
Hairy cell leukemia: I.M., S.C.: Induction dose is 3 million units/day for 16-24 weeks; maintenance: 3 million units 3 times/week
AIDS-related Kaposi's sarcoma: I.M., S.C.: Induction dose is 36 million units for 10-12 weeks; maintenance: 36 million units 3 times/week (may begin with dose escalation from 3-9-18 million units each day over 3 consecutive days followed by 36 million units daily for the remainder of the 10-12 weeks of induction)
Dosage Forms
Injection: 3 million units/mL (1 mL); 6 million units/mL (3 mL); 9 million units/mL (0.9 mL, 3 mL); 36 million units/mL (1 mL)
Powder for injection: 6 million units/mL when reconstituted

interferon alfa-2b
Brand Names Intron® A
Synonyms ifn-alpha 2; α-2-interferon; rIfn-α2
Therapeutic Category Antineoplastic Agent, Miscellaneous; Biological Response Modulator; Interferon
Use Induce hairy-cell leukemia remission; treatment of AIDS related Kaposi's sarcoma; condylomata acuminata; chronic hepatitis C
Usual Dosage Adults (refer to individual protocols):
Hairy cell leukemia: I.M., S.C.: 2 million units/m² 3 times/week

AIDS-related Kaposi's sarcoma: I.M., S.C.: 30 million units/m² 3 times/week or 50 million units/m² I.V. 5 days/week every other week
Condylomata acuminata: Intralesionally: 1 million units/lesion 3 times/week for 3 weeks; not to exceed 5 million units per treatment (maximum: 5 lesions at one time)

Chronic hepatitis C: I.M., S.C.: 3 million units 3 times/week for approximately a 6-month course
Dosage Forms Powder for injection, lyophilized: 3 million units, 5 million units, 10 million units, 18 million units, 25 million units, 50 million units

interferon alfa-n3
Brand Names Alferon® N
Therapeutic Category Antineoplastic Agent, Miscellaneous; Interferon
Use Intralesional treatment of refractory or recurring genital or venereal warts; useful in patients who do not respond or are not candidates for usual treatments; indications and dosage regimens are specific for a particular brand of interferon
Usual Dosage Adults: Inject 250,000 units (0.05 mL) in each wart twice weekly for a maximum of 8 weeks; therapy should not be repeated for at least 3 months after the initial 8-week course of therapy
Dosage Forms Injection: 5 million units (1 mL)

interferon beta-1b
Brand Names Betaseron®
Synonyms rIfn-b
Therapeutic Category Interferon
(Continued)

interferon beta-1b *(Continued)*

Use Reduce the frequency of clinical exacerbations in ambulatory patients with relapsing-remitting multiple sclerosis

Usual Dosage Adults: S.C.: 0.25 mg every other day

Dosage Forms Powder for injection, lyophilized: 0.3 mg [9.6 million units]

interferon gamma-1b

Brand Names Actimmune®

Therapeutic Category Biological Response Modulator

Use Reduce the frequency and severity of serious infections associated with chronic granulomatous disease

Usual Dosage Adults: S.C. (dosing is based on body surface (m^2)):

≤0.5: 1.5 mcg/kg/dose

>0.5: 50 mcg/m^2 (1.5 million units/m^2) 3 times/week

Dosage Forms Injection: 100 mcg [3 million units]

interleukin-2 *see* aldesleukin *on page 11*

Intralipid® *see* fat emulsion *on page 185*

intravascular perfluorochemical emulsion

Brand Names Fluosol®

Therapeutic Category Blood Modifiers

Use To prevent or diminish myocardial ischemia as manifested by decreased ventricular wall motion and global ejection fraction, occurring during percutaneous transluminal angioplasty (PTCA) in patients at high risk of ischemic complications of angioplasty.

Dosage Forms Emulsion, intravascular: 20% [200 mg/mL] (400 mL)

Intron® A *see* interferon alfa-2b *on previous page*

Intropin® Injection *see* dopamine hydrochloride *on page 155*

Inversine® *see* mecamylamine hydrochloride *on page 282*

iocetamic acid *see* radiological/contrast media (ionic) *on page 404*

iodamide meglumine *see* radiological/contrast media (ionic) *on page 404*

Iodex® Regular *see* povidone-iodine *on page 380*

iodinated glycerol (eye' oh di nay ted gli' ser ole)

Brand Names Iophen®; Par Glycerol®; R-Gen®

Therapeutic Category Expectorant

Use Mucolytic expectorant in adjunctive treatment of bronchitis, bronchial asthma, pulmonary emphysema, cystic fibrosis, or chronic sinusitis

Usual Dosage Oral:

Children: 30 mg 4 times/day

Adults: 60 mg 4 times/day

Dosage Forms Organically bound iodine in brackets

Elixir (Iophen™, Par Glycerol®, R-Gen®): 60 mg/5 mL [30 mg/5 mL] (120 mL, 480 mL)

Solution, oral (Iophen™): 50 mg/mL [25 mg/mL] (30 mL)

Tablet (Iophen™) 30 mg [15 mg]

iodinated glycerol and codeine

Brand Names Iophen-C®; IoTuss®; Par Glycerol C®; Tussi-Organidin®; Tussi-R-Gen®

Therapeutic Category Antitussive; Cough Preparation; Expectorant

Use Symptomatic relief of irritating, nonproductive cough associated with respiratory conditions such as bronchitis, bronchial asthma, tracheobronchitis, and the common cold

Usual Dosage Oral:
Children: 2.5-5 mL every 4 hours
Adults: 5-10 mL every 4 hours
Dosage Forms Liquid: Iodinated glycerol 30 mg and codeine phosphate 10 mg per 5 mL

iodinated glycerol and dextromethorphan
Brand Names Iophen® DM; IoTuss-DM®; Par Glycerol DM®; Tussi-Organidin® DM; Tussi-R-Gen DM®; Tusso-DM®
Therapeutic Category Antitussive; Cough Preparation; Expectorant
Use Symptomatic relief of irritating, nonproductive cough associated with respiratory tract conditions
Usual Dosage Oral:
Children: 2.5-5 mL every 4 hours
Adults: 5-10 mL every 4 hours
Dosage Forms Liquid: Iodinated glycerol 30 mg and dextromethorphan hydrobromide 10 mg per 5 mL (120 mL, 480 mL, 4000 mL)

iodine
Therapeutic Category Topical Skin Product
Use Preoperatively to reduce vascularity of the thyroid gland prior to thyroidectomy; management of thyrotoxic crisis or recurrent hyperthyroidism
Usual Dosage Apply topically as necessary to affected areas of skin
Dosage Forms
Solution: 2%
Tincture: 2%

iodipamide meglumine *see* radiological/contrast media (ionic) *on page 404*

iodochlorhydroxyquin *see* clioquinol *on page 106*

iodochlorhydroxyquin and hydrocortisone *see* clioquinol and hydrocortisone *on page 106*

Iodopen® *see* trace metals *on page 465*

iodoquinol (eye oh doe kwin' ole)
Brand Names Yodoxin®
Synonyms diiodohydroxyquin
Therapeutic Category Amebicide
Use Treatment of acute and chronic intestinal amebiasis; asymptomatic cyst passers; *Blastocystis hominis* infections
Usual Dosage Oral:
Children: 30-40 mg/kg/day in 3 divided doses for 20 days; not to exceed 1.95 g/day
Adults: 650 mg 3 times/day after meals for 20 days; not to exceed 2 g/day
Dosage Forms
Powder: 25 g
Tablet: 210 mg, 650 mg

iodoquinol and hydrocortisone
Brand Names Vytone® Topical
Therapeutic Category Antifungal Agent, Topical; Corticosteroid, Topical (Low Potency)
Use Treatment of eczema; infectious dermatitis; chronic eczematoid otitis externa; mycotic dermatoses
Usual Dosage Topical: Apply 3-4 times/day
Dosage Forms Cream: Iodoquinol 1% and hydrocortisone 1% (30 g)

iohexol *see* radiological/contrast media (non-ionic) *on page 406*

Ionamin® *see* phentermine hydrochloride *on page 363*

iopamidol *see* radiological/contrast media (non-ionic) *on page 406*

iopanoic acid *see* radiological/contrast media (ionic) *on page 404*

Iophen® *see* iodinated glycerol *on page 248*

Iophen-C® *see* iodinated glycerol and codeine *on page 248*

Iophen® DM *see* iodinated glycerol and dextromethorphan *on previous page*

Iopidine® *see* apraclonidine hydrochloride *on page 32*

iothalamate meglumine and iothalamate sodium *see* radiological/contrast media (ionic) *on page 404*

iothalamate sodium *see* radiological/contrast media (ionic) *on page 404*

IoTuss® *see* iodinated glycerol and codeine *on page 248*

IoTuss-DM® *see* iodinated glycerol and dextromethorphan *on previous page*

ioversol *see* radiological/contrast media (non-ionic) *on page 406*

I-Paracaine® Ophthalmic *see* proparacaine hydrochloride *on page 392*

ipecac syrup (ip' e kak)
Therapeutic Category Antidote, Emetic
Use Treatment of acute oral drug overdosage and in certain poisonings
Usual Dosage Oral:
Children:
6-12 months: 5-10 mL followed by 10-20 mL/kg of water; repeat dose one time if vomiting does not occur within 20 minutes
1-12 years: 15 mL followed by 10-20 mL/kg of water; repeat dose one time if vomiting does not occur within 20 minutes

Adults: 30 mL followed by 200-300 mL of water; repeat dose one time if vomiting does not occur within 20 minutes
Dosage Forms Syrup: 70 mg/mL (15 mL, 30 mL, 473 mL, 4000 mL)

I-Pentolate® *see* cyclopentolate hydrochloride *on page 120*

I-Phrine® Ophthalmic Solution *see* phenylephrine hydrochloride *on page 364*

I-Picamide® Ophthalmic *see* tropicamide *on page 476*

ipodate calcium *see* radiological/contrast media (ionic) *on page 404*

ipodate sodium *see* radiological/contrast media (ionic) *on page 404*

IPOL™ *see* poliovirus vaccine, inactivated *on page 374*

ipratropium bromide (i pra troe' pee um)
Brand Names Atrovent® Aerosol Inhalation; Atrovent® Inhalation Solution
Therapeutic Category Anticholinergic Agent; Bronchodilator
Use Bronchodilator used in bronchospasm associated with COPD, bronchitis, and emphysema
Usual Dosage Children >12 years and Adults: 2 inhalations 4 times/day up to 12 inhalations/24 hours
Dosage Forms Solution:
Inhalation: 18 mcg/actuation (14 g)
Nebulizing: 0.2% (2.5 mL)

iproveratril hydrochloride *see* verapamil hydrochloride *on page 486*

ipv *see* poliovirus vaccine, inactivated *on page 374*

Ircon® [OTC] *see* ferrous fumarate *on page 189*

iron dextran complex
Brand Names InFed™ Injection
Therapeutic Category Iron Salt
Use Treatment of microcytic hypochromic anemia resulting from iron deficiency in whom oral administration is infeasible or ineffective
Usual Dosage I.M., I.V.:

A 0.5 mL test dose (0.25 mL in infants) should be given prior to starting iron dextran therapy

Total replacement dosage of iron dextran (mL) = 0.0476 x weight (kg) x (Hb$_n$-Hb$_o$) + 1 mL/per 5 kg body weight (up to maximum of 14 mL)
Hb$_n$ = desired hemoglobin (g/dL)
Hb$_o$ = measured hemoglobin (g/dL)

Maximum daily dose:
Infants <5 kg: 25 mg iron
Children:
5-10 kg: 50 mg iron
10-50 kg: 100 mg iron
Adults >50 kg: 100 mg iron
Dosage Forms Injection: 50 mg/mL (2 mL, 10 mL)

isd see isosorbide dinitrate on page 254

isdn see isosorbide dinitrate on page 254

isg see immune globulin, intramuscular on page 243

Ismelin® see guanethidine monosulfate on page 218

ismn see isosorbide mononitrate on page 254

Ismo™ see isosorbide mononitrate on page 254

Ismotic® see isosorbide on page 254

isoamyl nitrite see amyl nitrite on page 27

isobamate see carisoprodol on page 77

Iso-Bid® see isosorbide dinitrate on page 254

Isocaine® HCl Injection see mepivacaine hydrochloride on page 288

Isocet® see butalbital compound on page 63

Isoclor® Expectorant see guaifenesin, pseudoephedrine, and codeine on page 217

Isoclor® Tablet see chlorpheniramine and pseudoephedrine on page 94

Isoclor® Timesules® see chlorpheniramine and pseudoephedrine on page 94

Isocult® for Bacteriuria see diagnostic aids (in vitro), urine on page 137

Isocult® for Neisseria gonorrhoeae see diagnostic aids (in vitro), other on page 137

Isocult® for Pseudomonas aeruginosa see diagnostic aids (in vitro), urine on page 137

Isocult® for Staphylococcus aureus see diagnostic aids (in vitro), other on page 137

Isocult® for Trichomonas vaginalis see diagnostic aids (in vitro), other on page 137

Isocult® Throat Streptococci see diagnostic aids (in vitro), other on page 137

Isodine® [OTC] see povidone-iodine on page 380

isoethadione see paramethadione on page 349

isoetharine (eye soe eth' a reen)
Brand Names Arm-a-Med® Isoetharine; Beta-2®; Bronkometer®; Bronkosol®; Dey-Lute® Isoetharine
Therapeutic Category Adrenergic Agonist Agent; Bronchodilator
(Continued)

251

isoetharine *(Continued)*

Use Bronchodilator in bronchial asthma and for reversible bronchospasm occurring with bronchitis and emphysema

Usual Dosage Treatments are usually not repeated more often than every 4 hours, except in severe cases, and may be repeated up to 5 times/day if necessary

Nebulizer: Children: 0.1-0.2 mg/kg/dose every 2-6 hours as needed; adult: 0.5 mL diluted in 2-3 mL normal saline or 4 inhalations of undiluted 1% solution

Dosage Forms

Aerosol, oral, as mesylate: 340 mcg/metered spray

Solution, inhalation, as hydrochloride: 0.062% (4 mL); 0.08% (3.5 mL); 0.1% (2.5 mL, 5 mL); 0.125% (4 mL); 0.167% (3 mL); 0.17% (3 mL); 0.2% (2.5 mL); 0.25% (2 mL, 3.5 mL); 0.5% (0.5 mL); 1% (0.5 mL, 0.25 mL, 10 mL, 14 mL, 30 mL)

isoflurane (eye soe flure' ane)

Brand Names Forane®

Therapeutic Category General Anesthetic

Use General induction and maintenance of anesthesia (inhalation)

Usual Dosage 1.5% to 3%

Dosage Forms Solution: 100 mL, 125 mL, 250 mL

isoflurophate (eye soe flure' oh fate)

Brand Names Floropryl® Ophthalmic

Synonyms dfp; diisopropyl fluorophosphate; dyflos; fluostigmin

Therapeutic Category Cholinergic Agent, Ophthalmic; Ophthalmic Agent, Miotic

Use Treat primary open-angle glaucoma and conditions that obstruct aqueous outflow and to treat accommodative convergent strabismus

Usual Dosage Adults: Ophthalmic:

Glaucoma: Instill $\frac{1}{4}$" strip in eye every 8-72 hours

Strabismus: Instill $\frac{1}{4}$" strip to each eye every night for 2 weeks then reduce to $\frac{1}{4}$" every other night to once weekly for 2 months

Dosage Forms Ointment, ophthalmic: 0.025% in polyethylene mineral oil gel (3.5 g)

Isollyl Improved® *see* butalbital compound *on page 63*

Isonate® *see* isosorbide dinitrate *on page 254*

isoniazid (eye soe nye' a zid)

Brand Names INH™; Laniazid®; Nydrazid®

Synonyms inh; isonicotinic acid hydrazide

Therapeutic Category Antitubercular Agent

Use Treatment of susceptible tuberculosis infections and prophylactically to those individuals exposed to tuberculosis

Usual Dosage Oral, I.M.:

Children: 10-20 mg/kg/day in 1-2 divided doses (maximum: 300 mg total dose)
Prophylaxis: 10 mg/kg/day given daily (up to 300 mg total dose) for 12 months

Adults: 5 mg/kg/day given daily (usual dose is 300 mg)
Disseminated disease: 10 mg/kg/day in 1-2 divided doses
Treatment should be continued for 9 months with rifampin or for 6 months with rifampin and pyrazinamide
Prophylaxis: 300 mg/day given daily for 12 months

American Thoracic Society and CDC currently recommend twice weekly therapy as part of a short-course regimen which follows 1-2 months of daily treatment for uncomplicated pulmonary tuberculosis in compliant patients
Children: 20-40 mg/kg/dose (up to 900 mg) twice weekly
Adults: 15 mg/kg/dose (up to 900 mg) twice weekly

Dosage Forms

Injection: 100 mg/mL (10 mL)

Syrup (orange flavor): 50 mg/5 mL (473 mL)

Tablet: 50 mg, 100 mg, 300 mg

isonicotinic acid hydrazide *see* isoniazid *on previous page*

isonipecaine hydrochloride *see* meperidine hydrochloride *on page 286*

isoprenaline hydrochloride *see* isoproterenol *on this page*

isopropamide iodide (eye soe proe' pa mide)
Brand Names Darbid®
Therapeutic Category Anticholinergic Agent; Antispasmodic Agent, Gastrointestinal
Use Adjunctive therapy for peptic ulcer, irritable bowel syndrome
Usual Dosage Children >12 years and Adults: Oral: 5-10 mg every 12 hours
Dosage Forms Tablet: 5 mg

isoproterenol (eye soe proe ter' e nole)
Brand Names Arm-a-Med® Isoproterenol; Dey-Dose® Isoproterenol; Dispos-a-Med® Iso-proterenol; Isuprel®; Medihaler-Iso®; Norisodrine®
Synonyms isoprenaline hydrochloride
Therapeutic Category Adrenergic Agonist Agent; Bronchodilator
Use Asthma or COPD (reversible airway obstruction); A-V nodal block; hemodynamically compromised bradyarrhythmias or atropine-resistant bradyarrhythmias, temporary use in 3rd degree A-V block until pacemaker insertion; low cardiac output; vasoconstrictive shock states
Usual Dosage
Children:
Bronchodilation: Inhalation 1-2 metered doses up to 5 times/day
Nebulization: 0.01 mL/kg; minimum dose: 0.1 mL; maximum dose: 0.5 mL diluted in 2-3 mL normal saline
I.V. infusion: 0.05-2 mcg/kg/minute; rate (mL/hour) = dose (mcg/kg/minute) x weight (kg) x 60 minutes/hour divided by concentration (mcg/mL)
Adults:
Bronchodilation: 1-2 inhalations 4-6 times/day
A-V nodal block: I.V. infusion: 2-20 mcg/minute
Dosage Forms
Inhalation: Aerosol: 0.2% [2 mg/mL = 1:500] (15 mL, 22.5 mL); 0.25% [2.5 mg/mL = 1:400] (15 mL)
Injection: 0.02% [0.2 mg/mL = 1:5000] (1 mL, 5 mL, 10 mL)
Solution for nebulization: 0.031% (4 mL); 0.062% (4 mL); 0.25% (0.5 mL, 30 mL); 0.5% (0.5 mL, 10 mL, 60 mL); 1% (10 mL)
Tablet, sublingual: 10 mg, 15 mg

isoproterenol and phenylephrine
Brand Names Duo-Medihaler® Aerosol
Therapeutic Category Adrenergic Agonist Agent
Use Treatment of bronchospasm associated with acute and chronic bronchial asthma, bronchitis, pulmonary emphysema, and bronchiectasis
Usual Dosage Daily maintenance: 1-2 inhalations 4-6 times/day, no more than 2 inhalations at any one time or more than 6 in any 1 hour within 24 hours
Dosage Forms Aerosol: Each actuation releases isoproterenol hydrochloride 0.16 mg and phenylephrine bitartrate 0.24 mg (15 mL, 22.5 mL)

Isoptin® *see* verapamil hydrochloride *on page 486*

Isopto® Atropine Ophthalmic *see* atropine sulfate *on page 38*

Isopto® Carbachol Ophthalmic *see* carbachol *on page 73*

Isopto® Carpine Ophthalmic *see* pilocarpine *on page 369*

Isopto® Frin Ophthalmic Solution *see* phenylephrine hydrochloride *on page 364*

Isopto® Homatropine Ophthalmic *see* homatropine hydrobromide *on page 226*

Isopto® Hyoscine Ophthalmic *see* scopolamine *on page 418*

Isopto® Plain [OTC] *see* artificial tears *on page 34*

Isopto® Tears [OTC] *see* artificial tears *on page 34*

Isordil® *see* isosorbide dinitrate *on this page*

isosorbide (eye soe sor' bide)

Brand Names Ismotic®

Therapeutic Category Diuretic, Osmotic; Ophthalmic Agent, Osmotic

Use Short-term emergency treatment of acute angle-closure glaucoma

Usual Dosage Adults: Oral: Initial: 1.5 g/kg with a usual range of 1-3 g/kg 2-4 times/day

Dosage Forms Solution: 45% [450 mg/mL] (220 mL)

isosorbide dinitrate (eye soe sor' bide)

Brand Names Dilatrate®-SR; Iso-Bid®; Isonate®; Isordil®; Isotrate®; Sorbitrate®

Synonyms isd; isdn

Therapeutic Category Antianginal Agent; Nitrate; Vasodilator, Coronary

Use Prevention and treatment of angina pectoris; for congestive heart failure; to relieve pain, dysphagia, and spasm in esophageal spasm with GE reflux

Usual Dosage Adults:
Oral: 5-30 mg 4 times/day or 40 mg every 6-12 hours in sustained-released dosage form
Chewable: 5-10 mg every 2-3 hours
Sublingual: 2.5-10 mg every 4-6 hours

Dosage Forms
Capsule, sustained release: 40 mg
Tablet:
Chewable: 5 mg, 10 mg
Oral: 5 mg, 10 mg, 20 mg, 30 mg
Sublingual: 2.5 mg, 5 mg, 10 mg
Sustained release: 40 mg

isosorbide mononitrate

Brand Names Imdur™; Ismo™; Monoket®

Synonyms ismn

Therapeutic Category Antianginal Agent; Vasodilator, Coronary

Use Long-acting metabolite of the vasodilator isosorbide dinitrate used for the prophylactic treatment of angina pectoris

Usual Dosage Oral: Adults:
Regular tablet: 20 mg twice daily separated by 7 hours; maintenance doses as high as 120 mg have been used
Extended release tablet: 30 mg ($^1/_2$ of 60 mg tablet) or 60 mg (given as a single tablet) once daily; after several days the dosage may be increased to 120 mg (given as two 60 mg tablets) once daily; the daily dose should be taken in the morning upon arising

Dosage Forms
Tablet (Ismo™, Monoket®): 10 mg, 20 mg
Tablet, extended release (Imdur™): 60 mg

isosulfan blue *see* radiological/contrast media (ionic) *on page 404*

Isotrate® *see* isosorbide dinitrate *on this page*

isotretinoin (eye soe tret' i noyn)

Brand Names Accutane®

Synonyms 13-*cis*-retinoic acid

Therapeutic Category Acne Products; Retinoic Acid Derivative; Vitamin A Derivative

Use Treatment of severe recalcitrant cystic and/or conglobate acne unresponsive to conventional therapy; used investigationally for the treatment of children with metastatic neuroblastoma or leukemia that does not respond to conventional therapy

Usual Dosage Oral:

Children: Maintenance therapy for neuroblastoma: 100-250 mg/m^2/day in 2 divided doses has been used investigationally

Children and Adults: 0.5-2 mg/kg/day in 2 divided doses for 15-20 weeks

Dosage Forms Capsule: 10 mg, 20 mg, 40 mg

Isovex® see ethaverine hydrochloride *on page 177*

Isovue® see radiological/contrast media (non-ionic) *on page 406*

isoxsuprine hydrochloride (eye sox' syoo preen)

Brand Names Vasodilan®

Therapeutic Category Vasodilator

Use Treatment of peripheral vascular diseases, such as arteriosclerosis obliterans and Raynaud's disease

Usual Dosage Adults: Oral: 10-20 mg 3-4 times/day

Dosage Forms Tablet: 10 mg, 20 mg

isradipine (is ra' di peen)

Brand Names DynaCirc®

Therapeutic Category Calcium Channel Blocker

Use Management of hypertension, alone or concurrently with thiazide-type diuretics

Usual Dosage Adults: Oral: Initial: 2.5 mg twice daily, if satisfactory response does not occur after 2-4 weeks the dose may be adjusted in increments of 5 mg/day at 2- to 4-week intervals up to a maximum of 20 mg/day

Dosage Forms Capsule: 2.5 mg, 5 mg

I-Sulfacet® Ophthalmic see sodium sulfacetamide *on page 431*

Isuprel® see isoproterenol *on page 253*

Itch-X® [OTC] see pramoxine hydrochloride *on page 381*

itraconazole (i tra koe' na zole)

Brand Names Sporanox® Oral

Therapeutic Category Antifungal Agent, Systemic

Use Treatment of susceptible fungal infections in immunocompromised and nonimmunocompromised patients including blastomycosis and histoplasmosis

Usual Dosage Adults: Oral: 200 mg once daily, if obvious improvement or there is evidence of progressive fungal disease, increase the dose in 100 mg increments to a maximum of 400 mg/day; doses >200 mg/day are given in 2 divided doses

Life-threatening: Loading dose: 200 mg give 3 times/day (600 mg/day) should be given for the first 3 days

Dosage Forms Capsule: 100 mg

I-Tropine® Ophthalmic see atropine sulfate *on page 38*

iudr see idoxuridine *on page 241*

ivig see immune globulin, intravenous *on page 243*

Janimine® Oral see imipramine *on page 242*

Japanese encephalitis virus vaccine, inactivated

Brand Names JE-VAX®

Therapeutic Category Vaccine, Inactivated Virus

Use Active immunization against Japanese encephalitis for persons spending a month or longer in endemic areas, especially if travel will include rural areas

(Continued)

Japanese encephalitis virus vaccine, inactivated *(Continued)*
Usual Dosage S.C. (given on days 0, 7, and 30):
Children 1-3 years: 3 doses of 0.5 mL; booster doses of 0.5 mL may given 2 years after primary immunization series

Children >3 years and Adults: 3 doses of 1 mL; booster doses of 1 mL may be given 2 years after primary immunization series
Dosage Forms Powder for injection, lyophilized: 1 mL, 10 mL

Jenamicin® Injection *see* gentamicin sulfate *on page 207*

JE-VAX® *see* Japanese encephalitis virus vaccine, inactivated *on previous page*

K+8® *see* potassium chloride *on page 378*

Kabikinase® *see* streptokinase *on page 436*

Kalcinate® *see* calcium gluconate *on page 68*

kanamycin sulfate *(kan a mye' sin)*
Brand Names Kantrex™
Therapeutic Category Antibiotic, Aminoglycoside
Use
Oral: Preoperative bowel preparation in the prophylaxis of infections and adjunctive treatment of hepatic coma (oral kanamycin is not indicated in the treatment of systemic infections)
Parenteral: Initial therapy of severe infections where the strain is thought to be susceptible in patients allergic to other antibiotics, or in mixed staphylococcal or gram-negative infections
Usual Dosage
Children: Infections: I.M., I.V.: 15 mg/kg/day in divided doses every 8-12 hours
Adults:
Infections: I.M., I.V.: 15 mg/kg/day in divided doses every 8-12 hours
Preoperative intestinal antisepsis: Oral: 1 g every 4-6 hours for 36-72 hours
Dosage Forms
Capsule: 500 mg
Injection:
Pediatric: 75 mg (2 mL)
Adults: 500 mg (2 mL); 1 g (3 mL)

Kantrex® *see* kanamycin sulfate *on this page*

Kaochlor® S-F *see* potassium chloride *on page 378*

Kaodene® [OTC] *see* kaolin and pectin *on this page*

kaolin and pectin
Brand Names Kaodene™ [OTC]; Kao-Spen™ [OTC]; Kapectolin® [OTC]
Synonyms pectin and kaolin
Therapeutic Category Antidiarrheal
Use Treatment of uncomplicated diarrhea
Usual Dosage Oral:
Children:
<6 years: Do not use
6-12 years: 30-60 mL after each loose stool
Adults: 60-120 mL after each loose stool
Dosage Forms Suspension, oral: Kaolin 975 mg and pectin 22 mg per 5 mL

kaolin and pectin with opium
Brand Names Parepectolin™
Therapeutic Category Antidiarrheal
Use Symptomatic relief of diarrhea

Usual Dosage Oral:
  Children:
      3-6 years: 7.5 mL with each loose bowel movement, not to exceed 30 mL in 12 hours
      6-12 years: 5-10 mL with each loose bowel movement, not to exceed 40 mL in 12 hours
  Children >12 years and Adults: 15-30 mL with each loose bowel movement, not to exceed
  120 mL in 12 hours
  Dosage Forms Suspension, oral: Kaolin 5.5 g, pectin 162 mg, and opium 15 mg per 30 mL
  [3.7 mL paregoric] (240 mL)

Kaon® *see* potassium gluconate *on page 379*

Kaon-CL® *see* potassium chloride *on page 378*

Kaopectate® **Maximum Strength Caplets** *see* attapulgite *on page 39*

Kaopectate® **Advanced Formula [OTC]** *see* attapulgite *on page 39*

Kaopectate® **II [OTC]** *see* loperamide hydrochloride *on page 272*

Kao-Spen® **[OTC]** *see* kaolin and pectin *on previous page*

Kapectolin PG® *see* hyoscyamine, atropine, scopolamine, kaolin, pectin, and opium
  on page 239

Kapectolin® **[OTC]** *see* kaolin and pectin *on previous page*

Karidium® *see* fluoride *on page 196*

Karigel® *see* fluoride *on page 196*

Karigel®**-N** *see* fluoride *on page 196*

Kasof® **[OTC]** *see* docusate *on page 153*

Kato® *see* potassium chloride *on page 378*

Kaybovite-1000® *see* cyanocobalamin *on page 119*

Kayexalate® *see* sodium polystyrene sulfonate *on page 430*

KCl *see* potassium chloride *on page 378*

K-Dur® *see* potassium chloride *on page 378*

Keflex® *see* cephalexin monohydrate *on page 84*

Keflin® **Injection** *see* cephalothin sodium *on page 84*

Keftab® *see* cephalexin monohydrate *on page 84*

Kefurox® **Injection** *see* cefuroxime *on page 83*

Kefzol® *see* cefazolin sodium *on page 79*

Kemadrin® *see* procyclidine hydrochloride *on page 389*

Kenacort® **Syrup** *see* triamcinolone *on page 467*

Kenacort® **Tablet** *see* triamcinolone *on page 467*

Kenalog® **Injection** *see* triamcinolone *on page 467*

Kenalog® **in Orabase**® *see* triamcinolone *on page 467*

Kenonel® *see* triamcinolone *on page 467*

Keralyt® **Gel** *see* salicylic acid and propylene glycol *on page 416*

Kerlone® **Oral** *see* betaxolol hydrochloride *on page 53*

Kestrone® *see* estrone *on page 175*

Ketalar® **Injection** *see* ketamine hydrochloride *on this page*

ketamine hydrochloride (keet' a meen)

  Brand Names Ketalar® Injection
  Therapeutic Category General Anesthetic
  Use Induction of anesthesia; short procedures; supplement nitrous oxide; dressing changes
  Usual Dosage
  Children:
      I.M.: 3-7 mg/kg
  (Continued)

ketamine hydrochloride *(Continued)*

I.V.: Range: 0.5-2 mg/kg, use smaller doses (0.5-1 mg/kg) for sedation for minor procedures; usual induction dosage: 1-2 mg/kg

Adults:
I.M.: 3-8 mg/kg
I.V.: Range: 1-4.5 mg/kg; usual induction dosage: 1-2 mg/kg

Children and Adults: Maintenance: Supplemental doses of $\frac{1}{3}$ to $\frac{1}{2}$ of initial dose
Dosage Forms Injection: 10 mg/mL (20 mL, 25 mL, 50 mL); 50 mg/mL (10 mL); 100 mg/mL (5 mL)

ketoconazole (kee toe koe' na zole)
Brand Names Nizoral® Oral; Nizoral® Topical
Therapeutic Category Antifungal Agent, Systemic; Antifungal Agent, Topical
Use Treatment of susceptible fungal infections, including candidiasis, oral thrush, blastomycosis, histoplasmosis, paracoccidioidomycosis, chronic mucocutaneous candidiasis, as well as certain recalcitrant cutaneous dermatophytoses; used topically for treatment of tinea corporis, tinea cruris, tinea versicolor and cutaneous candidiasis
Usual Dosage
Children: Oral: 5-10 mg/kg/day divided every 12-24 hours until lesions clear

Adults:
Oral: 200-400 mg/day as a single daily dose
Topical: Rub gently into the affected area once daily to twice daily for two weeks
Dosage Forms
Cream: 2% (15 g, 30 g, 60 g)
Shampoo: 2% (120 mL)
Tablet: 200 mg

Keto-Diastix® [OTC] *see* diagnostic aids (*in vitro*), urine *on page 137*

ketoprofen (kee toe proe' fen)
Brand Names Orudis®; Oruvail®
Therapeutic Category Analgesic, Non-Narcotic; Anti-inflammatory Agent; Nonsteroidal Anti-Inflammatory Agent (NSAID), Oral
Use Acute or long-term treatment of rheumatoid arthritis and osteoarthritis; primary dysmenorrhea; mild to moderate pain
Usual Dosage Oral:
Children 3 months to 14 years: Fever: 0.5-1 mg/kg

Children >12 years and Adults:
Rheumatoid arthritis or osteoarthritis: 50-75 mg 3-4 times/day up to a maximum of 300 mg/day
Mild to moderate pain: 25-50 mg every 6-8 hours up to a maximum of 300 mg/day
Dosage Forms
Capsule (Orudis®): 25 mg, 50 mg, 75 mg
Capsule, extended release (Oruvail®): 200 mg

ketorolac tromethamine (kee' toe role ak)
Brand Names Acular® Ophthalmic; Toradol® Injection; Toradol® Oral
Therapeutic Category Analgesic, Non-Narcotic; Anti-inflammatory Agent; Nonsteroidal Anti-Inflammatory Agent (NSAID), Oral; Nonsteroidal Anti-Inflammatory Agent (NSAID), Parenteral
Use Short-term management of pain; first parenteral NSAID for analgesia; 30 mg provides the analgesia comparable to 12 mg of morphine or 100 mg of meperidine
Usual Dosage Adults: Pain relief usually begins within 10 minutes
Oral: 10 mg every 4-6 hours for a maximum of 40 mg/day
I.M.: Initial: 30 mg then 15 mg every 6 hours thereafter, or 60 mg initially, then 30 mg every 6 hours thereafter; maximum dose in the first 24 hours: 150 mg with 120 mg/24 hours thereafter

Dosage Forms
Injection: 15 mg/mL (1 mL); 30 mg/mL (1 mL, 2 mL)
Solution, ophthalmic: 0.5% (5 mL)
Tablet: 10 mg

Ketostix® [OTC] *see* diagnostic aids (*in vitro*), urine *on page 137*

Key-Pred® Injection *see* prednisolone *on page 383*

Key-Pred-SP® Injection *see* prednisolone *on page 383*

KI *see* potassium iodide *on page 379*

K-Ide® *see* potassium bicarbonate and potassium citrate, effervescent *on page 377*

Kinesed® *see* hyoscyamine, atropine, scopolamine, and phenobarbital *on page 238*

Kinevac® *see* sincalide *on page 423*

Klerist-D® *see* chlorpheniramine and pseudoephedrine *on page 94*

Klonopin™ *see* clonazepam *on page 107*

K-Lor™ *see* potassium chloride *on page 378*

Klor-con® *see* potassium chloride *on page 378*

Klor-con®/EF *see* potassium bicarbonate and potassium citrate, effervescent *on page 377*

Klorvess® *see* potassium chloride *on page 378*

Klotrix® *see* potassium chloride *on page 378*

K-Lyte® *see* potassium bicarbonate and potassium citrate, effervescent *on page 377*

K-Lyte/CL® *see* potassium chloride *on page 378*

Koāte®-HP *see* antihemophilic factor (human) *on page 29*

Koāte®-HS *see* antihemophilic factor (human) *on page 29*

KoGENate® *see* antihemophilic factor (human) *on page 29*

Kolephrin® GG/DM [OTC] *see* guaifenesin and dextromethorphan *on page 214*

Kolyum® *see* potassium gluconate *on page 379*

Konakion® Injection *see* phytonadione *on page 368*

Kondon's Nasal® [OTC] *see* ephedrine sulfate *on page 167*

Konsyl-D® [OTC] *see* psyllium *on page 398*

Konsyl Fiber® [OTC] *see* calcium polycarbophil *on page 70*

Konsyl® [OTC] *see* psyllium *on page 398*

Konyne® 80 *see* factor ix complex (human) *on page 184*

Koromex® [OTC] *see* nonoxynol 9 *on page 331*

K-Phos® Neutral *see* potassium phosphate and sodium phosphate *on page 380*

K-Phos® Original *see* potassium acid phosphate *on page 377*

Kronofed-A-Jr® *see* chlorpheniramine and pseudoephedrine *on page 94*

K-Tab® *see* potassium chloride *on page 378*

Ku-Zyme® HP *see* pancrelipase *on page 346*

K-Vescent® *see* potassium bicarbonate and potassium citrate, effervescent *on page 377*

Kwelcof® *see* hydrocodone and guaifenesin *on page 230*

Kwell® Cream *see* lindane *on page 269*

Kwell® Lotion *see* lindane *on page 269*

Kwell® Shampoo *see* lindane *on page 269*

Kytril™ Injection *see* granisetron *on page 212*

Kytril™ Tablet *see* granisetron *on page 212*

***L*-3-hydroxytyrosine** *see* levodopa *on page 265*

LA-12® *see* hydroxocobalamin *on page 235*

labetalol hydrochloride (la bet' a lole)
Brand Names Normodyne® Injection; Normodyne® Oral; Trandate® Injection; Trandate® Oral
Synonyms ibidomide hydrochloride
Therapeutic Category Alpha-/Beta- Adrenergic Blocker
Use Treatment of mild to severe hypertension; I.V. for hypertensive emergencies
Usual Dosage
Children: Limited information regarding labetalol use in pediatric patients is currently available in literature. Some centers recommend initial oral doses of 4 mg/kg/day in 2 divided doses. Reported oral doses have started at 3 mg/kg/day and 20 mg/kg/day and have increased up to 40 mg/kg/day.

I.V., intermittent bolus doses of 0.3-1 mg/kg/dose have been reported

For treatment of pediatric hypertensive emergencies, initial continuous infusions of 0.4-1 mg/kg/hour with a maximum of 3 mg/kg/hour have been used.

Due to limited documentation of its use, labetalol should be initiated cautiously in pediatric patients with careful dosage adjustment and blood pressure monitoring
Adults:
Oral: Initial: 100 mg twice daily, may increase as needed every 2-3 days by 100 mg until desired response is obtained; usual dose: 200-400 mg twice daily; not to exceed 2.4 g/day
I.V.: 20 mg or 1-2 mg/kg whichever is lower, IVP over 2 minutes, may give 40-80 mg at 10-minute intervals, up to 300 mg total dose
I.V. infusion: Initial: 2 mg/minute; titrate to response
Dosage Forms
Injection: 5 mg/mL (20 mL, 40 mL, 60 mL)
Tablet: 100 mg, 200 mg, 300 mg

Labstix® [OTC] *see* diagnostic aids (*in vitro*), urine *on page 137*

Lac-Hydrin® *see* lactic acid with ammonium hydroxide *on next page*

Lactaid® [OTC] *see* lactase enzyme *on this page*

lactase enzyme (lak' tase)
Brand Names Dairy Ease® [OTC]; Lactaid® [OTC]; Lactrase® [OTC]
Therapeutic Category Nutritional Supplement
Use Help digest lactose in milk for patients with lactose intolerance
Usual Dosage
Capsule: 1-2 capsules taken with milk or meal; pretreat milk with 1-2 capsules per quart of milk
Liquid: 5-15 drops per quart of milk
Tablet: 1-3 tablets with meals
Dosage Forms
Caplet: 3000 FCC lactase units
Capsule: 250 mg
Liquid: 1250 neutral lactase units/5 drops
Tablet, chewable: 3300 FCC lactase units

lactic acid and salicylic acid *see* salicylic acid and lactic acid *on page 416*

lactic acid and sodium-PCA
Brand Names LactiCare® [OTC]
Synonyms sodium-pca and lactic acid
Therapeutic Category Topical Skin Product
Use Lubricate and moisturize the skin counteracting dryness and itching
Usual Dosage Apply as needed
Dosage Forms Lotion, topical: Lactic acid 5% and sodium-PCA 2.5% (240 mL)

lactic acid with ammonium hydroxide
Brand Names Lac-Hydrin®
Synonyms ammonium lactate
Therapeutic Category Topical Skin Product
Use Treatment of moderate to severe xerosis and ichthyosis vulgaris
Usual Dosage Shake well; apply to affected areas, use twice daily, rub in well
Dosage Forms Lotion: Lactic acid 12% with ammonium hydroxide (150 mL)

LactiCare-HC® see hydrocortisone on page 232
LactiCare® [OTC] see lactic acid and sodium-PCA on this page
Lactinex® [OTC] see lactobacillus on this page

lactobacillus (lak toe ba sil' us)
Brand Names Bacid® [OTC]; Lactinex® [OTC]; More-Dophilus™ [OTC]
Therapeutic Category Antidiarrheal
Use Uncomplicated diarrhea particularly that caused by antibiotic therapy; re-establish normal physiologic and bacterial flora of the intestinal tract
Usual Dosage Children and Adults: Oral:
Capsule: Take 2 capsules 2-4 times daily
Granules: 1 packet added to or taken with cereal, food, milk, fruit juice, or water, 3-4 times/day
Tablet, chewable: 4 tablets 3-4 times/day; may follow each dose with a small amount of milk, fruit juice, or water
Recontamination protocol for BMT unit: 1 packet 3 times/day for 6 doses for those patients who refuse yogurt.
Dosage Forms
Capsule: 50s, 100s
Granules: 1 g/packet (12 packets/box)
Powder: 12 oz
Tablet, chewable: 50's

lactoflavin see riboflavin on page 410
Lactrase® [OTC] see lactase enzyme on previous page

lactulose (lak' tyoo lose)
Brand Names Cephulac®; Cholac®; Chronulac®; Constilac®; Constulose®; Duphalac®; Enulose®; Evalose®; Hepalac®; Lactulose PSE®
Therapeutic Category Ammonium Detoxicant; Laxative, Miscellaneous
Use Adjunct in the prevention and treatment of portal-systemic encephalopathy; treatment of chronic constipation
Usual Dosage Oral:
Infants: 2.5-10 mL/day divided 3-4 times/day

Children: 40-90 mL/day divided 3-4 times/day

Adults:
Acute episodes of portal systemic encephalopathy: 30-45 mL at 1- to 2-hour intervals until laxative effect observed
Chronic therapy: 30-45 mL/dose 3-4 times/day; titrate dose to produce 2-3 soft stools per day
(Continued)

261

lactulose *(Continued)*

Rectal: 300 mL diluted with 700 mL of water or normal saline, and given via a rectal balloon catheter and retained for 30-60 minutes; may give every 4-6 hours
Dosage Forms Syrup: 10 g/15 mL (15 mL, 30 mL, 237 mL, 473 mL, 946 mL, 1890 mL)

Lactulose PSE® *see* lactulose *on previous page*

ladakamycin *see* azacitidine *on page 40*

Lamictal® *see* lamotrigine *on this page*

Lamisil® Topical *see* terbinafine hydrochloride *on page 447*

lamotrigine (la moe' tri jeen)
Brand Names Lamictal®
Synonyms ltg
Therapeutic Category Anticonvulsant, Miscellaneous
Use Partial/secondary generalized seizures, childhood epilepsy
Usual Dosage
Initial dose: 50-100 mg/day then titrate to daily maintenance dose of 100-400 mg/day in 1-2 divided daily doses
With concomitant valproic acid therapy: Start initial dose at 25 mg/day then titrate to maintenance dose of 50-200 mg/day in 1-2 divided daily doses
Dosage Forms Tablet: 25 mg, 50 mg, 100 mg

Lamprene® *see* clofazimine palmitate *on page 107*

Lanacort® [OTC] *see* hydrocortisone *on page 232*

Lanaphilic® Topical [OTC] *see* urea *on page 480*

Laniazid® *see* isoniazid *on page 252*

lanolin, cetyl alcohol, glycerin, and petrolatum
Brand Names Lubriderm® [OTC]
Therapeutic Category Topical Skin Product
Use Treatment of dry skin
Usual Dosage Topical: Apply to skin as necessary
Dosage Forms Lotion: 480 mL

Lanophyllin-GG® *see* theophylline and guaifenesin *on page 454*

Lanorinal® *see* butalbital compound *on page 63*

Lanoxicaps® *see* digoxin *on page 144*

Lanoxin® *see* digoxin *on page 144*

lansoprazole (lan soe' pra zole)
Brand Names Prevacid®
Therapeutic Category Gastric Acid Secretion Inhibitor
Use Short-term (4-8 weeks) treatment of severe erosive esophagitis (grade 2 or above), diagnosed by endoscopy and short-term treatment of symptomatic gastroesophageal reflux disease (GERD) poorly responsible to customary medical treatment; pathological hypersecretory conditions

Lanvisone® Topical *see* clioquinol and hydrocortisone *on page 106*

Largon® Injection *see* propiomazine hydrochloride *on page 393*

Lariam® *see* mefloquine hydrochloride *on page 284*

Larodopa® *see* levodopa *on page 265*

Lasix® *see* furosemide *on page 203*

Lassar's zinc paste *see* zinc oxide *on page 495*

latamoxef disodium *see* moxalactam disodium *on page 312*

***Latrodectus mactans* antivenin** *see* antivenin, black widow spider (equine) *on page 31*

Lavacol® [OTC] *see* alcohol, ethyl *on page 11*

Lax-Pills® [OTC] *see* phenolphthalein *on page 362*

LazerSporin-C® Otic *see* neomycin, polymyxin b, and hydrocortisone *on page 323*

/-bunolol hydrochloride *see* levobunolol hydrochloride *on next page*

l-carnitine *see* levocarnitine *on page 265*

lcd *see* coal tar *on page 110*

lcr *see* vincristine sulfate *on page 488*

l-deprenyl *see* selegiline hydrochloride *on page 420*

/-dopa *see* levodopa *on page 265*

Ledercillin® VK Oral *see* penicillin v potassium *on page 354*

Lederplex® [OTC] *see* vitamin b complex *on page 490*

Legatrin® [OTC] *see* quinine sulfate *on page 403*

Lente® Iletin® I *see* insulin preparations *on page 245*

Lente® Iletin® II *see* insulin preparations *on page 245*

Lente® Insulin *see* insulin preparations *on page 245*

Lente® L *see* insulin preparations *on page 245*

Lescol® *see* fluvastatin *on page 201*

Lessadale [OTC] *see* zinc oxide paste and cold cream *on page 496*

leucovorin calcium (loo koe vor' in)

Brand Names Wellcovorin® Injection; Wellcovorin® Oral

Synonyms calcium leucovorin; citrovorum factor; folinic acid; 5-formyl tetrahydrofolate

Therapeutic Category Antidote, Methotrexate; Folic Acid Derivative

Use Antidote for folic acid antagonists, prevention of hematopoietic effects of folic acid antagonists, treatment of megaloblastic anemias when folate is deficient as in infancy, sprue, pregnancy, and nutritional deficiency when oral folate therapy is not possible and I.V. folic acid cannot be used; in combination with fluorouracil in the treatment of malignancy

Usual Dosage Children and Adults:

Adjunctive therapy with antimicrobial agents (pyrimethamine): Oral: 2-15 mg/day for 3 days or until blood counts are normal or 5 mg every 3 days; doses of 6 mg/day are needed for patients with platelet counts <100,000/mm^3

Folate deficient megaloblastic anemia: I.M.: 1 mg/day

Megaloblastic anemia secondary to congenital deficiency of dihydrofolate reductase: I.M.: 3-6 mg/day

Rescue dose: I.V.: 10 mg/m^2 to start, then 10 mg/m^2 every 6 hours orally for 72 hours; if serum creatinine 24 hours after methotrexate is elevated 50% or more **or** the serum MTX concentration is >5 x 10^{-6}M, increase dose to 100 mg/m^2/dose every 3 hours until serum methotrexate level is less than 1 x 10^{-8}M

Dosage Forms
Injection: 3 mg/mL (1 mL)
Powder for injection: 25 mg, 50 mg, 100 mg, 350 mg
Powder for oral solution: 1 mg/mL (60 mL)
Tablet: 5 mg, 10 mg, 15 mg, 25 mg

Leukeran® *see* chlorambucil *on page 88*

Leukine™ *see* sargramostim *on page 418*

leuprolide acetate (loo proe' lide)
Brand Names Lupron™ Injection
Synonyms leuprorelin acetate
Therapeutic Category Antineoplastic Agent, Hormone (Gonadotropin Hormone-Releasing Antigen); Gonadotropin Releasing Hormone Analog
Use Palliative treatment of advanced prostate carcinoma, precocious puberty, endometriosis
Usual Dosage
  Children: S.C.: Precocious puberty: 20-45 mcg/kg/day

  Adults: Advanced prostatic carcinoma:
    S.C.: 1 mg/day **or**
    I.M. (suspension): 7.5 mg/dose given monthly

  Endometriosis: ≥18 years: I.M.: 3.75 mg/month for 6 months
Dosage Forms
  Injection: 5 mg/mL (2.8 mL)
  Powder for injection (depot):
    Depot™: 3.75 mg, 7.5 mg
    Depot-Ped™: 7.5 mg, 11.25 mg, 15 mg

leuprorelin acetate *see* leuprolide acetate *on this page*

leurocristine *see* vincristine sulfate *on page 488*

Leustatin™ *see* cladribine *on page 103*

levamisole hydrochloride (lee vam' i sole)
Brand Names Ergamisol™
Therapeutic Category Immune Modulator
Use Adjuvant treatment with fluorouracil in Dukes stage C colon cancer
Usual Dosage Oral: Initial: 50 mg every 8 hours for 3 days, then 50 mg every 8 hours for 3 days every 2 weeks (fluorouracil is always given concomitantly)
Dosage Forms Tablet, as base: 50 mg

levarterenol bitartrate *see* norepinephrine bitartrate *on page 331*

Levatol® *see* penbutolol sulfate *on page 352*

Levlen® *see* ethinyl estradiol and levonorgestrel *on page 178*

levobunolol hydrochloride (lee voe byoo' noe lole)
Brand Names AKBeta™ Ophthalmic; Betagan™ Liquifilm® Ophthalmic
Synonyms *l*-bunolol hydrochloride
Therapeutic Category Beta-Adrenergic Blocker, Ophthalmic
Use Lower intraocular pressure in chronic open-angle glaucoma or ocular hypertension
Usual Dosage Adults: 1-2 drops of 0.5% solution in eye(s) once daily or 1-2 drops of 0.25% solution twice daily
Dosage Forms Solution: 0.25% [2.5 mg/mL] (2 mL, 5 mL, 10 mL, 15 mL); 0.5% [5 mg/mL] (2 mL, 5 mL, 10 mL, 15 mL)

levocabastine hydrochloride (lee' voe kab as teen)
Brand Names Livostin™ Ophthalmic
Therapeutic Category Ophthalmic Agent, Miscellaneous
Use Temporary relief of the signs and symptoms of seasonal allergic conjunctivitis
Usual Dosage Adults: Ophthalmic: Instill one drop in affected eye 4 times daily for up to 2 weeks
Dosage Forms Suspension, ophthalmic: 0.05% (2.5 mL, 5 mL, 10 mL)

levocarnitine (lee voe kar' ni teen)
Brand Names Carnitor® Injection; Carnitor® Oral; Vitacarn® Oral
Synonyms l-carnitine
Therapeutic Category Dietary Supplement
Use Therapy in patients with primary systemic carnitine deficiency
Usual Dosage Oral:
Children: 50-100 mg/kg/day divided 2-3 times/day, maximum: 3 g/day; dosage must be individualized based upon patient response; higher dosages have been used

Adults: 1-3 g/day for 50 kg subject; start at 1 g/day, increase slowly assessing tolerance and response
Dosage Forms
Capsule: 250 mg
Injection: 1 g/5 mL (5 mL)
Liquid (cherry flavor): 100 mg/mL (10 mL)
Tablet: 330 mg

levodopa (lee voe doe' pa)
Brand Names Dopar®; Larodopa®
Synonyms L-3-hydroxytyrosine; l-dopa
Therapeutic Category Anti-Parkinson's Agent
Use Treatment of Parkinson's disease; used as a diagnostic agent for growth hormone deficiency
Usual Dosage Children: Oral (given as a single dose to evaluate growth hormone deficiency): 0.5 g/m^2
or
<30 lbs: 125 mg
30-70 lbs: 250 mg
>70 lbs: 500 mg
Dosage Forms
Capsule: 100 mg, 250 mg, 500 mg
Tablet: 100 mg, 250 mg, 500 mg

levodopa and carbidopa
Brand Names Sinemet®
Synonyms carbidopa and levodopa
Therapeutic Category Anti-Parkinson's Agent
Use Treatment of Parkinsonian syndrome
Usual Dosage Adults: Oral (carbidopa/levodopa): 75/300 to 150/1500 mg/day in 3-4 divided doses; can increase up to 200/2000 mg/day
Dosage Forms Tablet:
10/100: Carbidopa 10 mg and levodopa 100 mg
25/100: Carbidopa 25 mg and levodopa 100 mg
25/250: Carbidopa 25 mg and levodopa 250 mg
Sustained release: Carbidopa 25 mg and levodopa 100 mg; carbidopa 50 mg and levodopa 200 mg

Levo-Dromoran® *see* levorphanol tartrate *on next page*

levomepromazine *see* methotrimeprazine hydrochloride *on page 296*

levomethadyl acetate hydrochloride (lee voe meth' a dil)
Brand Names ORLAAM®
Therapeutic Category Analgesic, Narcotic
Use Management of opiate dependence
Usual Dosage Adults: Oral: 20-40 mg 3 times/week; range: 10 mg to as high as 140 mg 3 times/week
Dosage Forms Solution, oral: 10 mg/mL (474 mL)

levonorgestrel (lee' voe nor jess trel)
Brand Names Norplant® Implant
Therapeutic Category Contraceptive, Implant; Contraceptive, Progestin Only; Progestin
Use Prevention of pregnancy
Usual Dosage Each Norplant® silastic capsule releases 80 mcg of drug/day for 6-18 months, following which a rate of release of 25-30 mcg/day is maintained for ≤5 years.
Dosage Forms Capsule, subdermal implantation: 36 mg (6s)

levonorgestrel and ethinyl estradiol *see* ethinyl estradiol and levonorgestrel *on page 178*

Levophed® Injection *see* norepinephrine bitartrate *on page 331*

Levoprome® *see* methotrimeprazine hydrochloride *on page 296*

levorphanol tartrate (lee vor' fa nole)
Brand Names Levo-Dromoran®
Synonyms levorphan tartrate
Therapeutic Category Analgesic, Narcotic
Use Relief of moderate to severe pain; also used parenterally for preoperative sedation and an adjunct to nitrous oxide/oxygen anesthesia
Usual Dosage Adults: Oral, S.C.: 2 mg, up to 3 mg if necessary
Dosage Forms
Injection: 2 mg/mL (1 mL, 10 mL)
Tablet: 2 mg

levorphan tartrate *see* levorphanol tartrate *on this page*

Levo-T™ *see* levothyroxine sodium *on this page*

Levothroid® *see* levothyroxine sodium *on this page*

levothyroxine sodium (lee voe thye rox' een)
Formerly Known As Levoxine®
Brand Names Eltroxin®; Levo-T™; Levothroid®; Levoxyl™; Synthroid®
Synonyms L-thyroxine sodium; t₄ thyroxine sodium
Therapeutic Category Thyroid Product
Use Replacement or supplemental therapy in hypothyroidism, myxedema, coma or stupor
Usual Dosage
Children:
Oral:
0-6 months: 8-10 mcg/kg/day
6-12 months: 6-8 mcg/kg/day
1-5 years: 5-6 mcg/kg/day
6-12 years: 4-5 mcg/kg/day
>12 years: 2-3 mcg/kg/day
I.M., I.V.: 75% of the oral dose

Adults:
Oral: 12.5-50 mcg/day to start, then increase by 25-50 mcg/day at intervals of 2-4 weeks; average adult dose: 100-200 mcg/day
I.M., I.V.: 50% of the oral dose

Myxedema coma or stupor: I.V.: 200-500 mcg one time, then 100-300 mcg the next day if necessary
Dosage Forms
Powder for injection, lyophilized: 0.2 mg/vial (6 mL, 10 mL); 0.5 mg/vial (6 mL, 10 mL)
Tablet: 0.025 mg, 0.05 mg, 0.075 mg, 0.088 mg, 0.1 mg, 0.112 mg, 0.125 mg, 0.15 mg, 0.175 mg, 0.2 mg, 0.3 mg

Levoxine® *see* levothyroxine sodium *on this page*

Levoxyl™ *see* levothyroxine sodium *on previous page*

Levsin® *see* hyoscyamine sulfate *on page 239*

Levsinex® *see* hyoscyamine sulfate *on page 239*

Levsin/SL® *see* hyoscyamine sulfate *on page 239*

***l*-hyoscyamine sulfate** *see* hyoscyamine sulfate *on page 239*

Librax® *see* clidinium and chlordiazepoxide *on page 105*

Libritabs® *see* chlordiazepoxide *on page 89*

Librium® *see* chlordiazepoxide *on page 89*

Lice-Enz® [OTC] *see* pyrethrins *on page 400*

Lida-Mantle HC® Topical *see* lidocaine and hydrocortisone *on this page*

Lidex-E® Topical *see* fluocinonide *on page 195*

Lidex® Topical *see* fluocinonide *on page 195*

lidocaine and epinephrine

Brand Names Octocaine® Injection; Xylocaine® With Epinephrine
Therapeutic Category Local Anesthetic, Injectable
Use Local infiltration anesthesia
Usual Dosage Children (dosage varies with the anesthetic procedure): Use lidocaine concentrations of 0.5% or 1% (or even more dilute) to decrease possibility of toxicity; lidocaine dose should not exceed 4.5 mg/kg/dose; do not repeat within 2 hours
Dosage Forms Injection with epinephrine:
   1:200,000: Lidocaine hydrochloride 0.5% [5 mg/mL] (50 mL); 1% [10 mg/mL] (30 mL); 1.5% [15 mg/mL] (5 mL, 10 mL, 30 mL); 2% [20 mg/mL] (20 mL)
   1:100,000: Lidocaine hydrochloride 1% [10 mg/mL] (20 mL, 50 mL); 2% [20 mg/mL] (1.8 mL, 20 mL, 50 mL)
   1:50,000: Lidocaine hydrochloride 2% [20 mg/mL] (1.8 mL)

lidocaine and hydrocortisone

Brand Names Lida-Mantle HC® Topical
Therapeutic Category Corticosteroid, Topical (Low Potency); Local Anesthetic, Topical
Use Topical anti-inflammatory and anesthetic for skin disorders
Usual Dosage Topical: Apply 2-4 times/day
Dosage Forms Cream: Lidocaine 3% and hydrocortisone 0.5% (15 g, 30 g)

lidocaine and prilocaine

Brand Names EMLA® Topical
Therapeutic Category Analgesic, Topical; Antipruritic, Topical; Local Anesthetic, Topical
Use Topical anesthetic for use on normal intact skin to provide local analgesia for minor procedures such as I.V. cannulation or venipuncture; has also been used for painful procedures such as lumbar puncture and skin graft harvesting
Usual Dosage Children and Adults: Topical: Apply a thick layer of cream to intact skin and cover with an occlusive dressing; for minor procedures, apply 2.5 g/site for at least 60 minutes; for painful procedures, apply 2 g/10 cm^2 of skin and leave on for at least 2 hours
Dosage Forms Cream: Lidocaine 2.5% and prilocaine 2.5% [2 Tegaderm™ dressings] (5 g, 30 g)

lidocaine hydrochloride (lye' doe kane)

Brand Names Anestacon®; Dermaflex® Gel; Dilocaine®; Dr Scholl's® Cracked Heel Relief Cream [OTC]; Duo-Trach®; LidoPen®; Nervocaine®; Octocaine®; Xylocaine®; Zilactin-L® [OTC]
Synonyms lignocaine hydrochloride
Therapeutic Category Antiarrhythmic Agent, Class Ib; Local Anesthetic, Injectable; Local Anesthetic, Topical
(Continued)

lidocaine hydrochloride (Continued)

Use Local anesthetic and acute treatment of ventricular arrhythmias from myocardial infarction, cardiac manipulation, digitalis intoxication

Usual Dosage

Topical: Apply to affected area as needed; maximum: 3 mg/kg/dose; do not repeat within 2 hours

Injectable local anesthetic: Varies with procedure, degree of anesthesia needed, vascularity of tissue, duration of anesthesia required, and physical condition of patient; maximum: 4.5 mg/kg/dose; do not repeat within 2 hours

Children: Endotracheal, I.O., I.V.: Loading dose: 1 mg/kg; may repeat in 10-15 minutes to a maximum total dose of 5 mg/kg; after loading dose, start I.V. continuous infusion 20-50 mcg/kg/minute. Use 20 mcg/kg/minute in patients with shock, hepatic disease, mild congestive heart failure (CHF); moderate to severe CHF may require $\frac{1}{2}$ loading dose and lower infusion rates to avoid toxicity. Endotracheal doses should be diluted to 1-2 mL with normal saline prior to endotracheal administration and may need 2-3 times the I.V. dose.

Adults: Antiarrhythmic:

Endotracheal: Total dose: 5 mg/kg; follow with 0.5 mg/kg in 10 minutes if effective

I.M.: 300 mg may be repeated in 1-1$\frac{1}{2}$ hours

I.V.: Loading dose: 1 mg/kg/dose, then 50-100 mg bolus over 2-3 minutes; may repeat in 5-10 minutes up to 200-300 mg in a 1-hour period; continuous infusion of 20-50 mcg/kg/minute or 1-4 mg/minute; decrease the dose in patients with CHF, shock, or hepatic disease

Dosage Forms

Cream: 2% (56 g)

Gel, topical: 2% (30 mL); 2.5% (15 mL)

Injection: 0.5% [5 mg/mL] (50 mL); 1% [10 mg/mL] (2 mL, 5 mL, 10 mL, 20 mL, 30 mL, 50 mL); 1.5% [15 mg/mL] (20 mL); 2% [20 mg/mL] (2 mL, 5 mL, 10 mL, 20 mL, 30 mL, 50 mL); 4% [40 mg/mL] (5 mL); 10% [100 mg/mL] (10 mL); 20% [200 mg/mL] (10 mL, 20 mL)

Injection:

I.M. use: 10% [100 mg/mL] (3 mL, 5 mL)

Direct I.V.: 1% [10 mg/mL] (5 mL, 10 mL); 20 mg/mL (5 mL)

I.V. admixture, preservative free: 4% [40 mg/mL] (25 mL, 30 mL); 10% [100 mg/mL] (10 mL); 20% [200 mg/mL] (5 mL, 10 mL)

I.V. infusion, in D$_5$W: 0.2% [2 mg/mL] (500 mL); 0.4% [4 mg/mL] (250 mL, 500 mL, 1000 mL); 0.8% [8 mg/mL] (250 mL, 500 mL)

Liquid, topical: 2.5% (7.5 mL)

Liquid, viscous: 2% (20 mL, 100 mL)

Ointment, topical: 2.5% [OTC]; 5% (35 g)

Solution, topical: 2% (15 mL, 240 mL); 4% (50 mL)

LidoPen® see lidocaine hydrochloride on previous page

Lidox® see clidinium and chlordiazepoxide on page 105

lignocaine hydrochloride see lidocaine hydrochloride on previous page

Limbitrol® see amitriptyline and chlordiazepoxide on page 21

Lincocin® Injection see lincomycin hydrochloride on this page

Lincocin® Oral see lincomycin hydrochloride on this page

lincomycin hydrochloride (lin koe mye' sin)

Brand Names Lincocin® Injection; Lincocin® Oral; Lincorex® Injection

Therapeutic Category Antibiotic, Macrolide

Use Treatment of susceptible bacterial infections, mainly those caused by streptococci and staphylococci

Usual Dosage

Children >1 month:

Oral: 30-60 mg/kg/day in 3-4 divided doses

I.M.: 10 mg/kg every 12-24 hours

I.V.: 10-20 mg/kg/day in divided doses 2-3 times/day
Adults:
Oral: 500 mg every 6-8 hours
I.M.: 600 mg every 12-24 hours
I.V.: 600-1 g every 8-12 hours up to 8 g/day
Dosage Forms
Capsule: 250 mg, 500 mg
Injection: 300 mg/mL (2 mL, 10 mL)

Lincorex® Injection *see* lincomycin hydrochloride *on previous page*

lindane (lin' dane)
Brand Names G-well® Lotion; G-well® Shampoo; Kwell® Cream; Kwell® Lotion; Kwell® Shampoo; Scabene® Lotion; Scabene® Shampoo
Synonyms benzene hexachloride; gamma benzene hexachloride; hexachlorocyclohexane
Therapeutic Category Antiparasitic Agent, Topical; Pediculocide; Scabicidal Agent; Shampoos
Use Treatment of scabies (*Sarcoptes scabiei*) and pediculosis (*Pediculus capitis* – head lice, *Pediculus pubis* – crab lice)
Usual Dosage Children and Adults: Topical:
Scabies: Apply a thin layer of lotion and massage it on skin from the neck to the toes. For adults, bathe and remove the drug after 8-12 hours; for children, wash off 6 hours after application.

Pediculosis: 15-30 mL of shampoo is applied and lathered for 4-5 minutes; rinse hair thoroughly and comb with a fine tooth comb to remove nits; repeat treatment in 7 days if lice or nits are still present
Dosage Forms
Cream: 1% (60 g, 454 g)
Lotion: 1% (60 mL, 473 mL, 4000 mL)
Shampoo: 1% (60 mL, 473 mL, 4000 mL)

Lioresal® *see* baclofen *on page 44*

liothyronine sodium (lye oh thye' roe neen)
Brand Names Cytomel® Oral; Triostat™ Injection
Synonyms sodium *l*-tri-iodothyronine; t$_3$ thyronine sodium
Therapeutic Category Thyroid Product
Use Replacement or supplemental therapy in hypothyroidism, management of nontoxic goiter, chronic lymphocytic thyroiditis, as an adjunct in thyrotoxicosis and as a diagnostic aid
Usual Dosage
Mild hypothyroidism: 25 mcg/day; daily dosage may then be increased by 12.5 or 25 mcg/day every 1 or 2 weeks; maintenance: 25-75 mcg/day

Myxedema: 5mcg/day; may be increased by 5-10 mcg/day every 1-2 weeks; when 25 mcg is reached, dosage may often be increased by 12.5 or 25 mcg every 1 or 2 weeks; maintenance: 50-100 mcg/day

Cretinism: 5 mcg/day with a 5 mcg increment every 3-4 days until the desired response is achieved

Simple (nontoxic) goiter: 5 mcg/day; may be increased every week or two by 5 or 10 mcg; when 25 mcg/day is reached, dosage may be increased every week or two by 12.5 or 25 mcg; maintenance: 75 mcg/day

T$_3$ Suppression Test: I^{131} thyroid uptake is in the borderline-high range, administer 75-100 mcg/day for 7 days then repeat I^{131} thyroid uptake test

In the elderly or children: Start therapy with 5 mcg/day; increase only by 5 mcg increments at the recommended intervals
Dosage Forms
Injection: 10 mcg/mL (1 mL)
Tablet: 5 mcg, 25 mcg, 50 mcg

liotrix (lye' oh trix)
Brand Names Thyrolar®
Synonyms t_3/t_4 liotrix
Therapeutic Category Thyroid Hormone
Use Replacement or supplemental therapy in hypothyroidism
Usual Dosage
  Congenital hypothyroidism: Oral:
    Children (dose/day):
      0-6 months: 8-10 mcg/kg
      6-12 months: 6-8 mcg/kg
      1-5 years: 5-6 mcg/kg
      6-12 years: 4-5 mcg/kg
      >12 years: 2-3 mcg/kg
    Adults: 30 mg/day, increasing by 15 mg/day at 2- to 3-week intervals to a maximum of 180 mg/day
Dosage Forms Tablet: 30 mg, 60 mg, 120 mg, 180 mg [thyroid equivalent]

lipancreatin see pancrelipase on page 346

Lipidil® see fenofibrate on page 187

Liposyn® see fat emulsion on page 185

Lipovite® [OTC] see vitamin b complex on page 490

Liquaemin® see heparin on page 222

Liquibid® see guaifenesin on page 213

Liqui-Char® [OTC] see charcoal on page 86

liquid antidote see charcoal on page 86

Liquid Barosperse® see radiological/contrast media (ionic) on page 404

Liquid Pred® Oral see prednisone on page 384

Liqui-E® see tocophersolan on page 463

Liquipake® see radiological/contrast media (ionic) on page 404

Liquiprin® [OTC] see acetaminophen on page 2

lisinopril (lyse in' oh pril)
Brand Names Prinivil®; Zestril®
Therapeutic Category Angiotensin-Converting Enzyme (ACE) Inhibitors
Use Treatment of hypertension, either alone or in combination with other antihypertensive agents
Usual Dosage Adults: Oral: 10-40 mg/day in a single dose
Dosage Forms Tablet: 5 mg, 10 mg, 20 mg, 40 mg

lisinopril and hydrochlorothiazide
Brand Names Prinzide®; Zestoretic®
Therapeutic Category Antihypertensive
Dosage Forms Tablet:
  [12.5]-Lisinopril 20 mg and hydrochlorothiazide 12.5 mg
  [25]-lisinopril 20 mg and hydrochlorothiazide 25 mg

Listermint® with Fluoride [OTC] see fluoride on page 196

Lithane® see lithium on this page

lithium (lith' ee um)
Brand Names Eskalith®; Lithane®; Lithonate®; Lithotabs®
Therapeutic Category Antimanic Agent
Use Management of acute manic episodes, bipolar disorders, and depression

Usual Dosage Oral: Monitor serum concentrations and clinical response (efficacy and toxicity) to determine proper dose

Children: 15-60 mg/kg/day in 3-4 divided doses; dose not to exceed usual adult dosage
Adults: 300 mg 3-4 times/day; usual maximum maintenance dose: 2.4 g/day
Dosage Forms
Capsule, as carbonate: 150 mg, 300 mg, 600 mg
Syrup, as citrate: 300 mg/5 mL (5 mL, 10 mL, 480 mL)
Tablet, as carbonate: 300 mg
Tablet:
Controlled release, as carbonate: 450 mg
Slow release, as carbonate: 300 mg

Lithonate® *see* lithium *on previous page*
Lithostat® *see* acetohydroxamic acid *on page 6*
Lithotabs® *see* lithium *on previous page*
Livostin® Ophthalmic *see* levocabastine hydrochloride *on page 264*
LKV-Drops® [OTC] *see* vitamin, multiple (pediatric) *on page 491*

l-lysine hydrochloride
Brand Names Enisyl® [OTC]; Lycolan® Elixir [OTC]
Therapeutic Category Dietary Supplement
Use Improves utilization of vegetable proteins
Usual Dosage Adults: Oral: 334-1500 mg/day
Dosage Forms
Capsule: 500 mg
Elixir: 100 mg/15 mL with glycine 1800 mg/15 mL and alcohol 12%
Tablet: 312 mg, 334 mg, 500 mg, 1000 mg

8-*L*-lysine vasopressin *see* lypressin *on page 275*
LMD® *see* dextran *on page 133*
Lobac® *see* chlorzoxazone *on page 99*
Locoid® *see* hydrocortisone *on page 232*
Lodine® *see* etodolac *on page 182*
Lodosyn® *see* carbidopa *on page 74*

Iodoxamide tromethamine (loe dox' a mide)
Brand Names Alomide® Ophthalmic
Therapeutic Category Ophthalmic Agent, Miscellaneous
Use Symptomatic treatment of vernal keratoconjunctivitis, vernal conjunctivitis, and vernal keratitis
Usual Dosage Children >2 years and Adults: 1-2 drops in eye(s) 4 times daily for up to 3 months
Dosage Forms Solution, ophthalmic: 0.1% (10 mL)

Loestrin® *see* ethinyl estradiol and norethindrone *on page 178*
Lofene® *see* diphenoxylate and atropine *on page 149*
Logen® *see* diphenoxylate and atropine *on page 149*
Lomanate® *see* diphenoxylate and atropine *on page 149*

lomefloxacin hydrochloride (loe me flox' a sin)
Brand Names Maxaquin® Oral
Therapeutic Category Antibiotic, Quinolone
Use Quinolone antibiotic for skin and skin structure, lower respiratory and urinary tract infections, and sexually transmitted diseases
(Continued)

271

lomefloxacin hydrochloride (Continued)
Usual Dosage Oral: Adults: 400 mg once daily for 10-14 days
Dosage Forms Tablet: 400 mg

Lomodix® *see* diphenoxylate and atropine *on page 149*

Lomotil® *see* diphenoxylate and atropine *on page 149*

lomustine (loe mus' teen)
Brand Names CeeNU™ Oral
Synonyms ccnu
Therapeutic Category Antineoplastic Agent, Alkylating Agent (Nitrosourea)
Use Treatment of brain tumors, Hodgkin's and non-Hodgkin's lymphomas
Usual Dosage Refer to individual protocol. Oral:
  Children: 75-150 mg/m^2 as a single dose every 6 weeks. Subsequent doses are readjusted after initial treatment according to platelet and leukocyte counts

  Adults: 100-130 mg/m^2 as a single dose every 6 weeks; readjust after initial treatment according to platelet and leukocyte counts
Dosage Forms
  Capsule: 10 mg, 40 mg, 100 mg
  Dose Pack: 10 mg (2s); 100 mg (2s); 40 mg (2s)

Loniten® *see* minoxidil *on page 308*

Lonox® *see* diphenoxylate and atropine *on page 149*

Lo/Ovral® *see* ethinyl estradiol and norgestrel *on page 180*

loperamide hydrochloride (loe per' a mide)
Brand Names Diar-aid™ [OTC]; Imodium®; Imodium® A-D [OTC]; Kaopectate® II [OTC]; Pepto™ Diarrhea Control [OTC]
Therapeutic Category Antidiarrheal
Use Treatment of acute diarrhea and chronic diarrhea associated with inflammatory bowel disease; to decrease the volume of ileostomy discharge
Usual Dosage Oral:
  Children:
    Acute diarrhea: 0.4-0.8 mg/kg/day divided every 6-12 hours, maximum: 2 mg/dose
    Chronic diarrhea: 0.08-0.24 mg/kg/day divided 2-3 times/day, maximum: 2 mg/dose

  Adults: 4 mg (2 capsules) initially, followed by 2 mg after each loose stool, up to 16 mg/day (8 capsules)
Dosage Forms
  Caplet: 2 mg
  Capsule: 2 mg
  Liquid, oral: 1 mg/5 mL (60 mL, 90 mL, 120 mL)
  Tablet: 2 mg

Lopid® *see* gemfibrozil *on page 206*

lopremone *see* protirelin *on page 396*

Lopressor® *see* metoprolol *on page 303*

Loprox® *see* ciclopirox olamine *on page 101*

Lopurin® *see* allopurinol *on page 13*

Lorabid™ *see* loracarbef *on this page*

loracarbef (loe ra kar' bef)
Brand Names Lorabid™
Therapeutic Category Antibiotic, Carbacephem
Use Infections caused by susceptible organisms involving the respiratory tract, otitis media, sinusitis, skin and skin structure, bone and joint, and urinary tract and gynecologic as well as septicemia

Usual Dosage Oral:
  Acute otitis media: Children: 15 mg/kg twice a day for 10 days
  Urinary tract infections: Women: 200 mg once a day for 7 days
Dosage Forms
  Capsule: 200 mg
  Suspension, oral: 100 mg/5 mL (50 mL, 100 mL); 200 mg/5 mL (50 mL, 100 mL)

loratadine (lor at' a deen)
Brand Names Claritin®
Therapeutic Category Antihistamine
Use Perennial and seasonal allergic rhinitis and other allergic symptoms including urticaria
Usual Dosage Adults: Oral: 10 mg daily on an empty stomach
Dosage Forms Tablet: 10 mg

lorazepam (lor a' ze pam)
Brand Names Ativan®
Therapeutic Category Antianxiety Agent; Benzodiazepine; Hypnotic; Sedative
Use Management of anxiety, status epilepticus, preoperative sedation, and amnesia
Usual Dosage
  Anxiety and sedation:
    Infants and Children: Oral, I.V.: Usual: 0.05 mg/kg/dose (range: 0.02-0.09 mg/kg) every 4-8 hours
    Adults: Oral: 1-10 mg/day in 2-3 divided doses; usual dose: 2-6 mg/day in divided doses
  Insomnia: Adults: Oral: 2-4 mg at bedtime
  Preoperative: Adults:
    I.M.: 0.05 mg/kg administered 2 hours before surgery; maximum: 4 mg/dose
    I.V.: 0.044 mg/kg 15-20 minutes before surgery; usual maximum: 2 mg/dose
  Operative amnesia: Adults: I.V.: up to 0.05 mg/kg; maximum: 4 mg/dose
  Status epilepticus: I.V.:
    Neonates: 0.05 mg/kg over 2-5 minutes; may repeat in 10-15 minutes (see warning regarding benzyl alcohol)
    Infants and Children: 0.1 mg/kg slow I.V. over 2-5 minutes, do not exceed 4 mg/single dose; may repeat second dose of 0.05 mg/kg slow I.V. in 10-15 minutes if needed
    Adolescents: 0.07 mg/kg slow I.V. over 2-5 minutes; maximum: 4 mg/dose; may repeat in 10-15 minutes
    Adults: 4 mg/dose given slowly over 2-5 minutes; may repeat in 10-15 minutes; usual maximum dose: 8 mg
Dosage Forms
  Injection: 2 mg/mL (1 mL, 10 mL); 4 mg/mL (1 mL, 10 mL)
  Solution, oral concentrated, alcohol and dye free: 2 mg/mL (30 mL)
  Tablet: 0.5 mg, 1 mg, 2 mg

Lorcet® *see* hydrocodone and acetaminophen *on page 230*

Lorcet® 10/650 *see* hydrocodone and acetaminophen *on page 230*

Lorcet®-HD *see* hydrocodone and acetaminophen *on page 230*

Lorcet® Plus *see* hydrocodone and acetaminophen *on page 230*

Lorelco® *see* probucol *on page 387*

Loroxide® [OTC] *see* benzoyl peroxide *on page 50*

Lortab® ASA *see* hydrocodone and aspirin *on page 230*

losartan potassium (lo sar' tan)
Brand Names Cozaar®
Therapeutic Category Antihypertensive
Use Antihypertensive

Losec® *see* omeprazole *on page 336*

Lotensin® *see* benazepril hydrochloride *on page 47*

Lotrimin® *see* clotrimazole *on page 109*

Lotrimin AF® Cream [OTC] *see* clotrimazole *on page 109*

Lotrimin AF® Lotion [OTC] *see* clotrimazole *on page 109*

Lotrimin AF® Solution [OTC] *see* clotrimazole *on page 109*

Lotrimin AF® Powder [OTC] *see* miconazole *on page 305*

Lotrimin AF® Spray Liquid [OTC] *see* miconazole *on page 305*

Lotrimin AF® Spray Powder [OTC] *see* miconazole *on page 305*

Lotrisone® *see* betamethasone dipropionate and clotrimazole *on page 53*

lovastatin (loe' va sta tin)
Brand Names Mevacor®
Synonyms mevinolin; monacolin k
Therapeutic Category Antilipemic Agent; HMG-CoA Reductase Inhibitor
Use Adjunct to dietary therapy to decrease elevated serum total and LDL cholesterol concentrations in primary hypercholesterolemia
Usual Dosage Adults: Oral: Initial: 20 mg with evening meal, then adjust at 4-week intervals; maximum dose: 80 mg/day
Dosage Forms Tablet: 10 mg, 20 mg, 40 mg

Lovenox® Injection *see* enoxaparin sodium *on page 166*

Low-Quel® *see* diphenoxylate and atropine *on page 149*

loxapine (lox' a peen)
Brand Names Loxitane® I.M. Injection; Loxitane® Oral
Synonyms oxilapine succinate
Therapeutic Category Antipsychotic Agent
Use Management of psychotic disorders
Usual Dosage Adults:
  Oral: 10 mg twice daily, increase dose until psychotic symptoms are controlled; usual dose range: 60-100 mg/day in divided doses 2-4 times/day; dosages >250 mg/day are not recommended
  I.M.: 12.5-50 mg every 4-6 hours or longer as needed and change to oral therapy as soon as possible
Dosage Forms
  Capsule: 5 mg, 10 mg, 25 mg, 50 mg
  Concentrate, oral: 25 mg/mL (120 mL dropper bottle)
  Injection: 50 mg/mL (1 mL)

Loxitane® I.M. Injection *see* loxapine *on this page*

Loxitane® Oral *see* loxapine *on this page*

Lozol® *see* indapamide *on page 244*

l-pam *see* melphalan *on page 285*

lrh *see* gonadorelin *on page 211*

l-sarcolysin *see* melphalan *on page 285*

ltg *see* lamotrigine *on page 262*

L-thyroxine sodium *see* levothyroxine sodium *on page 266*

Lubriderm® [OTC] *see* lanolin, cetyl alcohol, glycerin, and petrolatum *on page 262*

Ludiomil® *see* maprotiline hydrochloride *on page 280*

Lufyllin® *see* dyphylline *on page 161*

Lugol's solution *see* potassium iodide *on page 379*

Luminal® *see* phenobarbital *on page 361*

Lung Check® *see* diagnostic aids (*in vitro*), other *on page 137*

Lupron® Injection *see* leuprolide acetate *on page 264*

Luride® *see* fluoride *on page 196*

Luride® Lozi-Tab® *see* fluoride *on page 196*

Luride®-SF Lozi-Tab® *see* fluoride *on page 196*

Lutrepulse® Injection *see* gonadorelin *on page 211*

Luvox® *see* fluvoxamine *on page 201*

Lycolan® Elixir [OTC] *see* l-lysine hydrochloride *on page 271*

Lymphazurin® *see* radiological/contrast media (ionic) *on page 404*

lymphocyte immune globulin, antithymocyte globulin (equine)
Brand Names Atgam®
Synonyms atg; horse anti-human thymocyte gamma globulin
Therapeutic Category Immunosuppressant Agent
Use Prevention and treatment of acute renal allograft rejection; treatment of moderate to severe aplastic anemia in patients not considered suitable candidates for bone marrow transplantation; prevention of graft-vs-host disease following bone marrow transplantation
Usual Dosage An intradermal skin test is recommended prior to administration of the initial dose of ATG. Use 0.1 mL of a 1:1000 dilution of ATG in normal saline

Aplastic anemia protocol: I.V.: 10-20 mg/kg/day for 8-14 days, then give every other day for 7 more doses

Rejection prevention: Children and Adults: I.V.: 15 mg/kg/day for 14 days, then give every other day for 7 more doses; initial dose should be administered within 24 hours before or after transplantation

Rejection treatment: Children and Adults: I.V. 10-15 mg/kg/day for 14 days, then give every other day for 7 more doses
Dosage Forms Injection: 50 mg/mL (5 mL)

Lyphocin® Injection *see* vancomycin hydrochloride *on page 483*

lypressin (lye press' in)
Brand Names Diapid® Nasal Spray
Synonyms 8-*L*-lysine vasopressin
Therapeutic Category Antidiuretic Hormone Analog
Use Control or prevent signs and complications of neurogenic diabetes insipidus
Usual Dosage Children and Adults: 1-2 sprays into one or both nostrils 4 times/day; approximately 2 USP posterior pituitary pressor units per spray
Dosage Forms Spray: 0.185 mg/mL (equivalent to 50 USP posterior pituitary units/mL) (8 mL)

Lysodren® *see* mitotane *on page 309*

Maalox Anti-Gas® [OTC] *see* simethicone *on page 423*

Maalox® [OTC] *see* aluminum hydroxide and magnesium hydroxide *on page 16*

Maalox® Therapeutic Concentrate [OTC] *see* aluminum hydroxide and magnesium hydroxide *on page 16*

Maalox® Plus [OTC] *see* aluminum hydroxide, magnesium hydroxide, and simethicone *on page 16*

Maalox® Daily Fiber Therapy [OTC] *see* psyllium *on page 398*

Macrobid® *see* nitrofurantoin *on page 329*

Macrodantin® *see* nitrofurantoin *on page 329*
Macrodex® *see* dextran *on page 133*

mafenide acetate (ma' fe nide)
Brand Names Sulfamylon® Topical
Therapeutic Category Antibacterial, Topical; Antibiotic, Topical
Use Adjunct in the treatment of second and third degree burns to prevent septicemia caused by susceptible organisms
Usual Dosage Children and Adults: Topical: Apply once or twice daily with a sterile gloved hand; apply to a thickness of approximately 16 mm; the burned area should be covered with cream at all times
Dosage Forms Cream, topical: 85 mg/g (60 g, 120 g, 435 g)

magaldrate (mag' al drate)
Brand Names Riopan® [OTC]
Synonyms hydromagnesium aluminate
Therapeutic Category Antacid
Use Symptomatic relief of hyperacidity associated with peptic ulcer, gastritis, peptic esophagitis and hiatal hernia
Usual Dosage Adults: Oral: 540-1080 mg between meals and at bedtime
Dosage Forms Suspension, oral: 540 mg/5 mL (360 mL)

magaldrate and simethicone
Brand Names Riopan Plus® [OTC]
Synonyms simethicone and magaldrate
Therapeutic Category Antacid; Antiflatulent
Use Relief of hyperacidity associated with peptic ulcer, gastritis, peptic esophagitis and hiatal hernia which are accompanied by symptoms of gas
Usual Dosage Adults: Oral: 5-10 mL between meals and at bedtime
Dosage Forms Suspension, oral: Magaldrate 480 mg and simethicone 20 mg per 5 mL (360 mL)

magnesia magma *see* magnesium hydroxide *on next page*

magnesium chloride
Brand Names Slow-Mag® [OTC]
Therapeutic Category Magnesium Salt
Use Correct or prevent hypomagnesemia
Usual Dosage I.V. in TPN:
Children: 2-10 mEq/day; the usual recommended pediatric maintenance intake of magnesium ranges from 0.2-0.6 mEq/kg/day. The dose of magnesium may also be based on the caloric intake; on that basis, 3-10 mEq/day of magnesium are needed; maximum maintenance dose: 8-16 mEq/day

Adults: 8-24 mEq/day
Dosage Forms
Injection: 200 mg/mL [1.97 mEq/mL] (30 mL, 50 mL)
Tablet: Elemental magnesium 64 mg

magnesium citrate
Brand Names Evac-Q-Mag® [OTC]
Synonyms citrate of magnesia
Therapeutic Category Laxative, Saline
Use To evacuate bowel prior to certain surgical and diagnostic procedures

Usual Dosage Cathartic: Oral:

Children:
> <6 years: 2-4 mL/kg given as a single daily dose or in divided doses
> 6-12 years: $\frac{1}{3}$ to $\frac{1}{2}$ bottle

Adults ≥12 years: $\frac{1}{2}$ to 1 full bottle
Dosage Forms Solution, oral: 300 mL

magnesium gluconate

Brand Names Magonate® [OTC]
Therapeutic Category Magnesium Salt
Use Dietary supplement for treatment of magnesium deficiencies
Usual Dosage The recommended dietary allowance (RDA) of magnesium is 4.5 mg/kg which is a total daily allowance of 350-400 mg for adult men and 280-300 mg for adult women. During pregnancy the RDA is 300 mg and during lactation the RDA is 355 mg. Average daily intakes of dietary magnesium have declined in recent years due to processing of food. The latest estimate of the average American dietary intake was 349 mg/day.

Dietary supplement: Oral:
> Children: 3-6 mg/kg/day in divided doses 3-4 times/day; maximum: 400 mg/day
> Adults: 27-54 mg 2-3 times/day or 100 mg 4 times/day

Dosage Forms Tablet: 500 mg [elemental magnesium 27 mg]

magnesium hydroxide

Brand Names Phillips'® Milk of Magnesia [OTC]
Synonyms magnesia magma; milk of magnesia; mom
Therapeutic Category Antacid; Laxative, Saline; Magnesium Salt
Use Short-term treatment of occasional constipation and symptoms of hyperacidity
Usual Dosage Oral:

Laxative:
> <2 years: 0.5 mL/kg/dose
> 2-5 years: 5-15 mL/day or in divided doses
> 6-12 years: 15-30 mL/day or in divided doses
> ≥12 years: 30-60 mL/day or in divided doses

Antacid:
> Children: 2.5-5 mL as needed
> Adults: 5-15 mL as needed

Dosage Forms
> Liquid: 390 mg/5 mL (10 mL, 15 mL, 20 mL, 30 mL, 100 mL, 120 mL, 180 mL, 360 mL, 720 mL)
> Liquid, concentrate: 10 mL equivalent to 30 mL milk of magnesia USP
> Suspension, oral: 2.5 g/30 mL (10 mL, 15 mL, 30 mL)
> Tablet: 300 mg, 600 mg

magnesium hydroxide and aluminum hydroxide *see* aluminum hydroxide and magnesium hydroxide *on page 16*

magnesium hydroxide and mineral oil emulsion

Brand Names Haley's M-O® [OTC]
Synonyms mom/mineral oil emulsion
Therapeutic Category Laxative, Lubricant; Laxative, Saline
Use Short-term treatment of occasional constipation
Dosage Forms Suspension, oral: Equivalent to magnesium hydroxide 24 mL/mineral oil emulsion 6 mL (30 mL unit dose)

magnesium oxide

Brand Names Maox®
Therapeutic Category Antacid
Use Short-term treatment of occasional constipation and symptoms of hyperacidity
(Continued)

277

magnesium oxide *(Continued)*
Usual Dosage Oral:
Antacid: 250 mg to 1.5 g with water or milk 4 times/day after meals and at bedtime
Laxative: 2-4 g at bedtime with full glass of water
Dosage Forms
Capsule: 140 mg
Tablet: 400 mg, 425 mg

magnesium sulfate
Synonyms epsom salts
Therapeutic Category Anticonvulsant, Miscellaneous; Electrolyte Supplement, Parenteral; Laxative, Saline; Magnesium Salt
Use Treatment and prevention of hypomagnesemia and in seizure prevention in severe pre-eclampsia or eclampsia, pediatric acute nephritis; also used as short-term treatment of constipation
Usual Dosage Dose represented as $MgSO_4$ unless stated otherwise
Hypomagnesemia:
Neonates: I.V.: 25-50 mg/kg/dose (0.2-0.4 mEq/kg/dose) every 8-12 hours for 2-3 doses
Children:
I.M., I.V.: 25-50 mg/kg/dose (0.2-0.4 mEq/kg/dose) every 4-6 hours for 3-4 doses, maximum single dose: 2000 mg (16 mEq), may repeat if hypomagnesemia persists (higher dosage up to 100 mg/kg/dose $MgSO_4$ I.V. has been used)
Oral: 100-200 mg/kg/dose 4 times/day
Maintenance: I.V.: 30-60 mg/kg/day (0.25-0.5 mEq/kg/day)
Adults: I.M., I.V.: 1 g every 6 hours for 4 doses or 250 mg/kg over a 4-hour period; for severe hypomagnesemia: 8-12 g $MgSO_4$/day in divided doses has been used; Oral: 3 g every 6 hours for 4 doses as needed

For management of seizures and hypertension: Children: I.M., I.V.: 20-100 mg/kg/dose every 4-6 hours as needed; in severe cases doses as high as 200 mg/kg/dose have been used

Cathartic: Oral:
Children: 0.25 g/kg/dose
Adults: 10-30 g
Dosage Forms
Granules: ~40 mEq magnesium/5 g (240 g)
Injection: 100 mg/mL (20 mL); 125 mg/mL (8 mL); 250 mg/mL (150 mL); 500 mg/mL (2 mL, 5 mL, 10 mL, 30 mL, 50 mL)
Solution, oral: 50% [500 mg/mL] (30 mL)

Magnevist® *see* radiological/contrast media (ionic) *on page 404*
Magonate® [OTC] *see* magnesium gluconate *on previous page*
Maigret-50 *see* phenylpropanolamine hydrochloride *on page 365*
Malatal® *see* hyoscyamine, atropine, scopolamine, and phenobarbital *on page 238*

malathion (mal a thye' on)
Brand Names Ovide™ Topical
Therapeutic Category Pediculocide
Use Treatment of head lice and their ova
Usual Dosage Sprinkle Ovide™ lotion on dry hair and rub gently until the scalp is thoroughly moistened; pay special attention to the back of the head and neck. Allow to dry naturally – use no heat and leave uncovered. After 8-12 hours, the hair should be washed with a non-medicated shampoo; rinse and use a fine-toothed comb to remove dead lice and eggs. If required, repeat with second application in 7-9 days. Further treatment is generally not necessary. Other family members should be evaluated to determine if infested and if so, receive treatment.
Dosage Forms Lotion: 0.5% (59 mL)

Mallamint® **[OTC]** *see* calcium carbonate *on page 66*

Mallazine® Eye Drops [OTC] *see* tetrahydrozoline hydrochloride *on page 452*

Mallergan-VC® With Codeine *see* promethazine, phenylephrine, and codeine *on page 391*

Malotuss® [OTC] *see* guaifenesin *on page 213*

malt soup extract
Brand Names Maltsupex® [OTC]
Therapeutic Category Laxative, Bulk-Producing
Use Short-term treatment of constipation
Usual Dosage Oral:
Infants >1 month:
   Breast fed: 1-2 teaspoonfuls in 2-4 oz of water or fruit juice 1-2 times/day
   Bottle fed: $1/2$ to 2 tablespoonfuls/day in formula for 3-4 days, then 1-2 teaspoonfuls/day
Children 2-11 years: 1-2 tablespoonfuls 1-2 times/day
Adults ≥12 years: 2 tablespoonfuls twice daily for 3-4 days, then 1-2 tablespoonfuls every evening
Dosage Forms
Liquid: Nondiastatic barley malt extract 16 g/15 mL
Powder: Nondiastatic barley malt extract 16 g/heaping tablespoonful
Tablet: Nondiastatic barley malt extract 750 mg

Maltsupex® [OTC] *see* malt soup extract *on this page*

Mandelamine® *see* methenamine *on page 293*

Mandol® *see* cefamandole nafate *on page 79*

mandrake *see* podophyllum resin *on page 374*

manganese *see* trace metals *on page 465*

mannitol (man' i tole)
Brand Names Osmitrol® Injection; Resectisol® Irrigation Solution
Synonyms *d*-mannitol
Therapeutic Category Diuretic, Osmotic
Use Reduction of increased intracranial pressure associated with cerebral edema; promotion of diuresis in the prevention and/or treatment of oliguria or anuria due to acute renal failure; reduction of increased intraocular pressure; promoting urinary excretion of toxic substances
Usual Dosage
Children:
   Test dose (to assess adequate renal function): 200 mg/kg over 3-5 minutes to produce a urine flow of at least 1 mL/kg/hour for 1-3 hours
   Initial: 0.5-1 g/kg
   Maintenance: 0.25-0.5 g/kg/hour given every 4-6 hours
Adults:
   Test dose: 12.5 g (200 mg/kg) over 3-5 minutes to produce a urine flow of at least 30-50 mL of urine per hour over the next 2-3 hours
   Initial: 0.5-1 g/kg
   Maintenance: 0.25-0.5 g/kg every 4-6 hours
Dosage Forms
Injection: 5% [50 mg/mL] (1000 mL); 10% [100 mg/mL] (500 mL, 1000 mL); 15% [150 mg/mL] (150 mL, 500 mL); 20% [200 mg/mL] (150 mL, 250 mL, 500 mL); 25% [250 mg/mL] (50 mL, 500 mL)
Solution, urogenital: 0.54% [5.4 mg/mL] (2000 mL)

Manoplax® *see* flosequinan *on page 193*

Mantoux *see* tuberculin tests *on page 477*

Maolate® *see* chlorphenesin carbamate *on page 93*
Maox® *see* magnesium oxide *on page 277*

maprotiline hydrochloride (ma proe' ti leen)
Brand Names Ludiomil®
Therapeutic Category Antidepressant, Tetracyclic
Use Treatment of depression and anxiety associated with depression
Usual Dosage Oral:
  Children 6-14 years: 10 mg/day, increase to a maximum daily dose of 75 mg

  Adults: 75 mg/day to start, increase by 25 mg every 2 weeks up to 150-225 mg/day; given in 3 divided doses or in a single daily dose
Dosage Forms Tablet: 25 mg, 50 mg, 75 mg

Marax® *see* theophylline, ephedrine, and hydroxyzine *on page 454*
Marazide® *see* benzthiazide *on page 50*
Marbaxin® *see* methocarbamol *on page 295*
Marcaine® *see* bupivacaine hydrochloride *on page 61*
Marcillin® *see* ampicillin *on page 26*
Marezine® [OTC] *see* cyclizine *on page 120*
Margesic® *see* butalbital compound *on page 63*
Margesic® H *see* hydrocodone and acetaminophen *on page 230*
Margesic® No. 3 *see* acetaminophen and codeine *on page 3*
Marinol® *see* dronabinol *on page 159*
Marmine® Injection *see* dimenhydrinate *on page 147*
Marmine® Oral [OTC] *see* dimenhydrinate *on page 147*
Marnal® *see* butalbital compound *on page 63*
Marpres® *see* hydralazine, hydrochlorothiazide, and reserpine *on page 228*
Marthritic® *see* salsalate *on page 417*

masoprocol (may so pro' kol)
Brand Names Actinex®
Therapeutic Category Topical Skin Product; Topical Skin Product, Acne
Use Treatment of actinic keratosis
Dosage Forms Cream: 10% (30 g)

Massé® Breast Cream [OTC] *see* glycerin, lanolin and peanut oil *on page 210*
Matulane® *see* procarbazine hydrochloride *on page 388*
Maxair™ Inhalation Aerosol *see* pirbuterol acetate *on page 372*
Maxaquin® Oral *see* lomefloxacin hydrochloride *on page 271*
Max-Caro® [OTC] *see* beta-carotene *on page 52*
Maxidex® *see* dexamethasone *on page 131*
Maxiflor® Topical *see* diflorasone diacetate *on page 143*
Maximum Strength Desenex® Antifungal Cream [OTC] *see* miconazole *on page 305*
Maximum Strength Nytol® [OTC] *see* diphenhydramine hydrochloride *on page 149*
Maxitrol® Ophthalmic *see* neomycin, polymyxin b, and dexamethasone *on page 322*
Maxivate® *see* betamethasone *on page 52*

Maxolon® *see metoclopramide on page 302*

Maxzide® *see hydrochlorothiazide and triamterene on page 229*

may apple *see podophyllum resin on page 374*

mch *see microfibrillar collagen hemostat on page 306*

m-cresyl acetate
Brand Names Cresylate®
Therapeutic Category Otic Agent, Anti-infective
Use Provides an acid medium; for external otitis infections caused by susceptible bacteria or fungus
Usual Dosage Otic: Instill 2-4 drops as required
Dosage Forms Solution: 25% with isopropanol 25%, chlorobutanol 1%, benzyl alcohol 1%, and castor oil 5% in propylene glycol (15 mL dropper bottle)

MCT Oil® [OTC] *see medium chain triglycerides on page 283*

MD-Gastroview® *see radiological/contrast media (ionic) on page 404*

measles and rubella vaccines, combined
Brand Names M-R-VAX® II
Synonyms rubella and measles vaccines, combined
Therapeutic Category Vaccine, Live Virus
Use Simultaneous immunization against measles and rubella
Usual Dosage S.C.: Inject into outer aspect of upper arm
Dosage Forms Injection: 1000 $TCID_{50}$ each of live attenuated measles virus vaccine and live rubella virus vaccine

measles, mumps and rubella vaccines, combined
Brand Names M-M-R® II
Synonyms mmr
Therapeutic Category Vaccine, Live Virus
Use Measles, mumps, and rubella prophylaxis
Usual Dosage S.C.: Inject in outer aspect of the upper arm to children ≥15 months of age; each dose contains 1000 $TCID_{50}$ (tissue culture infectious doses) of 5 attenuated measle virus vaccine, 5000 $TCID_{50}$ of live mumps virus vaccine and 1000 $TCID_{50}$ of live rubella virus vaccine
Dosage Forms Injection: 1000 $TCID_{50}$ each of measles virus vaccine and rubella virus vaccine, 5000 $TCID_{50}$ mumps virus vaccine

measles virus vaccine, live, attenuated
Brand Names Attenuvax®
Synonyms more attenuated enders strain; rubeola vaccine
Therapeutic Category Vaccine, Live Virus
Use Immunization against measles (rubeola) in persons ≥15 months of age
Usual Dosage Children >15 months and Adults: S.C.: 0.5 mL in outer aspect of the upper arm
Dosage Forms Injection: 1000 $TCID_{50}$/dose

Measurin® [OTC] *see aspirin on page 35*

Mebaral® *see mephobarbital on page 287*

mebendazole (me ben' da zole)
Brand Names Vermox®
Therapeutic Category Anthelmintic
Use Treatment of pinworms, whipworms, roundworms, and hookworms
(Continued)

281

mebendazole *(Continued)*
Usual Dosage Children and Adults: Oral:
Pinworms: Single chewable tablet; may need to repeat after 2 weeks

Whipworms, roundworms, hookworms: 1 tablet twice daily, morning and evening on 3 consecutive days; if patient is not cured within 3-4 weeks, a second course of treatment may be administered
Dosage Forms Tablet, chewable: 100 mg

mecamylamine hydrochloride (mek a mill' a meen)
Brand Names Inversine®
Therapeutic Category Ganglionic Blocking Agent
Use Treatment of moderately severe to severe hypertension and in uncomplicated malignant hypertension
Usual Dosage Adults: Oral: 2.5 mg twice daily after meals for 2 days; increased by increments of 2.5 mg at intervals of ≥ 2 days until desired blood pressure response is achieved
Dosage Forms Tablet: 2.5 mg

mechlorethamine hydrochloride (me klor eth' a meen)
Brand Names Mustargen® Hydrochloride
Synonyms HN_2; mustine; nitrogen mustard
Therapeutic Category Antineoplastic Agent, Alkylating Agent (Nitrogen Mustard)
Use Combination therapy of Hodgkin's disease, brain tumors, non-Hodgkin's lymphoma and malignant lymphomas; palliative treatment of bronchogenic, breast and ovarian carcinoma; may be used by intracavitary injection for treatment of metastatic tumors, pleural and other malignant effusions
Usual Dosage Refer to individual protocols
Children: MOPP: I.V.: 6 mg/m^2 on days 1 and 8 of a 28-day cycle

Adults:
I.V.: 0.4 mg/kg or 12-16 mg/m^2 for one dose or divided into 0.1 mg/kg/day for 4 days
Intracavitary: 10-20 mg or 0.2-0.4 mg/kg
Dosage Forms Powder for injection: 10 mg

Meclan® Topical *see* meclocycline sulfosalicylate *on this page*

meclizine hydrochloride (mek' li zeen)
Brand Names Antivert®; Antrizine®; Bonine® [OTC]; Dizmiss® [OTC]; Dramamine® II [OTC]; Meni-D®; Nico-Vert® [OTC]; Ru-Vert-M®; Vergon® [OTC]
Synonyms meclozine hydrochloride
Therapeutic Category Antiemetic; Antihistamine
Use Prevention and treatment of motion sickness; management of vertigo with diseases affecting the vestibular system
Usual Dosage Children >12 years and Adults: Oral:
Motion sickness: 25-50 mg 1 hour before travel, repeat dose every 24 hours if needed
Vertigo: 25-100 mg/day in divided doses
Dosage Forms
Capsule: 15 mg, 25 mg, 30 mg
Tablet: 12.5 mg, 25 mg, 50 mg
Tablet:
Chewable: 25 mg
Film coated: 25 mg

meclocycline sulfosalicylate (me kloe sye' kleen)
Brand Names Meclan® Topical
Therapeutic Category Antibiotic, Topical; Topical Skin Product, Acne
Use Topical treatment of inflammatory acne vulgaris

Usual Dosage Apply to affected areas twice daily
Dosage Forms Cream, topical: 1% (20 g, 45 g)

meclofenamate sodium (me kloe fen am' ate)
Brand Names Meclomen® Oral
Therapeutic Category Analgesic, Non-Narcotic; Anti-inflammatory Agent; Nonsteroidal Anti-Inflammatory Agent (NSAID), Oral
Use Treatment of inflammatory disorders
Usual Dosage Adults: Oral: 200-300 mg 3-4 times/day
Dosage Forms Capsule: 50 mg, 100 mg

Meclomen® Oral *see meclofenamate sodium on this page*

meclozine hydrochloride *see meclizine hydrochloride on previous page*

medicinal carbon *see charcoal on page 86*

medicinal charcoal *see charcoal on page 86*

Medigesic® *see butalbital compound on page 63*

Medihaler-Epi® *see epinephrine on page 167*

Medihaler Ergotamine™ *see ergotamine derivatives on page 169*

Medihaler-Iso® *see isoproterenol on page 253*

Medilax® [OTC] *see phenolphthalein on page 362*

Mediplast® Plaster [OTC] *see salicylic acid on page 416*

Medipren® [OTC] *see ibuprofen on page 240*

Medi-Quick® Ointment [OTC] *see bacitracin, neomycin, and polymyxin b on page 43*

Medi-Tuss® AC *see guaifenesin and codeine on page 214*

Medi-Tuss® [OTC] *see guaifenesin on page 213*

medium chain triglycerides
Brand Names MCT Oil® [OTC]
Synonyms triglycerides, medium chain
Therapeutic Category Nutritional Supplement
Use Dietary supplement for those who cannot digest long chain fats
Usual Dosage Oral: 15 mL 3-4 times/day
Dosage Forms Oil: 14 g/15 mL (960 mL)

Medralone® Injection *see methylprednisolone on page 300*

Medrol® Oral *see methylprednisolone on page 300*

medroxyprogesterone acetate (me drox' ee proe jess' te rone)
Brand Names Amen® Oral; Curretab® Oral; Cycrin® Oral; Depo-Provera® Injection; Provera® Oral
Synonyms acetoxymethylprogesterone; methylacetoxyprogesterone
Therapeutic Category Contraceptive, Progestin Only; Progestin
Use Endometrial carcinoma or renal carcinoma as well as secondary amenorrhea or abnormal uterine bleeding due to hormonal imbalance; prevention of pregnancy
Usual Dosage
Adolescents and Adults: Oral:
Amenorrhea: 5-10 mg/day for 5-10 days or 2.5 mg/day
Abnormal uterine bleeding: 5-10 mg for 5-10 days starting on day 16 or 21 of cycle
Accompanying cyclic estrogen therapy, postmenopausal: 2.5-10 mg the last 10-13 days of estrogen dosing each month
(Continued)

medroxyprogesterone acetate *(Continued)*

Adults:

Contraception: Deep I.M.: 150 mg every 3 months or 450 mg every 6 months

Endometrial or renal carcinoma: I.M.: 400-1000 mg/week

Dosing adjustment in hepatic impairment: Dose needs to be lowered in patients with alcoholic cirrhosis

Dosage Forms

Injection, suspension: 100 mg/mL (5 mL); 150 mg/mL (1 mL); 400 mg/mL (1 mL, 2.5 mL, 10 mL)

Tablet: 2.5 mg, 5 mg, 10 mg

medrysone (me' dri sone)

Brand Names HMS Liquifilm® Ophthalmic

Therapeutic Category Anti-inflammatory Agent, Ophthalmic; Corticosteroid, Ophthalmic

Use Treatment of allergic conjunctivitis, vernal conjunctivitis, episcleritis, ophthalmic epinephrine sensitivity reaction

Usual Dosage Children and Adults: Ophthalmic: 1 drop in conjunctival sac 2-4 times/day up to every 4 hours; may use every 1-2 hours during first 1-2 days

Dosage Forms Solution, ophthalmic: 1% (5 mL, 10 mL)

mefenamic acid (me fe nam' ik)

Brand Names Ponstel®

Therapeutic Category Analgesic, Non-Narcotic; Nonsteroidal Anti-Inflammatory Agent (NSAID), Oral

Use Short-term relief of mild to moderate pain including primary dysmenorrhea

Usual Dosage Children >14 years and Adults: Oral: 500 mg to start then 250 mg every 4 hours as needed; maximum therapy: 1 week

Dosage Forms Capsule: 250 mg

mefloquine hydrochloride (me' floe kwin)

Brand Names Lariam®

Therapeutic Category Antimalarial Agent

Use Treatment of acute malarial infections and prevention of malaria

Usual Dosage Adults: Oral:

Mild to moderate malaria infection: 5 tablets (1250 mg) as a single dose with at least 8 oz of water

Malaria prophylaxis: 1 tablet (250 mg) once weekly for 4 weeks, then 1 tablet every other week; start treatment 1 week prior to departure to an endemic area; to avoid development of malaria after return from an endemic area, continue prophylaxis for 4 additional weeks; for prolonged stays in an endemic area this prophylaxis be achieved by continuing the recommended dosage schedule, once weekly for 4 weeks, then once every other week, until traveler has taken 3 doses following return to a malaria-free area

Dosage Forms Tablet: 250 mg

Mefoxin® *see* cefoxitin sodium *on page 81*

Mega-B® [OTC] *see* vitamin b complex *on page 490*

Megace® *see* megestrol acetate *on this page*

Megaton™ [OTC] *see* vitamin b complex *on page 490*

megestrol acetate (me jess' trole)

Brand Names Megace®

Therapeutic Category Antineoplastic Agent, Hormone (Gonadotropin Hormone-Releasing Antigen); Progestin

Use Palliative treatment of breast and endometrial carcinomas, appetite stimulation and promotion of weight gain in cachexia

Usual Dosage Adults: Oral:
Breast carcinoma: 40 mg 4 times/day
Endometrial: 40-320 mg/day in divided doses
Dosage Forms
Suspension, oral: 40 mg/mL with alcohol 0.06% (240 mL)
Tablet: 20 mg, 40 mg

Melanex® *see* hydroquinone *on page 235*
Mellaril® *see* thioridazine *on page 457*
Mellaril-S® *see* thioridazine *on page 457*
Melpaque HP® *see* hydroquinone *on page 235*

melphalan (mel' fa lan)
Brand Names Alkeran®
Synonyms l-pam; l-sarcolysin; phenylalanine mustard
Therapeutic Category Antineoplastic Agent, Alkylating Agent (Nitrogen Mustard)
Use Palliative treatment of multiple myeloma and nonresectable epithelial ovarian carcinoma; neuroblastoma, rhabdomyosarcoma
Usual Dosage Refer to individual protocols
Children: I.V. (Investigational, distributed under the auspices of the NCI for authorized studies):
Pediatric rhabdomyosarcoma: 10-35 mg/m^2 bolus every 21-28 days
Chemoradiotherapy supported by marrow infusions for neuroblastoma: 70-140 mg/m^2 on day 7 and 6 before BMT

Adults: Oral:
Multiple myeloma: 6 mg/day or 10 mg/day for 7-10 days, or 0.15 mg/kg/day for 7 days
Ovarian carcinoma: 0.2 mg/kg/day for 5 days, repeat in 4-5 weeks
Dosage Forms
Powder for injection: 50 mg
Tablet: 2 mg

Melquin HP® *see* hydroquinone *on page 235*

menadiol sodium diphosphate (men a dye' ole)
Brand Names Synkayvite®
Synonyms vitamin k$_4$
Therapeutic Category Vitamin, Water Soluble
Use Prevention and treatment of hypoprothrombinemia caused by vitamin K deficiency secondary to oral anti-infective therapy and salicylates, inadequate absorption and synthesis of vitamin K due to lack of bile salts, eg, cystic fibrosis, obstructive jaundice, biliary fistula
Usual Dosage
Hypoprothrombinemia (vitamin K deficiency, liver disease or malabsorption): Oral, I.M., I.V., S.C.:
Term infants >1 month: 2.5-5 mg/dose; repeat every 12-24 hours as needed
Children: 5-10 mg/dose; repeat every 12-24 hours as needed
Adults: 5-15 mg/dose 1-2 times/day

Minimum daily requirement not well established
Infants: 1-5 mcg/kg/day
Adults: 0.03 mcg/kg/day
Dosage Forms
Injection: 5 mg/mL (1 mL); 10 mg/mL (1 mL); 37.5 mg/mL (2 mL)
Tablet: 5 mg

Menadol® [OTC] *see* ibuprofen *on page 240*
Menest® *see* estrogens, esterified *on page 175*

Meni-D® see meclizine hydrochloride on page 282

meningococcal polysaccharide vaccine, groups A, C, Y and W-135
Brand Names Menomune®-A/C/Y/W-135
Therapeutic Category Vaccine, Live Bacteria
Use Immunization against infection caused by Neisseria meningitidis groups A,C,Y, and W-135 in persons ≥2 years
Usual Dosage Do not inject intradermally or I.V.; inject S.C. only. The immunizing dose is one S.C. injection of 0.5 mL.
Dosage Forms Injection: 10 dose, 50 dose

Menomune®-A/C/Y/W-135 see meningococcal polysaccharide vaccine, groups A, C, Y and W-135 on this page

menotropins (men oh troe' pins)
Brand Names Pergonal®
Therapeutic Category Gonadotropin; Ovulation Stimulator
Use Used sequentially with hCG to induce ovulation and pregnancy in the infertile woman with functional anovulation; used with hCG in men to stimulate spermatogenesis in those with primary hypogonadotropic hypogonadism
Usual Dosage I.M.:
  Male: Following pretreatment with hCG, 1 ampul 3 times/week and hCG 2000 units twice weekly until sperm is detected in the ejaculate (4-6 months) then may be increased to 2 ampuls of menotropins 3 times/week

  Female: 1 ampul/day (75 units of FSH and LH) for 9-12 days followed by 10,000 units hCG 1 day after the last dose; repeated at least twice at same level before increasing dosage to 2 ampuls
Dosage Forms Injection: Follicle stimulating hormone activity 75 units and luteinizing hormone activity 75 units per 2 mL ampul; follicle stimulating hormone activity 150 units and luteinizing hormone activity 150 units per 2 mL ampul

mepenzolate bromide (me pen' zoe late)
Brand Names Cantil®
Therapeutic Category Anticholinergic Agent; Antispasmodic Agent, Gastrointestinal
Use Management of peptic ulcer disease; inhibit salivation and excessive secretions in respiratory tract preoperatively
Usual Dosage Adults: Oral: 25-50 mg 4 times/day with meal and at bedtime
Dosage Forms Tablet, with tartrazine: 25 mg

Mepergan® see meperidine and promethazine on this page

meperidine and promethazine
Brand Names Mepergan®
Therapeutic Category Analgesic, Narcotic
Use Management of moderate to severe pain
Usual Dosage Adults:
  Oral: One capsule every 4-6 hours
  I.M.: Inject 1-2 mL every 3-4 hours
Dosage Forms
  Capsule: Meperidine hydrochloride 50 mg and promethazine hydrochloride 25 mg
  Injection: Meperidine hydrochloride 25 mg and promethazine hydrochloride 25 per mL (2 mL, 10 mL)

meperidine hydrochloride (me per' i deen)
Brand Names Demerol®
Synonyms isonipecaine hydrochloride; pethidine hydrochloride
Therapeutic Category Analgesic, Narcotic

Use Management of moderate to severe pain; adjunct to anesthesia and preoperative sedation

Usual Dosage Doses should be titrated to appropriate analgesic effect; when changing route of administration, note that oral doses are about half as effective as parenteral dose

Children: Oral, I.M., I.V., S.C.: 1-1.5 mg/kg/dose every 3-4 hours as needed; 1-2 mg/kg as a single dose preoperative medication may be used; maximum 100 mg/dose

Adults: Oral, I.M., I.V.: S.C.: 50-150 mg/dose every 3-4 hours as needed

Dosage Forms
Injection:
Multiple dose vials: 50 mg/mL (30 mL); 100 mg/mL (20 mL)
Single dose: 10 mg/mL (5 mL, 10 mL, 30 mL); 25 mg/dose (0.5 mL, 1 mL); 50 mg/dose (1 mL); 75 mg/dose (1 mL, 1.5 mL); 100 mg/dose (1 mL)
Syrup: 50 mg/5 mL (500 mL)
Tablet: 50 mg, 100 mg

mephentermine sulfate (me fen' ter meen)
Brand Names Wyamine® Sulfate Injection
Therapeutic Category Adrenergic Agonist Agent; Sympathomimetic
Use Treatment of hypotension secondary to ganglionic blockade or spinal anesthesia; may be used as an emergency measure to maintain blood pressure until whole blood replacement becomes available
Usual Dosage
Hypotension: I.M., I.V.:
Children: 0.4 mg/kg
Adults: 0.5 mg/kg

Hypotensive emergency: I.V. infusion: 20-60 mg
Dosage Forms Injection: 15 mg/mL (2 mL, 10 mL); 30 mg/mL (10 mL)

mephenytoin (me fen' i toyn)
Brand Names Mesantoin®
Synonyms methoin; methylphenylethylhydantoin; phenantoin
Therapeutic Category Anticonvulsant, Hydantoin
Use Management of tonic-clonic seizures, partial seizures, partial seizures with motor symptoms, and partial seizures with complex symptomatology in patients refractory to less toxic anticonvulsants
Usual Dosage Oral:
Children: 3-15 mg/kg/day in 3 divided doses; usual maintenance dose: 100-400 mg/day in 3 divided doses

Adults: Initial dose: 50-100 mg/day given daily; increase by 50-100 mg at weekly intervals; usual maintenance dose: 200-600 mg/day in 3 divided doses; maximum: 800 mg/day
Dosage Forms Tablet: 100 mg

mephobarbital (me foe bar' bi tal)
Brand Names Mebaral®
Synonyms methylphenobarbital
Therapeutic Category Anticonvulsant, Barbiturate
Use Prophylactic management of tonic-clonic (grand mal) seizures and absence (petit mal) seizures
Usual Dosage Epilepsy: Oral:
Children: 4-10 mg/kg/day in 2-4 divided doses
Adults: 200-600 mg/day in 2-4 divided doses
Dosage Forms Tablet: 32 mg, 50 mg, 100 mg

Mephyton® Oral see phytonadione on page 368

mepivacaine hydrochloride (me piv' a kane)
Brand Names Carbocaine™ Injection; Isocaine® HCl Injection; Polocaine® Injection
Therapeutic Category Local Anesthetic, Injectable
Use Local anesthesia by nerve block; infiltration in dental procedures
Usual Dosage
Injectable local anesthetic: Varies with procedure, degree of anesthesia needed, vascularity of tissue, duration of anesthesia required, and physical condition of patient
Topical: Apply to affected area as needed
Dosage Forms Injection: 1% [10 mg/mL] (30 mL, 50 mL); 1.5% [15 mg/mL] (30 mL); 2% [20 mg/mL] (20 mL, 50 mL); 3% [30 mg/mL] (1.8 mL)

meprobamate (me proe ba' mate)
Brand Names Equanil™; Meprospan®; Miltown®; Neuramate®
Therapeutic Category Antianxiety Agent
Use Management of anxiety disorders
Usual Dosage Oral:
Children 6-12 years:
100-200 mg 2-3 times/day
Sustained release: 200 mg twice daily

Adults:
400 mg 3-4 times/day, up to 2400 mg/day
Sustained release; 400-800 mg twice daily
Dosage Forms
Capsule, sustained release: 200 mg, 400 mg
Tablet: 200 mg, 400 mg, 600 mg

meprobamate and aspirin see aspirin and meprobamate on page 36

Mepron® see atovaquone on page 37

Meprospan® see meprobamate on this page

merbromin (meer bro' min)
Brand Names Mercurochrome™
Therapeutic Category Topical Skin Product
Use Topical antiseptic
Usual Dosage Topical: Apply freely, until injury has healed
Dosage Forms Solution, topical: 2%

mercaptopurine (mer kap toe pyoor' een)
Brand Names Purinethol™
Synonyms 6-mercaptopurine; 6-mp
Therapeutic Category Antineoplastic Agent, Antimetabolite; Antineoplastic Agent, Purine
Use Treatment of leukemias
Usual Dosage Oral (refer to individual protocols):
Induction: 2.5 mg/kg/day for several weeks or more; if, after 4 weeks there is no improvement and no myelosuppression, increase dosage up to 5 mg/kg/day

Maintenance: 1.5-2.5 mg/kg/day
Dosage Forms Tablet: 50 mg

6-mercaptopurine see mercaptopurine on this page

mercuric oxide
Synonyms yellow mercuric oxide
Therapeutic Category Antibiotic, Ophthalmic
Use Treatment of irritation and minor infections of the eyelids

Usual Dosage Ophthalmic: Apply small amount to inner surface of lower eyelid once or twice daily
Dosage Forms Ointment, ophthalmic: 1%, 2% [OTC]

Mercurochrome® *see* merbromin *on previous page*
Merlenate® Topical [OTC] *see* undecylenic acid and derivatives *on page 479*
Mersol® [OTC] *see* thimerosal *on page 456*
Merthiolate® [OTC] *see* thimerosal *on page 456*
Meruvax® II *see* rubella virus vaccine, live *on page 415*

mesalamine (me sal' a meen)
Brand Names Asacol® Oral; Pentasa® Oral; Rowasa® Rectal
Synonyms 5-aminosalicylic acid; 5-asa; fisalamine; mesalazine
Therapeutic Category 5-Aminosalicylic Acid Derivative; Anti-inflammatory Agent, Rectal
Use Treatment of ulcerative colitis, proctosigmoiditis, and proctitis
Usual Dosage Adults (usual course of therapy is 3-6 weeks): Oral: 800 mg 3 times/day
Retention enema: 60 mL (4 g) at bedtime, retained over night, approximately 8 hours
Rectal suppository: Insert 1 suppository in rectum twice daily
Dosage Forms
Capsule, controlled release (Pentasa®): 250 mg
Suppository, rectal (Rowasa®): 500 mg
Suspension, rectal (Rowasa®): 4 g/60 mL (7s)
Tablet, enteric coated (Asacol®): 400 mg

mesalazine *see* mesalamine *on this page*
Mesantoin® *see* mephenytoin *on page 287*

mesna (mes' na)
Brand Names Mesnex™ Injection
Synonyms sodium 2-mercaptoethane sulfonate
Therapeutic Category Antidote, Cyclophosphamide-induced Hemorrhagic Cystitis; Antidote, Ifosfamide-induced Hemorrhagic Cystitis
Use Detoxifying agent used as a protectant against hemorrhagic cystitis induced by ifosfamide and cyclophosphamide
Usual Dosage Children and Adults (refer to individual protocols):
Ifosfamide: I.V.: 20% W/W of ifosfamide dose at time of administration and 4 and 8 hours after each dose of ifosfamide
Cyclophosphamide: I.V.: 20% W/W of cyclophosphamide dose prior to administration and 3, 6, 9, 12 hours after cyclophosphamide dose (total daily dose = 120% to 180% of cyclophosphamide dose)
Oral dose: 40% W/W of the antineoplastic agent dose in 3 doses at 4-hour intervals
Dosage Forms Injection: 100 mg/mL (2 mL, 4 mL, 10 mL)

Mesnex™ Injection *see* mesna *on this page*

mesoridazine besylate (mez oh rid' a zeen)
Brand Names Serentil®
Therapeutic Category Antipsychotic Agent; Phenothiazine Derivative
Use Symptomatic management of psychotic disorders, including schizophrenia, behavioral problems, alcoholism as well as reducing anxiety and tension occurring in neurosis
Usual Dosage Initial: 25 mg for most patients; may repeat dose in 30-60 minutes, if necessary; the usual optimum dosage range is 25-200 mg/day. Concentrate may be diluted just prior to administration with distilled water, acidified tap water, orange or grape juice; do not prepare and store bulk dilutions.
(Continued)

mesoridazine besylate (Continued)
Dosage Forms
Injection: 25 mg/mL (1 mL)
Liquid, oral: 25 mg/mL (118 mL)
Tablet: 10 mg, 25 mg, 50 mg, 100 mg

Mestinon® Injection see pyridostigmine bromide on page 400
Mestinon® Oral see pyridostigmine bromide on page 400

mestranol and norethindrone
Brand Names Norinyl® 1+50; Ortho-Novum™ 1/50
Synonyms norethindrone and mestranol
Therapeutic Category Contraceptive, Low Estrogen/Progestin; Contraceptive, Monophasic; Contraceptive, Oral; Progestin
Use Prevention of pregnancy; treatment of hypermenorrhea, endometriosis, female hypogonadism
Usual Dosage Contraception: Oral: 1 tablet daily, beginning on day 5 of menstrual cycle (first day of menstrual flow is day 1). With 20-tablet and 21-tablet packages, new dosing cycle begins 7 days after last tablet taken; with 28-tablet packages, dosage is 1 tablet daily without interruption; extra tablets are placebos or contain iron. If next menstrual period does not begin on schedule, rule out pregnancy before starting new dosing cycle; if menstrual period begins, start new dosing cycle 7 days after last tablet was taken. If all doses have been taken on schedule and 1 menstrual period is missed, continue dosing cycle; if 2 consecutive menstrual periods are missed, pregnancy test is required before new dosing cycle is started.
Dosage Forms Tablet: Mestranol 0.05 mg and norethindrone 1 mg (21s and 28s)

mestranol and norethynodrel
Brand Names Enovid®
Synonyms norethynodrel and mestranol
Therapeutic Category Contraceptive, Oral
Use Prevention of pregnancy; treatment of hypermenorrhea, endometriosis, female hypogonadism
Usual Dosage Adults: Female: Oral:
Endometriosis: 5-10 mg/day for 2 weeks beginning on day 5 of menstrual cycle; increase by 5-10 mg increments at 2-week intervals up to 20 mg/day for 6-9 months

Hypermenorrhea: 20-30 mg/day until bleeding is controlled, then reduce to 10 mg/day and continue through day 24 of cycle; administer 5-10 mg/day from day 5 through day 24 of next 2-3 cycles
Dosage Forms Tablet:
5: Mestranol 0.075 mg and norethynodrel 5 mg
10: Mestranol 0.150 mg and norethynodrel 9.85 mg

metacortandralone see prednisolone on page 383
Metahydrin® see trichlormethiazide on page 469
Metamucil® [OTC] see psyllium on page 398
Metamucil® Instant Mix [OTC] see psyllium on page 398
Metandren® see methyltestosterone on page 301
Metaprel® see metaproterenol sulfate on this page

metaproterenol sulfate (met a proe ter' e nol)
Brand Names Alupent®; Arm-a-Med® Metaproterenol; Dey-Dose® Metaproterenol; Metaprel®; Prometa®
Synonyms orciprenaline sulfate
Therapeutic Category Adrenergic Agonist Agent; Beta-2-Adrenergic Agonist Agent; Bronchodilator

Use Bronchodilator in reversible airway obstruction due to asthma or COPD; because of its delayed onset of action (one hour) and prolonged effect (4 or more hours), this may not be the drug of choice for assessing response to a bronchodilator

Usual Dosage

Oral:

Children:

<2 years: 0.4 mg/kg/dose given 3-4 times/day; in infants, the dose can be given every 8-12 hours

2-6 years: 1-2.6 mg/kg/day divided every 6-8 hours

6-9 years: 10 mg/dose given 3-4 times/day

Children >9 years and Adults: 20 mg/dose given 3-4 times/day

Inhalation: Children >12 years and Adults: 2-3 inhalations every 3-4 hours, up to 12 inhalations in 24 hours

Nebulizer:

Infants: 6 mg/dose administered over 5 minutes

Children <12 years: 0.01-0.02 mL/kg of 5% solution; diluted in 2-3 mL normal saline every 4-6 hours (may be given more frequently according to need), maximum dose: 15 mg/dose every 4-6 hours

Adolescents and Adults: 5-20 breaths of full strength 5% metaproterenol **or** 0.2 to 0.3 mL 5% metaproterenol in 2.5-3 mL normal saline nebulized every 4-6 hours (can be given more frequently according to need)

Dosage Forms

Aerosol, oral: 0.65 mg/dose (5 mL, 10 mL)

Solution for inhalation, preservative free: 0.4% [4 mg/mL] (2.5 mL); 0.6% [6 mg/mL] (2.5 mL); 5% [50 mg/mL] (10 mL, 30 mL)

Syrup: 10 mg/5 mL (480 mL)

Tablet: 10 mg, 20 mg

metaraminol bitartrate (met a ram' i nole)

Brand Names Aramine®

Therapeutic Category Adrenergic Agonist Agent

Use Acute hypotensive crisis in the treatment of shock

Usual Dosage Adults:

Prevention of hypotension: I.M., S.C.: 2-10 mg

Adjunctive treatment of hypotension: I.V.: 15-100 mg in 250-500 mL NS or 5% dextrose in water

Severe shock: I.V.: 0.5-5 mg direct I.V. injection then use I.M. dose

Dosage Forms Injection: 10 mg/mL (10 mL)

Metasep® [OTC] *see* parachlorometaxylenol *on page 348*

Metastron® Injection *see* strontium-89 chloride *on page 437*

metaxalone (me tax' a lone)

Brand Names Skelaxin®

Therapeutic Category Skeletal Muscle Relaxant

Use Relief of discomfort associated with acute, painful musculoskeletal conditions

Usual Dosage Children >12 years and Adults: Oral: 800 mg 3-4 times/day

Dosage Forms Tablet: 400 mg

methacholine chloride (meth a kol' leen)

Brand Names Provocholine®

Therapeutic Category Diagnostic Agent, Bronchial Airway Hyperactivity

Use Diagnosis of bronchial airway hyperactivity in subjects who do not have clinically apparent asthma

Usual Dosage The following is a suggested schedule for administration of methacholine challenge. Calculate cumulative units by multiplying number of breaths by concentration

(Continued)

methacholine chloride *(Continued)*

Vial	Serial Concentration (mg/mL)	No. of Breaths	Cumulative Units per Concentration	Total Cumulative Units
E	0.025	5	0.125	0.125
D	0.25	5	1.25	1.375
C	2.5	5	12.5	13.88
B	10	5	50	63.88
A	25	5	125	188.88

given. Total cumulative units is the sum of cumulative units for each concentration given. See table.

Dosage Forms Powder for reconstitution, inhalation: 100 mg/5 mL

methadone hydrochloride (meth' a done)
Brand Names Dolophine® Oral
Therapeutic Category Analgesic, Narcotic
Use Management of severe pain, used in narcotic detoxification maintenance programs
Usual Dosage Doses should be titrated to appropriate effects:
Children: Analgesia:
Oral, I.M., S.C.: 0.7 mg/kg/24 hours divided every 4-6 hours as needed or 0.1-0.2 mg/kg every 4-12 hours as needed; maximum: 10 mg/dose
I.V.: 0.1 mg/kg every 4 hours initially for 2-3 doses, then every 6-12 hours as needed; maximum: 10 mg/dose

Adults:
Analgesia: Oral, I.M., I.V., S.C.: 2.5-10 mg every 3-8 hours as needed, up to 5-20 mg every 6-8 hours
Detoxification: Oral: 15-40 mg/day
Maintenance of opiate dependence: Oral: 20-120 mg/day
Dosage Forms
Injection: 10 mg/mL (1 mL, 10 mL, 20 mL)
Solution:
Oral: 5 mg/5 mL (5 mL, 500 mL); 10 mg/5 mL (500 mL)
Oral, concentrate: 10 mg/mL (30 mL)
Tablet: 5 mg, 10 mg
Tablet, dispersible: 40 mg

methaminodiazepoxide hydrochloride *see* chlordiazepoxide *on page 89*

methamphetamine hydrochloride (meth am fet' a meen)
Brand Names Desoxyn®
Synonyms desoxyephedrine hydrochloride
Therapeutic Category Amphetamine; Central Nervous System Stimulant, Amphetamine
Use Narcolepsy; exogenous obesity; abnormal behavioral syndrome in children (minimal brain dysfunction)
Usual Dosage
Attention deficit disorder: Children >6 years: 2.5-5 mg 1-2 times/day, may increase by 5 mg increments weekly until optimum response is achieved, usually 20-25 mg/day

Exogenous obesity: Children >12 years and Adults: 5 mg, 30 minutes before each meal, 10-15 mg in morning; treatment duration should not exceed a few weeks
Dosage Forms
Tablet: 5 mg
Tablet, extended release (Gradumet®): 5 mg, 10 mg, 15 mg

methantheline bromide (meth an' tha leen)
Brand Names Banthine®
Synonyms methanthelinium bromide
Therapeutic Category Anticholinergic Agent; Antispasmodic Agent, Gastrointestinal
Use Adjunctive treatment of peptic ulcer, irritable bowel syndrome, pancreatitis, ureteral and urinary bladder spasm; to reduce duodenal motility during diagnostic radiologic procedures and treatment of an uninhibited neurogenic bladder
Usual Dosage Oral:
Neonates: 12.5 mg twice daily then 3 times/day

Children:
<1 year: 12.5-25 mg 4 times/day
>1 year: 12.5-50 mg 4 times/day

Adults: 50-100 mg every 6 hours
Dosage Forms Tablet: 50 mg

methanthelinium bromide *see* methantheline bromide *on this page*

methazolamide (meth a zoe' la mide)
Brand Names GlaucTabs®; Neptazane®
Therapeutic Category Carbonic Anhydrase Inhibitor; Diuretic, Carbonic Anhydrase Inhibitor
Use Adjunctive treatment of open-angle or secondary glaucoma; short-term therapy of narrow-angle glaucoma when delay of surgery is desired
Usual Dosage Adults: Oral: 50-100 mg 2-3 times/day
Dosage Forms Tablet: 25 mg, 50 mg

methdilazine hydrochloride (meth dill' a zeen)
Brand Names Tacaryl®
Therapeutic Category Antihistamine; Phenothiazine Derivative
Use Symptomatic relief of pruritus associated with urticaria; neuroallergic, atopic, contact, poison ivy or eczematous dermatitis; pruritus ani or drug rash
Usual Dosage Oral:
Children >3 years: 4 mg 2-4 times/day
Adults: 8 mg 2-4 times/day
Dosage Forms
Syrup: 4 mg/5 mL (473 mL)
Tablet: 8 mg
Tablet, chewable: 3.6 mg [methdilazine hydrochloride 4 mg]

methenamine (meth en' a meen)
Brand Names Hiprex®; Mandelamine®; Urex®
Synonyms hexamethylenetetramine
Therapeutic Category Antibiotic, Miscellaneous
Use Prophylaxis or suppression of recurrent urinary tract infections; urinary tract discomfort secondary to hypermotility
Usual Dosage Oral:
Children:
Hippurate: 6-12 years: 25-50 mg/kg/day divided every 12 hours
Mandelate: 50-75 mg/kg/day divided every 6 hours

Adults:
Hippurate: 1 g twice daily
Mandelate: 1 g 4 times/day after meals and at bedtime
Dosage Forms
Tablet, as hippurate (Hiprex®, Urex®): 1 g (Hiprex® contains tartrazine dye)
Tablet, as mandelate, enteric coated (Mandelamine®): 250 mg, 500 mg, 1 g

Methergine® *see* methylergonovine maleate *on page 299*

methicillin sodium (meth i sill' in)
Brand Names Staphcillin(R)
Synonyms dimethoxyphenyl penicillin sodium; sodium methicillin
Therapeutic Category Antibiotic, Penicillin
Use Treatment of susceptible bacterial infections such as osteomyelitis, septicemia, endocarditis, and CNS infections due to penicillinase-producing strains of *Staphylococcus*
Usual Dosage I.M., I.V.:
Neonates:
0-4 weeks, <1200 g: 50 mg/kg/day divided every 12 hours; meningitis: 100 mg/kg/day divided every 12 hours
Postnatal age <7 days:
1200-2000 g: 50 mg/kg/day divided every 12 hours; meningitis: 100 mg/kg/day divided every 12 hours
>2000 g: 75 mg/kg/day divided every 8 hours; meningitis: 150 mg/kg/day divided every 8 hours
Postnatal age >7 days:
1200-2000 g: 75 mg/kg/day divided every 8 hours; meningitis: 150 mg/kg/day divided every 8 hours
>2000 g: 100 mg/kg/day divided every 6 hours; meningitis: 200 mg/kg/day divided every 6 hours

Children: 150-200 mg/kg/day divided every 6 hours; 200-400 mg/kg/day divided every 4-6 hours has been used for treatment of severe infections; maximum dose: 12 g/day

Adults: 4-12 g/day in divided doses every 4-6 hours
Dosage Forms Powder for injection: 1 g, 4 g, 6 g, 10 g

methimazole (meth im' a zole)
Brand Names Tapazole(R)
Synonyms thiamazole
Therapeutic Category Antithyroid Agent
Use Palliative treatment of hyperthyroidism, to return the hyperthyroid patient to a normal metabolic state prior to thyroidectomy, and to control thyrotoxic crisis that may accompany thyroidectomy
Usual Dosage Oral:
Children: Initial: 0.4 mg/kg/day in 3 divided doses; maintenance: 0.2 mg/kg/day in 3 divided doses

Adults: Initial: 10 mg every 8 hours; maintenance dose ranges from 5-30 mg/day
Dosage Forms Tablet: 5 mg, 10 mg

methionine (me thye' oh neen)
Brand Names Pedameth(R)
Therapeutic Category Dietary Supplement
Use Treatment of diaper rash and control of odor, dermatitis and ulceration caused by ammoniacal urine
Usual Dosage Oral:
Children: Control of diaper rash: 75 mg in formula or other liquid 3-4 times/day for 3-5 days
Adults:
Control of odor in incontinent adults: 200-400 mg 3-4 times/day
Dietary supplement: 500 mg/day
Dosage Forms
Capsule: 200 mg, 300 mg, 500 mg
Liquid: 75 mg/5 mL (473 mL)
Tablet: 500 mg

methocarbamol (meth oh kar' ba mole)
Brand Names Delaxin®; Marbaxin®; Robaxin®; Robomol®
Therapeutic Category Skeletal Muscle Relaxant
Use Treatment of muscle spasm associated with acute painful musculoskeletal conditions; supportive therapy in tetanus
Usual Dosage
Children: Recommended **only** for use in tetanus I.V.: 15 mg/kg/dose or 500 mg/m²/dose, may repeat every 6 hours if needed; maximum dose: 1.8 g/m²/day for 3 days only

Adults: Muscle spasm:
    Oral: 1.5 g 4 times/day for 2-3 days, then decrease to 4-4.5 g/day in 3-6 divided doses
    I.M., I.V.: 1 g every 8 hours if oral not possible
Dosage Forms
Injection: 100 mg/mL in polyethylene glycol 50% (10 mL)
Tablet: 500 mg, 750 mg

methocarbamol and aspirin
Brand Names Robaxisal®
Therapeutic Category Skeletal Muscle Relaxant
Use Adjunct to rest, physical therapy, and other measures for the relief of discomfort associated with acute, painful musculoskeletal disorders
Usual Dosage Children >12 years and Adults: Oral: 2 tablets 4 times/day
Dosage Forms Tablet: Methocarbamol 400 mg and aspirin 325 mg

methohexital sodium (meth oh hex' i tal)
Brand Names Brevital® Sodium
Therapeutic Category Barbiturate; General Anesthetic; Sedative
Use Induction and maintenance of general anesthesia for short procedures
Usual Dosage Doses must be titrated to effect
Children:
    I.M.: Preop: 5-10 mg/kg/dose
    I.V.: Induction: 1-2 mg/kg/dose
    Rectal: Preop/induction: 20-35 mg/kg/dose; usual: 25 mg/kg/dose; give as 10% aqueous solution

Adults: I.V.: Induction: 50-120 mg to start; 20-40 mg every 4-7 minutes
Dosage Forms Injection: 500 mg, 2.5 g, 5 g

methoin see mephenytoin *on page 287*

methotrexate (meth oh trex' ate)
Brand Names Folex® PFS; Rheumatrex®
Synonyms amethopterin; mtx
Therapeutic Category Antineoplastic Agent, Antimetabolite
Use Treatment of trophoblastic neoplasms, leukemias, psoriasis, rheumatoid arthritis, osteosarcoma, non-Hodgkin's lymphoma
Usual Dosage Refer to individual protocols
Children:
    High-dose MTX for acute lymphocytic leukemia: I.V.: Loading dose of 200 mg/m² and a 24-hour infusion of 1200 mg/m²/day
    Induction of remission in acute lymphoblastic leukemias: Oral, I.M., I.V.: 3.3 mg/m²/day for 4-6 weeks
    Leukemia: Remission maintenance: Oral, I.M.: 20-30 mg/m² 2 times/week
    Juvenile rheumatoid arthritis: Oral: 5-15 mg/m²/week as a single dose or as 3 divided doses given 12 hours apart
    Osteosarcoma:
    I.T.: 10-15 mg/m² (maximum dose: 15 mg) by protocol
(Continued)
295

methotrexate *(Continued)*

I.V.: <12 years: 12 g/m^2 (12-18 g); >12 years: 8 g/m^2 (maximum dose: 18 g)
Non-Hodgkin's lymphoma: I.V.: 200-300 mg/m^2

Adults:
Trophoblastic neoplasms: Oral, I.M.: 15-30 mg/day for 5 days, repeat in 7 days for 3-5 courses
Rheumatoid arthritis: Oral: 7.5 mg once weekly or 2.5 mg every 12 hours for 3 doses/week; not to exceed 20 mg/week

Dosage Forms
Dose Pack: 2.5 mg (4 cards with 3 tablets each)
Injection, as sodium: 2.5 mg/mL (2 mL); 25 mg/mL (2 mL, 4 mL, 8 mL, 10 mL)
Injection, as sodium, preservative free: 25 mg/mL (2 mL, 4 mL, 8 mL, 10 mL)
Powder for injection, as sodium: 20 mg, 25 mg, 50 mg, 100 mg, 250 mg, 1000 mg
Tablet, as sodium: 2.5 mg

methotrimeprazine hydrochloride (meth oh trye mep' ra zeen)

Brand Names Levoprome®
Synonyms levomepromazine
Therapeutic Category Analgesic, Non-Narcotic; Phenothiazine Derivative; Sedative
Use Relief of moderate to severe pain in nonambulatory patients; for analgesia and sedation when respiratory depression is to be avoided, as in obstetrics; preanesthetic for producing sedation, somnolence and relief of apprehension and anxiety
Usual Dosage Adults: I.M.:
Sedation analgesia: 10-20 mg every 4-6 hours as needed

Preoperative medication: 2-20 mg, 45 minutes to 3 hours before surgery

Postoperative analgesia: 2.5-7.5 mg every 4-6 hours is suggested as necessary since residual effects of anesthetic may be present

Pre- and postoperative hypotension: I.M.: 5-10 mg
Dosage Forms Injection: 20 mg/mL (10 mL)

methoxamine hydrochloride (meth ox' a meen)

Brand Names Vasoxyl™
Therapeutic Category Adrenergic Agonist Agent
Use Treatment of hypotension occurring during general anesthesia; to terminate episodes of supraventricular tachycardia; treatment of shock
Usual Dosage Adults:
Emergencies: I.V.: 3-5 mg
Supraventricular tachycardia: I.V.: 10 mg
During spinal anesthesia: I.M.: 10-20 mg
Dosage Forms Injection: 20 mg/mL (1 mL)

methoxsalen (meth ox' a len)

Brand Names Oxsoralen™ Topical; Oxsoralen-Ultra® Oral
Synonyms methoxypsoralen; 8-mop
Therapeutic Category Psoralen
Use Symptomatic control of severe, recalcitrant, disabling psoriasis in conjunction with long wave ultraviolet radiation; induce repigmentation in vitiligo topical repigmenting agent in conjunction with controlled doses of ultraviolet A (UVA) or sunlight
Usual Dosage
Psoriasis: Adults: Oral: 10-70 mg 1$\frac{1}{2}$-2 hours before exposure to ultraviolet light, 2-3 times at least 48 hours apart; dosage is based upon patient's body weight and skin type

Vitiligo: Children >12 years and Adults:
Oral: 20 mg 2-4 hours before exposure to UVA light or sunlight
Topical: Apply lotion 1-2 hours before exposure to UVA light, no more than once weekly
Dosage Forms
Capsule: 10 mg
Lotion: 1% (30 mL)

methoxycinnamate and oxybenzone (ox i ben' zone)
Brand Names PreSun® 29 [OTC]; Ti-Screen® [OTC]
Synonyms sunscreen (paba-free)
Therapeutic Category Sunscreen
Use Reduce the chance of premature aging of the skin and skin cancer from overexposure to the sun
Dosage Forms Lotion:
SPF 15: 120 mL
SPF 29: 120 mL

methoxyflurane (meth ox ee flóo' rane)
Brand Names Penthrane®
Therapeutic Category General Anesthetic
Use Adjunct to provide anesthesia procedures under 4 hours in duration
Usual Dosage 0.3% to 0.8% for analgesia and anesthesia, with 0.1% to 2% for maintenance when used with nitrous oxide
Dosage Forms Liquid: 15 mL, 125 mL

methoxypsoralen see methoxsalen *on previous page*

methscopolamine bromide (meth skoe pol' a meen)
Brand Names Pamine®
Therapeutic Category Anticholinergic Agent; Antispasmodic Agent, Gastrointestinal
Use Adjunctive therapy in the treatment of peptic ulcer
Usual Dosage Oral: 2.5 mg 30 minutes before meals or food and 2.5-5 mg at bedtime
Dosage Forms Tablet: 2.5 mg

methsuximide (meth sux' i mide)
Brand Names Celontin®
Therapeutic Category Anticonvulsant, Succinimide
Use Control of absence (petit mal) seizures; useful adjunct in refractory, partial complex (psychomotor) seizures
Usual Dosage Oral:
Children: Initial: 10-15 mg/kg/day in 3-4 divided doses; increase weekly up to maximum of 30 mg/kg/day

Adults: 300 mg/day for the first week; may increase by 300 mg/day at weekly intervals up to 1.2 g in 2-4 divided doses/day
Dosage Forms Capsule: 150 mg, 300 mg

methyclothiazide (meth i kloe thye' a zide)
Brand Names Aquatensen®; Enduron®
Therapeutic Category Diuretic, Thiazide
Use Management of mild to moderate hypertension; treatment of edema in congestive heart failure and nephrotic syndrome
Usual Dosage Adults: Oral:
Edema: 2.5-10 mg/day
Hypertension: 2.5-5 mg/day
Dosage Forms Tablet: 2.5 mg, 5 mg

methyclothiazide and cryptenamine tannates
Brand Names Diutensin®
Synonyms cryptenamine tannates and methyclothiazide
Therapeutic Category Antihypertensive, Combination
(Continued)

methyclothiazide and cryptenamine tannates *(Continued)*
Use Management of hypertension
Usual Dosage Oral: 1-4 tablets/day
Dosage Forms Tablet: Methyclothiazide 2.5 mg and cryptenamine tannates 2 mg

methyclothiazide and deserpidine
Brand Names Enduronyl®; Enduronyl® Forte
Therapeutic Category Antihypertensive, Combination
Use Management of mild to moderately severe hypertension
Usual Dosage Oral: Individualized, normally 1-4 tablets/day
Dosage Forms Tablet: Methyclothiazide 5 mg and deserpidine 0.25 mg; methyclothiazide 5 mg and deserpidine 0.5 mg

methyclothiazide and pargyline
Brand Names Eutron®
Synonyms pargyline and methyclothiazide
Therapeutic Category Antihypertensive, Combination
Use Management of hypertension
Usual Dosage Oral: Individualized, normally 1-4 tablets/day
Dosage Forms Tablet: Methyclothiazide 5 mg and pargyline hydrochloride 25 mg

methylacetoxyprogesterone *see* medroxyprogesterone acetate *on page 283*

methylbenzethonium chloride (meth ill ben ze thoe' nee um)
Brand Names Diaparene® [OTC]; Puri-Clens™ [OTC]; Sween Cream® [OTC]
Therapeutic Category Topical Skin Product
Use Diaper rash and ammonia dermatitis
Usual Dosage Topical: Apply to area as needed
Dosage Forms
Cream: 0.1% (30 g, 60 g, 120 g)
Ointment, topical: 0.1% (30 g, 60 g, 120 g)
Powder: 0.055% (120 g, 270 g, 420 g)

methylcellulose (meth ill sell' yoo lose)
Brand Names Citrucel® [OTC]
Therapeutic Category Ophthalmic Agent, Miscellaneous
Use
Oral: Adjunct in treatment of constipation
Ophthalmic: Relief of dry eyes and ocular lubricant for artificial eyes and contact lenses
Usual Dosage
Children:
Oral: 5-10 mL 1-2 times/day
Ophthalmic: Instill 1-2 drops of 0.25% to 1% in eye(s) 3-4 times/day

Adults: Oral: 5-20 mL 3 times/day
Dosage Forms
Liquid: 450 mg/5 mL
Powder: 105 mg/g

methyldopa (meth ill doe' pa)
Brand Names Aldomet®
Synonyms methyldopate hydrochloride
Therapeutic Category Alpha-Adrenergic Inhibitors, Central
Use Management of moderate to severe hypertension

Usual Dosage
Children:
Oral: Initial: 10 mg/kg/day in 2-4 divided doses; increase every 2 days as needed to maximum dose of 65 mg/kg/day; do not exceed 3 g/day
I.V.: 5-10 mg/kg/dose every 6-8 hours

Adults:
Oral: Initial: 250 mg 2-3 times/day; increase every 2 days as needed; usual dose 1-1.5 g/day in 2-4 divided doses; maximum dose: 3 g/day
I.V.: 250-1000 mg every 6-8 hours

Dosage Forms
Injection, as methyldopate HCl: 50 mg/mL (5 mL, 10 mL)
Suspension, oral: 250 mg/5 mL (5 mL, 473 mL)
Tablet: 125 mg, 250 mg, 500 mg

methyldopa and chlorothiazide *see* chlorothiazide and methyldopa *on page 92*

methyldopa and hydrochlorothiazide
Brand Names Aldoril®
Synonyms hydrochlorothiazide and methyldopa
Therapeutic Category Antihypertensive, Combination
Use Management of moderate to severe hypertension
Usual Dosage Oral: 1 tablet 2-3 times/day for first 48 hours, then decrease or increase at intervals of not less than 2 days until an adequate response is achieved
Dosage Forms Tablet:
15: Methyldopa 250 mg and hydrochlorothiazide 15 mg
25: Methyldopa 250 mg and hydrochlorothiazide 25 mg
D50: Methyldopa 500 mg and hydrochlorothiazide 50 mg

methyldopate hydrochloride *see* methyldopa *on previous page*

methylene blue (meth' i leen)
Brand Names Urolene Blue® Oral
Therapeutic Category Antidote, Cyanide; Antidote, Drug Induced Methemoglobinemia
Use Antidote for cyanide poisoning and drug-induced methemoglobinemia, indicator dye, chronic urolithiasis
Usual Dosage
Children:
NADH-methemoglobin reductase deficiency: Oral: 1.5-5 mg/kg/day (maximum: 300 mg/day) given with 5-8 mg/kg/day of ascorbic acid
Methemoglobinemia: I.V.: 1-2 mg/kg over several minutes

Adults:
Genitourinary antiseptic: Oral: 55-130 mg 3 times/day (maximum: 390 mg/day)
Methemoglobinemia: I.V.: 1-2 mg/kg over several minutes; may be repeated in 1 hour if necessary

Dosage Forms
Injection: 10 mg/mL (1 mL, 10 mL)
Tablet: 55 mg, 65 mg

methylergometrine maleate *see* methylergonovine maleate *on this page*

methylergonovine maleate (meth ill er goe noe' veen)
Brand Names Methergine®
Synonyms methylergometrine maleate
Therapeutic Category Ergot Alkaloid
Use Prevention and treatment of postpartum and postabortion hemorrhage caused by uterine atony or subinvolution
(Continued)

methylergonovine maleate *(Continued)*
Usual Dosage Adults:
Oral: 0.2-0.4 mg every 6-12 hours for 2-7 days
I.M., I.V.: 0.2 mg every 2-4 hours for 5 doses then change to oral dosage
Dosage Forms
Injection: 0.2 mg/mL (1 mL)
Tablet: 0.2 mg

methylmorphine *see* codeine *on page 111*

methylphenidate hydrochloride (meth ill fen' i date)
Brand Names Ritalin®; Ritalin-SR®
Therapeutic Category Central Nervous System Stimulant, Nonamphetamine
Use Treatment of attention deficit disorder and symptomatic management of narcolepsy
Usual Dosage Oral:
Children ≥6 years: Attention deficit disorder: Initial: 0.3 mg/kg/dose or 2.5-5 mg/dose given before breakfast and lunch; increase by 0.1 mg/kg/dose or by 5-10 mg/day at weekly intervals; usual dose: 0.5-1 mg/kg/day; maximum dose: 2 mg/kg/day or 60 mg/day

Adults: Narcolepsy: 10 mg 2-3 times/day, up to 60 mg/day
Dosage Forms
Tablet: 5 mg, 10 mg, 20 mg
Tablet, sustained release: 20 mg

methylphenobarbital *see* mephobarbital *on page 287*
methylphenylethylhydantoin *see* mephenytoin *on page 287*
methylphenyl isoxazolyl penicillin *see* oxacillin sodium *on page 340*
methylphytyl napthoquinone *see* phytonadione *on page 368*

methylprednisolone (meth ill pred niss' oh lone)
Brand Names Adlone™ Injection; A-methaPred® Injection; depMedalone® Injection; Depoject™ Injection; Depo-Medrol® Injection; Depopred® Injection; D-Med® Injection; Duralone® Injection; Medralone™ Injection; Medrol™ Oral; M-Prednisol® Injection; Solu-Medrol® Injection
Synonyms 6-α-methylprednisolone
Therapeutic Category Adrenal Corticosteroid; Anti-inflammatory Agent; Corticosteroid, Systemic; Corticosteroid, Topical (Low Potency)
Use Primarily as an anti-inflammatory or immunosuppressant agent in the treatment of a variety of diseases including those of hematologic, allergic, inflammatory, neoplastic, and autoimmune origin
Usual Dosage Methylprednisolone sodium succinate is highly soluble and has a rapid effect by I.M. and I.V. routes. Methylprednisolone acetate has a low solubility and has a sustained I.M. effect.

Children:
Anti-inflammatory or immunosuppressive: Oral, I.M., I.V. (sodium succinate): 0.16-0.8 mg/kg/day or 5-25 mg/m²/day in divided doses every 6-12 hours
Status asthmaticus: I.V. (sodium succinate): Loading dose: 2 mg/kg/dose, then 0.5-1 mg/kg/dose every 6 hours for up to 5 days
Lupus nephritis:
I.V. (sodium succinate): 30 mg/kg every other day for 6 doses
Topical: Apply sparingly 2-4 times/day

Adults:
Anti-inflammatory or immunosuppressive: Oral: 4-48 mg/day to start, followed by gradual reduction in dosage to the lowest possible level consistent with maintaining an adequate clinical response
I.M. (sodium succinate): 10-80 mg/day once daily
I.M. (acetate): 40-120 mg every 1-2 weeks

I.V. (sodium succinate): 10-40 mg over a period of several minutes and repeated I.V. or I.M. at intervals depending on clinical response; when high dosages are needed, give 30 mg/kg over a period of 10-20 minutes and may be repeated every 4-6 hours for 48 hours

Status asthmaticus: I.V. (sodium succinate): Loading dose: 2 mg/kg/dose, then 0.5-1 mg/kg/dose every hours for up to 5 days

Lupus nephritis:

I.V. (sodium succinate): 1 g/day for 3 days

Topical: Apply sparingly 2-4 times/day

Intra-articular (acetate):

Large joints: 20-80 mg

Small joints: 4-10 mg

Intralesional (acetate): 20-60 mg

Dosage Forms

Injection, as sodium succinate: 40 mg (1 mL, 3 mL); 125 mg (2 mL, 5 mL); 500 mg (1 mL, 4 mL, 8 mL, 20 mL); 1000 mg (1 mL, 8 mL, 50 mL); 2000 mg (30.6 mL)

Injection, as acetate: 20 mg/mL (5 mL, 10 mL); 40 mg/mL (1 mL, 5 mL, 10 mL); 80 mg/mL (1 mL, 5 mL)

Ointment, topical, as acetate: 0.25% (30 g); 1% (30 g)

Tablet: 2 mg, 4 mg, 8 mg, 16 mg, 24 mg, 32 mg

Tablet, dose pack: 4 mg (21s)

6-α-methylprednisolone *see* methylprednisolone *on previous page*

methylrosaniline chloride *see* gentian violet *on page 207*

methyltestosterone (meth ill tess toss' te rone)

Brand Names Android®; Metandren®; Oreton® Methyl; Testred®; Virilon®

Therapeutic Category Androgen

Use

Male: Hypogonadism; delayed puberty; impotence and climacteric symptoms

Female: Palliative treatment of metastatic breast cancer; postpartum breast pain and/or engorgement

Usual Dosage Adults:

Male:

Oral: 10-40 mg/day

Buccal: 5-20 mg/day

Female:

Breast pain/engorgement:

Oral: 80 mg/day for 3-5 days

Buccal: 40 mg/day for 3-5 days

Breast cancer:

Oral: 200 mg/day

Buccal: 100 mg/day

Dosage Forms

Capsule: 10 mg

Tablet: 10 mg, 25 mg

Tablet, buccal: 5 mg, 10 mg

methysergide maleate (meth i ser' jide)

Brand Names Sansert®

Therapeutic Category Ergot Alkaloid

Use Prophylaxis of vascular headache

Usual Dosage Oral: 4-8 mg/day with meals; if no improvement is noted after 3 weeks, drug is unlikely to be beneficial; must not be given continuously for longer than 6 months, and a drug-free interval of 3-4 weeks must follow each 6-month course; dosage should be tapered over the 2-3 week period before drug discontinuation to avoid rebound headaches

Dosage Forms Tablet: 2 mg

Meticorten® Oral *see* prednisone *on page 384*
Metimyd® *see* sodium sulfacetamide and prednisolone *on page 431*

metipranolol hydrochloride (met i pran' oh lol)
Brand Names OptiPranolol® Ophthalmic
Therapeutic Category Beta-Adrenergic Blocker, Ophthalmic
Use Agent for lowering intraocular pressure
Usual Dosage Ophthalmic: Adults: 1 drop in the affected eye(s) twice daily
Dosage Forms Solution, ophthalmic: 0.3% (5 mL, 10 mL)

metoclopramide (met oh kloe pra' mide)
Brand Names Clopra®; Maxolon®; Octamide®; Reglan®
Therapeutic Category Antiemetic
Use Symptomatic treatment of diabetic gastric stasis, gastroesophageal reflux; prevention of nausea associated with chemotherapy or postsurgery and facilitates intubation of the small intestine
Usual Dosage
Children:
    Gastroesophageal reflux: Oral: 0.1 mg/kg/dose up to 4 times/day; efficacy of continuing metoclopramide beyond 12 weeks in reflux has not been determined; total daily dose should not exceed 0.5 mg/kg/day
    Gastrointestinal hypomotility: Oral, I.M., I.V.: 0.1 mg/kg/dose up to 4 times/day, not to exceed 0.5 mg/kg/day
    Antiemetic: I.V.: 1-2 mg/kg 30 minutes before chemotherapy and every 2-4 hours
    Facilitate intubation: I.V.: <6 years: 0.1 mg/kg; 6-14 years: 2.5-5 mg

Adults:
    Stasis/reflux: Oral: 10-15 mg/dose up to 4 times/day 30 minutes before meals or food and at bedtime; efficacy of continuing metoclopramide beyond 12 weeks in reflux has not been determined
    Gastrointestinal hypomotility: Oral, I.M., I.V.: 10 mg 30 minutes before each meal and at bedtime
    Antiemetic: I.V.: 1-2 mg/kg 30 minutes before chemotherapy and every 2-4 hours
    Facilitate intubation: I.V.: 10 mg
Dosage Forms
Injection: 5 mg/mL (2 mL, 10 mL, 30 mL, 50 mL, 100 mL)
Solution, oral, concentrated: 10 mg/mL (10 mL, 30 mL)
Syrup, sugar free: 5 mg/5 mL (10 mL, 480 mL)
Tablet: 5 mg, 10 mg

metocurine iodide (met oh kyoor' een)
Brand Names Metubine® Iodide
Synonyms dimethyl tubocurarine iodide
Therapeutic Category Neuromuscular Blocker Agent, Nondepolarizing
Use Adjunct to anesthesia to induce skeletal muscle relaxation
Usual Dosage
Children:
    Chronic respiratory paralysis in neonates: Start 0.25-0.5 mg/kg/dose (repeat once if paralysis is not achieved in 3 minutes); maintenance: repeat previous dose as soon as movement is observed. The dose should be titrated to achieve a dosage interval of 3-4 hours, then plateau at 10-20 mg/kg/24 hours
    Neuromuscular blockade for surgery: Initial: 0.2-0.4 mg/kg/dose; maintenance: 0.1-0.25 mg/kg/dose every 25-90 minutes

Adults:
    Surgery: 0.2-0.4 mg/kg (initial); supplement dose: 0.5-1 mg; use of anesthetics that potentiate effect of neuromuscular blocking drug requires less metocurine
    Electric shock therapy: 1.75-5.5 mg
Dosage Forms Injection: 2 mg/mL (20 mL)

metolazone (me tole' a zone)
Brand Names Mykrox®; Zaroxolyn®
Therapeutic Category Diuretic, Miscellaneous
Use Management of mild to moderate hypertension; treatment of edema in congestive heart failure and nephrotic syndrome; impaired renal function
Usual Dosage Oral:
Children: 0.2-0.4 mg/kg/day divided every 12-24 hours

Adults:
Edema: 5-20 mg/dose every 24 hours
Hypertension: 2.5-5 mg/dose every 24 hours
Dosage Forms Tablet:
Zaroxolyn®: 2.5 mg, 5 mg, 10 mg
Mykrox®: 0.5 mg

Metopirone® *see* metyrapone tartrate *on next page*

metoprolol (me toe' proe lole)
Brand Names Lopressor®; Toprol XL®
Therapeutic Category Beta-Adrenergic Blocker
Use Treatment of hypertension and angina pectoris; prevention of myocardial infarction; selective inhibitor of beta$_1$-adrenergic receptors
Usual Dosage Safety and efficacy in children have not been established.
Children: Oral: 1-5 mg/kg/24 hours divided twice daily; allow 3 days between dose adjustments

Adults:
Oral: 100-450 mg/day in 2-3 divided doses, begin with 50 mg twice daily and increase doses at weekly intervals to desired effect
I.V.: 5 mg every 2 minutes for 3 doses in early treatment of myocardial infarction; thereafter give 50 mg orally every 6 hours 15 minutes after last I.V. dose and continue for 48 hours; then administer a maintenance dose of 100 mg twice daily
Dosage Forms
Injection: 1 mg/mL (5 mL)
Tablet: 50 mg, 100 mg
Tablet, sustained release: 50 mg, 100 mg, 200 mg

Metreton® Ophthalmic *see* prednisolone *on page 383*

metrizamide *see* radiological/contrast media (non-ionic) *on page 406*

Metrodin® Injection *see* urofollitropin *on page 481*

MetroGel® Topical *see* metronidazole *on this page*

MetroGel®-Vaginal *see* metronidazole *on this page*

Metro I.V.® Injection *see* metronidazole *on this page*

metronidazole (me troe ni' da zole)
Brand Names Flagyl® Oral; MetroGel® Topical; MetroGel®-Vaginal; Metro I.V.® Injection; Protostat® Oral
Therapeutic Category Amebicide; Antibiotic, Anaerobic; Antibiotic, Topical; Antiprotozoal
Use Treatment of susceptible anaerobic bacterial and protozoal infections in the following conditions: amebiasis, symptomatic and asymptomatic trichomoniasis; skin and skin structure infections; CNS infections; intra-abdominal infections; systemic anaerobic infections; topically for the treatment of acne rosacea; treatment of antibiotic-associated pseudomembranous colitis (AAPC); bacterial vaginosis
Usual Dosage
Neonates: Anaerobic infections: Oral, I.V.:
0-4 weeks: <1200 g: 7.5 mg/kg every 48 hours
(Continued)

metronidazole *(Continued)*

Postnatal age <7 days:
  1200-2000 g: 7.5 mg/kg/day given every 24 hours
  >2000 g: 15 mg/kg/day in divided doses every 12 hours
Postnatal age >7 days:
  1200-2000 g: 15 mg/kg/day in divided doses every 12 hours
  >2000 g: 30 mg/kg/day in divided doses every 12 hours

Infants and Children:
  Amebiasis: Oral: 35-50 mg/kg/day in divided doses every 8 hours
  Other parasitic infections: Oral: 15-30 mg/kg/day in divided doses every 8 hours
  Anaerobic infections: Oral, I.V.: 30 mg/kg/day in divided doses every 6 hours
  Clostridium difficile (antibiotic-associated colitis): Oral: 20 mg/kg/day divided every 6 hours
  Maximum dose: 2 g/day

Adults:
  Amebiasis: Oral: 500-750 mg every 8 hours
  Other parasitic infections: Oral: 250 mg every 8 hours or 2 g as a single dose
  Anaerobic infections: Oral, I.V.: 30 mg/kg/day in divided doses every 6 hours; not to exceed 4 g/day
  AAPC: Oral: 250-500 mg 3-4 times/day for 10-14 days
  Topical: Apply a thin film twice daily to affected areas
  Vaginal: One applicatorful in vagina each morning and evening, as needed

Dosage Forms
Gel:
  Topical: 0.75% (30 g)
  Vaginal: 0.75% (70 g)
Injection, ready to use, in normal saline: 5 mg/mL (100 mL)
Powder for injection, as hydrochloride: 500 mg
Tablet: 250 mg, 500 mg

Metubine® Iodide *see* metocurine iodide *on page 302*

metyrapone tartrate *(me teer' a pone)*

Brand Names Metopirone®
Therapeutic Category Diagnostic Agent, Hypothalamic-Pituitary ACTH Function
Use Diagnostic test for hypothalamic-pituitary ACTH function

Unlabeled use: Controlling cortisol secretion in Cushing syndrome
Usual Dosage Discontinue all corticosteroid therapy prior to and during testing
Day 1: Control period: Collect 24-hour urine to measure 17-hydroxycorticosteroids (17-OHCS) or 17-ketogenic steroids (17-KGS)
Day 2: ACTH test: Standard ACTH test (ie, administer 50 units ACTH by infusion over 8 hours and measure 24-hour urinary steroids); if results indicate adequate response, proceed with test
Day 3 to 4: Rest period
Day 5: Administer metyrapone, preferably with milk or a snack
  Children: 15 mg/kg every 4 hours for 6 doses; use a minimal 250 mg single dose
  Adults: 750 mg every 4 hours for 6 doses; single dose is approximately equivalent to 15 mg/kg
Day 6: Determine 24-hour urinary steroids for effect
Dosage Forms Tablet: 250 mg

metyrosine *(me tye' roe seen)*

Brand Names Demser®
Therapeutic Category Tyrosine Hydroxylase Inhibitor
Use Short-term management of pheochromocytoma before surgery, long-term management when surgery is contraindicated or when malignant
Usual Dosage Children >12 years and Adults: Initial: 250 mg 4 times/day, increased by 250-500 mg/day up to 4 g/day; maintenance: 2-3 g/day in 4 divided doses; for preoperative preparation, give optimum effective dosage for 5-7 days
Dosage Forms Capsule: 250 mg

Mevacor® *see* lovastatin *on page 274*
mevinolin *see* lovastatin *on page 274*

mexiletine hydrochloride (mex' i le teen)
Brand Names Mexitil®
Therapeutic Category Antiarrhythmic Agent, Class Ib
Use Management of serious ventricular arrhythmias; suppression of PVCs
Usual Dosage Oral:
Children: Range: 1.4-5 mg/kg/dose (mean: 3.3 mg/kg/dose) given every 8 hours; start with lower initial dose and increase according to effects and serum concentrations

Adults: Initial: 200 mg every 8 hours (may load with 400 mg if necessary); adjust dose every 2-3 days; usual dose: 200-300 mg every 8 hours; maximum dose: 1.2 g/day (some patients respond to every 12-hour dosing)
Dosage Forms Capsule: 150 mg, 200 mg, 250 mg

Mexitil® *see* mexiletine hydrochloride *on this page*
Mezlin® *see* mezlocillin sodium *on this page*

mezlocillin sodium (mez loe sill' in)
Brand Names Mezlin®
Therapeutic Category Antibiotic, Penicillin
Use Treatment of infections caused by susceptible gram-negative aerobic bacilli (*Klebsiella*, *Proteus*, *Escherichia coli*, *Enterobacter*, *Pseudomonas aeruginosa*, *Serratia*) involving the skin and skin structure, bone and joint, respiratory tract, urinary tract, gastrointestinal tract, as well as septicemia
Usual Dosage I.M., I.V.:
Neonates:
Postnatal age <7 days: 150 mg/kg/day divided every 12 hours
Postnatal age >7 days: 225 mg/kg/day divided every 8 hours

Children: 200-300 mg/kg/day divided every 4-6 hours; maximum: 24 g/day
Adults:
Uncomplicated urinary tract infection: 1.5-2 g every 6 hours
Serious infections: 3-4 g every 4-6 hours
Dosage Forms Powder for injection: 1 g, 2 g, 3 g, 4 g, 20 g

Miacalcin® *see* calcitonin (salmon) *on page 65*
Micatin® Topical [OTC] *see* miconazole *on this page*

miconazole (mi kon' a zole)
Brand Names Breezee® Mist Antifungal [OTC]; Fungoid® Creme; Fungoid® HC Creme; Fungoid® Tincture; Lotrimin AF® Powder [OTC]; Lotrimin AF® Spray Liquid [OTC]; Lotrimin AF® Spray Powder [OTC]; Maximum Strength Desenex® Antifungal Cream [OTC]; Micatin® Topical [OTC]; Monistat-Derm™ Topical; Monistat i.v.™ Injection; Monistat™ Vaginal; Zeasorb-AF® Powder [OTC]
Therapeutic Category Antifungal Agent, Topical; Antifungal Agent, Vaginal
Use
I.V.: Treatment of severe systemic fungal infections and fungal meningitis that are refractory to standard treatment
Topical: Treatment of vulvovaginal candidiasis and a variety of skin and mucous membrane fungal infections
Usual Dosage
Children:
I.V.: 20-40 mg/kg/day divided every 8 hours
Topical: Apply twice daily for 2-4 weeks
Vaginal: Insert contents of one applicator of vaginal cream or 100 mg suppository at bedtime for 7 days, or 200 mg suppository at bedtime for 3 days
(Continued)

miconazole (Continued)

Adults:
    I.T.: 20 mg every 3-7 days
    I.V.: Candidiasis: 600-1800 mg/day divided every 8 hours
    Topical: Apply twice daily for 2-4 weeks
    Vaginal: Insert contents of one applicator of vaginal cream or 100 mg suppository at bedtime for 7 days, or 200 mg suppository at bedtime for 3 days
    Coccidioidomycosis: 1800-3600 mg/day divided every 8 hours
    Cryptococcosis: 1200-2400 mg/day divided every 8 hours
    Paracoccidioidomycosis: 200-1200 mg/day divided every 8 hours

Dosage Forms
Cream:
    Topical, as nitrate: 2% (15 g, 30 g, 56.7 g, 85 g)
    Vaginal, as nitrate: 2% (45 g is equivalent to 7 doses)
Cream with hydrocortisone 1% (Fungoid® HC Creme): 2%
Injection: 1% [10 mg/mL] (20 mL)
Lotion, as nitrate: 2% (30 mL, 60 mL)
Powder, topical: 2% (45 g, 90 g, 113 g)
Solution, topical: 2% with alcohol (7.39 mL, 29.57 mL)
Spray, topical: 2% (105 mL)
Suppository, vaginal, as nitrate: 100 mg (7s); 200 mg (3s)

MICRhoGAM™ see Rh$_o$(D) immune globulin on page 409

microfibrillar collagen hemostat
Brand Names Avitene®; Helistat®; Hemotene®
Synonyms mch
Therapeutic Category Hemostatic Agent
Use Adjunct to hemostasis when control of bleeding by ligature in ineffective or impractical
Usual Dosage Apply dry directly to source of bleeding
Dosage Forms
Fibrous: 1 g, 5 g
Nonwoven web: 70 mm x 70 mm x 1 mm; 70 mm x 35 mm x 1 mm

Micro-K® see potassium chloride on page 378

Micronase® see glyburide on page 209

microNefrin® see epinephrine on page 167

Micronor® see norethindrone on page 332

Microstix-3® see diagnostic aids (in vitro), urine on page 137

MicroTrak® HSV 1/HSV 2 Culture Identification/Typing Test see diagnostic aids (in vitro), blood on page 136

Mictrin® see hydrochlorothiazide on page 229

Midamor® see amiloride hydrochloride on page 19

midazolam hydrochloride (mid' ay zoe lam)
Brand Names Versed®
Therapeutic Category Benzodiazepine; Hypnotic; Sedative
Use Preoperative sedation and provide conscious sedation prior to diagnostic or radiographic procedures
Usual Dosage The dose of midazolam needs to be individualized based on the patient's age, underlying diseases, and concurrent medications. Personnel and equipment needed for standard respiratory resuscitation should be immediately available during midazolam administration.

Children:
    Preoperative sedation:
        I.M.: 0.07-0.08 mg/kg 30-60 minutes presurgery

I.V.: 0.035 mg/kg/dose, repeat over several minutes as required to achieve the desired sedative effect up to a total dose of 0.1-0.2 mg/kg

Conscious sedation during mechanical ventilation: I.V.: Loading dose: 0.05-0.2 mg/kg then follow with initial continuous infusion: 1-2 mcg/kg/minute; titrate to the desired effect; usual range: 0.4-6 mcg/kg/minute

Conscious sedation for procedures:

Oral, Intranasal: 0.2-0.4 mg/kg (maximum: 15 mg) 30-45 minutes before the procedure

I.V.: 0.05 mg/kg 3 minutes before procedure

Adolescents >12 years: I.V.: 0.5 mg every 3-4 minutes until effect achieved

Adults:

Preoperative sedation: I.M.: 0.07-0.08 mg/kg 30-60 minutes presurgery; usual dose: 5 mg

Conscious sedation: I.V.: Initial: 0.5-2 mg slow I.V. over at least 2 minutes; slowly titrate to effect by repeating doses every 2-3 minutes if needed; usual total dose: 2.5-5 mg; use decreased doses in elderly

Adults, healthy <60 years: Some patients respond to doses as low as 1 mg; no more than 2.5 mg should be administered over a period of 2 minutes. Additional doses of midazolam may be administered after a 2-minute waiting period and evaluation of sedation after each dose increment. A total dose >5 mg is generally not needed. If narcotics or other CNS depressants are administered concomitantly, the midazolam dose should be reduced by 30%.

Dosage Forms Injection: 1 mg/mL (2 mL, 5 mL, 10 mL); 5 mg/mL (1 mL, 2 mL, 5 mL, 10 mL)

Midol® PM [OTC] see acetaminophen and diphenhydramine on page 4

Midol® IB [OTC] see ibuprofen on page 240

Midrin® see acetaminophen and isometheptene mucate on page 4

mih see procarbazine hydrochloride on page 388

milk of magnesia see magnesium hydroxide on page 277

Milontin® see phensuximide on page 363

Milophene® see clomiphene citrate on page 107

milrinone lactate (mil' ri none)
Brand Names Primacor®
Therapeutic Category Cardiovascular Agent, Other
Use Short-term I.V. therapy of congestive heart failure
Usual Dosage Adults: I.V.: Loading dose: 50 mcg/kg administered over 10 minutes, then 0.375-0.75 mcg/kg/min as a continuous infusion for a total daily dose of 0.59-1.13 mg/kg
Dosage Forms Injection: 1 mg/mL (5 mL, 10 mL, 20 mL)

Miltown® see meprobamate on page 288

Mini-Gamulin® Rh see Rh₀(D) immune globulin on page 409

Minipress® see prazosin hydrochloride on page 383

Minitran® Patch see nitroglycerin on page 329

Minizide® see prazosin and polythiazide on page 382

Minocin® IV Injection see minocycline hydrochloride on this page

Minocin® Oral see minocycline hydrochloride on this page

minocycline hydrochloride (mi noe sye' kleen)
Brand Names Dynacin® Oral; Minocin® IV Injection; Minocin® Oral
Therapeutic Category Antibiotic, Tetracycline Derivative
Use Treatment of susceptible bacterial infections of both gram-negative and gram-positive organisms; acne
Usual Dosage
Children 8-12 years: 4 mg/kg stat, then 4 mg/kg/day (maximum: 200 mg/day) in divided doses every 12 hours

(Continued)

307

minocycline hydrochloride (Continued)

Adults:
    Infection: Oral, I.V.: 200 mg stat, 100 mg every 12 hours
    Acne: Oral: 50 mg 1-3 times/day
Dosage Forms
  Capsule: 50 mg, 100 mg
  Capsule (Dynacin®): 50 mg, 100 mg
  Capsule, pellet-filled (Minocin®): 50 mg, 100 mg
  Injection (Minocin® IV): 100 mg
  Suspension, oral (Minocin®)50 mg/5 mL (60 mL)

Minodyl® see minoxidil on this page

minoxidil (mi nox' i dill)

Brand Names Loniten®; Minodyl®; Rogaine®
Therapeutic Category Vasodilator
Use Management of severe hypertension; treatment of male pattern baldness (alopecia androgenetica)
Usual Dosage
  Children <12 years: Hypertension: Oral: Initial: 0.1-0.2 mg/kg once daily; maximum: 5 mg/day; increase gradually every 3 days; usual dosage: 0.25-1 mg/kg/day in 1-2 divided doses; maximum: 50 mg/day

  Adults:
      Hypertension: Oral: Initial: 5 mg once daily, increase gradually every 3 days; usual dose: 10-40 mg/day in 1-2 divided doses; maximum: 100 mg/day
      Alopecia: Topical: Apply twice daily
Dosage Forms
  Solution, topical: 2% = 20 mg/metered dose (60 mL)
  Tablet: 2.5 mg, 10 mg

Mintezol® see thiabendazole on page 455

Minute-Gel® see fluoride on page 196

Miochol® see acetylcholine chloride on page 6

Miostat® Intraocular see carbachol on page 73

misoprostol (mye soe prost' ole)

Brand Names Cytotec®
Therapeutic Category Prostaglandin
Use Prevention of NSAID induced gastric ulcers
Usual Dosage Oral: 200 mcg 4 times/day with food
Dosage Forms Tablet: 100 mcg, 200 mcg

Mithracin® see plicamycin on page 373

mithramycin see plicamycin on page 373

mitomycin (mye toe mye' sin)

Brand Names Mutamycin®
Synonyms mitomycin-c; mtc
Therapeutic Category Antineoplastic Agent, Antibiotic
Use Therapy of disseminated adenocarcinoma of stomach or pancreas in combination with other approved chemotherapeutic agents; bladder cancer
Usual Dosage Children and Adults (refer to individual protocols): I.V.: 10-20 mg/m^2/dose every 6-8 weeks, or 2 mg/m^2/day for 5 days, stop for 2 days then repeat; subsequent doses should be adjusted to platelet and leukocyte response.
Dosage Forms Powder for injection: 5 mg, 20 mg, 40 mg

mitomycin-c *see* mitomycin *on previous page*

mitotane (mye' toe tane)
Brand Names Lysodren®
Synonyms o,p'-ddd
Therapeutic Category Antiadrenal Agent; Antineoplastic Agent, Miscellaneous
Use Treatment of inoperable adrenal cortical carcinoma
Usual Dosage Adults: Oral: 8-10 g/day in 3-4 divided doses; dose is changed on basis of side effect with aim of giving as high a dose as tolerated
Dosage Forms Tablet: 500 mg

mitoxantrone hydrochloride (mye toe zan' trone)
Brand Names Novantrone®
Synonyms dhad
Therapeutic Category Antineoplastic Agent, Anthracycline; Antineoplastic Agent, Antibiotic

Use FDA approved for the treatment of acute nonlymphocytic leukemia (ANLL) in adults; mitoxantrone is also found to be very active against various leukemias, lymphoma, and breast cancer, and moderately active against pediatric sarcoma
Usual Dosage I.V. (refer to individual protocols):
Leukemias:
Children ≤2 years: 0.4 mg/kg/day once daily for 3-5 days
Children >2 years and Adults: 8-12 mg/m^2/day once daily for 5 days or 12 mg/m^2/day once daily for 3 days

Solid tumors:
Children: 18-20 mg/m^2 every 3-4 weeks
Adults: 12-14 mg/m^2 every 3-4 weeks
Dosage Forms Injection, as base: 2 mg/mL (10 mL, 12.5 mL, 15 mL)

Mitran® Oral *see* chlordiazepoxide *on page 89*
Mitrolan® Chewable Tablet [OTC] *see* calcium polycarbophil *on page 70*
Mivacron® *see* mivacurium chloride *on this page*

mivacurium chloride (mye va kyoo' ree um)
Brand Names Mivacron®
Therapeutic Category Neuromuscular Blocker Agent, Nondepolarizing
Use Produces skeletal muscle relaxation during surgery after induction of general anesthesia, increases pulmonary compliance during assisted respiration, facilitates endotracheal intubation
Usual Dosage I.V.:
Children 2-12 years: 0.2 mg/kg over 5-15 seconds; continuous infusion: 14 mcg/kg
Adults: Initial: 0.15 mg/kg administered over 5-15 seconds
Dosage Forms
Infusion, in D$_5$W: 0.5 mg/mL (50 mL)
Injection: 2 mg/mL (5 mL, 10 mL)

mmr *see* measles, mumps and rubella vaccines, combined *on page 281*
M-M-R® II *see* measles, mumps and rubella vaccines, combined *on page 281*
Moban® *see* molindone hydrochloride *on next page*
Moctanin® *see* monoctanoin *on next page*
Modane® Soft [OTC] *see* docusate *on page 153*
Modane® Plus [OTC] *see* docusate and phenolphthalein *on page 154*
Modane® [OTC] *see* phenolphthalein *on page 362*

Modane® Bulk [OTC] *see* psyllium *on page 398*
Modicon™ *see* ethinyl estradiol and norethindrone *on page 178*
modified Dakin's solution *see* sodium hypochlorite solution *on page 428*
modified Shohl's solution *see* sodium citrate and citric acid *on page 427*
Moducal® [OTC] *see* glucose polymers *on page 209*
Moduretic® *see* amiloride and hydrochlorothiazide *on page 19*
Moi-Stir® [OTC] *see* saliva substitute *on page 417*

molindone hydrochloride (moe lin' done)
Brand Names Moban®
Therapeutic Category Antipsychotic Agent
Use Management of psychotic disorder
Usual Dosage Oral: 50-75 mg/day; up to 225 mg/day
Dosage Forms
Concentrate, oral: 20 mg/mL (120 mL)
Tablet: 5 mg, 10 mg, 25 mg, 50 mg, 100 mg

Mol-Iron® [OTC] *see* ferrous sulfate *on page 189*
molybdenum *see* trace metals *on page 465*
Molypen® *see* trace metals *on page 465*
mom *see* magnesium hydroxide *on page 277*

mometasone furoate (moe met' a sone)
Brand Names Elocon® Topical
Therapeutic Category Corticosteroid, Topical (Medium Potency)
Use Relief of inflammatory and pruritic manifestations of corticosteroid-responsive dermatoses
Usual Dosage Apply to area once daily, do not use occlusive dressings
Dosage Forms
Cream: 0.1% (15 g, 45 g)
Lotion: 0.1% (30 mL, 60 mL)
Ointment, topical: 0.1% (15 g, 45 g)

mom/mineral oil emulsion *see* magnesium hydroxide and mineral oil emulsion *on page 277*
monacolin k *see* lovastatin *on page 274*
Monilia skin test *see* Candida albicans (Monilia) *on page 71*
Monistat-Derm™ Topical *see* miconazole *on page 305*
Monistat i.v.™ Injection *see* miconazole *on page 305*
Monistat™ Vaginal *see* miconazole *on page 305*
Monocid® *see* cefonicid sodium *on page 80*
Monoclate-P® *see* antihemophilic factor (human) *on page 29*
monoclonal antibody *see* muromonab-CD3 *on page 314*

monoctanoin (mon oh ock' ta noyn)
Brand Names Moctanin®
Synonyms monooctanoin
Therapeutic Category Gallstone Dissolution Agent
Use Solubilize cholesterol gallstones that are retained in the biliary tract after cholecystectomy
Usual Dosage Administer via T-tube into common bile duct at rate of 3-5 mL/hour at pressure of 10 mL water for 7-21 days
Dosage Forms Solution: 120 mL

Mono-Diff® *see* diagnostic aids (*in vitro*), blood *on page 136*

Monodox® Oral *see* doxycycline *on page 158*

Mono-Gesic® *see* salsalate *on page 417*

Monoket® *see* isosorbide mononitrate *on page 254*

Mononine® *see* factor ix complex (human) *on page 184*

monooctanoin *see* monoctanoin *on previous page*

Monopril® *see* fosinopril *on page 202*

Monospot® *see* diagnostic aids (*in vitro*), blood *on page 136*

Monosticon® Dri-Dot® *see* diagnostic aids (*in vitro*), blood *on page 136*

Mono-Sure® *see* diagnostic aids (*in vitro*), blood *on page 136*

Mono-Test® *see* diagnostic aids (*in vitro*), blood *on page 136*

8-mop *see* methoxsalen *on page 296*

more attenuated enders strain *see* measles virus vaccine, live, attenuated *on page 281*

More-Dophilus® [OTC] *see* lactobacillus *on page 261*

moricizine hydrochloride (mor i' siz een)
Brand Names Ethmozine®
Therapeutic Category Antiarrhythmic Agent, Class I
Use Treatment of ventricular tachycardia and life-threatening ventricular arrhythmias; a Class I antiarrhythmic agent
Usual Dosage Adults: Oral: 200-300 mg every 8 hours, adjust dosage at 150 mg/day at 3-day intervals
Dosage Forms Tablet: 200 mg, 250 mg, 300 mg

morphine sulfate
Brand Names Astramorph™ PF Injection; Duramorph® Injection; MS Contin® Oral; MSIR® Oral; OMS® Oral; Oramorph SR™ Oral; RMS® Rectal; Roxanol™ Oral; Roxanol SR™ Oral
Synonyms ms
Therapeutic Category Analgesic, Narcotic
Use Relief of moderate to severe acute and chronic pain; pain of myocardial infarction; relieves dyspnea of acute left ventricular failure and pulmonary edema; preanesthetic medication
Usual Dosage Doses should be titrated to appropriate effect; when changing routes of administration in chronically treated patients, please note that oral doses are approximately $\frac{1}{6}$ as effective as parenteral dose

Infants and Children:
Oral: Tablet and solution (prompt release): 0.2-0.5 mg/kg/dose every 4-6 hours as needed; tablet (controlled release): 0.3-0.6 mg/kg/dose every 12 hours
I.M., I.V., S.C.: 0.1-0.2 mg/kg/dose every 2-4 hours as needed; usual maximum: 15 mg/dose; may initiate at 0.05 mg/kg/dose
I.V., S.C. continuous infusion: Sickle cell or cancer pain: 0.025-2 mg/kg/hour; postoperative pain: 0.01-0.04 mg/kg/hour
Sedation/analgesia for procedures: I.V.: 0.05-0.1 mg/kg 5 minutes before the procedure

Adolescents >12 years: Sedation/analgesia for procedures: I.V.: 3-4 mg and repeat in 5 minutes if necessary

Adults:
Oral: Prompt release: 10-30 mg every 4 hours as needed; controlled release: 15-30 mg every 8-12 hours
I.M., I.V., S.C.: 2.5-20 mg/dose every 2-6 hours as needed; usual: 10 mg/dose every 4 hours as needed
I.V., S.C. continuous infusion: 0.8-10 mg/hour; may increase depending on pain relief/adverse effects; usual range up to 80 mg/hour
Epidural: Initial: 5 mg in lumbar region; if inadequate pain relief within 1 hour, give 1-2 mg, maximum dose: 10 mg/24 hours

(Continued)

morphine sulfate *(Continued)*

Intrathecal ($\frac{1}{10}$ of epidural dose): 0.2-1 mg/dose; repeat doses **not** recommended

Dosage Forms

Injection: 0.5 mg/mL (10 mL); 1 mg/mL (10 mL, 30 mL, 60 mL); 2 mg/mL (1 mL, 2 mL, 60 mL); 3 mg/mL (50 mL); 4 mg/mL (1 mL, 2 mL); 5 mg/mL (1 mL, 30 mL); 8 mg/mL (1 mL, 2 mL); 10 mg/mL (1 mL, 2 mL, 10 mL); 15 mg/mL (1 mL, 2 mL, 20 mL)

Injection:

Preservative free:

Astramorph™ PF, Duramorph®: 0.5 mg/mL (2 mL, 10 mL); 1 mg/mL (2 mL, 10 mL)

Infumorph™: 10 mg/mL (20 mL); 25 mg/mL (20 mL)

I.V. via PCA pump: 1 mg/mL (10 mL, 30 mL, 60 mL); 5 mg/mL (30 mL)

I.V. infusion preparation: 25 mg/mL (4 mL, 10 mL, 20 mL)

Solution, oral: 10 mg/5 mL (5 mL, 10 mL, 100 mL, 120 mL, 500 mL); 20 mg/5 mL (2.5 mL, 5 mL, 100 mL, 120 mL, 500 mL);

OMS®, Roxanol™: 20 mg/mL (30 mL, 120 mL, 240 mL)

Suppository, rectal (RMS®, Roxanol™): 5 mg, 10 mg, 20 mg, 30 mg

Tablet (MSIR®): 15 mg, 30 mg

Tablet:

Controlled release (MS Contin®, Roxanol SR™): 15 mg, 30 mg, 60 mg, 100 mg, 200 mg

Soluble: 10 mg, 15 mg, 30 mg

Sustained release (Oramorph SR™): 30 mg, 60 mg, 100 mg

morrhuate sodium *(mor' yoo ate)*

Brand Names Scleromate®

Therapeutic Category Sclerosing Agent

Use Treatment of small, uncomplicated varicose veins of the lower extremities

Usual Dosage I.V.:

Children 1-18 years: Esophageal hemorrhage: 2, 3, or 4 mL of 5% solution repeated every 3-4 days until bleeding is controlled, then every 6 weeks until varices obliterated

Adults: 50-250 mg, repeated at 5- to 7-day intervals (50-100 mg for small veins, 150-250 mg for large veins)

Dosage Forms Injection: 50 mg/mL (5 mL)

Motofen® *see* difenoxin and atropine *on page 143*

Motrin® *see* ibuprofen *on page 240*

Motrin® IB [OTC] *see* ibuprofen *on page 240*

Motrin® IB Sinus [OTC] *see* pseudoephedrine and ibuprofen *on page 398*

moxalactam disodium *(mox' a lak tam)*

Brand Names Moxam®

Synonyms latamoxef disodium

Therapeutic Category Antibiotic, Cephalosporin (Third Generation)

Use Treatment of serious respiratory, urinary, CNS, intra-abdominal, gynecologic, and skin infections; septicemia, bacteremia, and meningitis; third generation cephalosporin

Usual Dosage I.M., I.V.:

Neonates: 50 mg/kg every 8-12 hours

Children: 50 mg/kg every 6-8 hours; maximum recommended dose for children and neonates: 200 mg/kg/day up to 12 g/day

Adults: 2-6 g/day in divided doses every 8-12 hours for 5-10 days or up to 14 days; life-threatening infections: 4 g every 8 hours

Dosage Forms Injection: 1 g, 2 g, 10 g

Moxam® *see* moxalactam disodium *on this page*

6-mp *see* mercaptopurine *on page 288*

M-Prednisol® Injection *see* methylprednisolone *on page 300*

M-R-VAX® II *see* measles and rubella vaccines, combined *on page 281*

ms *see* morphine sulfate *on page 311*

MS Contin® Oral *see* morphine sulfate *on page 311*

MSIR® Oral *see* morphine sulfate *on page 311*

msta *see* mumps skin test antigen *on this page*

mtc *see* mitomycin *on page 308*

M.T.E.-4® *see* trace metals *on page 465*

M.T.E.-5® *see* trace metals *on page 465*

M.T.E.-6® *see* trace metals *on page 465*

mtx *see* methotrexate *on page 295*

Mucomyst® *see* acetylcysteine *on page 6*

Mucoplex® [OTC] *see* vitamin b complex *on page 490*

Mucosol® *see* acetylcysteine *on page 6*

Multe-Pak-4® *see* trace metals *on page 465*

multiple sulfonamides *see* sulfadiazine, sulfamethazine, and sulfamerazine *on page 440*

Multistix® [OTC] *see* diagnostic aids (*in vitro*), urine *on page 137*

Multitest CMI® *see* skin test antigens, multiple *on page 424*

multivitamins/fluoride *see* vitamin, multiple (pediatric) *on page 491*

Multi Vit® Drops [OTC] *see* vitamin, multiple (pediatric) *on page 491*

mumps skin test antigen
Synonyms msta
Therapeutic Category Diagnostic Agent, Skin Test
Use Assess the status of cell-mediated immunity
Usual Dosage Children and Adults: 0.1 mL intradermally into flexor surface of the forearm; examine reaction site in 24-48 hours; a positive reaction is ≥1.5 mm diameter induration
Dosage Forms Injection: 1 mL (10 tests)

Mumpsvax® *see* mumps virus vaccine, live, attenuated *on this page*

mumps virus vaccine, live, attenuated
Brand Names Mumpsvax®
Therapeutic Category Vaccine, Live Virus
Use Immunization against mumps in children ≥12 months and adults
Usual Dosage 1 vial (5000 units) S.C. in outer aspect of the upper arm
Dosage Forms Injection: Single dose

mupirocin (myoo peer' oh sin)
Brand Names Bactroban® Nasal Spray; Bactroban® Topical
Synonyms pseudomonic acid a
Therapeutic Category Antibiotic, Topical
Use Topical treatment of impetigo; nasal spray used to reduce nasal carriage in children
Usual Dosage Children and Adults: Topical: Apply small amount 3 times/day for 5 days
Dosage Forms
Ointment, topical: 2% (15 g)
Spray, nasal

Murine® Ear Drops [OTC] *see* carbamide peroxide *on page 74*

Murine® Plus Ophthalmic [OTC] *see* tetrahydrozoline hydrochloride *on page 452*

Muro 128® Ophthalmic [OTC] *see* sodium chloride *on page 426*

Murocoll-2® Ophthalmic *see* phenylephrine and scopolamine *on page 364*

muromonab-CD3 (myoo roe moe' nab)
  Brand Names Orthoclone™ OKT3
  Synonyms monoclonal antibody; okt3
  Therapeutic Category Immunosuppressant Agent
  Use Treatment of acute allograft rejection in renal transplant patients; effective in reversing acute hepatic, cardiac, and bone marrow transplant rejection episodes resistant to conventional treatment
  Usual Dosage I.V. (refer to individual protocols):
    Children <30 kg: 2.5 mg/day once daily for 10-14 days

    Adults: 5 mg/day once daily for 10-14 days

    Children and Adults: Methylprednisolone sodium succinate 1 mg/kg I.V. given prior to first muromonab-CD3 administration and I.V. hydrocortisone sodium succinate 50-100 mg given 30 minutes after administration are strongly recommended to decrease the incidence of reactions to the first dose; patient temperature should not exceed 37.8°C (100°F) at time of administration
  Dosage Forms Injection: 5 mg/5 mL

Mus-Lac® *see* chlorzoxazone *on page 99*

Mustargen® Hydrochloride *see* mechlorethamine hydrochloride *on page 282*

mustine *see* mechlorethamine hydrochloride *on page 282*

Mutamycin® *see* mitomycin *on page 308*

M.V.C.® 9 + 3 *see* vitamin, multiple (injectable) *on page 491*

M.V.I.®-12 *see* vitamin, multiple (injectable) *on page 491*

M.V.I.® Concentrate *see* vitamin, multiple (injectable) *on page 491*

M.V.I.® Pediatric *see* vitamin, multiple (injectable) *on page 491*

Myambutol® *see* ethambutol hydrochloride *on page 176*

Myapap® Drops [OTC] *see* acetaminophen *on page 2*

Mycelex® *see* clotrimazole *on page 109*

Mycelex®-G *see* clotrimazole *on page 109*

Mycifradin® Sulfate Oral *see* neomycin sulfate *on page 323*

Mycifradin® Sulfate Topical *see* neomycin sulfate *on page 323*

Mycitracin® [OTC] *see* bacitracin, neomycin, and polymyxin b *on page 43*

Mycobutin® Oral *see* rifabutin *on page 411*

Mycogen® II Topical *see* nystatin and triamcinolone *on page 335*

Mycolog®-II Topical *see* nystatin and triamcinolone *on page 335*

Myconel® Topical *see* nystatin and triamcinolone *on page 335*

Mycostatin® Oral *see* nystatin *on page 334*

Mycostatin® Topical *see* nystatin *on page 334*

Mycostatin® Vaginal *see* nystatin *on page 334*

Mydfrin® Ophthalmic Solution *see* phenylephrine hydrochloride *on page 364*

Mydriacyl® Ophthalmic *see* tropicamide *on page 476*

Mykrox® *see* metolazone *on page 303*

Mylanta Gas® [OTC] *see* simethicone *on page 423*

Mylanta®-II [OTC] *see* aluminum hydroxide, magnesium hydroxide, and simethicone *on page 16*

Mylanta® [OTC] *see* aluminum hydroxide, magnesium hydroxide, and simethicone *on page 16*

Mylanta® Natural Fiber Supplement [OTC] *see* psyllium *on page 398*

Myleran® *see* busulfan *on page 62*

Mylicon® [OTC] *see* simethicone *on page 423*

Mylosar® *see* azacitidine *on page 40*

Myminic® Syrup [OTC] *see* chlorpheniramine and phenylpropanolamine *on page 94*

Myminic® Expectorant [OTC] *see* guaifenesin and phenylpropanolamine *on page 215*

Myochrysine® *see* gold sodium thiomalate *on page 211*

Myoflex® [OTC] *see* triethanolamine salicylate *on page 470*

Myotonachol™ *see* bethanechol chloride *on page 53*

Myphetane DC® *see* brompheniramine, phenylpropanolamine, and codeine *on page 60*

Myphetapp® [OTC] *see* brompheniramine and phenylpropanolamine *on page 59*

Myprozine® Ophthalmic *see* natamycin *on page 320*

Mysoline® *see* primidone *on page 386*

Mytelase® Caplets® *see* ambenonium chloride *on page 17*

Mytrex® F Topical *see* nystatin and triamcinolone *on page 335*

Mytussin® AC *see* guaifenesin and codeine *on page 214*

Mytussin® DAC *see* guaifenesin, pseudoephedrine, and codeine *on page 217*

Mytussin® [OTC] *see* guaifenesin *on page 213*

Mytussin® DM [OTC] *see* guaifenesin and dextromethorphan *on page 214*

nabilone (na' bi lone
 Brand Names Cesamet®
 Therapeutic Category Antiemetic
 Use Treat nausea and vomiting associated with cancer chemotherapy
 Usual Dosage Oral:
   Children >4 years:
     <18 kg: 0.5 mg twice daily
     18-30 kg: 1 mg twice daily
     >30 kg: 1 mg 3 times/day

   Adults: 1-2 mg twice daily beginning 1-3 hours before chemotherapy is administered and continuing around the clock until 1 dose after chemotherapy is completed; maximum daily dose: 6 mg divided in 3 doses
 Dosage Forms Capsule: 1 mg

nabumetone (na byoo' me tone)
 Brand Names Relafen®
 Therapeutic Category Nonsteroidal Anti-Inflammatory Agent (NSAID), Oral
 Use Management of osteoarthritis and rheumatoid arthritis
 Usual Dosage Adults: Oral: 1000 mg/day; an additional 500-1000 mg may be needed in some patients to obtain more symptomatic relief; may be administered once or twice daily
 Dosage Forms Tablet: 500 mg, 750 mg

n-acetyl-p-aminophenol *see* acetaminophen *on page 2*

NaCl *see* sodium chloride *on page 426*

nadolol (nay doe' lole)
Brand Names Corgard™
Therapeutic Category Antianginal Agent; Beta-Adrenergic Blocker
Use Treatment of hypertension and angina pectoris; prevention of myocardial infarction; prophylaxis of migraine headaches
Usual Dosage Adults: Initial: 40 mg once daily; increase gradually; usual dosage: 40-80 mg/day; may need up to 240-320 mg/day; doses as high as 640 mg/day have been used
Dosage Forms Tablet: 20 mg, 40 mg, 80 mg, 120 mg, 160 mg

nafarelin acetate (naf' a re lin)
Brand Names Synarel™
Therapeutic Category Hormone, Posterior Pituitary; Luteinizing Hormone-Releasing Hormone Analog
Use Treatment of endometriosis, including pain and reduction of lesions
Usual Dosage Adults: 1 spray in 1 nostril each morning and evening for 6 months
Dosage Forms Solution, nasal: 2 mg/mL (10 mL)

Nafazair® Ophthalmic see naphazoline hydrochloride on page 319
Nafcil™ Injection see nafcillin sodium on this page

nafcillin sodium (naf sill' in)
Brand Names Nafcil™ Injection; Nallpen® Injection; Unipen® Injection; Unipen® Oral
Synonyms ethoxynaphthamido penicillin sodium
Therapeutic Category Antibiotic, Penicillin
Use Treatment of susceptible bacterial infections such as osteomyelitis, septicemia, endocarditis, and CNS infections due to penicillinase-producing strains of Staphylococcus
Usual Dosage
Neonates: I.M., I.V.:
　0-4 weeks: <1200 g: 50 mg/kg/day in divided doses every 12 hours
　<7 days:
　　1200-2000 g: 50 mg/kg/day in divided doses every 12 hours
　　>2000 g: 60 mg/kg/day in divided doses every 8 hours
　>7 days:
　　1200-2000 g: 75 mg/kg/day in divided doses every 8 hours
　　>2000 g: 100 mg/kg/day in divided doses every 6 hours

Children: I.M., I.V.:
　Mild to moderate infections: 50-100 mg/kg/day in divided doses every 6 hours
　Severe infections: 100-200 mg/kg/day in divided doses every 4-6 hours
　Maximum dose: 12 g/day
　Oral: 50-100 mg/kg/day divided every 6 hours

Adults:
　Oral: 250-500 mg every 4-6 hours, up to 1 g every 4-6 hours for more severe infections
　I.M.: 500 mg every 4-6 hours
　I.V.: 500-2000 mg every 4-6 hours
Dosage Forms
Capsule: 250 mg
Powder for injection: 500 mg, 1 g, 2 g, 4 g, 10 g
Tablet: 500 mg

naftifine hydrochloride (naf' ti feen)
Brand Names Naftin® Topical
Therapeutic Category Antifungal Agent, Topical
Use Topical treatment of tinea cruris and tinea corporis
Usual Dosage Adults: Topical: Apply twice daily
Dosage Forms
Cream: 1% (15 g, 30 g, 60 g)
Gel, topical: 1% (20 g, 40 g, 60 g)

Naftin® Topical *see* naftifine hydrochloride *on previous page*
NaHCO₃ *see* sodium bicarbonate *on page 426*

nalbuphine hydrochloride (nal' byoo feen)
Brand Names Nubain®
Therapeutic Category Analgesic, Narcotic
Use Relief of moderate to severe pain
Usual Dosage I.M., I.V., S.C.: 10 mg/70 kg every 3-6 hours
Dosage Forms Injection: 10 mg/mL (1 mL, 10 mL); 20 mg/mL (1 mL, 10 mL)

Naldecon® *see* chlorpheniramine, phenyltoloxamine, phenylpropanolamine and phenylephrine *on page 96*

Naldecon-EX® Children's Syrup [OTC] *see* guaifenesin and phenylpropanolamine *on page 215*

Naldecon® Senior EX [OTC] *see* guaifenesin *on page 213*

Naldecon® Senior DX [OTC] *see* guaifenesin and dextromethorphan *on page 214*

Naldecon® DX Adult Liquid [OTC] *see* guaifenesin, phenylpropanolamine, and dextromethorphan *on page 217*

Naldelate® *see* chlorpheniramine, phenyltoloxamine, phenylpropanolamine and phenylephrine *on page 96*

Nalfon® *see* fenoprofen calcium *on page 187*

Nalgest® *see* chlorpheniramine, phenyltoloxamine, phenylpropanolamine and phenylephrine *on page 96*

nalidixic acid (nal i dix' ik)
Brand Names NegGram®
Synonyms nalidixinic acid
Therapeutic Category Antibiotic, Quinolone
Use Urinary tract infections
Usual Dosage Oral:
   Children: 55 mg/kg/day divided every 6 hours; suppressive therapy is 33 mg/kg/day divided every 6 hours

   Adults: 1 g 4 times/day for 2 weeks; then suppressive therapy of 500 mg 4 times/day
Dosage Forms
   Suspension, oral (raspberry flavor): 250 mg/5 mL (473 mL)
   Tablet: 250 mg, 500 mg, 1 g

nalidixinic acid *see* nalidixic acid *on this page*

Nallpen® Injection *see* nafcillin sodium *on previous page*

***n*-allylnoroxymorphone hydrochloride** *see* naloxone hydrochloride *on this page*

naloxone hydrochloride (nal ox' one)
Brand Names Narcan® Injection
Synonyms *n*-allylnoroxymorphone hydrochloride
Therapeutic Category Antidote, Narcotic Agonist
Use Reverses CNS and respiratory depression in suspected narcotic overdose; neonatal opiate depression; coma of unknown etiology; used investigationally for shock, PCP and alcohol ingestion, and Alzheimer's disease
(Continued)

naloxone hydrochloride *(Continued)*

Usual Dosage I.M., I.V. (preferred), intratracheal, S.C. (give undiluted injection):

Neonates: Narcotic-induced asphyxia: 0.01-0.1 mg/kg every 2-3 minutes as needed; may need to repeat every 1-2 hours

Infants and Children: Postanesthesia narcotic reversal: 0.01 mg/kg; may repeat every 2-3 minutes as needed based on response

Opiate intoxication: Birth (including premature infants) to 5 years or <20 kg: 0.1 mg/kg; repeat every 2-3 minutes if needed; may need to repeat doses every 20-60 minutes
>5 years or ≥20 kg: 2 mg/dose; if no response, repeat every 2-3 minutes; may need to repeat doses every 20-60 minutes

Children and Adults: Continuous infusion: I.V.: If continuous infusion is required, calculate dosage/hour based on effective intermittent dose used and duration of adequate response seen, titrate dose

Adults: 0.4-2 mg every 2-3 minutes as needed; may need to repeat doses every 20-60 minutes; if no response is observed for a total of 10 mg, re-evaluate patient for possibility of a drug or disease process unresponsive to naloxone. **Note:** Use 0.1-0.2 mg increments in patients who are opioid dependent and in postoperative patients to avoid large cardiovascular changes

Dosage Forms
Injection: 0.4 mg/mL (1 mL, 2 mL, 10 mL); 1 mg/mL (2 mL, 10 mL)
Injection, neonatal: 0.02 mg/mL (2 mL)

Nalspan® *see* chlorpheniramine, phenyltoloxamine, phenylpropanolamine and phenylephrine *on page 96*

naltrexone hydrochloride (nal trex' one)

Brand Names Trexan™ Oral
Therapeutic Category Antidote, Narcotic Agonist
Use Adjunct to the maintenance of an opioid-free state in detoxified individual
Usual Dosage Do not give until patient is opioid-free for 7-10 days as required by urine analysis

Adults: Oral: 25 mg; if no withdrawal signs within 1 hour give another 25 mg; maintenance regimen is flexible, variable and individualized (50 mg/day to 100-150 mg 3 times/week)
Dosage Forms Tablet: 50 mg

nandrolone (nan' droe lone)

Brand Names Anabolin® Injection; Androlone®-D Injection; Androlone® Injection; Deca-Durabolin® Injection; Durabolin® Injection; Hybolin™ Decanoate Injection; Hybolin™ Improved Injection; Neo-Durabolic Injection
Therapeutic Category Androgen
Use Control of metastatic breast cancer; management of anemia of renal insufficiency
Usual Dosage
Children 2-13 years: 25-50 mg every 3-4 weeks

Adults:
Male: 100-200 mg/week
Female: 50-100 mg/week
Dosage Forms
Injection, as phenpropionate, in oil: 25 mg/mL (5 mL); 50 mg/mL (2 mL)
Injection, as decanoate, in oil: 50 mg/mL (1 mL, 2 mL); 100 mg/mL (1 mL, 2 mL); 200 mg/mL (1 mL)
Injection, repository, as decanoate: 50 mg/mL (2 mL); 100 mg/mL (2 mL); 200 mg/mL (2 mL)

naphazoline and antazoline

Brand Names Albalon-A® Ophthalmic; Antazoline-V® Ophthalmic; Vasocon-A® Ophthalmic
Therapeutic Category Ophthalmic Agent, Vasoconstrictor
Use Topical ocular congestion, irritation and itching

Usual Dosage Ophthalmic: 1-2 drops every 3-4 hours
Dosage Forms Solution: Naphazoline hydrochloride 0.05% and antazoline phosphate 0.5% (15 mL)

naphazoline and pheniramine
Brand Names Naphcon-A® Ophthalmic
Synonyms pheniramine and naphazoline
Therapeutic Category Ophthalmic Agent, Vasoconstrictor
Use Topical ocular vasoconstrictor
Usual Dosage Ophthalmic: 1-2 drops every 3-4 hours
Dosage Forms Solution, ophthalmic: Naphazoline hydrochloride 0.025% and pheniramine 0.3% (15 mL)

naphazoline hydrochloride (naf az' oh leen)
Brand Names AK-Con® Ophthalmic; Albalon® Liquifilm® Ophthalmic; Allerest® Eye Drops [OTC]; Clear Eyes® [OTC]; Comfort® Ophthalmic [OTC]; Degest® 2 Ophthalmic [OTC]; Estivin® II Ophthalmic [OTC]; I-Naphline® Ophthalmic; Nafazair® Ophthalmic; Naphcon Forte® Ophthalmic; Naphcon® Ophthalmic [OTC]; Opcon® Ophthalmic; Privine® Nasal [OTC]; VasoClear® Ophthalmic [OTC]; Vasocon Regular® Ophthalmic
Therapeutic Category Adrenergic Agonist Agent, Ophthalmic; Decongestant, Nasal; Nasal Agent, Vasoconstrictor; Ophthalmic Agent, Vasoconstrictor
Use Topical ocular vasoconstrictor; will temporarily relieve congestion, itching, and minor irritation, and to control hyperemia in patients with superficial corneal vascularity
Usual Dosage
Nasal:
    Children:
        <6 years: Not recommended (especially infants) due to CNS depression
        6-12 years: 1 spray of 0.05% into each nostril, repeat in 3 hours if necessary
        Children >12 years and Adults: 0.05%, instill 2 drops or sprays every 3-6 hours if needed; therapy should not exceed 3-5 days or more frequently than every 3 hours
Ophthalmic:
        Children <6 years: Not recommended for use due to CNS depression (especially in infants)
        Children >6 years and Adults: Instill 1-2 drops into conjunctival sac of affected eye(s) every 3-4 hours; therapy generally should not exceed 3-4 days
Dosage Forms Solution:
Nasal:
    Drops: 0.05% (20 mL)
    Spray: 0.05% (15 mL)
Ophthalmic: 0.012% (7.5 mL, 30 mL); 0.02% (15 mL); 0.03% (15 mL); 0.1% (15 mL)

Naphcon-A® Ophthalmic *see* naphazoline and pheniramine *on this page*
Naphcon Forte® Ophthalmic *see* naphazoline hydrochloride *on this page*
Naphcon® Ophthalmic [OTC] *see* naphazoline hydrochloride *on this page*
Naprosyn® *see* naproxen *on this page*

naproxen (na prox' en)
Brand Names Aleve® [OTC]; Anaprox®; Naprosyn®
Synonyms naproxen sodium
Therapeutic Category Analgesic, Non-Narcotic; Anti-inflammatory Agent; Nonsteroidal Anti-Inflammatory Agent (NSAID), Oral
Use Management of inflammatory disease and rheumatoid disorders (including juvenile rheumatoid arthritis); acute gout; mild to moderate pain; dysmenorrhea; fever
(Continued)

ALPHABETICAL LISTING OF DRUGS

naproxen *(Continued)*

Usual Dosage Oral (as naproxen):
Children >2 years:
Antipyretic or analgesic: 5-7 mg/kg/dose every 8-12 hours
Juvenile rheumatoid arthritis: 10 mg/kg/day, up to a maximum of 1000 mg/day divided twice daily

Adults:
Rheumatoid arthritis, osteoarthritis, and ankylosing spondylitis: 500-1000 mg/day in 2 divided doses
Mild to moderate pain or dysmenorrhea: Initial: 500 mg, then 250 mg every 6-8 hours; maximum: 1250 mg/day

Dosage Forms
Suspension, oral: 125 mg/5 mL (15 mL, 30 mL, 480 mL)
Tablet, as sodium (Anaprox™): 275 mg (250 mg base); 550 mg (500 mg base)
Tablet:
Aleve™: 200 mg
Naprosyn™: 250 mg, 375 mg, 500 mg

naproxen sodium *see* naproxen *on previous page*

Naqua® *see* trichlormethiazide *on page 469*

Narcan® Injection *see* naloxone hydrochloride *on page 317*

Nardil® *see* phenelzine sulfate *on page 360*

Nasabid® *see* guaifenesin and pseudoephedrine *on page 216*

Nasacort® *see* triamcinolone *on page 467*

Nasahist B® Injection *see* brompheniramine maleate *on page 59*

Nasalcrom® Nasal Solution *see* cromolyn sodium *on page 118*

Nasalide® Nasal Aerosol *see* flunisolide *on page 195*

Natabec® [OTC] *see* vitamin, multiple (prenatal) *on page 491*

Natabec® FA [OTC] *see* vitamin, multiple (prenatal) *on page 491*

Natabec® Rx *see* vitamin, multiple (prenatal) *on page 491*

Natacyn® Ophthalmic *see* natamycin *on this page*

Natalins® [OTC] *see* vitamin, multiple (prenatal) *on page 491*

Natalins® Rx *see* vitamin, multiple (prenatal) *on page 491*

natamycin (na ta mye' sin)

Brand Names Myprozine™ Ophthalmic; Natacyn® Ophthalmic
Synonyms pimaricin
Therapeutic Category Antifungal Agent, Ophthalmic
Use Treatment of blepharitis, conjunctivitis, and keratitis caused by susceptible fungi (*Aspergillus, Candida*), *Cephalosporium, Curvularia, Fusarium, Penicillium, Microsporum, Epidermophyton, Blastomyces dermatitidis, Coccidioides immitis, Cryptococcus neoformans, Histoplasma capsulatum, Sporothrix schenckii, Trichomonas vaginalis*
Usual Dosage Adults: 1 drop in conjunctival sac every 1-2 hours, after 3-4 days dose may be reduced to one drop 6-8 times/day; usual course of therapy: 2-3 weeks
Dosage Forms Suspension, ophthalmic: 5% (15 mL)

natural lung surfactant *see* beractant *on page 51*

Naturetin® *see* bendroflumethiazide *on page 47*

Naus-A-Way® [OTC] *see* phosphorated carbohydrate solution *on page 367*

Nausetrol® [OTC] *see* phosphorated carbohydrate solution *on page 367*

Navane® *see* thiothixene *on page 458*

N D Clear® *see* chlorpheniramine and pseudoephedrine *on page 94*

ND-Stat® Injection *see* brompheniramine maleate *on page 59*

Nebcin® Injection *see* tobramycin *on page 462*

NebuPent™ Inhalation *see* pentamidine isethionate *on page 355*

nedocromil sodium (ne doe kroe' mil)
Brand Names Tilade® Inhalation Aerosol
Therapeutic Category Antiasthmatic; Antihistamine, Inhalation
Use Maintenance therapy in patients with mild to moderate bronchial asthma
Usual Dosage Adults: Inhalation: 2 inhalations 4 times daily
Dosage Forms Aerosol: 1.75 mg/activation (16.2 g)

N.E.E.® 1/35 *see* ethinyl estradiol and norethindrone *on page 178*

nefazodone (nef ay' zoe done)
Brand Names Serzone®
Therapeutic Category Antidepressant, Monoamine Oxidase Inhibitor
Use Treatment of depression
Dosage Forms Tablet:

NegGram® *see* nalidixic acid *on page 317*

Neisseria gonorrhoeae *see* diagnostic aids (*in vitro*), other *on page 137*

Nelova™ *see* ethinyl estradiol and norethindrone *on page 178*

Nembutal® *see* pentobarbital *on page 356*

Neo-Calglucon® [OTC] *see* calcium glubionate *on page 68*

Neocidin® Ophthalmic Solution *see* neomycin, polymyxin b, and gramicidin *on next page*

Neo-Cortef® *see* neomycin and hydrocortisone *on next page*

NeoDecadron® *see* neomycin and dexamethasone *on this page*

Neo-Durabolic Injection *see* nandrolone *on page 318*

Neofed® [OTC] *see* pseudoephedrine *on page 397*

Neo-fradin® Oral *see* neomycin sulfate *on page 323*

Neoloid® [OTC] *see* castor oil *on page 78*

Neomixin® *see* bacitracin, neomycin, and polymyxin b *on page 43*

neomycin and dexamethasone
Brand Names NeoDecadron®
Synonyms dexamethasone and neomycin
Therapeutic Category Antibiotic, Ophthalmic; Corticosteroid, Ophthalmic
Use Treatment of steroid responsive inflammatory conditions of the palpebral and bulbar conjunctiva, lid, cornea, and anterior segment of the globe
Usual Dosage Apply thin coat 3-4 times/day until favorable response is observed, then reduce dose to one application/day
Dosage Forms
Cream: Neomycin sulfate 0.5% [5 mg/g] and dexamethasone 0.1% [1 mg/g] (15 g, 30 g)
Ointment, ophthalmic: Neomycin sulfate 0.35% [3.5 mg/g] and dexamethasone 0.05% [0.5 mg/g] (3.5 g)
Solution, ophthalmic: Neomycin sulfate 0.35% [3.5 mg/mL] and dexamethasone 0.1% [1 mg/mL] (15 mL)

neomycin and fluocinolone
Brand Names Neo-Synalar®
Therapeutic Category Antibiotic, Topical; Corticosteroid, Topical (Medium Potency)
Use Treatment of corticosteroid-responsive dermatoses with secondary infection
(Continued)

neomycin and fluocinolone *(Continued)*
Usual Dosage Topical: Apply to area in a thin film 2-4 times/day
Dosage Forms Cream: Neomycin sulfate 0.5% and fluocinolone acetonide 0.025% (15 g, 30 g, 60 g)

neomycin and hydrocortisone
Brand Names Neo-Cortef®
Therapeutic Category Antibiotic, Topical; Corticosteroid, Topical (Low Potency)
Use Treatment of susceptible topical bacterial infections with associated inflammation
Usual Dosage Topical: Apply to area in a thin film 2-4 times/day
Dosage Forms
Cream: Neomycin sulfate 0.5% and hydrocortisone 1% (20 g)
Ointment, topical: Neomycin sulfate 0.5% and hydrocortisone 0.5% (20 g); neomycin sulfate 0.5% and hydrocortisone 1% (20 g)
Solution, ophthalmic: Neomycin sulfate 0.5% and hydrocortisone 0.5% (5 mL)

neomycin and polymyxin b
Brand Names Neosporin® Cream [OTC]; Neosporin® G.U. Irrigant
Synonyms polymyxin b and neomycin
Therapeutic Category Antibiotic, Urinary Irrigation; Antibiotic, Topical
Use Short-term use as a continuous irrigant or rinse in the urinary bladder to prevent bacteriuria and gram-negative rod septicemia associated with the use of indwelling catheters; to help prevent infection in minor cuts, scrapes, and burns
Usual Dosage Children and Adults:
Topical: Apply cream 2-4 times/day
Bladder irrigation: Continuous irrigant or rinse in the urinary bladder for up to 10 days where 1 mL is added to 1 L of normal saline with administration rate adjusted to patient's urine output; usually no more than 1 L of irrigant is used per day
Dosage Forms
Cream: Neomycin sulfate 3.5 mg and polymyxin b sulfate 10,000 units per g (0.94 g, 15 g)
Solution, irrigant: Neomycin sulfate 40 mg and polymyxin b sulfate 200,000 units per mL (1 mL, 20 mL)

neomycin, polymyxin b, and dexamethasone
Brand Names AK-Trol® Ophthalmic; Dexacidin® Ophthalmic; Dexasporin® Ophthalmic; Infectrol® Ophthalmic; Maxitrol® Ophthalmic; Ocu-Trol® Ophthalmic
Therapeutic Category Antibiotic, Ophthalmic
Use Steroid-responsive inflammatory ocular conditions in which a corticosteroid is indicated and where bacterial infection or a risk of bacterial infection exists
Usual Dosage Children and Adults: Ophthalmic:
Ointment: Place a small amount ($\sim$ ½") in the affected eye 3-4 times/day or apply at bedtime as an adjunct with drops
Solution: Instill 1-2 drops into affected eye(s) every 4-6 hours; in severe disease drops may be used hourly and tapered to discontinuation
Dosage Forms
Ointment, ophthalmic: Neomycin sulfate 3.5 mg, polymyxin b sulfate 10,000 units, and dexamethasone 0.1% per g (3.5 g)
Suspension, ophthalmic: Neomycin sulfate 3.5 mg, polymyxin b sulfate 10,000 units, and dexamethasone 0.1% per mL (5 mL)

neomycin, polymyxin b, and gramicidin
Brand Names AK-Spore® Ophthalmic Solution; Neocidin® Ophthalmic Solution; Neosporin® Ophthalmic Solution; Neotricin® Ophthalmic Solution; Ocu-Spor-G® Ophthalmic Solution; Ocutricin® Ophthalmic Solution; Tri-Thalmic® Ophthalmic Solution
Therapeutic Category Antibiotic, Ophthalmic
Use Treatment of superficial ocular infection, infection prophylaxis in minor skin abrasions

Usual Dosage Ophthalmic: Drops: 1-2 drops 4-6 times/day or more frequently as required for severe infections

Dosage Forms Solution, ophthalmic: Polymyxin B sulfate 10,000 units, neomycin sulfate 1.75 mg, and gramicidin 0.025 mg per mL (1 mL, 2 mL, 10 mL)

neomycin, polymyxin b, and hydrocortisone

Brand Names AK-Spore H.C.® Otic; AntibiOtic® Otic; Bacticort® Otic; Cortatrigen® Otic; Cortisporin® Ophthalmic Suspension; Cortisporin® Otic; Cortisporin® Topical Cream; Drotic® Otic; LazerSporin-C® Otic; Octicair® Otic; Ocutricin® HC Otic; Otocort® Otic; Otomycin-HPN® Otic; Otosporin® Otic; PediOtic® Otic

Therapeutic Category Antibiotic, Ophthalmic; Antibiotic, Otic; Antibiotic, Topical; Corticosteroid, Ophthalmic; Corticosteroid, Otic; Corticosteroid, Topical (Low Potency)

Use Treatment of topical bacterial infections caused by susceptible bacteria and when the use of an anti-inflammatory is indicated

Usual Dosage Duration of use should be limited to 10 days unless otherwise directed by the physician

Adults and Children: Ophthalmic:
Ointment: Apply to the affected eye every 3-4 hours
Suspension: 1 drop every 3-4 hours

Children: Otic: Solution and suspension: 3 drops into affected ear 3-4 times/day
Adults: Otic: Solution and suspension: 4 drops into affected ear 3-4 times/day

Dosage Forms
Cream, topical: Neomycin sulfate 5 mg, polymyxin b sulfate 10,000 units, and hydrocortisone 10 mg per mL (7.5 g)
Solution, otic: Neomycin sulfate 5 mg, polymyxin b sulfate 10,000 units, and hydrocortisone 10 mg per mL (10 mL)
Suspension:
Ophthalmic: Neomycin sulfate 5 mg, polymyxin b sulfate 10,000 units, and hydrocortisone 10 mg per mL (7.5 mL)
Otic: Neomycin sulfate 5 mg, polymyxin b sulfate 10,000 units, and hydrocortisone 10 mg per mL (10 mL)

neomycin, polymyxin b, and prednisolone

Brand Names Poly-Pred® Liquifilm® Ophthalmic

Therapeutic Category Antibiotic, Ophthalmic; Corticosteroid, Ophthalmic

Use Steroid-responsive inflammatory ocular condition in which bacterial infection or a risk of bacterial ocular infection exists

Usual Dosage Children and Adults: Ophthalmic: Instill 1-2 drops every 3-4 hours; acute infections may require every 30-minute instillation initially with frequency of administration reduced as the infection is brought under control. To treat the lids: Instill 1-2 drops every 3-4 hours, close the eye and rub the excess on the lids and lid margins.

Dosage Forms Suspension: Neomycin sulfate 0.35%, polymyxin b sulfate 10,000 units, and prednisolone acetate 0.5% per mL (5 mL, 10 mL)

neomycin sulfate (nee oh mye' sin)

Brand Names Mycifradin® Sulfate Oral; Mycifradin® Sulfate Topical; Neo-fradin® Oral; Neo-Tabs® Oral

Therapeutic Category Ammonium Detoxicant; Antibiotic, Aminoglycoside; Antibiotic, Topical

Use Given orally to prepare GI tract for surgery; treat minor skin infections; treat diarrhea caused by *E. coli*; adjunct in the treatment of hepatic encephalopathy

Usual Dosage
Neonates: Oral: Necrotizing enterocolitis: 50-100 mg/kg/day divided every 6 hours

Children: Oral:
Preoperative intestinal antisepsis: 90 mg/kg/day divided every 4 hours for 2 days; or 25 mg/kg at 1 PM, 2 PM, and 11 PM on the day preceding surgery as an adjunct to mechanical cleansing of the intestine and in combination with erythromycin base

(Continued)

neomycin sulfate *(Continued)*

Hepatic coma: 50-100 mg/kg/day in divided doses every 6-8 hours or 2.5-7 g/m^2/day divided every 4-6 hours for 5-6 days not to exceed 12 g/day

Children and Adults: Topical: Apply ointment 1-4 times/day; topical solutions containing 0.1% to 1% neomycin have been used for irrigation

Adults: Oral:

Preoperative intestinal antisepsis: 1 g each hour for 4 doses then 1 g every 4 hours for 5 doses; or 1 g at 1 PM, 2 PM, and 11 PM on day preceding surgery as an adjunct to mechanical cleansing of the bowel and oral erythromycin; or 6 g/day divided every 4 hours for 2-3 days

Hepatic coma: 500-2000 mg every 6-8 hours or 4-12 g/day divided every 4-6 hours for 5-6 days

Chronic hepatic insufficiency: Oral: 4 g/day for an indefinite period

Dosage Forms

Cream: 0.5% (15 g)

Injection: 500 mg

Ointment, topical: 0.5% (15 g, 30 g, 120 g)

Solution, oral: 125 mg/5 mL (480 mL)

Tablet: 500 mg [base 300 mg]

neonatal trace metals *see* trace metals *on page 465*

Neopap® [OTC] *see* acetaminophen *on page 2*

Neoquess® Injection *see* dicyclomine hydrochloride *on page 142*

Neosar® Injection *see* cyclophosphamide *on page 121*

Neosporin® G.U. Irrigant *see* neomycin and polymyxin b *on page 322*

Neosporin® Ophthalmic Ointment *see* bacitracin, neomycin, and polymyxin b *on page 43*

Neosporin® Ophthalmic Solution *see* neomycin, polymyxin b, and gramicidin *on page 322*

Neosporin® Topical Ointment [OTC] *see* bacitracin, neomycin, and polymyxin b *on page 43*

Neosporin® Cream [OTC] *see* neomycin and polymyxin b *on page 322*

neostigmine *(nee oh stig' meen)*

Brand Names Prostigmin® Injection; Prostigmin® Oral

Therapeutic Category Antidote, Neuromuscular Blocking Agent; Cholinergic Agent; Diagnostic Agent, Myasthenia Gravis

Use Treatment of myasthenia gravis and to prevent and treat postoperative bladder distention and urinary retention; reversal of the effects of nondepolarizing neuromuscular blocking agents after surgery

Usual Dosage

Myasthenia gravis: Diagnosis: I.M.:

Children: 0.04 mg/kg as a single dose

Adults: 0.02 mg/kg as a single dose

Myasthenia gravis: Treatment:

Children:

I.M., I.V., S.C.: 0.01-.04 mg/kg every 2-4 hours

Oral: 2 mg/kg/day divided every 3-4 hours

Adults:

I.M., I.V., S.C.: 0.5-2.5 mg every 1-3 hours

Oral: 15 mg/dose every 3-4 hours

Reversal of nondepolarizing neuromuscular blockade after surgery in conjunction with atropine or glycopyrrolate: I.V.:

Infants: 0.025-0.1 mg/kg/dose

Children: 0.025-0.08 mg/kg/dose

Adults: 0.5-2.5 mg; total dose not to exceed 5 mg

Bladder atony: Adults: I.M., S.C.:
Prevention: 0.25 mg every 4-6 hours for 2-3 days
Treatment: 0.5-1 mg every 3 hours for 5 doses after bladder has emptied
Dosage Forms
Injection, as methylsulfate: 0.25 mg/mL (1 mL); 0.5 mg/mL (1 mL, 10 mL); 1 mg/mL (10 mL)
Tablet, as bromide: 15 mg

Neo-Synalar® *see* neomycin and fluocinolone *on page 321*

Neo-Synephrine® 12 Hour Nasal Solution [OTC] *see* oxymetazoline hydrochloride *on page 343*

Neo-Synephrine® Ophthalmic Solution *see* phenylephrine hydrochloride *on page 364*

Neo-Synephrine® Nasal Solution [OTC] *see* phenylephrine hydrochloride *on page 364*

Neo-Tabs® Oral *see* neomycin sulfate *on page 323*

Neothylline® *see* dyphylline *on page 161*

Neotrace-4® *see* trace metals *on page 465*

Neotricin® Ophthalmic Solution *see* neomycin, polymyxin b, and gramicidin *on page 322*

NeoVadrin® B Complex [OTC] *see* vitamin b complex *on page 490*

NeoVadrin® [OTC] *see* vitamin, multiple (prenatal) *on page 491*

Nephro-Calci® [OTC] *see* calcium carbonate *on page 66*

Nephrocaps® [OTC] *see* vitamin b complex with vitamin c and folic acid *on page 490*

Nephro-Fer™ [OTC] *see* ferrous fumarate *on page 189*

Nephrox Suspension [OTC] *see* aluminum hydroxide *on page 15*

Neptazane® *see* methazolamide *on page 293*

Nervocaine® *see* lidocaine hydrochloride *on page 267*

Nesacaine® *see* chloroprocaine hydrochloride *on page 91*

Nesacaine®-MPF *see* chloroprocaine hydrochloride *on page 91*

Nestrex® *see* pyridoxine hydrochloride *on page 400*

1-*n*-ethyl sisomicin *see* netilmicin sulfate *on this page*

netilmicin sulfate (ne til mye' sin)
Brand Names Netromycin® Injection
Synonyms 1-*n*-ethyl sisomicin
Therapeutic Category Antibiotic, Aminoglycoside
Use Short-term treatment of serious or life-threatening infections including septicemia, perito-
nitis, intra-abdominal abscess, lower respiratory tract infections, urinary tract infections, skin,
bone and joint infections caused by sensitive *Pseudomonas aeruginosa*, *Escherichia coli*,
Proteus, *Klebsiella*, *Serratia*, *Enterobacter*, *Citrobacter*, and *Staphylococcus*
Usual Dosage I.M., I.V.:
Neonates <6 weeks: 2-3.25 mg/kg/dose every 12 hours

Children 6 weeks to 12 years: 1-2.5 mg/kg/dose every 8 hours

Children >12 years and Adults: 1.5-2 mg/kg/dose every 8-12 hours
Dosage Forms
Injection: 100 mg/mL (1.5 mL)
Injection:
Neonatal: 10 mg/mL (2 mL)
Pediatric: 25 mg/mL (2 mL)

ALPHABETICAL LISTING OF DRUGS

Netromycin® Injection *see* netilmicin sulfate *on previous page*
Neucalm® *see* hydroxyzine *on page 237*
Neupogen® Injection *see* filgrastim *on page 191*
Neuramate® *see* meprobamate *on page 288*
Neurontin® *see* gabapentin *on page 203*
Neut® Injection *see* sodium bicarbonate *on page 426*
Neutra-Phos® *see* potassium phosphate and sodium phosphate *on page 380*
Neutrexin™ Injection *see* trimetrexate glucuronate *on page 473*
Neutrogena® Acne Mask [OTC] *see* benzoyl peroxide *on page 50*
Neutrogena® T/Derm *see* coal tar *on page 110*
New Decongestant® *see* chlorpheniramine, phenyltoloxamine, phenylpropanolamine and phenylephrine *on page 96*
NGT® Topical *see* nystatin and triamcinolone *on page 335*
Niacels™ [OTC] *see* niacin *on this page*

niacin (nye' a sin)
Brand Names Niacels™ [OTC]; Nicobid® [OTC]; Nicolar® [OTC]; Nicotinex [OTC]; Slo-Niacin" [OTC]
Synonyms nicotinic acid; vitamin b$_3$
Therapeutic Category Antilipemic Agent; Vitamin, Water Soluble
Use Adjunctive treatment of hyperlipidemias; peripheral vascular disease and circulatory disorders; treatment of pellagra; dietary supplement
Usual Dosage
Children: Pellagra: Oral, I.M., I.V.: 50-100 mg/dose 3 times/day
Oral: Recommended daily allowances:
0-1 year: 6-8 mg/day
2-6 years: 9-11 mg/day
7-10 years: 16 mg/day
>10 years: 15-18 mg/day

Adults: Oral:
Hyperlipidemia: 1.5-6 g/day in 3 divided doses with or after meals
Pellagra: 50 mg 3-10 times/day, maximum: 500 mg/day
Niacin deficiency: 10-20 mg/day, maximum: 100 mg/day
Dosage Forms
Capsule, timed release: 125 mg, 250 mg, 300 mg, 400 mg, 500 mg
Elixir: 50 mg/5 mL (473 mL, 4000 mL)
Injection: 100 mg/mL (30 mL)
Tablet: 25 mg, 50 mg, 100 mg, 250 mg, 500 mg
Tablet, timed release: 150 mg, 250 mg, 500 mg, 750 mg

niacinamide (nye a sin' a mide)
Synonyms nicotinamide
Therapeutic Category Vitamin, Water Soluble
Use Prophylaxis and treatment of pellagra
Usual Dosage Oral:
Children: Pellagra: 100-300 mg/day

Adults: 50 mg 3-10 times/day
Pellagra: 300-500 mg/day
Hyperlipidemias: 1-2 g 3 times/day
Dosage Forms Tablet: 50 mg, 100 mg, 125 mg, 250 mg, 500 mg

nicardipine hydrochloride (nye kar' de peen)
Brand Names Cardene"; Cardene" SR
Therapeutic Category Antianginal Agent; Calcium Channel Blocker
Use Chronic stable angina; management of essential hypertension

Usual Dosage Adults:
Oral: 40 mg 3 times/day (allow 3 days between dose increases)
Oral, sustained release: Initial: 30 mg twice daily, titrate up to 60 mg twice daily
I.V.: (Dilute to 0.1 mg/mL) Initial: 5 mg/hour increased by 2.5 mg/hour every 15 minutes to a maximum of 15 mg/hour
Oral to I.V. dose:
    20 mg every 8 hours = I.V. 0.5 mg/hour
    30 mg every 8 hours = I.V. 1.2 mg/hour
    40 mg every 8 hours = I.V. 2.2 mg/hour
Dosage Forms
Capsule: 20 mg, 30 mg
Capsule, sustained release: 30 mg, 45 mg, 60 mg
Injection: 2.5 mg/mL (10 mL)

Niclocide® *see niclosamide on this page*

niclosamide (ni kloe' sa mide)
Brand Names Niclocide®
Therapeutic Category Anthelmintic
Use Treatment of intestinal beef, fish, and dwarf tapeworm infections
Usual Dosage Oral:
Beef and fish tapeworm:
  Children:
    11-34 kg: 1 g as a single dose
    >34 kg: 1.5 g as a single dose
  Adults: 2 g (4 tablets) in a single dose

Dwarf tapeworm:
  Children:
    11-34 kg: 1 g chewed thoroughly in a single dose the first day, then 0.5 g/day for next 6 days
    >34 kg: 1.5 g in a single dose the first day, then 1 g/day for 6 days
  Adults: 2 g in a single daily dose for 7 days
Dosage Forms Tablet, chewable (vanilla flavor): 500 mg

Nicobid® [OTC] *see niacin on previous page*
Nicoderm® Patch *see nicotine on this page*
Nicolar® [OTC] *see niacin on previous page*
Nicorette® DS Gum *see nicotine on this page*
Nicorette® Gum *see nicotine on this page*
nicotinamide *see niacinamide on previous page*

nicotine (nik oh teen')
Brand Names Habitrol™ Patch; Nicoderm® Patch; Nicorette® DS Gum; Nicorette® Gum; Nicotrol® Patch; ProStep® Patch
Therapeutic Category Smoking Deterrent
Use Treatment aid to giving up smoking while participating in a behavioral modification program, under medical supervision
Usual Dosage
Gum: Chew 1 piece of gum when urge to smoke, up to 30 pieces/day; most patients require 10-12 pieces of gum/day
Transdermal patches: Apply new patch every 24 hours to nonhairy, clean, dry skin on the upper body or upper outer arm; each patch should be applied to a different site; start with the 21 mg/day or 22 mg/day patch, except those patients with stable coronary artery disease should start with 14 mg/day; most patients the dosage can be reduced after 6-8 weeks; progressively lower doses are used every 2 weeks, with complete nicotine elimination achieved after 10 weeks
(Continued)

nicotine *(Continued)*
Dosage Forms
Patch, transdermal:
Habitrol™: 21 mg/day; 14 mg/day; 7 mg/day (30 systems/box)
Nicoderm'": 21 mg/day; 14 mg/day; 7 mg/day (14 systems/box)
ProStep'": 22 mg/day; 11 mg/day (7 systems/box)
Pieces, chewing gum, as polacrilex: 2 mg/square (96 pieces/box); 4 mg/square (96 pieces/box)

Nicotinex [OTC] *see* niacin *on page 326*
nicotinic acid *see* niacin *on page 326*
Nicotrol® Patch *see* nicotine *on previous page*
Nico-Vert® [OTC] *see* meclizine hydrochloride *on page 282*
Nidryl® Oral [OTC] *see* diphenhydramine hydrochloride *on page 149*

nifedipine (nye fed' i peen)
Brand Names Adalat®; Adalat® CC; Procardia®; Procardia XL®
Therapeutic Category Antianginal Agent; Calcium Channel Blocker
Use Angina, hypertrophic cardiomyopathy, hypertension (sustained release only)
Usual Dosage Oral, S.L.:
Children:
Hypertensive emergencies: 0.25-0.5 mg/kg/dose
Hypertrophic cardiomyopathy: 0.6-0.9 mg/kg/24 hours in 3-4 divided doses

Adults: Initial: 10 mg 3 times/day as capsules or 30-60 mg once daily as sustained release tablet; maintenance: 10-30 mg 3-4 times/day (capsules); maximum: 180 mg/24 hours (capsules) or 120 mg/day (sustained release)
Dosage Forms
Capsule, liquid-filled (Adalat'", Procardia'"): 10 mg, 20 mg
Tablet, extended release (Adalat'" CC): 30 mg, 60 mg, 90 mg
Tablet, sustained release (Procardia XL'"): 30 mg, 60 mg, 90 mg

Niferex®-PN *see* vitamin, multiple (prenatal) *on page 491*
Niferex® [OTC] *see* polysaccharide-iron complex *on page 376*
Nilstat® Oral *see* nystatin *on page 334*
Nilstat® Topical *see* nystatin *on page 334*
Nilstat® Vaginal *see* nystatin *on page 334*
Nimbus® *see* diagnostic aids (*in vitro*), urine *on page 137*

nimodipine (nye moe' di peen)
Brand Names Nimotop'"
Therapeutic Category Calcium Channel Blocker
Use Improvement of neurological deficits due to spasm following subarachnoid hemorrhage from ruptured congenital intracranial aneurysms who are in good neurological condition postictus
Usual Dosage Adults: Oral: 60 mg every 4 hours for 21 days, start therapy within 96 hours after subarachnoid hemorrhage
Dosage Forms Capsule, liquid-filled: 30 mg

Nimotop® *see* nimodipine *on this page*
Nipent™ Injection *see* pentostatin *on page 357*
Nitro-Bid® I.V. Injection *see* nitroglycerin *on next page*
Nitro-Bid® Ointment *see* nitroglycerin *on next page*

Nitro-Bid® Oral *see* nitroglycerin *on this page*

Nitrocine® Oral *see* nitroglycerin *on this page*

Nitrodisc® Patch *see* nitroglycerin *on this page*

Nitro-Dur® Patch *see* nitroglycerin *on this page*

nitrofural *see* nitrofurazone *on this page*

nitrofurantoin (nye troe fyoor an' toyn)
Brand Names Furadantin®; Furalan®; Furan®; Furanite®; Macrobid®; Macrodantin®
Therapeutic Category Antibiotic, Miscellaneous
Use Prevention and treatment of urinary tract infections caused by susceptible gram-negative and some gram-positive organisms; *Pseudomonas, Serratia,* and most species of *Proteus* are generally resistant to nitrofurantoin
Usual Dosage Oral:
Children >1 month: 5-7 mg/kg/day divided every 6 hours; maximum: 400 mg/day
Chronic therapy: 1-2 mg/kg/day in divided doses every 12-24 hours; maximum dose: 400 mg/day

Adults: 50-100 mg/dose every 6 hours (not to exceed 400 mg/24 hours)
Prophylaxis: 50-100 mg/dose at bedtime
Dosage Forms
Capsule: 50 mg, 100 mg
Capsule:
Macrocrystal: 25 mg, 50 mg, 100 mg
Macrocrystal/monohydrate: 100 mg
Suspension, oral: 25 mg/5 mL (470 mL)

nitrofurazone (nye troe fyoor' a zone)
Brand Names Furacin® Topical
Synonyms nitrofural
Therapeutic Category Antibacterial, Topical
Use Antibacterial agent used in second and third degree burns and skin grafting
Usual Dosage Children and Adults: Topical: Apply once daily or every few days to lesion or place on gauze
Dosage Forms
Cream: 0.2% (4 g, 28 g)
Powder, topical: 0.2% (14 g)
Soluble dressing, topical: 0.2% (28 g, 56 g, 454 g, 480 g)

Nitrogard® Buccal *see* nitroglycerin *on this page*

nitrogen mustard *see* mechlorethamine hydrochloride *on page 282*

nitroglycerin (nye troe gli' ser in)
Brand Names Deponit® Patch; Minitran® Patch; Nitro-Bid® I.V. Injection; Nitro-Bid® Ointment; Nitro-Bid® Oral; Nitrocine® Oral; Nitrodisc® Patch; Nitro-Dur® Patch; Nitrogard® Buccal; Nitroglyn® Oral; Nitrolingual® Translingual Spray; Nitrol® Ointment; Nitrong® Oral Tablet; Nitrostat® Sublingual; Transdermal-NTG® Patch; Transderm-Nitro® Patch; Tridil® Injection
Synonyms glyceryl trinitrate; nitroglycerol; ntg
Therapeutic Category Antianginal Agent; Nitrate; Vasodilator, Coronary
Use Angina pectoris; I.V. for congestive heart failure (especially when associated with acute myocardial infarction); pulmonary hypertension; hypertensive emergencies occurring perioperatively (especially during cardiovascular surgery)
Usual Dosage Note: Hemodynamic and antianginal tolerance often develops within 24-48 hours of continuous nitrate administration

Children: Pulmonary hypertension: Continuous infusion: Start 0.25-0.5 mcg/kg/minute and titrate by 1 mcg/kg/minute at 20- to 60-minute intervals to desired effect; usual dose: 1-3 mcg/kg/minute; maximum: 5 mcg/kg/minute
(Continued)

329

nitroglycerin (Continued)

Adults:

Oral: 2.5-9 mg 2-4 times/day (up to 26 mg 4 times/day)

I.V.: 5 mcg/minute, increase by 5 mcg/minute every 3-5 minutes to 20 mcg/minute; if no response at 20 mcg/minute increase by 10 mcg/minute every 3-5 minutes, up to 200 mcg/minute

Sublingual: 0.2-0.6 mg every 5 minutes for maximum of 3 doses in 15 minutes; may also use prophylactically 5-10 minutes prior to activities which may provoke an attack

Ointment: 1" to 2" every 8 hours up to 4" to 5" every 4 hours

Patch, transdermal: 0.2-0.4 mg/hour initially and titrate to doses of 0.4-0.8 mg/hour; tolerance is minimized by using a patch on period of 12-14 hours and patch off period of 10-12 hours

Translingual: 1-2 sprays into mouth under tongue every 3-5 minutes for maximum of 3 doses in 15 minutes, may also be used 5-10 minutes prior to activities which may provoke an attack prophylactically

Buccal: Initial: 1 mg every 3-5 hours while awake (3 times/day); titrate dosage upward if angina occurs with tablet in place

May need to use nitrate-free interval (10-12 hours/day) to avoid tolerance development; tolerance may possibly be reversed with acetylcysteine; gradually decrease dose in patients receiving NTG for prolonged period to avoid withdrawal reaction

Dosage Forms

Capsule, sustained release: 2.5 mg, 6.5 mg, 9 mg

Injection: 0.5 mg/mL (10 mL); 0.8 mg/mL (10 mL); 5 mg/mL (1 mL, 5 mL, 10 mL, 20 mL); 10 mg/mL (5 mL, 10 mL)

Ointment, topical (Nitrol®): 2% [20 mg/g] (30 g, 60 g)

Patch, transdermal, topical: Systems designed to deliver 2.5, 5, 7.5, 10, or 15 mg NTG over 24 hours

Spray, translingual: 0.4 mg/metered spray (13.8 g)

Tablet:

Buccal, controlled release: 1 mg, 2 mg, 3 mg

Sublingual (Nitrostat®): 0.15 mg, 0.3 mg, 0.4 mg, 0.6 mg

Sustained release: 2.6 mg, 6.5 mg, 9 mg

nitroglycerol see nitroglycerin on previous page

Nitroglyn® Oral see nitroglycerin on previous page

Nitrolingual® Translingual Spray see nitroglycerin on previous page

Nitrol® Ointment see nitroglycerin on previous page

Nitrong® Oral Tablet see nitroglycerin on previous page

Nitropress® see nitroprusside sodium on this page

nitroprusside sodium (nye troe pruss' ide)

Brand Names Nitropress®

Synonyms sodium nitroferricyanide; sodium nitroprusside

Therapeutic Category Vasodilator

Use Management of hypertensive crises; congestive heart failure; used for controlled hypotension to reduce bleeding during surgery

Usual Dosage I.V.:

Children: Continuous infusion:

Initial: 1 mcg/kg/minute by continuous I.V. infusion; increase in increments of 1 mcg/kg/minute at intervals of 20-60 minutes; titrating to the desired response

Usual dose: 3 mcg/kg/minute; rarely need >4 mcg/kg/minute

Maximum: 10 mcg/kg/minute. Dilute 15 mg x weight (kg) to 250 mL D₅W, then dose in mcg/kg/minute = infusion rate in mL/hour

Adults: Begin at 5 mcg/kg/minute; increase in increments of 5 mcg/kg/minute (up to 20 mcg/kg/minute), then in increments of 10-20 mcg/kg/minute; titrating to the desired hemodynamic effect or the appearance of headache or nausea. When >500 mcg/kg is administered by prolonged infusion of faster than 2 mcg/kg/minute, cyanide is generated faster than an unaided patient can handle.

Dosage Forms Injection: 10 mg/mL (5 mL); 25 mg/mL (2 mL)

Nitrostat® Sublingual *see* nitroglycerin *on page 329*

Nix™ Creme Rinse *see* permethrin *on page 359*

nizatidine (ni za' ti deen)
Brand Names Axid®
Therapeutic Category Histamine-2 Antagonist
Use Treatment and maintenance of duodenal ulcer
Usual Dosage Adults: Active duodenal ulcer: Oral:
Treatment: 300 mg at bedtime or 150 mg twice daily
Maintenance: 150 mg/day
Dosage Forms Capsule: 150 mg, 300 mg

Nizoral® Oral *see* ketoconazole *on page 258*

Nizoral® Topical *see* ketoconazole *on page 258*

Nostrilla® [OTC] *see* oxymetazoline hydrochloride *on page 343*

n-methylhydrazine *see* procarbazine hydrochloride *on page 388*

Nolahist® [OTC] *see* phenindamine tartrate *on page 361*

Nolamine® *see* chlorpheniramine, phenindamine, and phenylpropanolamine *on page 95*

Nolex® LA *see* guaifenesin and phenylpropanolamine *on page 215*

Nolvadex® Oral *see* tamoxifen citrate *on page 445*

nonoxynol 9 (noe nox' ee nole)
Brand Names Because® [OTC]; Delfen® [OTC]; Emko® [OTC]; Encare® [OTC]; Gynol II® [OTC]; Intercept™ [OTC]; Koromex® [OTC]; Ramses® [OTC]; Semicid® [OTC]; Shur-Seal® [OTC]
Therapeutic Category Spermicide
Use Spermatocide in contraception
Usual Dosage Insert into vagina at least 15 minutes before intercourse
Dosage Forms Vaginal:
Cream: 2% (103.5 g)
Foam: 12.5% (60 g)
Jelly: 2% (81 g, 126 g)

No Pain-HP® [OTC] *see* capsaicin *on page 72*

noradrenaline acid tartrate *see* norepinephrine bitartrate *on this page*

Norcept-E® 1/35 *see* ethinyl estradiol and norethindrone *on page 178*

Norcet® *see* hydrocodone and acetaminophen *on page 230*

Norcuron® *see* vecuronium *on page 485*

nordeoxyguanosine *see* ganciclovir *on page 204*

Nordette® *see* ethinyl estradiol and levonorgestrel *on page 178*

Nordryl® Injection *see* diphenhydramine hydrochloride *on page 149*

Nordryl® Oral *see* diphenhydramine hydrochloride *on page 149*

norepinephrine bitartrate (nor ep i nef' rin)
Brand Names Levophed® Injection
Synonyms levarterenol bitartrate; noradrenaline acid tartrate
Therapeutic Category Adrenergic Agonist Agent; Alpha-Adrenergic Agonist
(Continued)

norepinephrine bitartrate *(Continued)*
Use Treatment of shock which persists after adequate fluid volume replacement
Usual Dosage I.V.:
  Children: Initial: 0.05-0.1 mcg/kg/minute, titrate to desired effect; rate (mL/hour) = dose (mcg/kg/minute) x weight (kg) x 60 minutes/hour divided by concentration (mcg/mL)
  Adults: 8-12 mcg/minute as an infusion; initiate at 4 mcg/minute and titrate to desired response
  Note: Dose stated in terms of norepinephrine base
Dosage Forms Injection: 1 mg/mL (4 mL)

Norethin™ 1/35E *see* ethinyl estradiol and norethindrone *on page 178*

norethindrone (nor eth in' drone)
Brand Names Aygestin®; Micronor®; Norlutate®; Norlutin®; NOR-Q.D.®
Synonyms norethisterone
Therapeutic Category Contraceptive, Oral; Contraceptive, Progestin Only; Progestin
Use Treatment of amenorrhea; abnormal uterine bleeding; endometriosis, oral contraceptive in combination with estrogens
Usual Dosage Adolescents and Adults: Oral:
  Amenorrhea and abnormal uterine bleeding: 2.5-10 mg on days 5-25 of menstrual cycle
  Endometriosis: 5 mg/day for 14 days; increase at increments of 2.5 mg/day every 2 weeks up to 15 mg/day
Dosage Forms
  Tablet: 0.35 mg, 5 mg
  Tablet, as acetate: 5 mg

norethindrone acetate and ethinyl estradiol *see* ethinyl estradiol and norethindrone *on page 178*

norethindrone and mestranol *see* mestranol and norethindrone *on page 290*

norethisterone *see* norethindrone *on this page*

norethynodrel and mestranol *see* mestranol and norethynodrel *on page 290*

Norflex® *see* orphenadrine citrate *on page 339*

norfloxacin (nor flox' a sin)
Brand Names Chibroxin™ Ophthalmic; Noroxin® Oral
Therapeutic Category Antibiotic, Quinolone
Use Complicated and uncomplicated urinary tract infections caused by susceptible gram-negative and gram-positive bacteria
Usual Dosage
  Oral: Adults: 400 mg twice daily for 7-21 days depending on infection
  Ophthalmic: Children >1 year and Adults: Instill 1-2 drops in affected eye(s) 4 times/day for up to 7 days
Dosage Forms
  Solution, ophthalmic: 0.3% [3 mg/mL] (5 mL)
  Tablet: 400 mg

Norgesic® *see* orphenadrine, aspirin and caffeine *on page 339*

Norgesic® Forte *see* orphenadrine, aspirin and caffeine *on page 339*

norgestimate and ethinyl estradiol *see* ethinyl estradiol and norgestimate *on page 179*

norgestrel (nor jess' trel)
Brand Names Ovrette®
Therapeutic Category Contraceptive, Oral; Progestin
Use Prevention of pregnancy; treatment of hypermenorrhea, endometriosis, female hypogonadism

Usual Dosage Administer daily, starting the first day of menstruation, take one tablet at the same time each day, every day of the year. If one dose is missed, take as soon as remembered, then next tablet at regular time; if two doses are missed, take one tablet and discard the other, then take daily at usual time; if three doses are missed, use an additional form of birth control until menses or pregnancy is ruled out
Dosage Forms Tablet: 0.075 mg

norgestrel and ethinyl estradiol *see* ethinyl estradiol and norgestrel *on page 180*

Norinyl® 1+35 *see* ethinyl estradiol and norethindrone *on page 178*

Norinyl® 1+50 *see* mestranol and norethindrone *on page 290*

Norisodrine® *see* isoproterenol *on page 253*

Norlestrin® *see* ethinyl estradiol and norethindrone *on page 178*

Norlutate® *see* norethindrone *on previous page*

Norlutin® *see* norethindrone *on previous page*

normal saline *see* sodium chloride *on page 426*

Normodyne® Injection *see* labetalol hydrochloride *on page 260*

Normodyne® Oral *see* labetalol hydrochloride *on page 260*

Noroxin® Oral *see* norfloxacin *on previous page*

Norpace® *see* disopyramide phosphate *on page 152*

Norplant® Implant *see* levonorgestrel *on page 266*

Norpramin® *see* desipramine hydrochloride *on page 130*

NOR-Q.D.® *see* norethindrone *on previous page*

Nor-tet® Oral *see* tetracycline *on page 451*

north American coral snake antivenin *see* antivenin (*Micrurus fulvius*) *on page 31*

north and south American antisnake-bite serum *see* antivenin polyvalent (*Crotalidae*) *on page 31*

nortriptyline hydrochloride (nor trip' ti leen)
Brand Names Aventyl® Hydrochloride; Pamelor®
Therapeutic Category Antidepressant, Tricyclic
Use Treatment of various forms of depression, often in conjunction with psychotherapy
Usual Dosage Oral:
   Adults: 25 mg 3-4 times/day up to 150 mg/day
   Elderly and Adolescents: 30-50 mg/day in divided doses
Dosage Forms
   Capsule: 10 mg, 25 mg, 50 mg, 75 mg
   Solution: 10 mg/5 mL (473 mL)

Norvasc® *see* amlodipine *on page 22*

Norzine® *see* thiethylperazine maleate *on page 456*

Nostril® Nasal Solution [OTC] *see* phenylephrine hydrochloride *on page 364*

Novacet® Topical *see* sulfur and sodium sulfacetamide *on page 442*

Novafed® *see* pseudoephedrine *on page 397*

Novafed® A *see* chlorpheniramine and pseudoephedrine *on page 94*

Novahistine® DH *see* chlorpheniramine, pseudoephedrine, and codeine *on page 97*

Novahistine® Expectorant *see* guaifenesin, pseudoephedrine, and codeine *on page 217*

Novahistine® Elixir [OTC] *see* chlorpheniramine and phenylephrine *on page 93*

Novantrone® *see* mitoxantrone hydrochloride *on page 309*

Novocain® Injection *see* procaine hydrochloride *on page 387*

Novolin® 70/30 *see* insulin preparations *on page 245*

Novolin® 70/30 PenFil® *see* insulin preparations *on page 245*

Novolin® L *see* insulin preparations *on page 245*

Novolin® N *see* insulin preparations *on page 245*

Novolin® N PenFil® *see* insulin preparations *on page 245*

Novolin® R *see* insulin preparations *on page 245*

Novolin® R PenFil® *see* insulin preparations *on page 245*

NP-27® [OTC] *see* tolnaftate *on page 464*

NPH Iletin® I *see* insulin preparations *on page 245*

NPH Insulin *see* insulin preparations *on page 245*

NPH-N *see* insulin preparations *on page 245*

ntg *see* nitroglycerin *on page 329*

NTZ® Long Acting Nasal Solution [OTC] *see* oxymetazoline hydrochloride *on page 343*

Nubain® *see* nalbuphine hydrochloride *on page 317*

Nucofed® *see* guaifenesin, pseudoephedrine, and codeine *on page 217*

Nucofed® Pediatric Expectorant *see* guaifenesin, pseudoephedrine, and codeine *on page 217*

Nucotuss® *see* guaifenesin, pseudoephedrine, and codeine *on page 217*

Nu-Iron® [OTC] *see* polysaccharide-iron complex *on page 376*

Nullo® [OTC] *see* chlorophyll *on page 90*

NuLYTELY® *see* polyethylene glycol-electrolyte solution *on page 375*

Numorphan® Injection *see* oxymorphone hydrochloride *on page 344*

Numorphan® Oral *see* oxymorphone hydrochloride *on page 344*

Nupercainal® Topical [OTC] *see* dibucaine *on page 140*

Nuprin® [OTC] *see* ibuprofen *on page 240*

Nuquin HP® *see* hydroquinone *on page 235*

Nuromax® Injection *see* doxacurium chloride *on page 156*

Nutracort® *see* hydrocortisone *on page 232*

Nutraplus® Topical [OTC] *see* urea *on page 480*

Nutropin® Injection *see* human growth hormone *on page 226*

Nydrazid® *see* isoniazid *on page 252*

nystatin (nye stat' in)
    Brand Names Mycostatin® Oral; Mycostatin® Topical; Mycostatin® Vaginal; Nilstat® Oral; Nilstat® Topical; Nilstat® Vaginal; Nystat-Rx®; Nystex® Oral; Nystex® Topical; O-V Staticin® Oral/Vaginal
    Therapeutic Category Antifungal Agent, Oral Nonabsorbed; Antifungal Agent, Topical; Antifungal Agent, Vaginal
    Use Treatment of susceptible cutaneous, mucocutaneous, and oral cavity fungal infections normally caused by the *Candida* species
    Usual Dosage
        Oral candidiasis:
            Neonates: 100,000 units 4 times/day or 50,000 units to each side of mouth 4 times/day
            Infants: 200,000 units 4 times/day or 100,000 units to each side of mouth 4 times/day
            Children and Adults: 400,000-600,000 units 4 times/day; troche: 200,000-400,000 units 4-5 times/day

Cutaneous candidal infections: Children and Adults: Topical: Apply 3-4 times/day

Intestinal infections: Adults: Oral: 500,000-1,000,000 units every 8 hours

Vaginal infections: Adults: Vaginal tablets: Insert 1-2 tablets/day at bedtime for 2 weeks

Dosage Forms
Cream: 100,000 units/g (15 g, 30 g)
Ointment, topical: 100,000 units/g (15 g, 30 g)
Powder, for preparation of oral suspension: 50 million units, 1 billion units, 2 billion units, 5 billion units
Powder, topical: 100,000 units/g (15 g)
Suspension, oral: 100,000 units/mL (5 mL, 60 mL, 480 mL)
Tablet:
    Oral: 500,000 units
    Vaginal: 100,000 units (15 and 30/box with applicator)
Troche: 200,000 units

nystatin and triamcinolone

Brand Names Dermacomb® Topical; Mycogen® II Topical; Mycolog®-II Topical; Myconel® Topical; Mytrex® F Topical; NGT® Topical; Nyst-Olone® II Topical; Tri-Statin® II Topical
Synonyms triamcinolone and nystatin
Therapeutic Category Antifungal Agent, Topical; Corticosteroid, Topical (Medium Potency)
Use Treatment of cutaneous candidiasis
Usual Dosage Topical: Apply twice daily
Dosage Forms
Cream: Nystatin 100,000 units and triamcinolone acetonide 0.1% (15 g, 30 g, 45 g, 60 g, 240 g)
Ointment, topical: Nystatin 100,000 units and triamcinolone acetonide 0.1% (15 g, 30 g, 60 g, 120 g)

Nystat-Rx® *see* nystatin *on previous page*

Nystex® Oral *see* nystatin *on previous page*

Nystex® Topical *see* nystatin *on previous page*

Nyst-Olone® II Topical *see* nystatin and triamcinolone *on this page*

Nytol® Oral [OTC] *see* diphenhydramine hydrochloride *on page 149*

Occlusal-HP Liquid *see* salicylic acid *on page 416*

Occucoat™ *see* hydroxypropyl methylcellulose *on page 236*

Ocean Nasal Mist [OTC] *see* sodium chloride *on page 426*

OCL® *see* polyethylene glycol-electrolyte solution *on page 375*

Octamide® *see* metoclopramide *on page 302*

Octicair® Otic *see* neomycin, polymyxin b, and hydrocortisone *on page 323*

Octocaine® *see* lidocaine hydrochloride *on page 267*

Octocaine® Injection *see* lidocaine and epinephrine *on page 267*

octreotide acetate (ok tree' oh tide)

Brand Names Sandostatin®
Therapeutic Category Antisecretory Agent; Somatostatin Analog
Use Control of symptoms in patients with metastatic carcinoid and vasoactive intestinal peptide-secreting tumors (VIPomas)
Usual Dosage Adults: S.C.: Initial: 50 mcg 1-2 times/day and titrate dose based on patient tolerance and response
Carcinoid: 100-600 mcg/day in 2-4 divided doses

VIPomas: 200-300 mcg/day in 2-4 divided doses

Diarrhea: Initial: I.V.: 50-100 mcg every 8 hours; increase by 100 mcg/dose at 48-hour intervals; maximum dose: 500 mcg every 8 hours
Dosage Forms Injection: 0.05 mg (1 mL); 0.1 mg (1 mL); 0.5 mg (1 mL)

Ocu-Carpine® Ophthalmic *see* pilocarpine *on page 369*

OcuClear® [OTC] *see* oxymetazoline hydrochloride *on page 343*

Ocufen® Ophthalmic *see* flurbiprofen sodium *on page 200*

Ocuflox™ Ophthalmic *see* ofloxacin *on this page*

Ocupress® Ophthalmic *see* carteolol hydrochloride *on page 77*

Ocusert Pilo-20® Ophthalmic *see* pilocarpine *on page 369*

Ocusert Pilo-40® Ophthalmic *see* pilocarpine *on page 369*

Ocu-Spor-G® Ophthalmic Solution *see* neomycin, polymyxin b, and gramicidin *on page 322*

Ocutricin® HC Otic *see* neomycin, polymyxin b, and hydrocortisone *on page 323*

Ocutricin® Ophthalmic Solution *see* neomycin, polymyxin b, and gramicidin *on page 322*

Ocutricin® Topical Ointment *see* bacitracin, neomycin, and polymyxin b *on page 43*

Ocu-Trol® Ophthalmic *see* neomycin, polymyxin b, and dexamethasone *on page 322*

Ocu-Tropine® Ophthalmic *see* atropine sulfate *on page 38*

ofloxacin (oh floks' a sin)
Brand Names Floxin® Injection; Floxin® Oral; Ocuflox™ Ophthalmic
Therapeutic Category Antibiotic, Quinolone
Use Quinolone antibiotic for skin and skin structure, lower respiratory and urinary tract infections and sexually transmitted diseases
Usual Dosage Adults:
   Oral, I.V.: 200-400 mg every 12 hours for 7-10 days for most infections or for 6 weeks for prostatitis
   Ophthalmic: Instill 1-2 drops in affected eye(s) every 2-4 hours for the first 2 days, then use 4 times daily for an additional 5 days
   Dosing adjustment/interval in renal impairment:
      Cl_{cr} 10-50 mL/minute: Administer 50% of normal dose or administer every 24 hours
      Cl_{cr} <10 mL/minute: Administer 25% of normal dose or administer 50% of normal dose every 24 hours
Dosage Forms
   Injection: 200 mg (50 mL); 400 mg (10 mL, 20 mL, 100 mL)
   Solution, ophthalmic: 0.3% (5 mL)
   Tablet: 200 mg, 300 mg, 400 mg

Ogen® *see* estropipate *on page 175*

okt3 *see* muromonab-CD3 *on page 314*

old tuberculin *see* tuberculin tests *on page 477*

oleovitamin a *see* vitamin a *on page 489*

oleum ricini *see* castor oil *on page 78*

olsalazine sodium (ole sal' a zeen)
Brand Names Dipentum®
Therapeutic Category 5-Aminosalicylic Acid Derivative; Anti-inflammatory Agent
Use Maintenance of remission of ulcerative colitis in patients intolerant to sulfasalazine
Usual Dosage Adults: Oral: 1 g daily in 2 divided doses
Dosage Forms Capsule: 250 mg

omeprazole (oh me' pray zol)
Formerly Known As Losec®
Brand Names Prilosec™
Therapeutic Category Gastric Acid Secretion Inhibitor

Use Short-term (4-8 weeks) treatment of severe erosive esophagitis (grade 2 or above), diagnosed by endoscopy and short-term treatment of symptomatic gastroesophageal reflux disease (GERD) poorly responsible to customary medical treatment; pathological hypersecretory conditions

Usual Dosage Adults: Oral:

Active duodenal ulcer: 20 mg/day for 4-8 weeks

GERD or severe erosive esophagitis: 20 mg/day for 4-8 weeks

Pathological hypersecretory conditions: 60 mg once daily to start; doses up to 120 mg 3 times/day have been administered; administer daily doses >80 mg in divided doses

Dosage Forms Capsule: 20 mg

OmniHIB® *see* hemophilus b conjugate vaccine *on page 222*

Omnipaque® *see* radiological/contrast media (non-ionic) *on page 406*

Omnipen® *see* ampicillin *on page 26*

Omnipen®-N *see* ampicillin *on page 26*

OMS® Oral *see* morphine sulfate *on page 311*

Oncaspar® *see* pegaspargase *on page 351*

Oncovin® Injection *see* vincristine sulfate *on page 488*

ondansetron hydrochloride (on dan' se tron)

Brand Names Zofran® Injection; Zofran® Oral
Therapeutic Category Antiemetic
Use May be prescribed for patients who are refractory to or have severe adverse reactions to standard antiemetic therapy; also for young patients (ie, <45 years of age who are more likely to develop extrapyramidal reactions to high-dose metoclopramide) who are to receive highly emetogenic chemotherapeutic agents
Usual Dosage I.V. (the I.V. product has been used orally successfully. Dosage should be calculated based on weight):

Children >3 years and Adults: 0.15 mg/kg/dose infused 30 minutes before the start of emetogenic chemotherapy, with subsequent doses administered 4 and 8 hours after the first dose; decreased effectiveness has been reported when administered for prolonged therapy, eg, more than 3 doses

Adults:
>80 kg: 12 mg IVPB
45-80 kg: 8 mg IVPB
<45 kg: 0.15 mg/kg/dose IVPB

Dosage Forms
Injection: 2 mg/mL (20 mL); 32 mg (single-dose vials)
Tablet: 4 mg, 8 mg

Ony-Clear® Nail *see* triacetin *on page 467*

op-cck *see* sincalide *on page 423*

Opcon® Ophthalmic *see* naphazoline hydrochloride *on page 319*

o,p'-ddd *see* mitotane *on page 309*

Ophthacet® Ophthalmic *see* sodium sulfacetamide *on page 431*

Ophthaine® Ophthalmic *see* proparacaine hydrochloride *on page 392*

Ophthalgan® Ophthalmic *see* glycerin *on page 210*

Ophthetic® Ophthalmic *see* proparacaine hydrochloride *on page 392*

Ophthochlor® Ophthalmic *see* chloramphenicol *on page 88*

Ophthocort® Ophthalmic *see* chloramphenicol, polymyxin b, and hydrocortisone *on page 89*

opium alkaloids
Brand Names Pantopon®
Therapeutic Category Analgesic, Narcotic
Use Relief of severe pain
Usual Dosage Adults: I.M., S.C.: 5-20 mg every 4-5 hours
Dosage Forms Injection: 20 mg/mL (1 mL)

opium and belladonna *see* belladonna and opium *on page 46*

opium tincture
Synonyms deodorized opium tincture; dto
Therapeutic Category Analgesic, Narcotic; Antidiarrheal
Use Treatment of diarrhea or relief of pain
Usual Dosage Oral:
  Children:
    Diarrhea: 0.005-0.01 mL/kg/dose every 3-4 hours
    Analgesia: 0.01-0.02 mL/kg/dose every 3-4 hours

  Adults: 0.6 mL 4 times/day
Dosage Forms Liquid: 10% [0.6 mL equivalent to morphine 6 mg]

Optigene® Ophthalmic [OTC] *see* tetrahydrozoline hydrochloride *on page 452*

Optimine® *see* azatadine maleate *on page 41*

OptiPranolol® Ophthalmic *see* metipranolol hydrochloride *on page 302*

Optiray® *see* radiological/contrast media (non-ionic) *on page 406*

Optised® Ophthalmic [OTC] *see* phenylephrine and zinc sulfate *on page 364*

opv *see* poliovirus vaccine, live (trivalent, oral) *on page 374*

Orabase®-B [OTC] *see* benzocaine *on page 48*

Orabase® HCA *see* hydrocortisone *on page 232*

Orabase®-O [OTC] *see* benzocaine *on page 48*

Orabase® With Benzocaine [OTC] *see* benzocaine, gelatin, pectin, and sodium carboxymethylcellulose *on page 49*

Orabase® Plain [OTC] *see* gelatin, pectin, and methylcellulose *on page 206*

Oracit® *see* sodium citrate and citric acid *on page 427*

Oragest SR® *see* chlorpheniramine and phenylpropanolamine *on page 94*

Oragrafin® Calcium *see* radiological/contrast media (ionic) *on page 404*

Oragrafin® Sodium *see* radiological/contrast media (ionic) *on page 404*

Orajel® Brace-Aid Oral Anesthetic [OTC] *see* benzocaine *on page 48*

Orajel® Brace-Aid Rinse [OTC] *see* carbamide peroxide *on page 74*

Orajel® Mouth-Aid [OTC] *see* benzocaine *on page 48*

Orajel® Maximum Strength [OTC] *see* benzocaine *on page 48*

Oraminic® II Injection *see* brompheniramine maleate *on page 59*

Oramorph SR™ Oral *see* morphine sulfate *on page 311*

Orap™ *see* pimozide *on page 370*

Orasone® Oral *see* prednisone *on page 384*

Orazinc® Oral [OTC] *see* zinc sulfate *on page 496*

orciprenaline sulfate *see* metaproterenol sulfate *on page 290*

Ordine AT® Extended Release Capsule *see* caramiphen and phenylpropanolamine *on page 73*

Oretic® *see* hydrochlorothiazide *on page 229*

Oreton® Methyl *see* methyltestosterone *on page 301*

Orexin® [OTC] *see* vitamin b complex *on page 490*

Orex® [OTC] *see* saliva substitute *on page 417*

Orimune® *see* poliovirus vaccine, live (trivalent, oral) *on page 374*

Orinase® Diagnostic Injection *see* tolbutamide *on page 463*

Orinase® Oral *see* tolbutamide *on page 463*

ORLAAM® *see* levomethadyl acetate hydrochloride *on page 265*

Ormazine *see* chlorpromazine hydrochloride *on page 97*

Ornade® Spansule® *see* chlorpheniramine and phenylpropanolamine *on page 94*

Ornidyl® Injection *see* eflornithine hydrochloride *on page 164*

orphenadrine, aspirin and caffeine
Brand Names Norgesic® Forte; Norgesic®
Therapeutic Category Analgesic, Non-Narcotic; Skeletal Muscle Relaxant
Use Relief of discomfort associated with skeletal muscular conditions
Usual Dosage Oral: 1-2 tablets 3-4 times/day
Dosage Forms
  Tablet: Orphenadrine citrate 25 mg, aspirin 385 mg, and caffeine 30 mg
  Tablet (Norgesic® Forte): Orphenadrine citrate 50 mg, aspirin 770 mg, and caffeine 60 mg

orphenadrine citrate (or fen' a dreen)
Brand Names Norflex®
Therapeutic Category Skeletal Muscle Relaxant
Use Treatment of muscle spasm associated with acute painful musculoskeletal conditions; supportive therapy in tetanus
Usual Dosage Adults:
  Oral: 100 mg twice daily
  I.M., I.V.: 60 mg every 12 hours
Dosage Forms
  Injection: 30 mg/mL (2 mL, 10 mL)
  Tablet: 100 mg
  Tablet, sustained release: 100 mg

Ortho-Cept™ *see* ethinyl estradiol and desogestrel *on page 177*

Orthoclone® OKT3 *see* muromonab-CD3 *on page 314*

Ortho-Cyclen® *see* ethinyl estradiol and norgestimate *on page 179*

Ortho® Dienestrol Vaginal *see* dienestrol *on page 143*

Ortho-Est® *see* estropipate *on page 175*

Ortho-Novum™ 1/35 *see* ethinyl estradiol and norethindrone *on page 178*

Ortho-Novum™ 1/50 *see* mestranol and norethindrone *on page 290*

Ortho-Novum™ 7/7/7 *see* ethinyl estradiol and norethindrone *on page 178*

Ortho-Novum™ 10/11 *see* ethinyl estradiol and norethindrone *on page 178*

Ortho™ Tri-Cyclen® *see* ethinyl estradiol and norgestimate *on page 179*

Or-Tyl® Injection *see* dicyclomine hydrochloride *on page 142*

Orudis® *see* ketoprofen *on page 258*

Oruvail® *see* ketoprofen *on page 258*

Os-Cal® 500 [OTC] *see* calcium carbonate *on page 66*

Osmitrol® Injection *see* mannitol *on page 279*

Osmoglyn® Ophthalmic *see* glycerin *on page 210*

Osteocalcin® *see* calcitonin (salmon) *on page 65*

Otic Domeboro® *see* aluminum acetate and acetic acid *on page 15*

Otobiotic® Otic *see* polymyxin b and hydrocortisone *on page 375*

Otocalm® Ear *see* antipyrine and benzocaine *on page 30*

Otocort® Otic *see* neomycin, polymyxin b, and hydrocortisone *on page 323*

Otomycin-HPN® Otic *see* neomycin, polymyxin b, and hydrocortisone *on page 323*

Otosporin® Otic *see* neomycin, polymyxin b, and hydrocortisone *on page 323*

Otrivin® Nasal [OTC] *see* xylometazoline hydrochloride *on page 493*

Ovcon® *see* ethinyl estradiol and norethindrone *on page 178*

Ovide™ Topical *see* malathion *on page 278*

Ovral® *see* ethinyl estradiol and norgestrel *on page 180*

Ovrette® *see* norgestrel *on page 332*

O-V Staticin® Oral/Vaginal *see* nystatin *on page 334*

OvuKIT® Acetest® [OTC] *see* diagnostic aids (*in vitro*), urine *on page 137*

OvuQUICK® *see* diagnostic aids (*in vitro*), urine *on page 137*

oxacillin sodium (ox a sill' in)

Brand Names Bactocill® Injection; Bactocill® Oral; Prostaphlin® Injection; Prostaphlin® Oral
Synonyms methylphenyl isoxazolyl penicillin; sodium oxacillin
Therapeutic Category Antibiotic, Penicillin
Use Treatment of susceptible bacterial infections such as osteomyelitis, septicemia, endocarditis, and CNS infections due to penicillinase-producing strains of *Staphylococcus*
Usual Dosage
Neonates: I.M., I.V.:
Postnatal age <7 days:
<2000 g: 25 mg/kg/dose every 12 hours
>2000 g: 25 mg/kg/dose every 8 hours
Postnatal age >7 days:
<1200 g: 25 mg/kg/dose every 12 hours
1200-2000 g: 30 mg/kg/dose every 8 hours
>2000 g: 37.5 mg/kg/dose every 6 hours
Infants and Children: I.M., I.V.: 150-200 mg/kg/day in divided doses every 6 hours; maximum dose: 12 g/day
Infants and Children: Oral: 50-100 mg/kg/day divided every 6 hours
Adults:
Oral: 500-1000 mg every 4-6 hours for at least 5 days
I.M., I.V.: 250 mg to 2 g/dose every 4-6 hours
Dosage Forms
Capsule: 250 mg, 500 mg
Powder for injection: 250 mg, 500 mg, 1 g, 2 g, 4 g, 10 g
Powder for oral solution: 250 mg/5 mL (100 mL)

oxamniquine (ox am' ni kwin)

Brand Names Vansil™
Therapeutic Category Anthelmintic
Use Treat all stages of *Schistosoma mansoni* infection
Usual Dosage Oral:
Children <30 kg: 20 mg/kg in 2 divided doses of 10 mg/kg at 2- to 8-hour intervals
Adults: 12-15 mg/kg as a single dose
Dosage Forms Capsule: 250 mg

Oxandrine® *see* oxandrolone *on this page*

oxandrolone (ox an' droe lone)
Brand Names Oxandrine®
Therapeutic Category Androgen
Use Treatment of catabolic or tissue-depleting processes
Usual Dosage Adults: Oral: 2.5 mg 2-4 times daily
Dosage Forms Tablet: 2.5 mg

oxaprozin (ox a proe' zin)
Brand Names Daypro™
Therapeutic Category Nonsteroidal Anti-Inflammatory Agent (NSAID), Oral
Use Acute and long-term use in the management of signs and symptoms of osteoarthritis and rheumatoid arthritis
Usual Dosage Adults: Oral (individualize the dosage to the lowest effective dose to minimize adverse effects):
Osteoarthritis: 600-1200 mg once daily
Rheumatoid arthritis: 1200 mg once daily
Maximum dose: 1800 mg/day or 26 mg/kg (whichever is lower) in divided doses
Dosage Forms Tablet: 600 mg

oxazepam (ox a' ze pam)
Brand Names Serax®
Therapeutic Category Benzodiazepine
Use Treatment of anxiety and management of alcohol withdrawal; may also be used as an anticonvulsant in management of simple partial seizures
Usual Dosage Oral:
Children: 1 mg/kg/day has been administered

Adults:
Anxiety: 10-30 mg 3-4 times/day
Alcohol withdrawal: 15-30 mg 3-4 times/day
Hypnotic: 15-30 mg
Dosage Forms
Capsule: 10 mg, 15 mg, 30 mg
Tablet: 15 mg

oxiconazole nitrate (ox i kon' a zole)
Brand Names Oxistat® Topical
Therapeutic Category Antifungal Agent, Topical
Use Treatment of tinea pedis, tinea cruris, and tinea corporis
Usual Dosage Topical: Apply once daily to affected areas for 2 weeks to 1 month
Dosage Forms
Cream: 1% (15 g, 30 g, 60 g)
Lotion: 1% (30 mL)

oxilapine succinate *see* loxapine *on page 274*

Oxistat® Topical *see* oxiconazole nitrate *on this page*

oxpentifylline *see* pentoxifylline *on page 357*

Oxsoralen® Topical *see* methoxsalen *on page 296*

Oxsoralen-Ultra® Oral *see* methoxsalen *on page 296*

oxtriphylline (ox trye' fi lin)
Brand Names Choledyl®
Synonyms choline theophyllinate
Therapeutic Category Antiasthmatic; Bronchodilator; Theophylline Derivative
(Continued)

oxtriphylline *(Continued)*

Use Bronchodilator in symptomatic treatment of asthma and reversible bronchospasm
Usual Dosage Oral:
Children:
1-9 years: 6.2 mg/kg/dose every 6 hours
9-16 years: 4.7 mg/kg/dose every 6 hours

Adults: 4.7 mg/kg every 8 hours; sustained release: administer every 12 hours
Dosage Forms
Elixir: 100 mg/5 mL (5 mL, 10 mL, 473 mL)
Syrup: 50 mg/5 mL (473 mL)
Tablet: 100 mg, 200 mg
Tablet, sustained release: 400 mg, 600 mg

Oxy-5® [OTC] *see* benzoyl peroxide *on page 50*

Oxy-5® Tinted [OTC] *see* benzoyl peroxide *on page 50*

oxybutynin chloride (ox i byoo' ti nin)

Brand Names Ditropan®
Therapeutic Category Antispasmodic Agent, Urinary
Use Antispasmodic for neurogenic bladder
Usual Dosage Oral:
Children:
1-5 years: 0.2 mg/kg/dose 2-4 times/day
>5 years: 5 mg twice daily, up to 5 mg 3 times/day

Adults: 5 mg 2-3 times/day up to 5 mg 4 times/day maximum
Dosage Forms
Syrup: 5 mg/5 mL (473 mL)
Tablet: 5 mg

Oxycel® *see* cellulose, oxidized *on page 84*

oxychlorosene sodium (ox i klor' oh seen)

Brand Names Clorpactin® WCS-90
Therapeutic Category Antibiotic, Topical
Use Treating localized infections
Usual Dosage Topical (0.1% to 0.5% solutions): Apply by irrigation, instillation, spray, soaks, or wet compresses
Dosage Forms Powder for solution: 2 g, 5 g

oxycodone and acetaminophen

Brand Names Percocet®; Roxicet® 5/500; Roxilox®; Tylox®
Synonyms acetaminophen and oxycodone
Therapeutic Category Analgesic, Narcotic; Antipyretic
Use Management of moderate to severe pain
Usual Dosage Oral (doses should be titrated to appropriate analgesic effects):
Children: Oxycodone: 0.05-0.15 mg/kg/dose to 5 mg/dose (maximum) every 4-6 hours as needed

Adults: 1-2 tablets every 4-6 hours as needed for pain
Maximum daily dose of acetaminophen: 8 g/day, in alcoholics: 4 g/day
Dosage Forms
Caplet: Oxycodone hydrochloride 5 mg and acetaminophen 500 mg
Capsule: Oxycodone hydrochloride 5 mg and acetaminophen 500 mg
Solution, oral: Oxycodone hydrochloride 5 mg and acetaminophen 325 mg per 5 mL (5 mL, 500 mL)
Tablet: Oxycodone hydrochloride 5 mg and acetaminophen 325 mg

oxycodone and aspirin
Brand Names Codoxy®; Percodan®; Percodan®-Demi; Roxiprin®
Therapeutic Category Analgesic, Narcotic; Antipyretic
Use Relief of moderate to moderately severe pain
Usual Dosage Oral (based on oxycodone combined salts):
Children: 0.05-0.15 mg/kg/dose every 4-6 hours as needed; maximum: 5 mg/dose (1 tablet Percodan® or 2 tablets Percodan®-Demi/dose) **or**
Alternatively:
6-12 years: Percodan®-Demi: $^1/_4$ tablet every 6 hours as needed for pain
>12 years: $^1/_2$ tablet every 6 hours as needed for pain

Adults: Percodan®: 1 tablet every 6 hours as needed for pain or Percodan®-Demi: 1-2 tablets every 6 hours as needed for pain
Dosage Forms Tablet:
Percodan®: Oxycodone hydrochloride 4.5 mg, oxycodone terephthalate 0.38 mg, and aspirin 325 mg
Percodan®-Demi: Oxycodone hydrochloride 2.25 mg, oxycodone terephthalate 0.19 mg, and aspirin 325 mg

oxycodone hydrochloride (ox i koe' done)
Brand Names Roxicodone™
Synonyms dihydrohydroxycodeinone
Therapeutic Category Analgesic, Narcotic
Use Management of moderate to severe pain, normally used in combination with non-narcotic analgesics
Usual Dosage
Children:
6-12 years: 1.25 mg every 6 hours as needed
>12 years: 2.5 mg every 6 hours as needed

Adults: 5 mg every 6 hours as needed
Dosage Forms
Liquid, oral: 5 mg/5 mL (500 mL)
Solution, oral concentrate: 20 mg/mL (30 mL)
Tablet: 5 mg

oxymetazoline hydrochloride (ox i met az' oh leen)
Brand Names Afrin® Nasal Solution [OTC]; Allerest® 12 Hour Nasal Solution [OTC]; Chlorphed®-LA Nasal Solution [OTC]; Dristan® Long Lasting Nasal Solution [OTC]; Duration® Nasal Solution [OTC]; Neo-Synephrine® 12 Hour Nasal Solution [OTC]; Nōstrilla® [OTC]; NTZ® Long Acting Nasal Solution [OTC]; OcuClear® [OTC]; Sinarest® 12 Hour Nasal Solution; Vicks® Sinex® Long-Acting Nasal Solution [OTC]; 4-Way® Long Acting Nasal Solution [OTC]
Therapeutic Category Adrenergic Agonist Agent; Decongestant, Nasal; Vasoconstrictor, Nasal; Vasoconstrictor, Ophthalmic
Use Symptomatic relief of nasal mucosal congestion and adjunctive therapy of middle ear infections, associated with acute or chronic rhinitis, the common cold, sinusitis, hay fever or other allergies
Usual Dosage
Intranasal:
Children 2-5 years: 0.025% solution: Instill 2-3 drops in each nostril twice daily
Children ≥6 years and Adults: 0.05% solution: Instill 2-3 drops or 2-3 sprays into each nostril twice daily

Ophthalmic: Adults: Instill 1-2 drops into affected eye(s) every 6 hours
Dosage Forms
Nasal solution:
Drops:
Afrin® Children's Nose Drops: 0.025% (20 mL)
Afrin®, NTZ® Long Acting Nasal Solution: 0.05% (15 mL, 20 mL)
Spray: Afrin®, Allerest® 12 Hours, Chlorphed®-LA, Dristan® Long Lasting, Duration®, 4-Way® Long Acting, Genasal®, Nasal Relief®, Neo-Synephrine® 12 Hour, Nōstrilla®,
(Continued)

oxymetazoline hydrochloride *(Continued)*
NTZ® Long Acting Nasal Solution, Sinex® Long-Acting, Twice-A-Day®: 0.05% (15 mL, 30 mL)
Ophthalmic solution (OcuClear®, Visine® L.R.): 0.025% (15 mL, 30 mL)

oxymetholone (ox i meth' oh lone)
Brand Names Anadrol®
Therapeutic Category Anabolic Steroid
Use Anemias caused by the administration of myelotoxic drugs
Usual Dosage Erythropoietic effects: 1-5 mg/kg/day in 1 daily dose; maximum: 100 mg/day
Dosage Forms Tablet: 50 mg

oxymorphone hydrochloride (ox i mor' fone)
Brand Names Numorphan® Injection; Numorphan® Oral
Therapeutic Category Analgesic, Narcotic
Use Management of moderate to severe pain and preoperatively as a sedative and a supplement to anesthesia
Usual Dosage Adults:
I.M., S.C.: Initial: 0.5 mg, then 1-1.5 mg every 4-6 hours as needed
I.V.: Initial: 0.5 mg
Rectal: 5 mg every 4-6 hours
Dosage Forms
Injection: 1 mg (1 mL); 1.5 mg/mL (1 mL, 10 mL)
Suppository, rectal: 5 mg

oxyphenbutazone (ox i fen byoo' ta zone)
Therapeutic Category Analgesic, Non-Narcotic; Nonsteroidal Anti-Inflammatory Agent (NSAID), Oral
Use Management of inflammatory disorders, as an analgesic in the treatment of mild to moderate pain and as an antipyretic; I.V. form used as an alternate to surgery in management of patent ductus arteriosus in premature neonates; acute gouty arthritis
Usual Dosage Adults: Oral:
Rheumatoid arthritis: 100-200 mg 3-4 times/day until desired effect, then reduce dose to not exceeding 400 mg/day

Acute gouty arthritis: Initial: 400 mg then 100 mg every 4 hours until acute attack subsides
Dosage Forms Tablet: 100 mg

oxyphencyclimine hydrochloride (ox i fen sye' kli meen)
Brand Names Daricon®
Therapeutic Category Anticholinergic Agent; Antispasmodic Agent, Gastrointestinal
Use Adjunctive treatment of peptic ulcer
Usual Dosage Adults: Oral: 10 mg twice daily or 5 mg 3 times/day
Dosage Forms Tablet: 10 mg

oxytetracycline and polymyxin b
Brand Names Terramycin® Ophthalmic Ointment; Terramycin® w/ Polymyxin B Sulfate
Synonyms polymyxin b and oxytetracycline
Therapeutic Category Antibiotic, Ophthalmic
Use Treatment of superficial ocular infections involving the conjunctiva and/or cornea
Usual Dosage
Topical: Apply ½" of ointment onto the lower lid of affected eye 2-4 times/day
Vaginal: Insert one in vagina twice daily for 2-4 days
Dosage Forms
Ointment, ophthalmic/otic: Oxytetracycline hydrochloride 5 mg and polymyxin b 10,000 units per g (3.75 g)
Tablet, vaginal: Oxytetracycline hydrochloride 100 mg and polymyxin b 100,000 units (10s)

oxytetracycline hydrochloride (ox i tet ra sye' kleen)
Brand Names Terramycin® I.M. Injection; Terramycin® Oral; Uri-Tet® Oral
Therapeutic Category Antibiotic, Tetracycline Derivative
Use Treatment of susceptible bacterial infections; both gram-positive and gram-negative, as well as *Rickettsia* and *Mycoplasma* organisms
Usual Dosage
Oral:
Children: 40-50 mg/kg/day in divided doses every 6 hours (maximum: 2 g/24 hours)
Adults: 250-500 mg/dose every 6 hours

I.M.:
Children >8 years: 15-25 mg/kg/day (maximum: 250 mg/dose) in divided doses every 8-12 hours
Adults: 250-500 mg every 24 hours or 300 mg/day divided every 8-12 hours
Dosage Forms
Capsule: 250 mg
Injection, with lidocaine 2%: 5% [50 mg/mL] (2 mL, 10 mL); 12.5% [125 mg/mL] (2 mL)

oxytocin (ox i toe' sin)
Brand Names Pitocin® Injection; Syntocinon® Injection; Syntocinon® Nasal Spray
Synonyms pit
Therapeutic Category Oxytocic Agent
Use Induce labor at term; control postpartum bleeding; nasal preparation used to promote milk letdown in lactating females
Usual Dosage Adults:
Induction of labor: I.V.: 0.001-0.002 unit/minute; increase by 0.001-0.002 every 15-30 minutes until contraction pattern has been established

Postpartum bleeding: I.V.: 0.001-0.002 units/minute as needed

Promotion of milk letdown: Intranasal: 1 spray or 3 drops in one or both nostrils 2-3 minutes before breast feeding
Dosage Forms
Injection: 10 units/mL (1 mL, 10 mL)
Solution, nasal: 40 units/mL (2 mL, 5 mL)

Oyst-Cal 500 [OTC] *see* calcium carbonate *on page 66*

Oystercal® 500 *see* calcium carbonate *on page 66*

paclitaxel (pack li tax' el)
Brand Names Taxol®
Therapeutic Category Antineoplastic Agent, Antimicrotubular
Use Treatment of metastatic carcinoma of the ovary after failure of first-line or subsequent chemotherapy
Usual Dosage Adults: I.V.: 135 mg/m^2 over 24 hours every 3 weeks
Dosage Forms Injection: 6 mg/mL (5 mL)

Palmitate-A® 5000 [OTC] *see* vitamin a *on page 489*

PALS® [OTC] *see* chlorophyll *on page 90*

2-pam *see* pralidoxime chloride *on page 381*

Pamelor® *see* nortriptyline hydrochloride *on page 333*

pamidronate disodium (pa mi droe' nate)
Brand Names Aredia™
Therapeutic Category Antidote, Hypercalcemia; Biphosphonate Derivative
Use Symptomatic treatment of Paget's disease and heterotopic ossification due to spinal cord injury or after total hip replacement, hypercalcemia associated with malignancy
(Continued)

pamidronate disodium (Continued)

Usual Dosage Drug must be diluted properly before administration and infused slowly (at least over 2 hours)

Adults: I.V.:
> Moderate cancer related hypercalcemia (12-13 mg/dL): 60-90 mg given as a slow infusion over 2-24 hours;
> Severe cancer-related hypercalcemia (>13.5 mg/dL): 90 mg as a slow infusion over 2-24 hours
>> A period of 7 days should elapse before the use of second course; repeat infusions every 2-3 weeks have been suggested, however, could be administered every 2-3 months according to the degree and of severity of hypercalcemia and/or the type of malignancy

Paget's disease: 60 mg as a single 2-24 hour infusion
Dosage Forms Powder for injection, lyophilized: 30 mg, 60 mg

Pamine® see methscopolamine bromide on page 297

Panacet® 5/500 see hydrocodone and acetaminophen on page 230

Panadol® [OTC] see acetaminophen on page 2

Panasal® 5/500 see hydrocodone and aspirin on page 230

Pancrease® see pancrelipase on this page

Pancrease® MT 4 see pancrelipase on this page

Pancrease® MT 10 see pancrelipase on this page

Pancrease® MT 16 see pancrelipase on this page

pancreatin (pan' kree a tin)

Brand Names Creon℠; Donnazyme℠; Hi-Vegi-Lip®
Therapeutic Category Pancreatic Enzyme
Use Replacement therapy in symptomatic treatment of malabsorption syndrome caused by pancreatic insufficiency
Usual Dosage Enteric coated microspheres: The following dosage recommendations are only an approximation for initial dosages. The actual dosage will depend on the digestive requirements of the individual patient.

Children:
> <1 year: 2000 units of lipase with meals/feedings
> 1-6 years: 4000-8000 units of lipase with meals and 4,000 units with snacks
> 7-12 years: 4000-12,000 units of lipase with meals and snacks

Adults: 4000-16,000 units of lipase with meals and with snacks
Dosage Forms
Capsule, enteric coated microspheres (Creon®): Lipase 8000 units, amylase 30,000 units, protease 13,000 units and pancreatin 300 mg
Tablet:
> Donnazyme℠: Lipase 1000 units, amylase 12,500 units, protease 12,500 units and pancreatin 500 mg
> Hi-Vegi-Lip℠: Lipase 4800 units, amylase 60,000 units, protease 60,000 units and pancreatin 2400 mg

pancrelipase (pan kre li' pase)

Brand Names Cotazym℠; Cotazym-S℠; Creon 10®; Creon 20®; Ilozyme®; Ku-Zyme® HP; Pancrease℠; Pancrease℠ MT 4; Pancrease® MT 10; Pancrease® MT 16; Protilase®; Ultrase® MT12; Ultrase℠ MT20; Ultrase℠ MT24; Viokase®; Zymase®
Synonyms lipancreatin
Therapeutic Category Pancreatic Enzyme
Use Replacement therapy in symptomatic treatment of malabsorption syndrome caused by pancreatic insufficiency

Usual Dosage Oral:
Powder: Actual dose depends on the digestive requirements of the patient
Children <1 year: Start with $^1/_8$ teaspoonful with feedings

Enteric coated microspheres and microtablets: The following dosage recommendations are only an approximation for initial dosages. The actual dosage will depend on the digestive requirements of the individual patient.
Children <1 year: 2000 units of lipase with meals/feedings
Children 1-6 years: 4000-8000 units of lipase with meals and 4000 units with snacks
Children 7-12 years: 4000-12,000 units of lipase with meals and snacks
Adults: 4000-16,000 units of lipase with meals and with snacks

Dosage Forms
Capsule:
Cotazym®: Lipase 8000 units, protease 30,000 units, amylase 30,000 units
Ku-Zyme® HP: Lipase 8000 units, protease 30,000 units, amylase 30,000 units
Ultrase® MT12: Lipase 12,000 units, protease 39,000 units, amylase 39,000 units
Ultrase® MT20: Lipase 20,000 units, protease 65,000 units, amylase 65,000 units
Ultrase® MT24: Lipase 24,000 units, protease 78,000 units, amylase 78,000 units
Enteric coated microspheres (Pancrease®): Lipase 4000 units, protease 25,000 units, amylase 20,000 units
Enteric coated microtablets:
Pancrease® MT 4: Lipase 4000 units, protease 12,000 units, amylase 12,000 units
Pancrease® MT 10: Lipase 10,000 units, protease 30,000 units, amylase 30,000 units
Pancrease® MT 16: Lipase 16,000 units, protease 48,000 units, amylase 48,000 units
Enteric coated spheres:
Cotazym-S®: Lipase 5000 units, protease 20,000 units, amylase 20,000 units
Pancrelipase, Protilase®: Lipase 4000 units, protease 25,000 units, amylase 20,000 units
Zymase®: Lipase 12,000 units, protease 24,000 units, amylase 24,000 units
Delayed release:
Creon 10®: Lipase 10,000 units, protease 37,500 units, amylase 33,200 units
Creon 20®: Lipase 20,000 units, protease 75,000 units, amylase 66,400 units
Powder (Viokase®): Lipase 16,800 units, protease 70,000 units, amylase 70,000 units per 0.7 g
Tablet:
Ilozyme®: Lipase 11,000 units, protease 30,000 units, amylase 30,000 units
Viokase®: Lipase 8000 units, protease 30,000 units, amylase 30,000 units

pancuronium bromide (pan kyoo roe' nee um)
Brand Names Pavulon®
Therapeutic Category Neuromuscular Blocker Agent, Nondepolarizing; Skeletal Muscle Relaxant
Use Produces skeletal muscle relaxation during surgery after induction of general anesthesia, increases pulmonary compliance during assisted respiration, facilitates endotracheal intubation
Usual Dosage I.V.:
Neonates: ≤1 month: Initial: 0.03 mg/kg/dose repeated twice at 5- to 10-minute intervals as needed; maintenance: 0.03-0.09 mg/kg/dose every 30 minutes to 4 hours as needed

Infants >1 month, Children, and Adults: 0.04-0.1 mg/kg; maintenance dose: 0.02-0.1 mg/kg/dose every 30-60 minutes as needed
Dosage Forms Injection: 1 mg/mL (10 mL); 2 mg/mL (2 mL, 5 mL)

Panhematin® *see* hemin *on page 222*
Panmycin® Oral *see* tetracycline *on page 451*
PanOxyl®-AQ *see* benzoyl peroxide *on page 50*
PanOxyl® [OTC] *see* benzoyl peroxide *on page 50*
Panscol® Lotion [OTC] *see* salicylic acid *on page 416*
Panscol® Ointment [OTC] *see* salicylic acid *on page 416*

Panthoderm® Cream [OTC] *see* dexpanthenol *on page 133*

Pantopon® *see* opium alkaloids *on page 338*

pantothenic acid
Synonyms calcium pantothenate; vitamin b_5
Therapeutic Category Vitamin, Water Soluble
Use Pantothenic acid deficiency
Usual Dosage Adults: Oral: Recommended daily dose 4-7 mg/day
Dosage Forms Tablet: 25 mg, 50 mg, 100 mg, 218 mg, 250 mg, 500 mg, 545 mg, 1000 mg

pantothenyl alcohol *see* dexpanthenol *on page 133*

papaverine hydrochloride (pa pav' er een)
Brand Names Cerespan® Oral; Genabid® Oral; Pavabid® Oral; Pavased® Oral; Pavatine®
Oral; Paverolan™ Oral
Therapeutic Category Vasodilator
Use Relief of peripheral and cerebral ischemia associated with arterial spasm
Usual Dosage
Children: I.M., I.V.: 1.5 mg/kg 4 times/day

Adults:
Oral: 100-300 mg 3-5 times/day
Oral, sustained release: 150-300 mg every 12 hours
I.M., I.V.: 30-120 mg every 3 hours as needed
Dosage Forms
Capsule, sustained release: 150 mg
Injection: 30 mg/mL (2 mL, 10 mL)
Tablet: 30 mg, 60 mg, 100 mg, 150 mg, 200 mg, 300 mg
Tablet, timed release: 200 mg

para-aminosalicylate sodium
Synonyms aminosalicylate sodium; pas
Therapeutic Category Analgesic, Non-Narcotic; Salicylate
Use Adjunctive treatment of tuberculosis
Usual Dosage Oral:
Children: 240-360 mg/kg/day in 3-4 divided doses
Adults: 12-15 g/day in 3-4 divided doses
Dosage Forms Tablet: 500 mg

parabromdylamine *see* brompheniramine maleate *on page 59*

paracetaldehyde *see* paraldehyde *on next page*

paracetamol *see* acetaminophen *on page 2*

parachlorometaxylenol
Brand Names Metasep® [OTC]
Synonyms pcmx
Therapeutic Category Antiseborrheic Agent, Topical
Use Aid in relief of dandruff and associated conditions
Usual Dosage Massage to a foamy lather, allow to remain on hair for 5 minutes, rinse thoroughly and repeat
Dosage Forms Shampoo: 2% with isopropyl alcohol 9%

Paradione® *see* paramethadione *on next page*

Paraflex® *see* chlorzoxazone *on page 99*

Parafon Forte™ DSC *see* chlorzoxazone *on page 99*

Paral® *see* paraldehyde *on this page*

paraldehyde (par al' de hyde)
Brand Names Paral®
Synonyms paracetaldehyde
Therapeutic Category Anticonvulsant, Miscellaneous; Hypnotic; Sedative
Use Treatment of status epilepticus and tetanus induced seizures; has been used as a sedative/hypnotic and in the treatment of alcohol withdrawal symptoms (delirium tremens)
Usual Dosage Oral, rectal:
Children: 0.15-0.3 mL/kg
Adults:
  Hypnotic: 10-30 mL
  Sedative: 5-10 mL
Oral: Dilute in milk or iced fruit juice to mask taste and odor
Rectal: Mix paraldehyde 2:1 with oil (cottonseed or olive)

Dosing adjustment in hepatic impairment: Dosage may need to be reduced
Dosage Forms Liquid, oral or rectal: 1 g/mL (30 mL)

paramethad *see* paramethadione *on this page*

paramethadione (par a meth a dye' one)
Brand Names Paradione®
Synonyms isoethadione; paramethad
Therapeutic Category Anticonvulsant, Oxazolidinedione
Use To control absence (petit mal) seizures refractory to other drugs
Usual Dosage Oral:
Children: 300-900 mg/day in 3-4 equally divided doses
Adults: 900 mg to 2.4 g/day in 3-4 equally divided doses
Dosage Forms Capsule: 150 mg, 300 mg

Paraplatin® *see* carboplatin *on page 76*

Parathar™ Injection *see* teriparatide *on page 448*

Par Decon® *see* chlorpheniramine, phenyltoloxamine, phenylpropanolamine and phenylephrine *on page 96*

paregoric (par e gor' ik)
Synonyms camphorated tincture of opium
Therapeutic Category Analgesic, Narcotic; Antidiarrheal
Use Treatment of diarrhea or relief of pain; neonatal opiate withdrawal
Usual Dosage
Neonatal opiate withdrawal: Oral: 3-6 drops every 3-6 hours as needed, or initially 0.2 mL every 3 hours; increase dosage by approximately 0.05 mL every 3 hours until withdrawal symptoms are controlled; it is rare to exceed 0.7 mL/dose. Stabilize withdrawal symptoms for 3-5 days, then gradually decrease dosage over a 2- to 4-week period.

Children: 0.25-0.5 mL/kg 1-4 times/day

Adults: 5-10 mL 1-4 times/day
Dosage Forms Liquid: 2 mg morphine equivalent/5 mL [equivalent to 20 mg opium powder] (5 mL, 60 mL, 473 mL, 4000 mL)

Paremyd® Ophthalmic *see* hydroxyamphetamine and tropicamide *on page 235*

Parepectolin® *see* kaolin and pectin with opium *on page 256*

Par Glycerol® *see* iodinated glycerol *on page 248*

ALPHABETICAL LISTING OF DRUGS

Par Glycerol C® *see* iodinated glycerol and codeine *on page 248*

Par Glycerol DM® *see* iodinated glycerol and dextromethorphan *on page 249*

pargyline and methyclothiazide *see* methyclothiazide and pargyline *on page 298*

Parhist SR® *see* chlorpheniramine and phenylpropanolamine *on page 94*

Parlodel® *see* bromocriptine mesylate *on page 58*

Parnate® *see* tranylcypromine sulfate *on page 466*

paromomycin sulfate (par oh moe mye' sin)
Brand Names Humatin®
Therapeutic Category Amebicide
Use Treatment of acute and chronic intestinal amebiasis; preoperatively to suppress intestinal flora; tapeworm infestations; rid bowel of nitrogen forming bacteria in hepatic coma
Usual Dosage Oral:
Intestinal amebiasis: Children and Adults: 25-35 mg/kg/day in 3 divided doses for 5-10 days

Tapeworm (fish, dog, bovine, porcine):
Children: 11 mg/kg every 15 minutes for 4 doses
Adults: 1 g every 15 minutes for 4 doses

Hepatic coma: Adults: 4 g/day in 2-4 divided doses for 5-6 days

Dwarf tapeworm: Children and Adults: 45 mg/kg/dose every day for 5-7 days
Dosage Forms Capsule: 250 mg

paroxetine (pa rox' e teen)
Brand Names Paxil®
Therapeutic Category Antidepressant; Serotonin Antagonist
Use Treatment of depression
Usual Dosage Adults: Oral: 20 mg once daily, preferably in the morning
Dosage Forms Tablet: 20 mg, 30 mg

Parsidol® *see* ethopropazine hydrochloride *on page 181*

Partuss® LA *see* guaifenesin and phenylpropanolamine *on page 215*

pas *see* para-aminosalicylate sodium *on page 348*

Paser® *see* aminosalicylic acid *on page 21*

Pathilon® *see* tridihexethyl chloride *on page 469*

Pathocil® *see* dicloxacillin sodium *on page 141*

Pavabid® Oral *see* papaverine hydrochloride *on page 348*

Pavased® Oral *see* papaverine hydrochloride *on page 348*

Pavatine® Oral *see* papaverine hydrochloride *on page 348*

Paverolan® Oral *see* papaverine hydrochloride *on page 348*

Pavulon® *see* pancuronium bromide *on page 347*

Paxil® *see* paroxetine *on this page*

Paxipam® *see* halazepam *on page 219*

PBZ® *see* tripelennamine *on page 474*

PBZ-SR® *see* tripelennamine *on page 474*

PCE® Oral *see* erythromycin *on page 170*

pcmx *see* parachlorometaxylenol *on page 348*

pectin and kaolin *see* kaolin and pectin *on page 256*

Pedameth® *see* methionine *on page 294*

PediaCare® Oral *see* pseudoephedrine *on page 397*

Pediacof® *see* chlorpheniramine, phenylephrine, and codeine *on page 95*

Pediaflor® *see* fluoride *on page 196*

PediaPatch Transdermal Patch [OTC] *see* salicylic acid *on page 416*

Pediapred® Oral *see* prednisolone *on page 383*

Pediatric Triban® *see* trimethobenzamide hydrochloride *on page 472*

Pediazole® *see* erythromycin and sulfisoxazole *on page 171*

Pedi-Boro® [OTC] *see* aluminum acetate and calcium acetate *on page 15*

Pedi-Cort V® Topical *see* clioquinol and hydrocortisone *on page 106*

Pedi-Dri Topical *see* undecylenic acid and derivatives *on page 479*

PediOtic® Otic *see* neomycin, polymyxin b, and hydrocortisone *on page 323*

Pedi-Pro Topical [OTC] *see* undecylenic acid and derivatives *on page 479*

Pedituss® *see* chlorpheniramine, phenylephrine, and codeine *on page 95*

Pedte-Pak-5® *see* trace metals *on page 465*

Pedtrace-4® *see* trace metals *on page 465*

PedvaxHIB™ *see* hemophilus b conjugate vaccine *on page 222*

pegademase bovine (peg a' de mase)
Brand Names Adagen™
Therapeutic Category Enzyme, Replacement Therapy
Use Enzyme replacement therapy for adenosine deaminase (ADA) deficiency in patients with severe combined immunodeficiency disease (SCID) who can not benefit from bone marrow transplant
Usual Dosage Children: I.M.: Dose given every 7 days, 10 units/kg the first dose, 15 units/kg the second dose, and 20 units/kg the third; maintenance dose: 20 units/kg/week is recommended depending on patient's ADA level
Dosage Forms Injection: 250 units/mL (1.5 mL)

Peganone® *see* ethotoin *on page 181*

pegaspargase (pes as' par jase)
Brand Names Oncaspar®
Synonyms peg-l-asparaginase
Therapeutic Category Antineoplastic Agent, Miscellaneous
Use Acute lymphoblastic leukemia in patients who require L-asparaginase in their treatment regimen, but have developed hypersensitivity to the native forms of L-asparaginase
Usual Dosage Refer to individual protocols; I.M. administration may decrease the risk of anaphylaxis; dose must be individualized based upon clinical response and tolerance of the patient.
I.M., I.V.: 2000 units/m^2 every 14 days
Dosage Forms Injection, preservative free: 750 units/mL

peg-es *see* polyethylene glycol-electrolyte solution *on page 375*

peg-l-asparaginase *see* pegaspargase *on this page*

pemoline (pem' oh leen)
Brand Names Cylert®
Synonyms phenylisohydantoin; pio
Therapeutic Category Central Nervous System Stimulant, Nonamphetamine
Use Treatment of attention deficit disorder with hyperactivity (ADDH); narcolepsy
Usual Dosage
Children: <6 years: Not recommended.
(Continued)

pemoline *(Continued)*

Children ≥6 years and Adults: Initial: 37.5 mg given once daily in the morning, increase by 18.75 mg/day at weekly intervals; effective dose range: 56.25-75 mg/day; maximum: 112.5 mg/day; dosage range: 0.5-3 mg/kg/24 hours

Dosage Forms
Tablet: 18.75 mg, 37.5 mg, 75 mg
Tablet, chewable: 37.5 mg

penbutolol sulfate *(pen byoo' toe lole)*

Brand Names Levatol'"'
Therapeutic Category Beta-Adrenergic Blocker
Use Treatment of mild to moderate arterial hypertension
Usual Dosage Adults: Oral: Initial: 20 mg once daily, full effect of a 20 or 40 mg dose is seen by the end of a 2-week period, doses of 40-80 mg have been tolerated but have shown little additional antihypertensive effects
Dosage Forms Tablet: 20 mg

Penecort® *see* hydrocortisone *on page 232*

Penetrex™ Oral *see* enoxacin *on page 166*

penicillamine *(pen i sill' a meen)*

Brand Names Cuprimine'®'; Depen'®'
Synonyms d-3-mercaptovaline; β,β-dimethylcysteine; d-penicillamine
Therapeutic Category Antidote, Copper Toxicity; Antidote, Lead Toxicity; Chelating Agent, Oral
Use Treatment of Wilson's disease, cystinuria, adjunct in the treatment of rheumatoid arthritis; lead poisoning, primary biliary cirrhosis
Usual Dosage Oral:
Rheumatoid arthritis:
Children: Initial: 3 mg/kg/day (≤250 mg/day) for 3 months, then 6 mg/kg/day (≤500 mg/day) in divided doses twice daily for 3 months to a maximum of 10 mg/kg/day in 3-4 divided doses
Adults: 125-250 mg/day, may increase dose at 1- to 3-month intervals up to 1-1.5 g/day

Wilson's disease (doses titrated to maintain urinary copper excretion >1 mg/day):
Infants <6 months: 250 mg/dose once daily
Children <12 years: 250 mg/dose 2-3 times/day
Adults: 250 mg 4 times/day

Cystinuria:
Children: 30 mg/kg/day in 4 divided doses
Adults: 1-4 g/day in divided doses every 6 hours

Lead poisoning (continue until blood lead level is <60 mcg/dL):
Children: 25-40 mg/kg/day in 3 divided doses
Adults: 250 mg/dose every 8-12 hours

Primary biliary cirrhosis: 250 mg/day to start, increase by 250 mg every 2 weeks up to a maintenance dose of 1 g/day, usually given 250 mg 4 times/day

Arsenic poisoning: Children: 100 mg/kg/day in divided doses every 6 hours for 5 days; maximum: 1 g/day

Dosage Forms
Capsule: 125 mg, 250 mg
Tablet: 250 mg

penicillin g benzathine

Brand Names Bicillin'"' L-A Injection; Permapen'"' Injection
Synonyms benzathine benzylpenicillin; benzathine penicillin g; benzylpenicillin benzathine
Therapeutic Category Antibiotic, Penicillin

Use Active against most gram-positive organisms; some gram-negative organisms such as *Neisseria gonorrhoeae* and some anaerobes and spirochetes; used only for the treatment of mild to moderately severe infections caused by organisms susceptible to low concentrations of penicillin g, or for prophylaxis of infections caused by these organisms

Usual Dosage I.M.: Give undiluted injection, very slowly released from site of injection, providing uniform levels over 2-4 weeks; higher doses result in more sustained rather than higher levels. Use a penicillin g benzathine-penicillin g procaine combination to achieve early peak levels in acute infections

Neonates >1200 g: 50,000 units as a single dose

Infants and Children:
> Group A streptococcal upper respiratory infection: 25,000 units/kg as a single dose; maximum: 1.2 million units
> Prophylaxis of recurrent rheumatic fever: 25,000 units/kg every 3-4 weeks; maximum: 1.2 million units/dose
> Early syphilis: 50,000 units/kg as a single injection; maximum: 2.4 million units
> Syphilis of more than 1-year duration: 50,000 units/kg every week for 3 doses; maximum: 2.4 million units/dose

Adults:
> Group A streptococcal upper respiratory infection: 1.2 million units as a single dose
> Prophylaxis of recurrent rheumatic fever: 1.2 million units every 3-4 weeks or 600,000 units twice monthly; a single dose of 600,000 to 1,2000,000 units is effective in the prevention of rheumatic fever secondary to streptococcal pharyngitis
> Early syphilis: 2.4 million units as a single dose
> Syphilis of more than 1-year duration: 2.4 million units once weekly for 3 doses

Dosage Forms Injection: 300,000 units/mL (10 mL); 600,000 units/mL (1 mL, 2 mL, 4 mL)

penicillin g benzathine and procaine combined
Brand Names Bicillin® C-R 900/300 Injection; Bicillin® C-R Injection
Synonyms penicillin g procaine and benzathine combined
Therapeutic Category Antibiotic, Penicillin
Use Active against most gram-positive organisms, mostly streptococcal and pneumococcal
Usual Dosage I.M.:
Children:
> <30 lb: 600,000 units in a single dose
> 30-60 lb: 900,000 units to 1.2 million units in a single dose

Children >60 lb and Adults: 2.4 million units in a single dose

Dosage Forms
Injection:
> 300,000 units [150,000 units each of penicillin g benzathine and penicillin g procaine] (10 mL)
> 600,000 units [300,000 units each penicillin g benzathine and penicillin g procaine] (1 mL)
> 1,200,000 units [600,000 units each penicillin g benzathine and penicillin g procaine] (2 mL)
> 2,400,000 units [1,200,000 units each penicillin g benzathine and penicillin g procaine] (4 mL)

Injection: Penicillin g benzathine 900,000 units and penicillin g procaine 300,000 units per dose (2 mL)

penicillin g, parenteral
Brand Names Pfizerpen® Injection
Synonyms benzylpenicillin potassium; benzylpenicillin sodium; crystalline penicillin; penicillin g potassium; penicillin g sodium
Therapeutic Category Antibiotic, Penicillin
Use Active against most gram-positive organisms except *Staphylococcus aureus*; some gram-negative such as *Neisseria gonorrhoeae* and some anaerobes and spirochetes; although ceftriaxone is now the drug of choice for lyme disease and gonorrhea
Usual Dosage I.M., I.V.:
Neonates:
> Postnatal age <7 days:
> > <2000 g: 25,000 units/kg/dose every 12 hours; meningitis: 50,000 units/kg/dose every 12 hours

(Continued)

penicillin g, parenteral (Continued)

>2000 g: 20,000 units/kg/dose every 8 hours; meningitis: 50,000 units/kg/dose every 8 hours

Postnatal age >7 days:

<1200 g: 25,000 units/kg/dose every 12 hours; meningitis: 50,000 units/kg/dose every 12 hours

1200-2000 g: 25,000 units/kg/dose every 8 hours; meningitis: 75,000 units/kg/dose every 8 hours

>2000 g: 25,000 units/kg/dose every 6 hours; meningitis: 50,000 units/kg/dose every 6 hours

Infants and Children (sodium salt is preferred in children): 100,000-250,000 units/kg/day in divided doses every 4 hours; maximum: 4.8 million units/24 hours

Severe infections: Up to 400,000 units/kg/day in divided doses every 4 hours; maximum dose: 24 million units/day

Adults: 2-24 million units/day in divided doses every 4 hours

Dosage Forms

Injection, as sodium: 5 million units

Injection:

Frozen premixed, as potassium: 1 million units, 2 million units, 3 million units

Powder, as potassium: 1 million units, 5 million units, 10 million units, 20 million units

penicillin g potassium see penicillin g, parenteral on previous page

penicillin g procaine and benzathine combined see penicillin g benzathine and procaine combined on previous page

penicillin g procaine, aqueous

Brand Names Crysticillin" A.S. Injection; Pfizerpen®-AS Injection; Wycillin® Injection

Synonyms appg; aqueous procaine penicillin g; procaine benzylpenicillin; procaine penicillin g

Therapeutic Category Antibiotic, Penicillin

Use Moderately severe infections due to *Neisseria gonorrhoeae*, *Treponema pallidum* and other penicillin g-sensitive microorganisms that are susceptible to low but prolonged serum penicillin concentrations

Usual Dosage I.M.:

Newborns: 50,000 units/kg/day given every day (avoid using in this age group since sterile abscesses and procaine toxicity occur more frequently with neonates than older patients)

Children: 25,000-50,000 units/kg/day in divided doses 1-2 times/day; not to exceed 4.8 million units/24 hours

Gonorrhea: 100,000 units/kg one time (in 2 injection sites) along with probenecid 25 mg/kg (maximum: 1 g) orally 30 minutes prior to procaine penicillin

Adults: 0.6-4.8 million units/day in divided doses 1-2 times/day

Uncomplicated gonorrhea: 1 g probenecid orally, then 4.8 million units procaine penicillin divided into 2 injection sites 30 minutes later. When used in conjunction with an aminoglycoside for the treatment of endocarditis caused by susceptible *S. viridans*: 1.2 million units every 6 hours for 2-4 weeks

Dosage Forms Injection, suspension: 300,000 units/mL (10 mL); 500,000 units/mL (1.2 mL); 600,000 units/mL (1 mL, 2 mL, 4 mL)

penicillin g sodium see penicillin g, parenteral on previous page

penicillin v potassium

Brand Names Beepen-VK" Oral; Betapen"-VK Oral; Ledercillin® VK Oral; Pen.Vee® K Oral; Robicillin" VK Oral; V-Cillin K" Oral; Veetids" Oral

Synonyms pen vk; phenoxymethyl penicillin

Therapeutic Category Antibiotic, Penicillin

Use Treatment of moderate to severe susceptible bacterial infections involving the respiratory tract, skin and urinary tract; prophylaxis of pneumococcal infections and rheumatic fever; otitis media and sinusitis

Usual Dosage Oral:

Systemic infections:

Children <12 years: 25-50 mg/kg/day in divided doses every 6-8 hours; maximum dose: 3 g/day

Children >12 years and Adults: 125-500 mg every 6-8 hours

Prophylaxis of pneumococcal infections:

Children <5 years: 125 mg twice daily

Children ≥5 years: 250 mg twice daily

Prophylaxis of recurrent rheumatic fever:

Children <5 years: 125 mg

Children ≥5 years and Adults: 250 mg twice daily

Dosage Forms

Powder for oral solution: 125 mg/5 mL (3 mL, 100 mL, 150 mL, 200 mL); 250 mg/5 mL (100 mL, 150 mL, 200 mL)

Tablet: 125 mg, 250 mg, 500 mg

penicilloyl-polylysine see benzylpenicilloyl-polylysine on page 51

Pentacef™ see ceftazidime on page 82

pentaerythritol tetranitrate (pen ta er ith' ri tole te tra nye' trate)

Brand Names Duotrate®; Peritrate®; Peritrate® SA

Synonyms petn

Therapeutic Category Antianginal Agent; Nitrate; Vasodilator, Coronary

Use Prophylactic long-term management of angina pectoris

Usual Dosage Adults: Oral: 10-20 mg 4 times/day (160 mg/day) up to 40 mg 4 times/day before or after meals and at bedtime; administer sustained release preparation every 12 hours; maximum daily dose: 240 mg

Dosage Forms

Capsule: sustained release: 15 mg, 30 mg

Tablet: 10 mg, 20 mg, 40 mg

Tablet, sustained release: 80 mg

pentagastrin (pen ta gas' trin)

Brand Names Peptavlon®

Therapeutic Category Diagnostic Agent, Gastric Acid Secretory Function

Use Evaluate gastric acid secretory function in pernicious anemia, gastric carcinoma; in suspected duodenal ulcer or Zollinger-Ellison tumor

Usual Dosage Adults: S.C.: 6 mcg/kg

Dosage Forms Injection: 0.25 mg/mL (2 mL)

Pentam-300® Injection see pentamidine isethionate on this page

pentamidine isethionate (pen tam' i deen eye se thi' o nate)

Brand Names NebuPent™ Inhalation; Pentam-300® Injection

Therapeutic Category Antibiotic, Miscellaneous

Use Treatment and prevention of pneumonia caused by *Pneumocystis carinii* (PCP); treatment of trypanosomiasis

Usual Dosage

Children:

Treatment: I.M., I.V. (I.V. preferred): 4 mg/kg/day once daily for 14-21 days

(Continued)

pentamidine isethionate *(Continued)*

Prevention:
I.M., I.V.: 4 mg/kg monthly or biweekly
Inhalation (aerosolized pentamidine in children ≥5 years): 300 mg/dose given every 3 weeks or monthly via Respirgard™ II inhaler (8 mg/kg dose has also been used in children <5 years)
Treatment of trypanosomiasis: I.V.: 4 mg/kg/day once daily for 10 days

Adults:
Treatment: I.M., I.V. (I.V. preferred): 4 mg/kg/day once daily for 14 days
Prevention: Inhalation: 300 mg every 4 weeks via Respirgard® II nebulizer

Dosage Forms
Inhalation: 300 mg
Powder for injection, lyophilized: 300 mg

Pentasa® Oral *see* mesalamine *on page 289*

Pentaspan® *see* pentastarch *on this page*

pentastarch *(pen' ta starch)*
Brand Names Pentaspan™
Therapeutic Category Blood Modifiers
Use Adjunct in leukapheresis to improve the harvesting and increase the yield of leukocytes by centrifugal means

pentazocine *(pen taz' oh seen)*
Brand Names Talwin™; Talwin™ NX
Therapeutic Category Analgesic, Narcotic
Use Relief of moderate to severe pain; has also been used as a sedative prior to surgery and as a supplement to surgical anesthesia
Usual Dosage
Children: I.M., S.C.:
5-8 years: 15 mg
8-14 years: 30 mg

Children >12 years and Adults: Oral: 50 mg every 3-4 hours; may increase to 100 mg/dose if needed, but should not exceed 600 mg/day

Adults:
I.M., S.C.: 30-60 mg every 3-4 hours, not to exceed total daily dose of 360 mg
I.V.: 30 mg every 3-4 hours
Dosage Forms
Injection, as lactate: 30 mg/mL (1 mL, 1.5 mL, 2 mL, 10 mL)
Tablet, scored: Pentazocine hydrochloride 50 mg and naloxone hydrochloride 0.5 mg

pentazocine compound
Brand Names Talacen™; Talwin™ Compound
Therapeutic Category Analgesic, Narcotic
Use Relief of moderate to severe pain; has also been used as a sedative prior to surgery and as a supplement to surgical anesthesia
Usual Dosage Adults: Oral: 2 tablets 3-4 times/day
Dosage Forms Tablet:
Talacen™: Pentazocine hydrochloride 25 mg and acetaminophen 650 mg
Talwin™ Compound: Pentazocine hydrochloride 12.5 mg and aspirin 325 mg

Penthrane® *see* methoxyflurane *on page 297*

pentobarbital *(pen toe bar' bi tal)*
Brand Names Nembutal™
Synonyms pentobarbital sodium
Therapeutic Category Barbiturate; Sedative

Use Short-term treatment of insomnia; preoperative sedation; high-dose barbiturate coma for treatment of increased intracranial pressure or status epilepticus unresponsive to other therapy

Usual Dosage

Children:

Sedative: Oral: 2-6 mg/kg/day divided in 3 doses; maximum: 100 mg/day

Hypnotic: I.M.: 2-6 mg/kg; maximum: 100 mg/dose

Rectal:

2 months to 1 year (10-20 lb): 30 mg

1-4 years (20-40 lb): 30-60 mg

5-12 years (40-80 lb): 60 mg

12-14 years (80-110 lb): 60-120 mg **or**

<4 years: 3-6 mg/kg/dose

>4 years: 1.5-3 mg/kg/dose

Preoperative/preprocedure sedation: $\geq$6 months:

Oral, I.M., rectal: 2-6 mg/kg; maximum: 100 mg/dose

I.V.: 1-3 mg/kg to a maximum of 100 mg until asleep

Children 5-12 years: Conscious sedation prior to a procedure: I.V.: 2 mg/kg 5-10 minutes before procedures, may repeat one time

Adolescents: Conscious sedation: Oral, I.V.: 100 mg prior to a procedure

Children and Adults: Barbiturate coma in head injury patients: I.V.: Loading dose: 5-10 mg/kg given slowly over 1-2 hours; monitor blood pressure and respiratory rate; Maintenance infusion: Initial: 1 mg/kg/hour; may increase to 2-3 mg/kg/hour; maintain burst suppression on EEG

Adults:

Hypnotic:

Oral: 100-200 mg at bedtime or 20 mg 3-4 times/day for daytime sedation

I.M.: 150-200 mg

I.V.: Initial: 100 mg, may repeat every 1-3 minutes up to 200-500 mg total dose

Rectal: 120-200 mg at bedtime

Preoperative sedation: I.M.: 150-200 mg

Dosage Forms

Capsule, as sodium: 50 mg, 100 mg

Elixir: 18.2 mg/5 mL (473 mL, 4000 mL)

Injection, as sodium: 50 mg/mL (1 mL, 2 mL, 20 mL, 50 mL)

Suppository, rectal (C-III): 30 mg, 60 mg, 120 mg, 200 mg

pentobarbital sodium *see* pentobarbital *on previous page*

Pentolair® *see* cyclopentolate hydrochloride *on page 120*

pentostatin (pen' toe stat in)

Brand Names Nipent™ Injection

Synonyms dcf; 2'-deoxycoformycin

Therapeutic Category Antineoplastic Agent, Antimetabolite; Antineoplastic Agent, Nonirritant

Use Treatment of adult patients with alpha-interferon-refractory hairy cell leukemia; significant antitumor activity in various lymphoid neoplasms has been demonstrated; pentostatin also is known as 2'-deoxycoformycin; it is a purine analogue capable of inhibiting adenosine deaminase

Usual Dosage Refractory hairy cell leukemia: Adults: I.V.: 4 mg/m^2 every other week

Dosage Forms Powder for injection: 10 mg

Pentothal® Sodium *see* thiopental sodium *on page 457*

pentoxifylline (pen tox i' fi leen)

Brand Names Trental"

Synonyms oxpentifylline

Therapeutic Category Blood Viscosity Reducer Agent

(Continued)

pentoxifylline *(Continued)*

Use Symptomatic management of peripheral vascular disease, mainly intermittent claudication

Usual Dosage Adults: Oral: 400 mg 3 times/day with meals; may reduce to 400 mg twice daily if GI or CNS side effects occur

Dosage Forms Tablet, controlled release: 400 mg

Pentrax® [OTC] *see* coal tar *on page 110*

Pen.Vee® K Oral *see* penicillin v potassium *on page 354*

pen vk *see* penicillin v potassium *on page 354*

Pepcid® I.V. *see* famotidine *on page 185*

Pepcid® Oral *see* famotidine *on page 185*

Peptavlon® *see* pentagastrin *on page 355*

Pepto-Bismol® [OTC] *see* bismuth subsalicylate *on page 55*

Pepto® Diarrhea Control [OTC] *see* loperamide hydrochloride *on page 272*

Perchloracap® *see* radiological/contrast media (ionic) *on page 404*

Percocet® *see* oxycodone and acetaminophen *on page 342*

Percodan® *see* oxycodone and aspirin *on page 343*

Percodan®-Demi *see* oxycodone and aspirin *on page 343*

Percogesic® [OTC] *see* acetaminophen and phenyltoloxamine *on page 4*

Perdiem® Plain [OTC] *see* psyllium *on page 398*

pergolide mesylate *(per' go lide)*

Brand Names Permax"

Therapeutic Category Anti-Parkinson's Agent; Ergot Alkaloid

Use Adjunctive treatment to levodopa/carbidopa in the management of Parkinson's Disease

Usual Dosage Adults: Oral: Start with 0.05 mg/day for 2 days, then increase dosage by 0.1 or 0.15 mg/day every 3 days over next 12 days, increase dose by 0.25 mg/day every 3 days until optimal therapeutic dose is achieved

Dosage Forms Tablet: 0.05 mg, 0.25 mg, 1 mg

Pergonal® *see* menotropins *on page 286*

Periactin® *see* cyproheptadine hydrochloride *on page 122*

Peri-Colace® [OTC] *see* docusate and casanthranol *on page 154*

Peridex® Oral Rinse *see* chlorhexidine gluconate *on page 90*

perindopril erbumine *(per in' doe pril)*

Brand Names Aceon"

Therapeutic Category Antihypertensive

Use Treatment of hypertension

Usual Dosage Adults: Oral: 4 mg once daily; usual range is 4-8 mg/day, maximum of 16 mg/day

Dosage Forms Tablet: 2 mg, 4 mg, 8 mg

Peritrate® *see* pentaerythritol tetranitrate *on page 355*

Peritrate® SA *see* pentaerythritol tetranitrate *on page 355*

Permapen® Injection *see* penicillin g benzathine *on page 352*

Permax® *see* pergolide mesylate *on this page*

permethrin (per meth' rin)
Brand Names Elimite™ Cream; Nix™ Creme Rinse
Therapeutic Category Antiparasitic Agent, Topical; Scabicidal Agent
Use Single application treatment of infestation with *Pediculus humanus capitis* (head louse) and its nits, or *Sarcoptes scabiei* (scabies)
Usual Dosage
  Head lice: Children >2 months and Adults: Topical: After hair has been washed with shampoo, rinsed with water and towel dried, apply a sufficient volume to saturate the hair and scalp. Leave on hair for 10 minutes before rinsing off with water; remove remaining nits.

  Scabies: Apply cream from head to toe; leave on for 8-14 hours before washing off with water
Dosage Forms
  Cream: 5% (60 g)
  Creme rinse: 1% (60 mL with comb)

Permitil® Oral *see* fluphenazine *on page 199*
Pernox® [OTC] *see* sulfur and salicylic acid *on page 442*
Peroxin A5® *see* benzoyl peroxide *on page 50*
Peroxin A10® *see* benzoyl peroxide *on page 50*

perphenazine (per fen' a zeen)
Brand Names Trilafon®
Therapeutic Category Antiemetic; Antipsychotic Agent; Phenothiazine Derivative
Use Symptomatic management of psychotic disorders, as well as severe nausea and vomiting
Usual Dosage
  Children:
    Psychoses: Oral:
      1-6 years: 4-6 mg/day in divided doses
      6-12 years: 6 mg/day in divided doses
      >12 years: 4-16 mg 2-4 times/day
      I.M.: 5 mg every 6 hours
    Nausea/vomiting: I.M.: 5 mg every 6 hours

  Adults:
    Psychoses:
      Oral: 4-16 mg 2-4 times/day not to exceed 64 mg/day
      I.M.: 5 mg every 6 hours up to 15 mg/day in ambulatory patients and 30 mg/day in hospitalized patients
    Nausea/vomiting:
      Oral: 8-16 mg/day in divided doses up to 24 mg/day
      I.M.: 5-10 mg every 6 hours as necessary up to 15 mg/day in ambulatory patients and 30 mg/day in hospitalized patients
      I.V. (severe): 1 mg at 1- to 2-minute intervals up to a total of 5 mg
Dosage Forms
  Concentrate, oral: 16 mg/5 mL (118 mL)
  Injection: 5 mg/mL (1 mL)
  Tablet: 2 mg, 4 mg, 8 mg, 16 mg

perphenazine and amitriptyline *see* amitriptyline and perphenazine *on page 21*
Persa-Gel® *see* benzoyl peroxide *on page 50*
Persantine® *see* dipyridamole *on page 151*
Pertofrane® *see* desipramine hydrochloride *on page 130*
Pertussin® CS [OTC] *see* dextromethorphan hydrobromide *on page 135*
Pertussin® ES [OTC] *see* dextromethorphan hydrobromide *on page 135*

pertussis immune globulin, human
Brand Names Hypertussis™
Therapeutic Category Immune Globulin
Dosage Forms Injection: 1.25 mL

pethidine hydrochloride *see* meperidine hydrochloride *on page 286*

petn *see* pentaerythritol tetranitrate *on page 355*

pfa *see* foscarnet *on page 202*

Pfizerpen®-AS Injection *see* penicillin g procaine, aqueous *on page 354*

Pfizerpen® Injection *see* penicillin g, parenteral *on page 353*

pge₁ *see* alprostadil *on page 14*

pge₂ *see* dinoprostone *on page 148*

pgf₂ₐ *see* dinoprost tromethamine *on page 148*

Phanatuss® [OTC] *see* guaifenesin and dextromethorphan *on page 214*

Pharmaflur® *see* fluoride *on page 196*

Phazyme® [OTC] *see* simethicone *on page 423*

Phenameth® DM *see* promethazine with dextromethorphan *on page 391*

Phenameth® Oral *see* promethazine hydrochloride *on page 390*

phenantoin *see* mephenytoin *on page 287*

Phenazine® Injection *see* promethazine hydrochloride *on page 390*

phenazopyridine hydrochloride (fen az oh peer' i deen)
Brand Names Azo-Standard™; Geridium™; Prodium® [OTC]; Pyridiate®; Pyridium®
Synonyms phenylazo diamino pyridine hydrochloride
Therapeutic Category Analgesic, Urinary; Local Anesthetic, Urinary
Use Symptomatic relief of urinary burning, itching, frequency and urgency in association with urinary tract infection or following urologic procedures
Usual Dosage Oral:
Children 6-12 years: 12 mg/kg/day in 3 divided doses administered after meals for 2 days
Adults: 100-200 mg 3-4 times/day for 2 days
Dosage Forms Tablet:
Azo-Standard™, Geridium™, Pyridiate™, Pyridium™:100 mg, 200 mg
Prodium™: 95 mg

Phen DH® w/Codeine *see* chlorpheniramine, pseudoephedrine, and codeine *on page 97*

Phendry® Oral [OTC] *see* diphenhydramine hydrochloride *on page 149*

phenelzine sulfate (fen' el zeen)
Brand Names Nardil™
Therapeutic Category Antidepressant, Monoamine Oxidase Inhibitor
Use Symptomatic treatment of atypical, nonendogenous or neurotic depression
Usual Dosage Adults: Oral: 15 mg 3 times/day; may increase to 60-90 mg/day during early phase of treatment, then reduce to dose for maintenance therapy slowly after maximum benefit is obtained; takes 2-4 weeks for a significant response to occur
Dosage Forms Tablet: 15 mg

Phenerbel-S® *see* belladonna, phenobarbital, and ergotamine tartrate *on page 46*

Phenergan® Injection *see* promethazine hydrochloride *on page 390*

Phenergan® Oral *see* promethazine hydrochloride *on page 390*

Phenergan® Rectal see promethazine hydrochloride on page 390

Phenergan® VC see promethazine and phenylephrine on page 390

Phenergan® VC With Codeine see promethazine, phenylephrine, and codeine on page 391

Phenergan® with Codeine see promethazine and codeine on page 390

Phenergan® with Dextromethorphan see promethazine with dextromethorphan on page 391

Phenetron® Oral see chlorpheniramine maleate on page 95

Phenhist® Expectorant see guaifenesin, pseudoephedrine, and codeine on page 217

phenindamine tartrate (fen in' dah meen)
Brand Names Nolahist® [OTC]
Therapeutic Category Antihistamine
Use Treatment of perennial and seasonal allergic rhinitis and chronic urticaria
Usual Dosage Oral:
Children <6 years: As directed by physician
Children 6 to <12 years: 12.5 mg every 4-6 hours, up to 75 mg/24 hours
Adults: 25 mg every 4-6 hours, up to 150 mg/24 hours
Dosage Forms Tablet: 25 mg

pheniramine and naphazoline see naphazoline and pheniramine on page 319

pheniramine, phenylpropanolamine, and pyrilamine
Brand Names Triaminic® Oral Infant Drops
Therapeutic Category Antihistamine/Decongestant Combination
Use Symptomatic relief of nasal congestion and postnasal drip as well as allergic rhinitis
Usual Dosage Infants <1 year: Drops: 0.05 mL/kg/dose 4 times/day
Dosage Forms Drops: Pheniramine maleate 10 mg, phenylpropanolamine hydrochloride 20 mg, and pyrilamine maleate 10 mg per mL (15 mL)

phenobarbital (fee noe bar' bi tal)
Brand Names Barbita®; Luminal®; Solfoton®
Synonyms phenobarbitone; phenylethylmalonylurea
Therapeutic Category Anticonvulsant, Barbiturate; Barbiturate; Hypnotic; Sedative
Use Management of generalized tonic-clonic (grand mal) and partial seizures; prevention of febrile seizures in infants and young children; sedation; may also be used for prevention and treatment of neonatal hyperbilirubinemia and lowering of bilirubin in chronic cholestasis
Usual Dosage
Children:
Sedation: Oral: 2 mg/kg 3 times/day
Hypnotic: I.M., I.V., S.C.: 3-5 mg/kg at bedtime
Hyperbilirubinemia: <12 years: Oral: 3-8 mg/kg/day in 2-3 divided doses; doses up to 12 mg/kg/day have been used
Preoperative sedation: Oral, I.M., I.V.: 1-3 mg/kg 1-1.5 hours before procedure

Anticonvulsant: Status epilepticus: **Loading dose: I.V.:**
Neonates: 15-20 mg/kg in a single or divided dose
Infants, Children and Adults: 15-18 mg/kg in a single or divided dose; usual maximum loading dose: 20 mg/kg; in select patients may give additional 5 mg/kg/dose every 15-30 minutes until seizure is controlled or a total dose of 30 mg/kg is reached

Anticonvulsant maintenance dose: Oral, I.V.:
Neonates: 3-4 mg/kg/day in 1-2 divided doses; assess serum concentrations; increase to 5 mg/kg/day if needed (usually by second week of therapy)
Infants: 5-6 mg/kg/day in 1-2 divided doses
Children:
1-5 years: 6-8 mg/kg/day in 1-2 divided doses

(Continued)

phenobarbital (Continued)

      5-12 years: 4-6 mg/kg/day in 1-2 divided doses
      Children >12 years and Adults: 1-3 mg/kg/day in divided doses

Adults:
    Sedation: Oral, I.M.: 30-120 mg/day in 2-3 divided doses
    Hypnotic: Oral, I.M., I.V., S.C.: 100-320 mg at bedtime
    Hyperbilirubinemia: Oral: 90-180 mg/day in 2-3 divided doses
    Preoperative sedation: I.M.: 100-200 mg 1-1$\frac{1}{2}$ hours before procedure

Dosage Forms
Capsule: 16 mg
Elixir: 15 mg/5 mL (5 mL, 10 mL, 20 mL); 20 mg/5 mL (3.75 mL, 5 mL, 7.5 mL, 120 mL, 473 mL, 946 mL, 4000 mL)
Injection, as sodium: 30 mg/mL (1 mL); 60 mg/mL (1 mL); 65 mg/mL (1 mL); 130 mg/mL (1 mL)
Powder for injection: 120 mg
Tablet: 8 mg, 15 mg, 16 mg, 30 mg, 32 mg, 60 mg, 65 mg, 100 mg

phenobarbitone see phenobarbital on previous page

phenol

Brand Names Baker's P&S Topical [OTC]; Cĕpastat® [OTC]; Chloraseptic® Oral [OTC]
Synonyms carbolic acid
Therapeutic Category Pharmaceutical Aid
Use Relief of sore throat pain, mouth, gum, and throat irritations
Usual Dosage Allow to dissolve slowly in mouth; may be repeated every 2 hours as needed
Dosage Forms
Liquid, topical (Baker's P&S): 1% with sodium chloride, liquid paraffin oil and water (120 mL, 240 mL)
Lozenge:
    Cĕpastat'": 1.45% with menthol and eucalyptus oil
    Cĕpastat'" Cherry: 0.72% with menthol and eucalyptus oil
    Chloraseptic'": 32.5 mg total phenol, sugar, corn syrup
Mouthwash (Chloraseptic®): 1.4% with thymol, sodium borate, menthol, and glycerin (180 mL)
Solution (Liquified Phenol): 88% [880 mg/mL]

Phenolax® [OTC] see phenolphthalein on this page

phenolphthalein (fee nole thay' leen)

Brand Names Alophen Pills® [OTC]; Espotabs® [OTC]; Evac-U-Gen® [OTC]; Evac-U-Lax® [OTC]; Ex-Lax'" [OTC]; Feen-a-Mint'" [OTC]; Lax-Pills® [OTC]; Medilax® [OTC]; Modane® [OTC]; Phenolax'" [OTC]; Prulet® [OTC]
Therapeutic Category Laxative, Stimulant
Use Stimulant laxative
Usual Dosage Oral:
Children: 15-60 mg
Adults: 60-200 mg preferably at bedtime
Dosage Forms
Gum: 97.2 mg
Tablet: 60 mg, 90 mg, 97.2 mg, 130 mg
Tablet, chewable: 65 mg, 90 mg, 97.2 mg, 120 mg
Wafer: 64.8 mg
Wafer, chewable: 80 mg

phenol red see phenolsulfonphthalein on next page

phenolsulfonphthalein (fee nole sul fon thay' leen)
Synonyms phenol red; psp
Therapeutic Category Diagnostic Agent, Kidney Function
Use Evaluation of renal blood flow to aid in the determination of renal function
Usual Dosage I.M., I.V.: 6 mg
Dosage Forms Injection: 6 mg/mL (1 mL)

phenoxybenzamine hydrochloride (fen ox ee ben' za meen)
Brand Names Dibenzyline®
Therapeutic Category Alpha-Adrenergic Blocking Agent, Oral; Antihypertensive; Vasodilator, Coronary
Use Symptomatic management of pheochromocytoma; treatment of hypertensive crisis caused by sympathomimetic amines
Usual Dosage Oral:
Children: Initial: 0.2 mg/kg (maximum: 10 mg) once daily, increase by 0.2 mg/kg increments; usual maintenance dose: 0.4-1.2 mg/kg/day every 6-8 hours, maximum single dose: 10 mg
Adults: 10-40 mg every 8-12 hours
Dosage Forms Capsule: 10 mg

phenoxymethyl penicillin see penicillin v potassium on page 354

phensuximide (fen sux' i mide)
Brand Names Milontin®
Therapeutic Category Anticonvulsant, Succinimide
Use Control of absence (petit mal) seizures
Usual Dosage Children and Adults: Oral: 0.5-1 g 2-3 times/day
Dosage Forms Capsule: 500 mg

phentermine hydrochloride (fen' ter meen)
Brand Names Adipex-P®; Fastin®; Ionamin®; Zantryl®
Therapeutic Category Anorexiant
Use Short-term adjunct in exogenous obesity
Usual Dosage Children and Adults: Oral: 8 mg 3 times/day 30 minutes before meals or food or 15-37.5 mg/day before breakfast
Dosage Forms
Capsule: 15 mg, 18.75 mg, 30 mg, 37.5 mg
Capsule, resin complex: 15 mg, 30 mg
Tablet: 8 mg, 37.5 mg

phentolamine mesylate (fen tole' a meen)
Brand Names Regitine®
Therapeutic Category Alpha-Adrenergic Blocking Agent, Parenteral; Alpha-Adrenergic Inhibitors, Central; Antidote, Extravasation; Antihypertensive; Diagnostic Agent, Pheochromocytoma; Vasodilator, Coronary
Use Diagnosis of pheochromocytoma and to control or prevent paroxysmal hypertension prior to and during pheochromocytomectomy; as treatment of dermal necrosis after extravasation of drugs with alpha-adrenergic effects (norepinephrine, dopamine, epinephrine)
Usual Dosage
Treatment of extravasation: Infiltrate area S.C. with small amount of solution made by diluting 5-10 mg in 10 mL 0.9% NaCl within 12 hours of extravasation; for children use 0.1-0.2 mg/kg up to a maximum of 10 mg
Children: I.M., I.V.:
Diagnosis of pheochromocytoma: 0.05-0.1 mg/kg/dose, maximum single dose: 5 mg
Hypertension: 0.05-0.1 mg/kg/dose given 1-2 hours before procedure; repeat as needed until hypertension is controlled; maximum single dose: 5 mg
(Continued)
363

phentolamine mesylate *(Continued)*
Adults: I.M., I.V.:
Diagnosis of pheochromocytoma: 5 mg
Hypertension: 5 mg given 1-2 hours before procedure
Dosage Forms Injection: 5 mg/mL (1 mL)

phenylalanine mustard *see* melphalan *on page 285*

phenylazo diamino pyridine hydrochloride *see* phenazopyridine hydrochloride *on page 360*

phenylephrine and chlorpheniramine *see* chlorpheniramine and phenylephrine *on page 93*

phenylephrine and cyclopentolate *see* cyclopentolate and phenylephrine *on page 120*

phenylephrine and scopolamine
Brand Names Murocoll-2® Ophthalmic
Synonyms scopolamine and phenylephrine
Therapeutic Category Ophthalmic Agent, Mydriatic
Use Mydriasis, cycloplegia and to break posterior synechiae in iritis
Usual Dosage Ophthalmic: Instill 1-2 drops into eye(s); repeat in 5 minutes
Dosage Forms Solution, ophthalmic: Phenylephrine hydrochloride 10% and scopolamine hydrobromide 0.3% (7.5 mL)

phenylephrine and zinc sulfate
Brand Names Optised™ Ophthalmic [OTC]; Phenylzin® Ophthalmic [OTC]; Zincfrin® Ophthalmic [OTC]
Therapeutic Category Ophthalmic Agent, Miscellaneous
Use Soothe, moisturize, and remove redness due to minor eye irritation
Usual Dosage Ophthalmic: Instill 1-2 drops in eye(s) 2-4 times/day as needed
Dosage Forms Solution, ophthalmic: Phenylephrine hydrochloride 0.12% and zinc sulfate 0.25% (15 mL)

phenylephrine hydrochloride (fen ill ef' rin)
Brand Names AK-Dilate™ Ophthalmic Solution; AK-Nefrin® Ophthalmic Solution; Alconefrin® Nasal Solution [OTC]; Doktors™ Nasal Solution [OTC]; I-Phrine® Ophthalmic Solution; Isopto® Frin Ophthalmic Solution; Mydfrin™ Ophthalmic Solution; Neo-Synephrine® Nasal Solution [OTC]; Neo-Synephrine® Ophthalmic Solution; Nostril® Nasal Solution [OTC]; Prefrin™ Ophthalmic Solution; Relief™ Ophthalmic Solution; Rhinall® Nasal Solution [OTC]; Sinarest® Nasal Solution [OTC]; St. Joseph® Measured Dose Nasal Solution [OTC]; Vicks® Sinex® Nasal Solution [OTC]
Therapeutic Category Adrenergic Agonist Agent; Adrenergic Agonist Agent, Ophthalmic; Alpha-Adrenergic Blocking Agent, Ophthalmic; Nasal Agent, Vasoconstrictor; Ophthalmic Agent, Mydriatic
Use Treatment of hypotension, vascular failure in shock; as a vasoconstrictor in regional analgesia; symptomatic relief of nasal and nasopharyngeal mucosal congestion; as a mydriatic in ophthalmic procedures and treatment of wide-angle glaucoma
Usual Dosage
Ophthalmic procedures:
Infants <1 year: Instill 1 drop of 2.5% 15-30 minutes before procedures
Children and Adults: Instill 1 drop of 2.5% or 10% solution, may repeat in 10-60 minutes as needed

Nasal decongestant:
Children:
2-6 years: Instill 1 drop every 2-4 hours of 0.125% solution as needed
6-12 years: Instill 1-2 sprays or instill 1-2 drops every 4 hours of 0.25% solution as needed

Children >12 years and Adults: Instill 1-2 sprays or instill 1-2 drops every 4 hours of 0.25% to 0.5% solution as needed; 1% solution may be used in adult in cases of extreme nasal congestion; do not use nasal solutions more than 3 days

Hypotension/shock:
Children:
I.M., S.C.: 0.1 mg/kg/dose every 1-2 hours as needed (maximum: 5 mg)
I.V. bolus: 5-20 mcg/kg/dose every 10-15 minutes as needed
I.V. infusion: 0.1-0.5 mcg/kg/minute; the concentration and rate of infusion can be calculated using the following formulas: Dilute 0.6 mg x weight (kg) to 100 mL; then the dose in mcg/kg/minute = 0.1 x the infusion rate in mL/hour
Adults:
I.M., S.C.: 2-5 mg/dose every 1-2 hours as needed (initial dose should not exceed 5 mg)
I.V. bolus: 0.1-0.5 mg/dose every 10-15 minutes as needed (initial dose should not exceed 0.5 mg)
I.V. infusion: 10 mg in 250 mL D_5W or NS (1:25,000 dilution) (40 mcg/mL); start at 100-180 mcg/minute (2-5 mL/minute; 50-90 drops/minute) initially. When blood pressure is stabilized, maintenance rate: 40-60 mcg/minute (20-30 drops/minute)

Paroxysmal supraventricular tachycardia: I.V.:
Children: 5-10 mcg/kg/dose over 20-30 seconds
Adults: 0.25-0.5 mg/dose over 20-30 seconds

Dosage Forms
Injection (Neo-Synephrine®): 1% [10 mg/mL] (1 mL)
Nasal solution:
Drops:
Neo-Synephrine®: 0.125% (15 mL)
Alconefrin® 12: 0.16% (30 mL)
Alconefrin® 25, Neo-Synephrine®, Children's Nostril®, Rhinall®: 0.25% (15 mL, 30 mL, 40 mL)
Alconefrin®, Neo-Synephrine®: 0.5% (15 mL, 30 mL)
Spray:
Alconefrin® 25, Neo-Synephrine®, Rhinall®: 0.25% (15 mL, 30 mL, 40 mL)
Neo-Synephrine®, Nostril®, Sinex®: 0.5% (15 mL, 30 mL)
Neo-Synephrine®: 1% (15 mL)
Ophthalmic solution:
AK-Nefrin®, Isopto® Frin, Prefrin™ Liquifilm®, Relief®: 0.12% (0.3 mL, 15 mL, 20 mL)
AK-Dilate®, Mydfrin®, Neo-Synephrine®, Phenoptic®: 2.5% (2 mL, 3 mL, 5 mL, 15 mL)
AK-Dilate®, Neo-Synephrine®, Neo-Synephrine® Viscous: 10% (1 mL, 2 mL, 5 mL, 15 mL)

phenylethylmalonylurea see phenobarbital on page 361

Phenylfenesin® L.A. see guaifenesin and phenylpropanolamine on page 215

phenylisohydantoin see pemoline on page 351

phenylpropanolamine and brompheniramine see brompheniramine and phenylpropanolamine on page 59

phenylpropanolamine and caramiphen see caramiphen and phenylpropanolamine on page 73

phenylpropanolamine and chlorpheniramine see chlorpheniramine and phenylpropanolamine on page 94

phenylpropanolamine and guaifenesin see guaifenesin and phenylpropanolamine on page 215

phenylpropanolamine and hydrocodone see hydrocodone and phenylpropanolamine on page 231

phenylpropanolamine hydrochloride (fen ill proe pa nole' a meen)
Brand Names Acutrim® Precision Release® [OTC]; Control® [OTC]; Dexatrim® [OTC]; Maigret-50; Propadrine; Propagest® [OTC]; Stay Trim® Diet Gum [OTC]; Westrim® LA [OTC]
Synonyms dl-norephedrine hydrochloride; ppa
(Continued)

phenylpropanolamine hydrochloride (Continued)

Therapeutic Category Adrenergic Agonist Agent; Anorexiant; Decongestant; Nasal Agent, Vasoconstrictor

Use Anorexiant and nasal decongestant

Usual Dosage Oral:

Children: Decongestant:

2-6 years: 6.25 mg every 4 hours

6-12 years: 12.5 mg every 4 hours not to exceed 75 mg/day

Adults:

Decongestant: 25 mg every 4 hours or 50 mg every 8 hours, not to exceed 150 mg/day

Anorexic: 25 mg 3 times/day 30 minutes before meals or 75 mg (timed release) once daily in the morning

Precision release: 75 mg after breakfast

Dosage Forms

Capsule: 37.5 mg

Capsule, timed release: 25 mg, 75 mg

Tablet: 25 mg

Tablet:

Precision release: 75 mg

Timed release: 75 mg

phenyltoloxamine, phenylpropanolamine, and acetaminophen

Brand Names Sinubid™

Therapeutic Category Analgesic, Non-Narcotic; Antihistamine/Decongestant Combination; Antipyretic

Use Intermittent symptomatic treatment of nasal congestion in sinus or other frontal headache; allergic rhinitis, vasomotor rhinitis, coryza; facial pain and pressure of acute and chronic sinusitis

Usual Dosage Oral:

Children 6-12 years: $\frac{1}{2}$ tablet every 12 hours (twice daily)

Adults: 1 tablet every 12 hours (twice daily)

Dosage Forms Tablet: Phenyltoloxamine citrate 22 mg, phenylpropanolamine hydrochloride 25 mg, and acetaminophen 325 mg

Phenylzin® Ophthalmic [OTC] *see* phenylephrine and zinc sulfate *on page 364*

phenytoin (fen' i toyn)

Brand Names Dilantin™; Diphenylan Sodium®

Synonyms diphenylhydantoin; dph

Therapeutic Category Antiarrhythmic Agent, Class Ib; Anticonvulsant, Hydantoin

Use Management of generalized tonic-clonic (grand mal), simple partial and complex partial seizures; prevention of seizures following head trauma/neurosurgery; ventricular arrhythmias, including those associated with digitalis intoxication; beneficial effects in the treatment of migraine or trigeminal neuralgia in some patients

Usual Dosage

Status epilepticus: I.V.:

Neonates: Loading dose: 15-20 mg/kg in a single or divided dose; maintenance, anticonvulsant: Initial: 5 mg/kg/day in 2 divided doses; usual dose: 5-8 mg/kg/day in 2 divided doses; some patients may require dosing every 8 hours

Infants and Children: Loading dose: 15-18 mg/kg in a single or divided dose; maintenance, anticonvulsant: Initial: 5 mg/kg/day in 2 divided doses, usual doses:

6 months to 3 years: 8-10 mg/kg/day

4-6 years: 7.5-9 mg/kg/day

7-9 years: 7-8 mg/kg/day

10-16 years: 6-7 mg/kg/day, some patients may require every 8 hours dosing

Adults: Loading dose: 15-18 mg/kg in a single or divided dose; maintenance, anticonvulsant: usual: 300 mg/day or 5-6 mg/kg/day in 3 divided doses or 1-2 divided doses using extended release

Anticonvulsant: Children and Adults: Oral: Loading dose: 15-20 mg/kg; based on phenytoin serum concentrations and recent dosing history; administer oral loading dose in 3 divided doses given every 2-4 hours to decrease GI adverse effects and to ensure complete oral absorption; maintenance dose: same as I.V.

Arrhythmias:

Children and Adults: Loading dose: I.V.: 1.25 mg/kg IVP every 5 minutes may repeat up to total loading dose: 15 mg/kg

Children: Maintenance dose: Oral, I.V.: 5-10 mg/kg/day in 2 divided doses

Adults: Maintenance dose: Oral: 250 mg 4 times/day for 1 day, 250 mg twice daily for 2 days, then maintenance at 300-400 mg/day in divided doses 1-4 times/day

Dosage Forms
Capsule, as sodium:
Extended: 30 mg, 100 mg
Prompt: 30 mg, 100 mg
Injection, as sodium: 50 mg/mL (2 mL, 5 mL)
Suspension, oral: 30 mg/5 mL (5 mL, 240 mL); 125 mg/5 mL (5 mL, 240 mL)
Tablet, chewable: 50 mg

phenytoin with phenobarbital

Brand Names Dilantin® With Phenobarbital

Therapeutic Category Anticonvulsant, Barbiturate; Anticonvulsant, Hydantoin

Use Management of generalized tonic-clonic (grand mal), simple partial and complex partial seizures

Usual Dosage Children and Adults: Oral: Loading dose: 15-20 mg/kg; based on phenytoin serum concentrations and recent dosing history; administer oral loading dose in 3 divided doses given every 2-4 hours to decrease GI adverse effects and to ensure complete oral absorption

Dosage Forms Capsule: Phenytoin 100 mg and phenobarbital 15 mg; phenytoin 100 mg and phenobarbital 30 mg

Pherazine® VC see promethazine and phenylephrine on page 390

Pherazine® w/DM see promethazine with dextromethorphan on page 391

Pherazine® With Codeine see promethazine and codeine on page 390

Phicon® [OTC] see pramoxine hydrochloride on page 381

Phillips'® LaxCaps® [OTC] see docusate and phenolphthalein on page 154

Phillips'® Milk of Magnesia [OTC] see magnesium hydroxide on page 277

pHisoHex® see hexachlorophene on page 224

Phos-Flur® see fluoride on page 196

PhosLo® see calcium acetate on page 66

Phosphaljel® [OTC] see aluminum phosphate on page 17

phosphate, potassium see potassium phosphate on page 380

Phospholine Iodide® Ophthalmic see echothiophate iodide on page 162

phosphonoformic acid see foscarnet on page 202

phosphorated carbohydrate solution

Brand Names Emecheck® [OTC]; Emetrol® [OTC]; Naus-A-Way® [OTC]; Nausetrol® [OTC]

Therapeutic Category Antiemetic

Use Relieve nausea associated with upset stomach that occurs with intestinal flu, pregnancy, food indiscretions, and emotional upsets

Usual Dosage

Morning sickness: 15-30 mL on arising; repeat every 3 hours or when nausea threatens

Motion sickness and vomiting due to drug therapy: 5 mL doses for young children; 15 mL doses for older children and adults

(Continued)

phosphorated carbohydrate solution (Continued)

Regurgitation in infants: 5 or 10 mL, 10-15 minutes before each feeding; in refractory cases: 10-15 mL, 30 minutes before each feeding

Vomiting due to psychogenic factors:

Children: 5-10 mL; repeat dose every 15 minutes until distress subsides; do not take for more than 1 hour

Adults: 15-30 mL; repeat dose every 15 minutes until distress subsides; do not take for more than 1 hour

Dosage Forms Liquid, oral: Fructose, dextrose, and orthophosphoric acid (120 mL, 480 mL, 4000 mL)

Phrenilin® see butalbital compound on page 63

Phrenilin® Forte® see butalbital compound on page 63

p-hydroxyampicillin see amoxicillin trihydrate on page 24

Phyllocontin® see aminophylline on page 20

phylloquinone see phytonadione on this page

physostigmine (fye zoe stig' meen)

Brand Names Antilirium® Injection

Synonyms eserine salicylate

Therapeutic Category Antidote, Anticholinergic Agent; Cholinergic Agent; Cholinergic Agent, Ophthalmic

Use Reverse toxic CNS effects caused by anticholinergic drugs; used as miotic in treatment of glaucoma

Usual Dosage

Children: Reserve for life-threatening situations only: I.V.: 0.01-0.03 mg/kg/dose; may repeat after 15-20 minutes to a maximum total dose of 2 mg

Adults:

I.M., I.V., S.C.: 0.5-2 mg to start, repeat every 20 minutes until response occurs or adverse effect occurs

I.M., I.V. to reverse the anticholinergic effects of atropine or scopolamine given as pre-anesthetic medications: Give twice the dose, on a weight basis of the anticholinergic drug

Ophthalmic: 1-2 drops of 0.25% or 0.5% solution every 4-8 hours (up to 4 times/day); the ointment can be instilled at night

Dosage Forms

Injection, as salicylate: 1 mg/mL (2 mL)

Ointment, ophthalmic: 0.25% (3.5 g, 3.7 g)

phytomenadione see phytonadione on this page

phytonadione (fye toe na dye' one)

Brand Names AquaMEPHYTON® Injection; Konakion® Injection; Mephyton® Oral

Synonyms methylphytyl napthoquinone; phylloquinone; phytomenadione; vitamin k_1

Therapeutic Category Vitamin, Fat Soluble

Use Prevention and treatment of hypoprothrombinemia caused by drug-induced or anticoagulant-induced vitamin K deficiency, hemorrhagic disease of the newborn

Usual Dosage I.V. route should be restricted for emergency use only

Hemorrhagic disease of the newborn:

Prophylaxis: I.M., S.C.: 0.5-1 mg within 1 hour of birth

Treatment: I.M., S.C.: 1-2 mg/dose/day

Oral anticoagulant overdose:

Infants: I.M., I.V., S.C.: 1-2 mg/dose every 4-8 hours

Children and Adults: Oral, I.M., I.V., S.C.: 2.5-10 mg/dose; rarely up to 25-50 mg has been used; may repeat in 6-8 hours if given by I.M., I.V., S.C. route; may repeat 12-48 hours after oral route

Vitamin K deficiency: Due to drugs, malabsorption or decreased synthesis of vitamin K
  Infants and Children:
    Oral: 2.5-5 mg/24 hours
    I.M., I.V.: 1-2 mg/dose as a single dose
  Adults:
    Oral: 5-25 mg/24 hours
    I.M., I.V.: 10 mg

Minimum daily requirement: Not well established
  Infants: 1-5 mcg/kg/day
  Adults: 0.03 mcg/kg/day

Dosage Forms
Injection:
  Aqueous colloidal: 2 mg/mL (0.5 mL); 10 mg/mL (1 mL, 2.5 mL, 5 mL)
  Aqueous (I.M. only): 2 mg/mL (0.5 mL); 10 mg/mL (1 mL)
Tablet: 5 mg

Pilagan® Ophthalmic *see pilocarpine on this page*

Pilocar® Ophthalmic *see pilocarpine on this page*

pilocarpine (pye loe kar' peen)

Brand Names Adsorbocarpine® Ophthalmic; Akarpine® Ophthalmic; Isopto® Carpine Ophthalmic; Ocu-Carpine® Ophthalmic; Ocusert Pilo-20® Ophthalmic; Ocusert Pilo-40® Ophthalmic; Pilagan® Ophthalmic; Pilocar® Ophthalmic; Pilopine HS® Ophthalmic; Piloptic® Ophthalmic; Pilostat® Ophthalmic; Salagen® Oral

Therapeutic Category Cholinergic Agent; Cholinergic Agent, Ophthalmic; Ophthalmic Agent, Miotic

Use
Ophthalmic: Management of chronic simple glaucoma, chronic and acute angle-closure glaucoma; counter effects of cycloplegics
Oral: Symptomatic treatment of xerostomia caused by salivary gland hypofunction resulting from radiotherapy for cancer of the head and neck

Usual Dosage Ophthalmic: Adults:
Nitrate solution: Shake well before using; instill 1-2 drops 2-4 times/day
Hydrochloride solution:
  Instill 1-2 drops up to 6 times/day; adjust the concentration and frequency as required to control elevated intraocular pressure
  To counteract the mydriatic effects of sympathomimetic agents: Instill 1 drop of a 1% solution in the affected eye
Gel: Instill 0.5" ribbon into lower conjunctival sac once daily at bedtime
Ocular systems: Systems are labeled in terms of mean rate of release of pilocarpine over 7 days; begin with 20 mcg/hour at night and adjust based on response

Oral: Adults: 5 mg 3 times daily, titration up to 10 mg 3 times daily may be considered for patients who have not responded adequately

Dosage Forms
Gel, ophthalmic, as hydrochloride (Pilopine HS®): 4% (3.5 g)
Ocular therapeutic system (Ocusert® Pilo): Releases 20 or 40 mcg per hour for 1 week (8s)
Solution, ophthalmic, as hydrochloride (Adsorbocarpine®, Akarpine®, Isopto® Carpine, Pilagan®, Pilocar®, Piloptic®, Pilostat®): 0.25% (15 mL); 0.5% (15 mL, 30 mL); 1% (1 mL, 2 mL, 15 mL, 30 mL); 2% (1 mL, 2 mL, 15 mL, 30 mL); 3% (15 mL, 30 mL); 4% (1 mL, 2 mL, 15 mL, 30 mL); 6% (15 mL, 30 mL); 8% (2 mL); 10% (15 mL)
Solution, ophthalmic, as nitrate (Pilagan®): 1% (15 mL); 2% (15 mL); 4% (15 mL)
Tablet: 5 mg

pilocarpine and epinephrine

Brand Names E-Pilo-x® Ophthalmic; P$_x$E$_x$® Ophthalmic
Therapeutic Category Ophthalmic Agent, Miotic
Use Treatment of glaucoma; counter effect of cycloplegics
(Continued)

pilocarpine and epinephrine *(Continued)*
Usual Dosage Ophthalmic: Instill 1-2 drops up to 6 times/day
Dosage Forms Solution, ophthalmic: Epinephrine bitartrate 1% and pilocarpine hydrochloride 1%, 2%, 4%, 6% (15 mL)

Pilopine HS® Ophthalmic *see* pilocarpine *on previous page*

Piloptic® Ophthalmic *see* pilocarpine *on previous page*

Pilostat® Ophthalmic *see* pilocarpine *on previous page*

Pima® *see* potassium iodide *on page 379*

pimaricin *see* natamycin *on page 320*

pimozide (pi' moe zide)
Brand Names Orap™
Therapeutic Category Neuroleptic Agent
Use Suppression of severe motor and phonic tics in patients with Tourette's disorder
Usual Dosage Children >12 years and Adults: Oral: Initial: 1-2 mg/day, then increase dosage as needed every other day; range is usually 7-16 mg/day, maximum dose: 20 mg/day or 0.3 mg/kg/day should not be exceeded
Dosage Forms Tablet: 2 mg

pindolol (pin' doe lole)
Brand Names Visken®
Therapeutic Category Beta-Adrenergic Blocker
Use Management of hypertension
Usual Dosage Oral: 5 mg twice daily
Dosage Forms Tablet: 5 mg, 10 mg

Pin-Rid® [OTC] *see* pyrantel pamoate *on page 399*

Pin-X® [OTC] *see* pyrantel pamoate *on page 399*

pio *see* pemoline *on page 351*

pipecuronium bromide (pi pe kure oh' nee um)
Brand Names Arduan®
Therapeutic Category Neuromuscular Blocker Agent, Nondepolarizing
Use Adjunct to general anesthesia, to provide skeletal muscle relaxation during surgery and to provide skeletal muscle relaxation for endotracheal intubation; recommended only for procedures anticipated to last 90 minutes or longer
Usual Dosage I.V.:
Children:
3 months to 1 year: Adult dosage
1-14 years: May be less sensitive to effects

Adults: Dose is individualized based on ideal body weight, ranges are 85-100 mcg/kg initially to a maintenance dose of 5-25 mcg/kg
Dosage Forms Injection: 10 mg (10 mL)

piperacillin sodium (pi per' a sill in)
Brand Names Pipracil®
Therapeutic Category Antibiotic, Penicillin
Use Treatment of carbenicillin or ticarcillin-resistant *Pseudomonas aeruginosa* infections in combination with an aminoglycoside which are susceptible to piperacillin
Usual Dosage
Neonates: I.M., I.V.: 100 mg/kg/dose every 12 hours

Infants and Children: I.M., I.V.: 200-300 mg/kg/day in divided doses every 4-6 hours; maximum dose: 24 g/day

Higher doses have been used in cystic fibrosis: 350-500 mg/kg/day in divided doses every 4 hours

Adults:
    I.M.: 2-3 g/dose every 6-12 hours I.M.; maximum 24 g/24 hours
    I.V.: 3-4 g/dose every 4-6 hours; maximum 24 g/24 hours
Dosage Forms Powder for injection: 2 g, 3 g, 4 g, 40 g

piperacillin sodium and tazobactam sodium
Brand Names Zosyn™
Therapeutic Category Antibiotic, Penicillin
Use Treatment of infections of lower respiratory tract, urinary tract, skin and skin structures, gynecologic, bone and joint infections, and septicemia caused by susceptible organisms. Tazobactam expands activity of piperacillin to include beta-lactamase producing strains of *S. aureus*, *H. influenzae*, *Enterobacteriaceae*, *Pseudomonas*, *Klebsiella*, *Citrobacter*, *Serratia*, *Bacteroides*, and other gram-negative anaerobes.
Usual Dosage Adults: I.V.: 3.375 g (3 g piperacillin/0.375 g tazobactam) every 6 hours
Dosing interval in renal impairment:
    Cl_{cr} >40 mL/minute: No change
    Cl_{cr} 20-40 mL/minute: Administer 2.25 g every 6 hours
    Cl_{cr} <20 mL/minute: Administer 2.25 g every 8 hours
Hemodialysis: Administer 2.25 g every 8 hours with an additional dose of 0.75 g after each dialysis
Dosage Forms Injection: Piperacillin sodium 2 g and tazobactam sodium 0.25 g; piperacillin sodium 3 g and tazobactam sodium 0.375 g; piperacillin sodium 4 g and tazobactam sodium 0.5 g (vials at an 8:1 ratio of piperacillin sodium to tazobactam sodium)

piperazine citrate (pi' per a zeen)
Brand Names Vermizine®
Therapeutic Category Anthelmintic
Use Treatment of pinworm and roundworm infections (used as an alternative to first-line agents, mebendazole, or pyrantel pamoate)
Usual Dosage Oral:
Pinworms: Children and Adults: 65 mg/kg/day as a single daily dose for 7 days, in severe infections, repeat course after a 1-week interval; not to exceed 2.5 g/day

Roundworms:
    Children: 75 mg/kg/day as a single daily dose for 2 days; maximum: 3.5 g/day;
    Adults: 3.5 g/day for 2 days (in severe infections, repeat course, after a 1-week interval)
Dosage Forms
Syrup: 500 mg/5 mL (473 mL, 4000 mL)
Tablet: 250 mg

piperazine estrone sulfate *see* estropipate *on page 175*

pipobroman (pi poe broe' man)
Brand Names Vercyte®
Therapeutic Category Antineoplastic Agent, Alkylating Agent
Use Treat polycythemia vera; chronic myelocytic leukemia
Usual Dosage Children >15 years and Adults: Oral:
Polycythemia: 1 mg/kg/day for 30 days; may increase to 1.5-3 mg/kg until hematocrit reduced to 50% to 55%; maintenance: 0.1-0.2 mg/kg/day

Myelocytic leukemia: 1.5-2.5 mg/kg/day until WBC drops to 10,000 mm^3 then start maintenance 7-175 mg/day; stop if WBC falls below 3000/mm^3 or platelets fall below 150,000/mm^3
Dosage Forms Tablet: 25 mg

Pipracil® *see* piperacillin sodium *on previous page*

pirbuterol acetate (peer byoo' ter ole)
Brand Names Maxair™ Inhalation Aerosol
Therapeutic Category Beta-2-Adrenergic Agonist Agent; Bronchodilator
Use Prevention and treatment of reversible bronchospasm including asthma
Usual Dosage Children >12 years and Adults: 2 inhalations every 4-6 hours for prevention; two inhalations at an interval of at least 1-3 minutes, followed by a third inhalation in treatment of bronchospasm, not to exceed 12 inhalations/day
Dosage Forms Aerosol, oral: 0.2 mg/actuation (25.6 g)

piroxicam (peer ox' i kam)
Brand Names Feldene®
Therapeutic Category Analgesic, Non-Narcotic; Anti-inflammatory Agent; Nonsteroidal Anti-Inflammatory Agent (NSAID), Oral
Use Management of inflammatory disorders; symptomatic treatment of acute and chronic rheumatoid arthritis, osteoarthritis, and ankylosing spondylitis
Usual Dosage Oral:
Children: 0.2-0.3 mg/kg/day once daily; maximum dose: 15 mg/day

Adults: 10-20 mg/day once daily; although associated with increases in GI adverse effects, doses >20 mg/day have been used (ie, 30-40 mg/day)

Therapeutic efficacy of the drug should not be assessed for at least two weeks after initiation of therapy or adjustment of dosage
Dosage Forms Capsule: 10 mg, 20 mg

p-isobutylhydratropic acid *see ibuprofen on page 240*

pit *see oxytocin on page 345*

Pitocin® Injection *see oxytocin on page 345*

Pitressin® Injection *see vasopressin on page 484*

pit vipers antivenin *see antivenin polyvalent (Crotalidae) on page 31*

pix carbonis *see coal tar on page 110*

Placidyl® *see ethchlorvynol on page 177*

plague vaccine
Therapeutic Category Vaccine, Inactivated Bacteria
Use Vaccination of persons at high risk exposure to plaque
Usual Dosage Three I.M. doses: First dose 1 mL, second dose (0.2 mL) 1 month later, third dose (0.2 mL) 5 months after the second dose; booster doses (0.2 mL) at 1- to 2-year intervals if exposure continues
Dosage Forms Injection: 2 mL, 20 mL

plantago seed *see psyllium on page 398*

plantain seed *see psyllium on page 398*

Plaquenil® *see hydroxychloroquine sulfate on page 236*

Plasbumin® *see albumin human on page 10*

Plasmanate® *see plasma protein fraction on this page*

Plasma-Plex® *see plasma protein fraction on this page*

plasma protein fraction
Brand Names Plasmanate®; Plasma-Plex®; Plasmatein®; Protenate®
Therapeutic Category Blood Product Derivative
Use Plasma volume expansion and maintenance of cardiac output in the treatment of certain types of shock or impending shock
Usual Dosage I.V.: 250-1500 mL/day
Dosage Forms Injection: 5% (50 mL, 250 mL, 500 mL)

Plasmatein® *see plasma protein fraction on previous page*

Platinol® *see cisplatin on page 103*

Platinol®-AQ *see cisplatin on page 103*

Plendil® *see felodipine on page 187*

plicamycin (plye kay mye' sin)
Brand Names Mithracin®
Synonyms mithramycin
Therapeutic Category Antidote, Hypercalcemia; Antineoplastic Agent, Antibiotic
Use Malignant testicular tumors, in the treatment of hypercalcemia and hypercalciuria of malignancy; Paget's disease
Usual Dosage Refer to individual protocols. Adults: I.V. (dose based on ideal body weight): Testicular cancer: 25-50 mcg/kg/day or every other day for 5-10 days

Blastic chronic granulocytic leukemia: 25 mcg/kg over 2-4 hours every other day for 3 weeks

Hypercalcemia: 15-25 mcg/kg/day once daily for 3-4 days or 25 mcg/kg every 48-72 hours; additional courses of therapy may be given at intervals of 1 week or more if the initial course is unsuccessful. Reduce dose to 12.5 mcg/kg in patients with pre-existing hepatic or renal impairment

Paget's disease: 15 mcg/kg/day once daily for 10 days
Dosage Forms Powder for injection: 2.5 mg

pneumococcal vaccine, polyvalent
Brand Names Pneumovax® 23; Pnu-Imune® 23
Therapeutic Category Vaccine, Inactivated Bacteria
Use Immunity to pneumococcal lobar pneumonia and bacteremia in individuals ≥2 years of age who are at high risk of morbidity and mortality from pneumococcal infection
Usual Dosage Children >2 years and Adults: I.M., S.C.: 0.5 mL
Revaccination should be considered if ≥6 years since initial vaccination; revaccination is recommended in patients who received 14-valent pneumococcal vaccine and are at highest risk (asplenic) for fatal infection, or at ≥6 years in patients with nephrotic syndrome, renal failure, or transplant recipients, or 3-5 years in children with nephrotic syndrome, asplenia or sickle cell disease
Dosage Forms Injection: 25 mcg each of 23 polysaccharide isolates/0.5 mL dose (0.5 mL, 1 mL, 5 mL)

Pneumomist® *see guaifenesin on page 213*

Pneumovax® 23 *see pneumococcal vaccine, polyvalent on this page*

Pnu-Imune® 23 *see pneumococcal vaccine, polyvalent on this page*

Pod-Ben-25® *see podophyllum resin on next page*

Podocon-25® *see podophyllum resin on next page*

podofilox (po do fil' ox)
Brand Names Condylox®
Therapeutic Category Keratolytic Agent
Use Treatment of external genital warts
Usual Dosage Adults: Apply twice daily (morning and evening) for 3 consecutive days, then withhold use for 4 consecutive days; repeat this cycle may be repeated up to 4 times until there is no visible wart tissue
Dosage Forms Solution, topical: 0.5% (3.5 mL)

Podofin® *see podophyllum resin on next page*

podophyllin and salicylic acid
Brand Names Verrex-C&M®

Synonyms salicylic acid and podophyllin

Therapeutic Category Keratolytic Agent

Use Topical treatment of benign growths including external genital and perianal warts, papillomas, fibroids

Usual Dosage Topical: Apply daily with applicator, allow to dry; remove necrotic tissue before each application

Dosage Forms Solution, topical: Podophyllum 10% and salicylic acid 30% with penederm 0.5% (7.5 mL)

podophyllum resin po dof' fill um)
Brand Names Pod-Ben-25®; Podocon-25®; Podofin®

Synonyms mandrake; may apple

Therapeutic Category Keratolytic Agent

Use Topical treatment of benign growths including external genital and perianal warts, papillomas, fibroids

Usual Dosage Topical:

Children and Adults: 10% to 25% solution in compound benzoin tincture; apply drug to dry surface, use 1 drop at a time allowing drying between drops until area is covered; total volume should be limited to <0.5 mL per treatment session

Condylomata acuminatum: 25% solution is applied daily; use a 10% solution when applied to or near mucous membranes

Verrucae: 25% solution is applied 3-5 times/day directly to the wart

Dosage Forms Liquid, topical: 25% in benzoin (5 mL, 7.5 mL, 30 mL)

Point-Two® *see* fluoride *on page 196*

Poladex® *see* dexchlorpheniramine maleate *on page 133*

Polaramine® *see* dexchlorpheniramine maleate *on page 133*

Polargen® *see* dexchlorpheniramine maleate *on page 133*

poliomyelitis vaccine *see* poliovirus vaccine, inactivated *on this page*

poliovirus vaccine, inactivated
Brand Names IPOL™

Synonyms ipv; poliomyelitis vaccine; Salk vaccine

Therapeutic Category Vaccine, Live Virus and Inactivated Virus

Use Active immunization for the prevention of poliomyelitis

Usual Dosage

S.C.: 3 doses of 0.5 mL; the first 2 doses should be administered at an interval of 8 weeks; the third dose should be given at least 6 and preferably 12 months after the second dose

Booster dose: All children who have received the 3 dose primary series in infancy and early childhood should receive a booster dose of 0.5 mL before entering school. However, if the third dose of the primary series is administered on or after the fourth birthday, a fourth (booster) dose is not required at school entry.

Dosage Forms Injection: Suspension of three types of poliovirus (Types 1, 2 and 3) grown in human diploid cell cultures (0.5 mL)

poliovirus vaccine, live (trivalent, oral)
Brand Names Orimune®

Synonyms opv; Sabin vaccine; topv

Therapeutic Category Vaccine, Live Virus

Use Poliovirus immunization

Usual Dosage Oral:

Infants: 0.5 mL dose at age 2 months, 4 months, and 18 months; optional dose may be given at 6 months in areas where poliomyelitis is endemic

Older Children, Adolescents and Adults: Two 0.5 mL doses 8 weeks apart; third dose of 0.5 mL 6-12 months after second dose; a reinforcing dose of 0.5 mL should be given before entry to school, in children who received the third primary dose before their fourth birthday
Dosage Forms Solution, oral: Mixture of type 1, 2, and 3 viruses in monkey kidney tissue (0.5 mL)

Polocaine® Injection *see* mepivacaine hydrochloride *on page 288*

Polycillin® *see* ampicillin *on page 26*

Polycillin-N® *see* ampicillin *on page 26*

Polycillin-PRB® *see* ampicillin and probenecid *on page 26*

Polycitra® *see* sodium citrate and potassium citrate mixture *on page 428*

Polycitra®-K *see* potassium citrate and citric acid *on page 379*

Polycose® [OTC] *see* glucose polymers *on page 209*

polyestradiol phosphate (pol ee ess tra dye' ole)
Therapeutic Category Estrogen Derivative
Use Palliative treatment of advanced, inoperable carcinoma of the prostate
Usual Dosage Adults: I.M.: 40 mg every 2-4 weeks or less frequently
Dosage Forms Powder for injection: 40 mg

polyethylene glycol-electrolyte solution (pol ee eth' i leen gly' kol)
Brand Names Co-Lav®; Colovage®; CoLyte®; Go-Evac®; GoLYTELY®; NuLYTELY®; OCL®
Synonyms electrolyte lavage solution; peg-es
Therapeutic Category Laxative, Bowel Evacuant
Use Bowel cleansing prior to GI examination
Usual Dosage The recommended dose for adults is 4 L of solution prior to gastrointestinal examination, as ingestion of this dose produces a satisfactory preparation in >95% of patients. Ideally the patient should fast for approximately 3-4 hours prior to administration, but in no case should solid food be given for at least 2 hours before the solution is given. The solution is usually administered orally, but may be given via nasogastric tube to patients who are unwilling or unable to drink the solution.

Children: Oral administration: 25-40 mL/kg/hour for 4-10 hours

Adults:

  Oral administration: At a rate of 240 mL (8 oz) every 10 minutes, until 4 liters are consumed or the rectal effluent is clear; rapid drinking of each portion is preferred to drinking small amounts continuously

  Nasogastric tube administration: At the rate of 20-30 mL/minute (1.2-1.8 L/hour); the first bowel movement should occur approximately one hour after the start of administration

Dosage Forms Powder, for oral solution: PEG 3350 236 g, sodium sulfate 22.74 g, sodium bicarbonate 6.74 g, sodium chloride 5.86 g and potassium chloride 2.97 g (2000 mL, 4000 mL, 4800 mL, 6000 mL)

Polygam® *see* immune globulin, intravenous *on page 243*

Polygam® S/D *see* immune globulin, intravenous *on page 243*

Poly-Histine CS® *see* brompheniramine, phenylpropanolamine, and codeine *on page 60*

Polymox® *see* amoxicillin trihydrate *on page 24*

polymyxin b and hydrocortisone
Brand Names Otobiotic® Otic; Pyocidin-Otic®
Therapeutic Category Antibacterial, Otic; Corticosteroid, Otic
Use Treatment of superficial bacterial infections of external ear canal
(Continued)

polymyxin b and hydrocortisone *(Continued)*

Usual Dosage Otic: Instill 4 drops 3-4 times/day
Dosage Forms Solution, otic: Polymyxin b sulfate 10,000 units and hydrocortisone 0.5% [5 mg/mL] per mL (10 mL, 15 mL)

polymyxin b and neomycin *see* neomycin and polymyxin b *on page 322*

polymyxin b and oxytetracycline *see* oxytetracycline and polymyxin b
on page 344

polymyxin b and trimethoprim *see* trimethoprim and polymyxin b *on page 473*

polymyxin b sulfate (pol i mix' in)

Brand Names Aerosporin® Injection
Therapeutic Category Antibiotic, Ophthalmic; Antibiotic, Topical
Use
Parenteral: Has mainly been replaced by less toxic antibiotics; reserved for life-threatening infections caused by organisms resistant to the preferred drugs
Topical: Wound irrigation and bladder instillation against *Pseudomonas aeruginosa*; used occasionally for gut decontamination
Usual Dosage
Infants <2 years:
I.M.: 25,000-40,000 units/kg/day divided every 6 hours
I.V.: 15,000-45,000 units/kg/day by continuous I.V. infusion or divided every 12 hours

Children ≥2 years and Adults:
I.M.: 25,000-30,000 units/kg/day divided every 4-6 hours
I.V.: 15,000-25,000 units/kg/day divided every 12 hours or by continuous infusion
Total daily dose should not exceed 2,000,000 units/day
Bladder irrigation: Continuous irrigant or rinse in the urinary bladder for up to 10 days using 20 mg (equal to 200,000 units) added to 1 L of normal saline; usually no more than 1 L of irrigant is used per day unless urine flow rate is high; administration rate is adjusted to patient's urine output
Topical irrigation or topical solution: 0.1% to 0.3% solution used to irrigate infected wounds; should not exceed 2 million units/day in adults
Gut sterilization: Oral: 100,000-200,000 units/kg/day divided every 6-8 hours
Ophthalmic: A concentration of 0.1% to 0.25% is administered as 1-3 drops every hour, then increasing the interval as response indicates
Dosage Forms
Injection: 500,000 units
Powder for ophthalmic solution: 500,000 units

polymyxin e *see* colistin sulfate *on page 113*

Poly-Pred® Liquifilm® Ophthalmic *see* neomycin, polymyxin b, and prednisolone
on page 323

polysaccharide-iron complex

Brand Names Hytinic® [OTC]; Niferex® [OTC]; Nu-Iron® [OTC]
Therapeutic Category Iron Salt
Use Prevention and treatment of iron deficiency anemias
Usual Dosage
Children: 3 mg/kg 3 times/day
Adults: 200 mg 3-4 times/day
Dosage Forms
Capsule: Elemental iron 150 mg
Elixir: Elemental iron 100 mg/5 mL (240 mL)
Tablet: Elemental iron 50 mg

Polysporin® Ophthalmic *see* bacitracin and polymyxin b *on page 43*

Polysporin® Topical *see* bacitracin and polymyxin b *on page 43*

Polytar® [OTC] *see* coal tar *on page 110*

polythiazide (pol i thye' a zide)
Brand Names Renese®
Therapeutic Category Diuretic, Thiazide
Use Adjunctive therapy in treatment of edema and hypertension
Usual Dosage Adults: Oral: 1-4 mg/day
Dosage Forms Tablet: 1 mg, 2 mg, 4 mg

Polytrim® Ophthalmic *see* trimethoprim and polymyxin b *on page 473*

Poly-Vi-Flor® *see* vitamin, multiple (pediatric) *on page 491*

polyvinyl alcohol *see* artificial tears *on page 34*

Poly-Vi-Sol® [OTC] *see* vitamin, multiple (pediatric) *on page 491*

Pondimin® *see* fenfluramine hydrochloride *on page 187*

Ponstel® *see* mefenamic acid *on page 284*

Pontocaine® Injection *see* tetracaine hydrochloride *on page 450*

Pontocaine® Topical *see* tetracaine hydrochloride *on page 450*

Pontocaine® With Dextrose Injection *see* tetracaine with dextrose *on page 451*

Porcelana® [OTC] *see* hydroquinone *on page 235*

Pork NPH Iletin® II *see* insulin preparations *on page 245*

Pork Regular Iletin® II *see* insulin preparations *on page 245*

Posture® [OTC] *see* calcium phosphate, dibasic *on page 70*

Potasalan® *see* potassium chloride *on next page*

potassium acetate
Therapeutic Category Electrolyte Supplement, Parenteral; Potassium Salt
Use Potassium deficiency, hypokalemia; to avoid chloride when high concentration of potassium is needed
Usual Dosage I.V. infusion:
Children: Not to exceed 3 mEq/kg/day

Adults: Up to 150 mEq/day administered at a rate up to 20 mEq/hour; maximum concentration: 40 mEq/L
Dosage Forms Injection: 2 mEq/mL (20 mL, 50 mL, 100 mL); 4 mEq/mL (50 mL)

potassium acid phosphate
Brand Names K-Phos® Original
Therapeutic Category Electrolyte Supplement, Oral; Potassium Salt; Urinary Acidifying Agent
Use Acidify the urine and lower urinary calcium concentration; reduces odor and rash caused by ammoniacal urine
Usual Dosage Adults: Oral: 1000 mg dissolved in 6-8 oz of water 4 times/day with meals and at bedtime
Dosage Forms Tablet, sodium free: 500 mg [potassium 3.67 mEq]

potassium bicarbonate and potassium citrate, effervescent
Brand Names Effer-K™; K-Ide®; Klor-con®/EF; K-Lyte®; K-Vescent®
Synonyms potassium citrate and potassium bicarbonate, effervescent
Therapeutic Category Electrolyte Supplement, Oral; Potassium Salt
Use Treatment or prevention of hypokalemia
(Continued)

potassium bicarbonate and potassium citrate, effervescent
(Continued)

Usual Dosage Oral:
Children: 1-4 mEq/kg/24 hours as required to maintain normal serum potassium

Adults:
Prevention: 16-24 mEq/day in 2-4 divided doses
Treatment: 40-100 mEq/day in 2-4 divided doses

Dosage Forms
Capsule, extended release: 8 mEq, 10 mEq
Powder for oral solution: 15 mEq/packet; 20 mEq/packet; 25 mEq/packet
Tablet, effervescent: 25 mEq, 50 mEq

potassium chloride
Brand Names Cena-K®; Gen-K®; K+8®; Kaochlor® S-F; Kaon-CL®; Kato®; K-Dur®; K-Lor™; Klor-con®; Klorvess®; Klotrix®; K-Lyte/CL®; K-Tab®; Micro-K®; Potasalan®; Rum-K®; Slow-K®
Synonyms KCl
Therapeutic Category Electrolyte Supplement, Oral; Electrolyte Supplement, Parenteral; Potassium Salt
Use Treatment or prevention of hypokalemia
Usual Dosage I.V. doses should be incorporated into the patient's maintenance I.V. fluids, intermittent I.V. potassium administration should be reserved for severe depletion situations in patients undergoing EKG monitoring.

Normal daily requirement: Oral, I.V.:
Newborns: 2-6 mEq/kg/day
Children: 2-3 mEq/kg/day
Adults: 40-80 mEq/day

Prevention during diuretic therapy: Oral:
Children: 1-2 mEq/kg/day in 1-2 divided doses
Adults: 20-40 mEq/day in 1-2 divided doses

Treatment: Oral, I.V.:
Children: 2-3 mEq/kg/day
Adults: 40-100 mEq/day

I.V. intermittent infusion:
Children: Dose should not exceed 0.5 mEq/kg/hour, not to exceed 20 mEq/hour
Adults: 10-20 mEq/hour, not to exceed 40 mEq/hour and 150 mEq/day

Dosage Forms
Capsule, controlled release, micro encapsulated (Micro-K®): 600 mg [8 mEq]; 750 mg [10 mEq]
Injection: 1.5 mEq/mL, 2 mEq/mL, 3 mEq/mL
Liquid, oral: 10 mEq/15 mL, 15 mEq/15 mL, 20 mEq/15 mL, 30 mEq/15 mL, 40 mEq/15 mL, 45 mEq/15 mL
Powder, oral: 15 mEq, 20 mEq, 25 mEq packet
Tablet:
Effervescent, as potassium chloride: 25 mEq
Effervescent, as potassium bicarbonate: 20 mEq, 25 mEq, 50 mEq
Sustained release, microcrystalloids (K-Dur®): 750 mg [10 mEq]; 1500 mg [20 mEq]
Wax matrix:
Kaon-Cl®: 500 mg [6.7 mEq]
K+8®: 600 mg [8 mEq]
Slow-K®: 600 mg [8 mEq]; 750 mg [10 mEq]

potassium citrate
Brand Names Urocit®-K
Therapeutic Category Alkalinizing Agent Oral
Use Prevention of uric acid nephrolithiasis; prevention of calcium renal stones in patients with hypocitraturia; urinary alkalizer when sodium citrate is contraindicated
Usual Dosage Oral: Adults: 10-20 mEq three times daily with meals up to 100 mEq/day
Dosage Forms Tablet: 540 mg [5 mEq], 1080 mg [10 mEq]

potassium citrate and citric acid
Brand Names Polycitra®-K
Therapeutic Category Electrolyte Supplement, Oral; Potassium Salt
Use Treatment of metabolic acidosis; alkalinizing agent in conditions where long-term mainte-
nance of an alkaline urine is desirable
Dosage Forms
Crystals for reconstitution: Potassium citrate 3300 mg and citric acid 1002 mg per packet
Solution, oral: Potassium citrate 1100 mg and citric acid 334 mg per 5 mL

potassium citrate and potassium bicarbonate, effervescent *see* potassium
bicarbonate and potassium citrate, effervescent *on page 377*

potassium gluconate
Brand Names Kaon®; Kolyum®
Therapeutic Category Electrolyte Supplement, Oral; Potassium Salt
Use Potassium deficiency, hypopotassemia
Usual Dosage Oral:
Normal daily requirement:
Children: 2-3 mEq/kg/day
Adults: 40-80 mEq/day

Prevention during diuretic therapy:
Children: 1-2 mEq/kg/day in 1-2 divided doses
Adults: 20-40 mEq/kg/day in 1-2 divided doses

Treatment of hypokalemia:
Children: 2-3 mEq/kg/day in 2-4 divided doses
Adults: 40-100 mEq/day in 2-4 divided doses
Dosage Forms
Liquid, sugar free (Kaon®): 20 mEq/15 mL
Powder (Kolyum®): Potassium 20 mEq and chloride 3.4 mEq (potassium gluconate and po-
tassium chloride combination) per packet
Tablet: 500 mg, 595 mg

potassium iodide
Brand Names Pima®; Potassium Iodide Enseals®; SSKI®; Thyro-Block®
Synonyms KI; Lugol's solution; strong iodine solution
Therapeutic Category Antithyroid Agent; Expectorant
Use Facilitate bronchial drainage and cough; to reduce thyroid vascularity prior to thyroidecto-
my and management of thyrotoxic crisis; block thyroidal uptake of radioactive isotopes of io-
dine in a radiation emergency

Usual Dosage Oral:
Adults RDA: 130 mcg

Expectorant:
Children: 60-250 mg every 6-8 hours; maximum single dose: 500 mg
Adults: 300-1000 mg 2-3 times/day, may increase to 1-1.5 g 3 times/day

Preoperative thyroidectomy: Children and Adults: 50-250 mg 3 times/day (2-6 drops strong
iodine solution); give for 10 days before surgery

Thyrotoxic crisis:
Infants <1 year: $\frac{1}{2}$ adult dosage
Children and Adults: 300 mg = 6 drops SSKI® every 8 hours

Graves' disease in neonates: 1 drop of Lugol's solution every 8 hours

Sporotrichosis:
Oral: Initial:
Preschool: 50 mg/dose 3 times/day
Children: 250 mg/dose 3 times/day
Adults: 500 mg/dose 3 times/day
Oral increase 50 mg/dose daily
(Continued)

potassium iodide *(Continued)*

Maximum dose:
Preschool: 500 mg/dose 3 times/day
Children and Adults: 1-2 g/dose 3 times/day
Continue treatment for 4-6 weeks after lesions have completely healed

Dosage Forms
Solution, oral:
SSKI": 1 g/mL (30 mL, 240 mL, 473 mL)
Lugol's solution, strong iodine: 100 mg/mL with iodine 50 mg/mL (120 mL)
Syrup: 325 mg/5 mL
Tablet: 130 mg

Potassium Iodide Enseals® *see* potassium iodide *on previous page*

potassium perchlorate *see* radiological/contrast media (ionic) *on page 404*

potassium phosphate

Synonyms phosphate, potassium
Therapeutic Category Electrolyte Supplement, Oral; Electrolyte Supplement, Parenteral; Phosphate Salt; Potassium Salt
Use Source of potassium and phosphorus in parenteral nutrition and large volume I.V. fluids; treatment of conditions associated with excessive renal phosphate and potassium loss, inadequate GI absorption of these electrolytes, or inadequate phosphate and potassium in the diet
Usual Dosage I.V. doses should be incorporated into the patient's maintenance I.V. fluids; intermittent I.V. infusion should be reserved for severe depletion situations in patients undergoing continuous EKG monitoring. It is difficult to determine total body phosphorus deficit, the following dosages are empiric guidelines:
Dosage Forms Injection: Potassium 4.4 mEq and phosphate 3 mmol per mL (15 mL)

potassium phosphate and sodium phosphate

Brand Names K-Phos" Neutral; Neutra-Phos®; Uro-KP-Neutral®
Synonyms sodium phosphate and potassium phosphate
Therapeutic Category Electrolyte Supplement, Oral; Phosphate Salt; Potassium Salt
Use Treatment of conditions associated with excessive renal phosphate loss or inadequate GI absorption of phosphate
Usual Dosage All dosage forms to be mixed in 6-8 oz of water prior to administration
Children: 2-3 mmol phosphate/kg/24 hours given 4 times/day
Adults: 100-150 mmol phosphate/24 hours in divided doses after meals and at bedtime; 1-8 tablets or capsules/day, given 4 times/day
Dosage Forms
Powder, concentrate: Phosphate 8 mmol, sodium 7.125 mEq, and potassium 7.125 mEq per 75 mL when reconstituted
Tablet: Phosphate 8 mmol, sodium 13 mEq, and potassium 1.1 mEq (114 mg of phosphorus)

povidone-iodine *(poe' vi done)*

Brand Names Betadine® [OTC]; Efodine® [OTC]; Iodex® Regular; Isodine® [OTC]
Therapeutic Category Antibacterial, Topical
Use External antiseptic with broad microbicidal spectrum against bacteria, fungi, viruses, protozoa, and yeasts
Usual Dosage Apply as needed for treatment and prevention of susceptible microbial infections
Dosage Forms
Aerosol: 5% (90 mL)
Cleanser, topical: 7.5% (30 mL, 120 mL)
Concentrate:
Whirlpool: 10% (3840 mL)
Perineal wash: 10% (240 mL)

Douche: 10% (0.5 oz/packet 240 mL)
Foam, topical: 10% (250 g)
Gel, vaginal: 10% (3 oz)
Mouthwash: 0.5% (180 mL)
Ointment, topical: 10% (0.9 g foil packet, 0.94 g, 28 g, 480 g)
Pads, antiseptic gauze: 10% (3" x 9", 5" x 9")
Scrub, surgical: 7.5% (480 mL, 946 mL)
Shampoo: 7.5% (120 mL)
Solution:
    Swab aid: 10% (100s)
    Swabsticks, 4": 10%
    Topical: 10% (240 mL, 480 mL, 946 mL)
Suppository, vaginal: 10%

ppa *see* phenylpropanolamine hydrochloride *on page 365*

ppd *see* tuberculin tests *on page 477*

ppl *see* benzylpenicilloyl-polylysine *on page 51*

pralidoxime chloride (pra li dox' eem)
Brand Names Protopam®
Synonyms 2-pam; 2-pyridine aldoxime methochloride
Therapeutic Category Antidote, Anticholinesterase; Antidote, Organophosphate Poisoning
Use Reverse muscle paralysis with toxic exposure to organophosphate anticholinesterase pesticides and chemicals; control of overdose of drugs used to treat myasthenia gravis
Usual Dosage Poisoning: I.V.:
    Children: 20-50 mg/kg/dose; repeat in 1-2 hours if muscle weakness has not been relieved, then at 10- to 12-hour intervals if cholinergic signs recur

    Adults: 1-2 g; repeat in 1-2 hours if muscle weakness has not been relieved, then at 10- to 12-hour intervals if cholinergic signs recur
Dosage Forms Injection: 20 mL vial containing 1 g pralidoxime chloride with one 20 mL ampul diluent, disposable syringe, needle, and alcohol swab

PrameGel® [OTC] *see* pramoxine hydrochloride *on this page*

Pramet® FA *see* vitamin, multiple (prenatal) *on page 491*

Pramilet® FA *see* vitamin, multiple (prenatal) *on page 491*

Pramosone® *see* pramoxine and hydrocortisone *on this page*

pramoxine and hydrocortisone
Brand Names Enzone®; Pramosone®; Proctofoam®-HC; Zone-A Forte®
Synonyms hydrocortisone and pramoxine
Therapeutic Category Anti-inflammatory Agent; Corticosteroid, Topical (Low Potency); Local Anesthetic, Topical
Use Treatment of severe anorectal or perianal inflammation
Usual Dosage Apply to affected areas 3-4 times/day
Dosage Forms
    Cream, topical: Pramoxine hydrochloride 1% and hydrocortisone acetate 0.5% (30 g); pramoxine hydrochloride 1% and hydrocortisone acetate 1%
    Foam, rectal: Pramoxine hydrochloride 1% and hydrocortisone acetate 1% (10 g)
    Lotion, topical: Pramoxine hydrochloride 1% and hydrocortisone 0.25%; pramoxine hydrochloride 1% and hydrocortisone 2.5%; pramoxine hydrochloride 2.5% and hydrocortisone 1% (37.5 mL, 120 mL, 240 mL)

pramoxine hydrochloride (pra mox' een)
Brand Names Itch-X® [OTC]; Phicon® [OTC]; PrameGel® [OTC]; Prax® [OTC]; Proctofoam® [OTC]; Tronolane® [OTC]; Tronothane® [OTC]
Therapeutic Category Local Anesthetic, Topical
(Continued)
381

pramoxine hydrochloride *(Continued)*
Use Temporary relief of pain and itching associated with anogenital pruritus or irritation; dermatosis, minor burns or hemorrhoids
Usual Dosage Apply as directed, usually every 3-4 hours
Dosage Forms
Aerosol foam: 1% in an anesthetic mucoadhesive foam base (15 g)
Cream: 0.5% (30 g, 60 g); 1% (28.4 g, 113.4 g)
Gel, topical: 1% (37.5 g)
Liquid, topical: 1% (118 mL)
Lotion: 1% (15 mL, 20 mL, 240 mL)
Spray: 1% (60 mL)

Pravachol® *see* pravastatin sodium *on this page*

pravastatin sodium (pra' va stat in)
Brand Names Pravachol®
Therapeutic Category Antilipemic Agent; HMG-CoA Reductase Inhibitor
Use Adjunct to diet for the reduction of elevated total and LDL-cholesterol levels in patients with hypercholesterolemia (Type IIa and IIb)
Usual Dosage Adults: Oral: 10-20 mg once daily at bedtime
Dosage Forms Tablet: 10 mg, 20 mg, 40 mg

Prax® **[OTC]** *see* pramoxine hydrochloride *on previous page*

prazepam (pra' ze pam)
Brand Names Centrax®
Therapeutic Category Antianxiety Agent; Anticonvulsant, Benzodiazepine; Benzodiazepine
Use Treatment of anxiety and management of alcohol withdrawal; may also be used as an anticonvulsant in management of simple partial seizures
Usual Dosage Adults: Oral: 30 mg/day in divided doses
Dosage Forms
Capsule: 5 mg, 10 mg, 20 mg
Tablet: 5 mg, 10 mg

praziquantel (pray zi kwon' tel)
Brand Names Biltricide®
Therapeutic Category Anthelmintic
Use Treatment of all stages of schistosomiasis caused by all *Schistosoma* species pathogenic to humans; also active in the treatment of clonorchiasis, opisthorchiasis, cysticercosis, and many intestinal tapeworms
Usual Dosage Children and Adults: Oral:
Schistosomiasis: 20 mg/kg/dose 2-3 times/day for 1 day at 4- to 6-hour intervals

Flukes: 25 mg/kg/dose every 8 hours for 1-2 days

Cysticercosis: 50 mg/kg/day divided every 8 hours for 14 days

Tapeworms: 10-20 mg/kg as a single dose (25 mg/kg for *H. nana*)
Dosage Forms Tablet, tri-scored: 600 mg

prazosin and polythiazide
Brand Names Minizide®
Therapeutic Category Antihypertensive, Combination
Use Management of mild to moderate hypertension
Usual Dosage Adults: Oral: 1 capsule 2-3 times/day
Dosage Forms Capsule:
1: Prazosin 1 mg and polythiazide 0.5 mg
2: Prazosin 2 mg and polythiazide 0.5 mg
5: Prazosin 5 mg and polythiazide 0.5 mg

prazosin hydrochloride (pra' zoe sin)
Brand Names Minipress®
Synonyms furazosin
Therapeutic Category Alpha-Adrenergic Blocking Agent, Oral; Antihypertensive; Vasodilator, Coronary
Use Hypertension, severe congestive heart failure (in conjunction with diuretics and cardiac glycosides)
Usual Dosage Oral:
Children: Initial: 5 mcg/kg/dose (to assess hypotensive effects); usual dosing interval every 6 hours; increase dosage gradually up to maintenance of 25-150 mcg/kg/day divided every 6 hours

Adults: Initial: 1 mg/dose 2-3 times/day; usual maintenance dose: 3-15 mg/day in divided doses 2-4 times/day; maximum daily dose: 20 mg
Dosage Forms Capsule: 1 mg, 2 mg, 5 mg

Predaject® Injection see prednisolone on this page

Predalone Injection see prednisolone on this page

Predcor-TBA® Injection see prednisolone on this page

Pred Forte® Ophthalmic see prednisolone on this page

Pred-G® Ophthalmic see prednisolone and gentamicin on next page

Pred Mild® Ophthalmic see prednisolone on this page

prednicarbate (pred' ni kar bate)
Brand Names Dermatop®
Therapeutic Category Corticosteroid, Topical (Medium Potency)
Use Relief of inflammatory and pruritic manifestations of corticosteroid-responsive dermatoses
Dosage Forms Cream: 0.1% (15 g, 60 g)

Prednicen-M® Oral see prednisone on next page

prednisolone (pred niss' oh lone)
Brand Names AK-Pred® Ophthalmic; Articulose-50® Injection; Delta-Cortef® Oral; Econopred® Ophthalmic; Econopred® Plus Ophthalmic; Hydeltrasol® Injection; Hydeltra-T.B.A.® Injection; Inflamase® Forte Ophthalmic; Inflamase® Mild Ophthalmic; Key-Pred® Injection; Key-Pred-SP® Injection; Metreton® Ophthalmic; Pediapred® Oral; Predaject® Injection; Predalone Injection; Predcor-TBA® Injection; Pred Forte® Ophthalmic; Pred Mild® Ophthalmic; Prednisol® TBA Injection; Prelone® Oral
Synonyms deltahydrocortisone; metacortandralone
Therapeutic Category Adrenal Corticosteroid; Anti-inflammatory Agent; Corticosteroid, Ophthalmic; Corticosteroid, Systemic
Use Treatment of palpebral and bulbar conjunctivitis; corneal injury from chemical, radiation, thermal burns, or foreign body penetration; endocrine disorders, rheumatic disorders, collagen diseases, dermatologic diseases, allergic states, ophthalmic diseases, respiratory diseases, hematologic disorders, neoplastic diseases, edematous states, and gastrointestinal diseases; useful in patients with inability to activate prednisone (liver disease)
Usual Dosage Dose depends upon condition being treated and response of patient; dosage for infants and children should be based on severity of the disease and response of the patient rather than on strict adherence to dosage indicated by age, weight, or body surface area. Consider alternate day therapy for long-term therapy. Discontinuation of long-term therapy requires gradual withdrawal by tapering the dose.

Children:
Acute asthma:
Oral: 1-2 mg/kg/day in divided doses 1-2 times/day for 3-5 days
I.V.: 2-4 mg/kg/day divided 3-4 times/day
(Continued)

383

prednisolone *(Continued)*

Anti-inflammatory or immunosuppressive dose: Oral, I.V.: 0.1-2 mg/kg/day in divided doses 1-4 times/day

Nephrotic syndrome: Oral: Initial: 2 mg/kg/day (maximum: 80 mg/day) in divided doses 3-4 times/day until urine is protein free for 5 days (maximum: 28 days); if proteinuria persists, use 4 mg/kg/dose every other day for an additional 28 days (maximum: 120 mg/day); maintenance: 2 mg/kg/dose every other day for 28 days (maximum: 80 mg/dose); then taper over 4-6 weeks

Adults:

Oral, I.V.: 5-60 mg/day

Ophthalmic suspension: 1-2 drops into conjunctival sac every hour during day, every 2 hours at night until favorable response is obtained, then use 1 drop every 4 hours

Dosage Forms

Injection, as acetate: 25 mg/mL (10 mL, 30 mL); 50 mg/mL (10 mL, 30 mL); 100 mg/mL (10 mL)

Injection, as sodium phosphate: 20 mg/mL (2 mL, 5 mL, 10 mL)

Injection, as tebutate: 20 mg/mL (1 mL, 5 mL, 10 mL)

Liquid, oral, as sodium phosphate: 5 mg/5 mL (120 mL)

Solution, ophthalmic, as sodium phosphate: 0.125% (5 mL, 10 mL, 15 mL); 0.5% (5 mL)

Suspension, ophthalmic, as acetate: 0.12% (5 mL, 10 mL); 0.125% (5 mL, 10 mL); 1% (1 mL, 5 mL, 10 mL, 15 mL)

Syrup: 15 mg/5 mL (240 mL)

Tablet: 5 mg

prednisolone acetate and sodium sulfacetamide *see* sodium sulfacetamide and prednisolone *on page 431*

prednisolone and gentamicin

Brand Names Pred-G™ Ophthalmic

Synonyms gentamicin and prednisolone

Therapeutic Category Antibiotic, Ophthalmic; Corticosteroid, Ophthalmic

Use Treatment of steroid responsive inflammatory conditions and superficial ocular infections due to strains of microorganisms susceptible to gentamicin

Usual Dosage Children and Adults: Ophthalmic: 1 drop 2-4 times/day; during the initial 24-48 hours, the dosing frequency may be increased if necessary

Dosage Forms

Ointment, ophthalmic: Prednisolone acetate 0.6% and gentamicin sulfate 0.3% (3.5 g)

Suspension, ophthalmic: Prednisolone acetate 1% and gentamicin sulfate 0.3% (5 mL)

Prednisol® TBA Injection *see* prednisolone *on previous page*

prednisone *(pred' ni sone)*

Brand Names Deltasone™ Oral; Liquid Pred™ Oral; Meticorten® Oral; Orasone® Oral; Predni-cen-M™ Oral; Sterapred™ Oral

Synonyms deltacortisone; deltadehydrocortisone

Therapeutic Category Adrenal Corticosteroid; Anti-inflammatory Agent; Corticosteroid, Systemic

Use Treatment of a variety of diseases including adrenocortical insufficiency, hypercalcemia, rheumatic and collagen disorders, dermatologic, ocular, respiratory, gastrointestinal and neoplastic diseases, organ transplantation and a variety of diseases including those of hematologic, allergic, inflammatory, and autoimmune in origin

Usual Dosage Dose depends upon condition being treated and response of patient; dosage for infants and children should be based on severity of the disease and response of the patient rather than on strict adherence to dosage indicated by age, weight, or body surface area. Consider alternate day therapy for long-term therapy. Discontinuation of long-term therapy requires gradual withdrawal by tapering the dose.

Children: Oral: 0.05-2 mg/kg/day (anti-inflammatory or immunosuppressive dose) divided 1-4 times/day

Acute asthma: Oral: 1-2 mg/kg/day in divided doses 1-2 times/day for 3-5 days

Nephrotic syndrome: Oral: Initial: 2 mg/kg/day (maximum: of 80 mg/day) in divided doses 3-4 times/day until urine is protein free for 5 days (maximum: 28 days); if proteinuria persists, use 4 mg/kg/dose every other day (maximum: 120 mg/day) for an additional 28 days; maintenance: 2 mg/kg/dose every other day for 28 days (maximum: 80 mg/day); then taper over 4-6 weeks

Children and Adults: Physiologic replacement: 4-5 mg/m^2/day

Adults: Oral: 5-60 mg/day in divided doses 1-4 times/day

Dosage Forms

Solution:

Concentrate: 5 mg/mL (5 mL, 30 mL)

Oral: 5 mg/5 mL (10 mL, 20 mL, 500 mL)

Syrup: 5 mg/5 mL (120 mL, 240 mL)

Tablet: 1 mg, 2.5 mg, 5 mg, 10 mg, 20 mg, 50 mg

Prefrin™ Ophthalmic Solution *see* phenylephrine hydrochloride *on page 364*

pregnenedione *see* progesterone *on page 389*

Pregnosis® *see* diagnostic aids (*in vitro*), urine *on page 137*

Pregnospia® II *see* diagnostic aids (*in vitro*), urine *on page 137*

Pregnyl® *see* chorionic gonadotropin *on page 101*

Prehist® *see* chlorpheniramine and phenylephrine *on page 93*

Prelone® Oral *see* prednisolone *on page 383*

Premarin® *see* estrogens, conjugated *on page 174*

Premarin® With Methyltestosterone Oral *see* estrogens with methyltestosterone *on page 175*

prenatal vitamins *see* vitamin, multiple (prenatal) *on page 491*

Prenavite® [OTC] *see* vitamin, multiple (prenatal) *on page 491*

Pre-Par® *see* ritodrine hydrochloride *on page 413*

Prepcat® *see* radiological/contrast media (ionic) *on page 404*

Pre-Pen® *see* benzylpenicilloyl-polylysine *on page 51*

Prepidil® Vaginal Gel *see* dinoprostone *on page 148*

PreSun® 29 [OTC] *see* methoxycinnamate and oxybenzone *on page 297*

Pretz-D® [OTC] *see* ephedrine sulfate *on page 167*

Prevacid® *see* lansoprazole *on page 262*

Prevident® *see* fluoride *on page 196*

prilocaine (pril' oh kane)

Brand Names Citanest® Forte; Citanest" Plain

Therapeutic Category Local Anesthetic, Injectable

Use In dentistry for infiltration anesthesia and for nerve block anesthesia

Usual Dosage Dose varies with procedure, desired depth, and duration of anesthesia, desired muscle relaxation, vascularity of tissues, physical condition, and age of patient

Dosage Forms Injection:

Citanest® Plain: 4% (1.8 mL)

Citanest® Forte: 4% with epinephrine bitartrate 1:200,000 (1.8 mL)

Prilosec™ *see* omeprazole *on page 336*

primaclone *see* primidone *on next page*

Primacor® *see* milrinone lactate *on page 307*

primaquine and chloroquine *see* chloroquine and primaquine *on page 91*

primaquine phosphate (prim' a kween)
Synonyms prymaccone
Therapeutic Category Antimalarial Agent
Use Provide radical cure of *P. vivax* or *P. ovale* malaria after a clinical attack has been confirmed by blood smear or serologic titer and postexposure prophylaxis
Usual Dosage Oral:
Children: 0.3 mg base/kg/day once daily for 14 days not to exceed 15 mg/day or 0.9 mg base/kg once weekly for 8 weeks not to exceed 45 mg base/week

Adults: 15 mg/day (base) once daily for 14 days or 45 mg base once weekly for 8 weeks
Dosage Forms Tablet: 26.3 mg [15 mg base]

Primatene® Mist [OTC] *see* epinephrine *on page 167*
Primaxin® *see* imipenem/cilastatin *on page 242*

primidone (pri' mi done)
Brand Names Mysoline "
Synonyms desoxyphenobarbital; primaclone
Therapeutic Category Anticonvulsant, Barbiturate
Use Prophylactic management of partial seizures with complex symptomatology (psychomotor seizures), generalized tonic-clonic, and akinetic seizure
Usual Dosage Oral:
Children: 0.3 mg base/kg/day once daily for 14 days (not to exceed 15 mg/day) or 0.9 mg base/kg once weekly for 8 weeks not to exceed 45 mg base/week

Adults: 15 mg/day (base) once daily for 14 days or 45 mg base once weekly for 8 weeks
Dosage Forms
Suspension, oral: 250 mg/5 mL (240 mL)
Tablet: 50 mg, 250 mg

Principen® *see* ampicillin *on page 26*
Prinivil® *see* lisinopril *on page 270*
Prinzide® *see* lisinopril and hydrochlorothiazide *on page 270*
Priscoline® Injection *see* tolazoline hydrochloride *on page 463*
Privine® Nasal [OTC] *see* naphazoline hydrochloride *on page 319*
Proampacin® *see* ampicillin and probenecid *on page 26*
Proaqua® *see* benzthiazide *on page 50*
Probalan® *see* probenecid *on this page*
Pro-Banthine® *see* propantheline bromide *on page 392*
Proben-C® *see* colchicine and probenecid *on page 112*

probenecid (proe ben' e sid)
Brand Names Benemid "; Probalan "
Therapeutic Category Adjuvant Therapy, Penicillin Level Prolongation; Uric Acid Lowering Agent
Use Prevention of gouty arthritis; hyperuricemia; prolong serum levels of penicillin/cephalosporin
Usual Dosage Oral:
Children:
<2 years: Not recommended
2-14 years: Prolong penicillin serum levels: 25 mg/kg starting dose, then 40 mg/kg/day given 4 times/day
Gonorrhea: <45 kg: 25 mg/kg x 1 (maximum: 1 g/dose) 30 minutes before penicillin, ampicillin or amoxicillin

Adults:
Hyperuricemia with gout: 250 mg twice daily for one week; increase to 500 mg 2 times/day; may increase by 500 mg/month, if needed, to maximum of 2-3 g/day (dosages

may be decreased by 500 mg every 6 months if serum urate concentrations are controlled)
Prolong penicillin serum levels: 500 mg 4 times/day
Gonorrhea: 1 g 30 minutes before penicillin, ampicillin or amoxicillin
Dosage Forms Tablet: 500 mg

probenecid and colchicine *see* colchicine and probenecid *on page 112*

probucol (proe' byoo kole)
Brand Names Lorelco®
Synonyms biphenabid
Therapeutic Category Antilipemic Agent
Use Adjunct to dietary therapy to decrease elevated serum total and LDL cholesterol concentrations in primary hypercholesterolemia
Usual Dosage Oral:
Children:
<27 kg: 250 mg twice daily with meals
>27 kg: 500 mg twice daily with meals

Adults: 500 mg twice daily administered with the morning and evening meals
Dosage Forms Tablet: 250 mg, 500 mg

procainamide hydrochloride (proe kane a' mide)
Brand Names Procan® SR; Pronestyl®; Pronestyl-SR®
Synonyms procaine amide hydrochloride
Therapeutic Category Antiarrhythmic Agent, Class Ia
Use Ventricular tachycardia, premature ventricular contractions, paroxysmal atrial tachycardia, and atrial fibrillation; to prevent recurrence of ventricular tachycardia, paroxysmal supraventricular tachycardia, atrial fibrillation or flutter
Usual Dosage Must be titrated to patient's response
Children:
Oral: 15-50 mg/kg/24 hours divided every 3-6 hours; maximum 4 g/24 hours
I.M.: 20-30 mg/kg/24 hours divided every 4-6 hours in divided doses; maximum 4 g/24 hours
I.V.: Load: 3-6 mg/kg/dose over 5 minutes not to exceed 100 mg/dose; may repeat every 5-10 minutes to maximum of 15 mg/kg/load; maintenance as continuous I.V. infusion: 20-80 mcg/kg/minute; maximum: 2 g/24 hours

Adults:
Oral: 250-500 mg/dose every 3-6 hours or 500 mg to 1 g every 6 hours sustained release; usual dose: 50 mg/kg/24 hours or 2-4 g/24 hours
I.V.: Load: 50-100 mg/dose, repeated every 5-10 minutes until patient controlled; or load with 15-18 mg/kg, maximum loading dose: 1-1.5 g; maintenance: 2-6 mg/minute continuous I.V. infusion, usual maintenance: 3-4 mg/minute
Dosage Forms
Capsule: 250 mg, 375 mg, 500 mg
Injection: 100 mg/mL (10 mL); 500 mg/mL (2 mL)
Tablet: 250 mg, 375 mg, 500 mg
Tablet, sustained release: 250 mg, 500 mg, 750 mg, 1000 mg

procaine amide hydrochloride *see* procainamide hydrochloride *on this page*
procaine benzylpenicillin *see* penicillin g procaine, aqueous *on page 354*

procaine hydrochloride
Brand Names Novocain® Injection
Therapeutic Category Local Anesthetic, Injectable
Use Produce spinal anesthesia and epidural and peripheral nerve block by injection and infiltration methods
(Continued)
387

procaine hydrochloride *(Continued)*
Usual Dosage Dose varies with procedure, desired depth, and duration of anesthesia, desired muscle relaxation, vascularity of tissues, physical condition, and age of patient
Dosage Forms Injection: 1% [10 mg/mL] (2 mL, 6 mL, 30 mL, 100 mL); 2% [20 mg/mL] (30 mL, 100 mL); 10% (2 mL)

procaine penicillin g *see* penicillin g procaine, aqueous *on page 354*
Pro-Cal-Sof® [OTC] *see* docusate *on page 153*
Procan® SR *see* procainamide hydrochloride *on previous page*

procarbazine hydrochloride (proe kar' ba zeen)
Brand Names Matulane®
Synonyms ibenzmethyzin; mih; n-methylhydrazine
Therapeutic Category Antineoplastic Agent, Miscellaneous
Use Treatment of Hodgkin's disease, non-Hodgkin's lymphoma, brain tumor, bronchogenic carcinoma
Usual Dosage Refer to individual protocols. Oral:
Children: 50-100 mg/m^2/day once daily; doses as high as 100-200 mg/m^2/day once daily have been used for neuroblastoma and medulloblastoma

Adults: Initial: 2-4 mg/kg/day in single or divided doses for 7 days then increase dose to 4-6 mg/kg/day until response is obtained or leukocyte count decreased <4000/mm^3 or the platelet count decreased <100,000/mm^3; maintenance: 1-2 mg/kg/day
Dose reductions are necessary in patients with reduced renal function, reduced hepatic function, and/or bone marrow disorders
Dosage Forms Capsule: 50 mg

Procardia® *see* nifedipine *on page 328*
Procardia XL® *see* nifedipine *on page 328*

prochlorperazine (proe klor per' a zeen)
Brand Names Compazine®
Therapeutic Category Antiemetic; Antipsychotic Agent; Phenothiazine Derivative
Use Management of nausea and vomiting; acute and chronic psychosis
Usual Dosage
Children: Oral, rectal:
>10 kg: 0.4 mg/kg/24 hours in 3-4 divided doses; **or**
9-14 kg: 2.5 mg every 12-24 hours as needed; maximum: 7.5 mg/day
14-18 kg: 2.5 mg every 8-12 hours as needed; maximum: 10 mg/day
18-39 kg: 2.5 mg every 8 hours or 5 mg every 12 hours as needed; maximum: 15 mg/day
I.M.: 0.1-0.15 mg/kg/dose; usual: 0.13 mg/kg/dose; change to oral as soon as possible
I.V.: Not recommended
Adults:
Oral: 5-10 mg 3-4 times/day; usual maximum: 40 mg/day; doses up to 150 mg/day may be required in some patients
I.M.: 5-10 mg every 3-4 hours; usual maximum: 40 mg/day; doses up to 10-20 mg every 4-6 hours may be required in some patients
I.V.: 2.5-10 mg; maximum 10 mg/dose or 40 mg/day; may repeat dose every 3-4 hours as needed
Rectal: 25 mg twice daily
Dosage Forms
Capsule, sustained action, as maleate: 10 mg, 15 mg, 30 mg
Injection, as edisylate: 5 mg/mL (2 mL, 10 mL)
Suppository, rectal: 2.5 mg, 5 mg, 25 mg (12/box)
Syrup, as edisylate: 5 mg/5 mL (120 mL)
Tablet, as maleate: 5 mg, 10 mg, 25 mg

Procrit® *see* epoetin alfa *on page 168*

Proctocort™ *see* hydrocortisone *on page 232*

Proctofoam®-HC *see* pramoxine and hydrocortisone *on page 381*

Proctofoam® [OTC] *see* pramoxine hydrochloride *on page 381*

procyclidine hydrochloride (proe sye' kli deen)
Brand Names Kemadrin®
Therapeutic Category Anticholinergic Agent; Anti-Parkinson's Agent
Use Relieve symptoms of Parkinsonian syndrome and drug-induced extrapyramidal symptoms
Usual Dosage Adults: Oral: 2-2.5 mg 3 times/day after meals; if tolerated, gradually increase dose to 4-5 mg 3 times/day
Dosage Forms Tablet: 5 mg

Pro-Depo® Injection *see* hydroxyprogesterone caproate *on page 236*

Prodium® [OTC] *see* phenazopyridine hydrochloride *on page 360*

Prodrox® Injection *see* hydroxyprogesterone caproate *on page 236*

Profasi® HP *see* chorionic gonadotropin *on page 101*

Profenal® Ophthalmic *see* suprofen *on page 443*

Profilate® OSD *see* antihemophilic factor (human) *on page 29*

Profilnine® Heat-Treated *see* factor ix complex (human) *on page 184*

progesterone (proe jess' ter one)
Brand Names Gesterol®
Synonyms pregnenedione; progestin
Therapeutic Category Progestin
Use Endometrial carcinoma or renal carcinoma as well as secondary amenorrhea or abnormal uterine bleeding due to hormonal imbalance
Usual Dosage Adults: I.M.: 5-10 mg/day for 6-8 days
Dosage Forms Injection, in oil: 50 mg/mL (10 mL)

progestin *see* progesterone *on this page*

Proglycem® Oral *see* diazoxide *on page 140*

Prograf® *see* tacrolimus *on page 445*

ProHIBiT® *see* hemophilus b conjugate vaccine *on page 222*

Prolastin® Injection *see* alpha₁-proteinase inhibitor (human) *on page 13*

Proleukin® *see* aldesleukin *on page 11*

Prolixin Decanoate® Injection *see* fluphenazine *on page 199*

Prolixin Enanthate® Injection *see* fluphenazine *on page 199*

Prolixin® Injection *see* fluphenazine *on page 199*

Prolixin® Oral *see* fluphenazine *on page 199*

Proloprim® *see* trimethoprim *on page 473*

promazine hydrochloride (proe' ma zeen)
Brand Names Sparine®
Therapeutic Category Antipsychotic Agent; Phenothiazine Derivative
Use Treatment of psychoses
Usual Dosage Oral, I.M.:
Children >12 years: Antipsychotic: 10-25 mg every 4-6 hours
(Continued)

promazine hydrochloride *(Continued)*

Adults:
    Psychosis: 10-200 mg every 4-6 hours not to exceed 1000 mg/day
    Antiemetic: 25-50 mg every 4-6 hours as needed

Dosage Forms
Injection: 25 mg/mL (10 mL); 50 mg/mL (1 mL, 2 mL, 10 mL)
Tablet: 25 mg, 50 mg, 100 mg

Prometa® *see metaproterenol sulfate on page 290*

promethazine and codeine

Brand Names Phenergan® with Codeine; Pherazine® With Codeine; Prothazine-DC®
Therapeutic Category Antihistamine; Antitussive; Cough Preparation
Use Temporary relief of coughs and upper respiratory symptoms associated with allergy or the common cold
Usual Dosage Oral (in terms of codeine):
Children: 1-1.5 mg/kg/day every 4 hours as needed; maximum: 30 mg/day **or**
    2-6 years: 1.25-2.5 mL every 4-6 hours or 2.5-5 mg/dose every 4-6 hours as needed; maximum: 30 mg codeine/day
    6-12 years: 2.5-5 mL every 4-6 hours as needed or 5-10 mg/dose every 4-6 hours as needed; maximum: 60 mg codeine/day

Adults: 10-20 mg/dose every 4-6 hours as needed; maximum: 120 mg codeine/day; or 5-10 mL every 4-6 hours as needed
Dosage Forms Syrup: Promethazine hydrochloride 6.25 mg and codeine phosphate 10 mg per 5 mL (120 mL, 180 mL, 473 mL)

promethazine and phenylephrine

Brand Names Phenergan® VC; Pherazine® VC
Therapeutic Category Antihistamine/Decongestant Combination
Use Temporary relief of upper respiratory symptoms associated with allergy or the common cold
Usual Dosage Oral:
Children:
    2-6 years: 1.25 mL every 4-6 hours, not to exceed 7.5 mL in 24 hours
    6-12 years: 2.5 mL every 4-6 hours, not to exceed 15 mL in 24 hours

Children >12 years and Adults: 5 mL every 4-6 hours, not to exceed 30 mL in 24 hours
Dosage Forms Liquid: Promethazine hydrochloride 6.25 mg and phenylephrine hydrochloride 5 mg per 5 mL (120 mL, 180 mL, 240 mL, 480 mL, 4000 mL)

promethazine hydrochloride *(proe meth' a zeen)*

Brand Names Anergan® Injection; Phenameth® Oral; Phenazine® Injection; Phenergan® Injection; Phenergan® Oral; Phenergan® Rectal; Prometh® Injection; Prorex® Injection; Prothazine® Injection; Prothazine® Oral; V-Gan® Injection
Therapeutic Category Antiemetic; Antihistamine; Phenothiazine Derivative; Sedative
Use Symptomatic treatment of various allergic conditions, antiemetic, motion sickness, and as a sedative
Usual Dosage
Children:
    Antihistamine: Oral: 0.1 mg/kg/dose every 6 hours during the day and 0.5 mg/kg/dose at bedtime as needed
    Antiemetic: Oral, I.M., I.V., rectal: 0.25-1 mg/kg 4-6 times/day as needed
    Motion sickness: Oral: 0.5 mg/kg 30 minutes to 1 hour before departure, then every 12 hours as needed
    Sedation: Oral, I.M., I.V., rectal: 0.5-1 mg/kg/dose every 6 hours as needed

Adults:
Antihistamine:
Oral: 25 mg at bedtime or 12.5 mg 3 times/day
I.M., I.V., rectal: 25 mg, may repeat in 2 hours
Antiemetic: Oral, I.M., I.V., rectal: 12.5-25 mg every 4 hours as needed
Motion sickness: Oral: 25 mg 30 minutes to 1 hour before departure, then every 12 hours as needed
Sedation: Oral, I.M., I.V., rectal: 25-50 mg/dose

Dosage Forms
Injection: 25 mg/mL (1 mL, 10 mL); 50 mg/mL (1 mL, 10 mL)
Suppository, rectal: 12.5 mg, 25 mg, 50 mg
Syrup: 6.25 mg/5 mL (5 mL, 120 mL, 240 mL, 480 mL, 4000 mL); 25 mg/5mL (120 mL, 480 mL, 4000 mL)
Tablet: 12.5 mg, 25 mg, 50 mg

promethazine, phenylephrine, and codeine

Brand Names Mallergan-VC® With Codeine; Phenergan® VC With Codeine
Therapeutic Category Antihistamine/Decongestant Combination; Antitussive; Cough Preparation
Use Temporary relief of coughs and upper respiratory symptoms including nasal congestion
Usual Dosage Oral:
Children (expressed in terms of codeine dosage): 1-1.5 mg/kg/day every 4 hours, maximum: 30 mg/day **or**
<2 years: Not recommended
2 to 6 years:
Weight 25 lb: 1.25-2.5 mL every 4-6 hours, not to exceed 6 mL/24 hours
Weight 30 lb: 1.25-2.5 mL every 4-6 hours, not to exceed 7 mL/24 hours
Weight 35 lb: 1.25-2.5 mL every 4-6 hours, not to exceed 8 mL/24 hours
Weight 40 lb: 1.25-2.5 mL every 4-6 hours, not to exceed 9 mL/24 hours
6 to <12 years: 2.5-5 mL every 4-6 hours, not to exceed 15 mL/24 hours

Adults: 5 mL every 4-6 hours, not to exceed 30 mL/24 hours
Dosage Forms Liquid: Promethazine hydrochloride 6.25 mg, phenylephrine hydrochloride 5 mg, and codeine phosphate 10 mg per 5 mL with alcohol 7% (120 mL, 240 mL, 480 mL, 4000 mL)

promethazine with dextromethorphan

Brand Names Phenameth® DM; Phenergan® with Dextromethorphan; Pherazine® w/DM
Therapeutic Category Antitussive; Cough Preparation
Use Temporary relief of coughs and upper respiratory symptoms associated with allergy or the common cold
Usual Dosage Oral:
Children:
2-6 years: 1.25-2.5 mL every 4-6 hours up to 10 mL in 24 hours
6-12 years: 2.5-5 mL every 4-6 hours up to 20 mL in 24 hours

Adults: 5 mL every 4-6 hours up to 30 mL in 24 hours
Dosage Forms Syrup: Promethazine hydrochloride 6.25 mg and dextromethorphan hydrobromide 15 mg per 5 mL with alcohol 7% (120 mL, 480 mL, 4000 mL)

Prometh® Injection *see* promethazine hydrochloride *on previous page*

Promit® *see* dextran 1 *on page 134*

Pronestyl® *see* procainamide hydrochloride *on page 387*

Pronestyl-SR® *see* procainamide hydrochloride *on page 387*

Propacet® *see* propoxyphene and acetaminophen *on page 393*

Propadrine *see* phenylpropanolamine hydrochloride *on page 365*

propafenone hydrochloride (proe pa feen' one)
Brand Names Rythmol™
Therapeutic Category Antiarrhythmic Agent, Class Ic
Use Life-threatening ventricular arrhythmias; an oral sodium channel blocker similar to encainide and flecainide; in clinical trials was used effectively to treat atrial flutter, atrial fibrillation and other arrhythmias, but are not labeled indications; can worsen or even cause new ventricular arrhythmias (proarrhythmic effect)
Usual Dosage Adults: Oral: 150 mg every 8 hours, up to 300 mg every 8 hours
Dosage Forms Tablet: 150 mg, 225 mg, 300 mg

Propagest® [OTC] *see* phenylpropanolamine hydrochloride *on page 365*

propantheline bromide (proe pan' the leen)
Brand Names Pro-Banthine®
Therapeutic Category Antispasmodic Agent, Gastrointestinal
Use Adjunctive treatment of peptic ulcer, irritable bowel syndrome, pancreatitis, ureteral and urinary bladder spasm; to reduce duodenal motility during diagnostic radiologic procedures
Usual Dosage Oral:
Antisecretory:
Children: 1-2 mg/kg/day in 3-4 divided doses
Elderly patients: 7.5 mg 3 times/day before meals and at bedtime

Antispasmodic:
Children: 2-3 mg/kg/day in divided doses every 4-6 hours and at bedtime
Adults: 15 mg 3 times/day before meals or food and 30 mg at bedtime
Dosage Forms Tablet: 7.5 mg, 15 mg

proparacaine and fluorescein
Brand Names Fluoracaine™ Ophthalmic
Therapeutic Category Diagnostic Agent, Ophthalmic Dye; Local Anesthetic, Ophthalmic
Use Anesthesia for tonometry, gonioscopy; suture removal from cornea; removal of corneal foreign body; cataract extraction, glaucoma surgery
Usual Dosage
Tonometry, gonioscopy, suture removal: Adults: Instill 1-2 drops 0.5% solution in eye just prior to procedure

Ophthalmic surgery: Children and Adults: Instill 1 drop of 0.5% solution in eye every 5-10 minutes for 5-7 doses
Dosage Forms Solution: Proparacaine hydrochloride 0.5% and fluorescein sodium 0.25% (2 mL, 5 mL)

proparacaine hydrochloride (proe par' a kane)
Brand Names AK-Taine™ Ophthalmic; Alcaine™ Ophthalmic; I-Paracaine® Ophthalmic; Opthaine™ Ophthalmic; Ophthetic™ Ophthalmic
Synonyms proxymetacaine
Therapeutic Category Local Anesthetic, Ophthalmic
Use Anesthesia for tonometry, gonioscopy; suture removal from cornea; removal of corneal foreign body; cataract extraction, glaucoma surgery; short operative procedure involving the cornea and conjunctiva
Usual Dosage Children and Adults:
Ophthalmic surgery: Instill 1 drop of 0.5% solution in eye every 5-10 minutes for 5-7 doses

Tonometry, gonioscopy, suture removal: Instill 1-2 drops 0.5% solution in eye just prior to procedure
Dosage Forms Ophthalmic, solution: 0.5% (2 mL, 15 mL)

Propine® Ophthalmic *see* dipivefrin hydrochloride *on page 151*

propiomazine hydrochloride (proe pee oh' ma zeen)
Brand Names Largon® Injection
Therapeutic Category Antianxiety Agent; Antiemetic; Phenothiazine Derivative; Sedative
Use Relief of restlessness, nausea and apprehension before and during surgery or during labor
Usual Dosage I.M., I.V.:
 Children: 0.55-1.1 mg/kg
 Adults: 10-40 mg prior to procedure, additional may be repeated at 3-hour intervals
Dosage Forms Injection: 20 mg/mL (1 mL)

Proplex® T *see* factor ix complex (human) *on page 184*

propofol (proe' po fole)
Brand Names Diprivan® Injection
Therapeutic Category General Anesthetic
Use Induction or maintenance of anesthesia for inpatient or outpatient surgery
Usual Dosage Dosage must be individualized and titrated to the desired clinical effect; however, as a general guideline:

No pediatric dose has been established

Induction: I.V.:
 Adults ≤55 years, and/or ASA I or II patients: 2-2.5 mg/kg of body weight (approximately 40 mg every 10 seconds until onset of induction)
 Elderly, debilitated, hypovolemic, and/or ASA III or IV patients: 1-1.5 mg/kg of body weight (approximately 20 mg every 10 seconds until onset of induction)

Maintenance: I.V. infusion:
 Adults ≤55 years, and/or ASA I or II patients: 0.1-0.2 mg/kg of body weight/minute (6-12 mg/kg of body weight/hour)
 Elderly, debilitated, hypovolemic, and/or ASA III or IV patients: 0.05-0.1 mg/kg of body weight/minute (3-6 mg/kg of body weight/hour)

I.V. intermittent: 25-50 mg increments, as needed
Dosage Forms Injection: 10 mg/mL (20 mL)

propoxyphene (proe pox' i feen)
Brand Names Darvon®; Darvon-N®; Dolene®
Synonyms dextropropoxyphene
Therapeutic Category Analgesic, Narcotic
Use Management of mild to moderate pain
Usual Dosage Adults: Oral:
 Hydrochloride: 65 mg every 3-4 hours as needed for pain; maximum: 390 mg/day
 Napsylate: 100 mg every 4 hours as needed for pain; maximum: 600 mg/day
Dosage Forms
 Capsule, as hydrochloride: 65 mg
 Tablet, as napsylate: 100 mg

propoxyphene and acetaminophen
Brand Names Darvocet-N®; Darvocet-N® 100; E-Lor®; Genagesic®; Propacet®; Wygesic®
Synonyms propoxyphene hydrochloride and acetaminophen; propoxyphene napsylate and acetaminophen
Therapeutic Category Analgesic, Narcotic; Antipyretic
Use Management of mild to moderate pain
Usual Dosage Adults:
 Darvocet-N®: 1-2 tablets every 4 hours as needed; maximum: 600 mg propoxyphene napsylate/day
 Darvocet-N® 100: 1 tablet every 4 hours as needed; maximum: 600 mg propoxyphene napsylate/day
 (Continued)

propoxyphene and acetaminophen (Continued)

Dosage Forms Tablet:
Darvocet-N": Propoxyphene napsylate 50 mg and acetaminophen 325 mg
Darvocet-N" 100: Propoxyphene napsylate 100 mg and acetaminophen 650 mg
E-Lor", Genagesic", Wygesic": Propoxyphene hydrochloride 65 mg and acetaminophen 650 mg

propoxyphene and aspirin

Brand Names Bexophene®; Darvon® Compound-65 Pulvules®
Synonyms propoxyphene hydrochloride and aspirin; propoxyphene napsylate and aspirin
Therapeutic Category Analgesic, Narcotic; Antipyretic
Use Management of mild to moderate pain
Usual Dosage Oral: 1-2 capsules every 4 hours as needed
Dosage Forms
Capsule: Propoxyphene hydrochloride 65 mg and aspirin 389 mg with caffeine 32.4 mg
Tablet (Darvon-N" with A.S.A.): Propoxyphene napsylate 100 mg and aspirin 325 mg

propoxyphene hydrochloride and acetaminophen see propoxyphene and acetaminophen on previous page

propoxyphene hydrochloride and aspirin see propoxyphene and aspirin on this page

propoxyphene napsylate and acetaminophen see propoxyphene and acetaminophen on previous page

propoxyphene napsylate and aspirin see propoxyphene and aspirin on this page

propranolol and hydrochlorothiazide

Brand Names Inderide"
Therapeutic Category Antihypertensive, Combination
Use Management of hypertension
Usual Dosage Dose is individualized
Dosage Forms
Capsule, long acting (Inderide" LA):
80/50 Propranolol hydrochloride 80 mg and hydrochlorothiazide 50 mg
120/50 Propranolol hydrochloride 120 mg and hydrochlorothiazide 50 mg
160/50 Propranolol hydrochloride 160 mg and hydrochlorothiazide 50 mg
Tablet (Inderide"):
40/25 Propranolol hydrochloride 40 mg and hydrochlorothiazide 25 mg
80/25 Propranolol hydrochloride 80 mg and hydrochlorothiazide 25 mg

propranolol hydrochloride (proe pran' oh lole)

Brand Names Betachron E-R®; Inderal®; Inderal® LA
Therapeutic Category Antianginal Agent; Antiarrhythmic Agent, Class Ib; Antiarrhythmic Agent, Class II; Beta-Adrenergic Blocker
Use Management of hypertension, angina pectoris, pheochromocytoma, essential tremor, tetralogy of Fallot cyanotic spells, and arrhythmias (such as atrial fibrillation and flutter, A-V nodal re-entrant tachycardias, and catecholamine-induced arrhythmias); prevention of myocardial infarction, migraine headache; symptomatic treatment of hypertrophic subaortic stenosis
Usual Dosage
Tachyarrhythmias:
Oral:
Children: Initial: 0.5-1 mg/kg/day in divided doses every 6-8 hours; titrate dosage upward every 3-7 days; usual dose: 2-4 mg/kg/day; higher doses may be needed; do not exceed 16 mg/kg/day or 60 mg/day
Adults: 10-80 mg/dose every 6-8 hours

I.V.:
Children: 0.01-0.1 mg/kg slow IVP over 10 minutes; maximum dose: 1 mg
Adults: 1 mg/dose slow IVP; repeat every 5 minutes up to a total of 5 mg

Hypertension: Oral:
Children: Initial: 0.5-1 mg/kg/day in divided doses every 6-12 hours; increase gradually every 3-7 days; maximum: 2 mg/kg/24 hours
Adults: Initial: 40 mg twice daily or 60-80 mg once daily as sustained release capsules; increase dosage every 3-7 days; usual dose: ≤320 mg divided in 2-3 doses/day or once daily as sustained release; maximum daily dose: 640 mg

Migraine headache prophylaxis: Oral:
Children: 0.6-1.5 mg/kg/day **or**
≤35 kg: 10-20 mg 3 times/day
>35 kg: 20-40 mg 3 times/day
Adults: Initial: 80 mg/day divided every 6-8 hours; increase by 20-40 mg/dose every 3-4 weeks to a maximum of 160-240 mg/day given in divided doses every 6-8 hours; if satisfactory response not achieved within 6 weeks of starting therapy, drug should be withdrawn gradually over several weeks

Tetralogy spells: Children: Oral: 1-2 mg/kg/day every 6 hours as needed, may increase by 1 mg/kg/day to a maximum of 5 mg/kg/day, or if refractory may increase slowly to a maximum of 10-15 mg/kg/day

Thyrotoxicosis:
Neonates: Oral: 2 mg/kg/day in divided doses every 6-12 hours; occasionally higher doses may be required
Adolescents and Adults: Oral: 10-40 mg/dose every 6 hours
Adults: I.V.: 1-3 mg/dose slow IVP as a single dose

Adults: Oral:
Angina: 80-320 mg/day in doses divided 2-4 times/day or 80-160 mg of sustained release once daily
Pheochromocytoma: 30-60 mg/day in divided doses
Myocardial infarction prophylaxis: 180-240 mg/day in 3-4divided doses
Hypertrophic subaortic stenosis: 20-40 mg 3-4 times/day
Essential tremor: 40 mg twice daily initially; maintenance doses: usually 120-320 mg/day

Dosage Forms
Capsule, sustained action: 60 mg, 80 mg, 120 mg, 160 mg
Injection: 1 mg/mL (1 mL)
Solution, oral (strawberry-mint flavor): 4 mg/mL (5 mL, 500 mL); 8 mg/mL (5 mL, 500 mL)
Solution, oral, concentrate: 80 mg/mL (30 mL)
Tablet: 10 mg, 20 mg, 40 mg, 60 mg, 80 mg, 90 mg

Propulsid® see cisapride on page 102

propylene glycol and salicylic acid see salicylic acid and propylene glycol on page 416

propylhexedrine (proe pill hex' e dreen)
Brand Names Benzedrex® [OTC]
Therapeutic Category Decongestant
Use Topical nasal decongestant
Usual Dosage Inhale through each nostril while blocking the other
Dosage Forms Inhaler: 250 mg

propyliodone see radiological/contrast media (ionic) on page 404

2-propylpentanoic acid see valproic acid and derivatives on page 482

propylthiouracil (proe pill thye oh yoor' a sill)
Synonyms ptu
Therapeutic Category Antithyroid Agent
Use Palliative treatment of hyperthyroidism as an adjunct to ameliorate hyperthyroidism in preparation for surgical treatment or radioactive iodine therapy and in the management of thyrotoxic crisis
(Continued)

propylthiouracil *(Continued)*

Usual Dosage Oral:
Neonates: 5-10 mg/kg/day in divided doses every 8 hours

Children: Initial: 5-7 mg/kg/day in divided doses every 8 hours or
  6-10 years: 50-150 mg/day
  >10 years: 150-300 mg/day
  Maintenance: $\frac{1}{3}$ to $\frac{2}{3}$ of the initial dose in divided doses every 8-12 hours

Adults: Initial: 300-450 mg/day in divided doses every 8 hours; maintenance: 100-150 mg/day in divided doses every 8-12 hours

Dosage Forms Tablet: 50 mg

2-propylvaleric acid *see* valproic acid and derivatives *on page 482*

Prorex® Injection *see* promethazine hydrochloride *on page 390*

Proscar® Oral *see* finasteride *on page 192*

Pro-Sof® Plus [OTC] *see* docusate and casanthranol *on page 154*

ProSom™ *see* estazolam *on page 173*

prostaglandin e₁ *see* alprostadil *on page 14*

prostaglandin e₂ *see* dinoprostone *on page 148*

prostaglandin f₂ alpha *see* dinoprost tromethamine *on page 148*

Prostaphlin® Injection *see* oxacillin sodium *on page 340*

Prostaphlin® Oral *see* oxacillin sodium *on page 340*

ProStep® Patch *see* nicotine *on page 327*

Prostigmin® Injection *see* neostigmine *on page 324*

Prostigmin® Oral *see* neostigmine *on page 324*

Prostin/15M® *see* carboprost tromethamine *on page 76*

Prostin E₂® Vaginal Suppository *see* dinoprostone *on page 148*

Prostin F₂ Alpha® *see* dinoprost tromethamine *on page 148*

Prostin VR Pediatric® Injection *see* alprostadil *on page 14*

protamine sulfate *(proe' ta meen)*

Therapeutic Category Antidote, Heparin
Use Treatment of heparin overdosage; neutralize heparin during surgery or dialysis procedures
Usual Dosage Children and Adults: I.V.: 1 mg of protamine neutralizes 90 USP units of heparin (lung) and 115 USP units of heparin (intestinal); heparin neutralization occurs within 5 minutes following I.V. injection; administer 1 mg for each 100 units of heparin given in preceding 3-4 hours up to a maximum dose of 50 mg
Dosage Forms Injection: 10 mg/mL (5 mL, 10 mL, 25 mL)

Protectol® Medicated Powder [OTC] *see* calcium undecylenate *on page 70*

Protenate® *see* plasma protein fraction *on page 372*

Prothazine-DC® *see* promethazine and codeine *on page 390*

Prothazine® Injection *see* promethazine hydrochloride *on page 390*

Prothazine® Oral *see* promethazine hydrochloride *on page 390*

Protilase® *see* pancrelipase *on page 346*

protirelin *(proe tye' re lin)*

Brand Names Relefact TRH Injection; Thypinone Injection
Synonyms lopremone
Therapeutic Category Diagnostic Agent, Thyroid Function

Use Adjunct in the diagnostic assessment of thyroid function, and an adjunct to other diagnostic procedures in assessment of patients with pituitary or hypothalamic dysfunction; also causes release of prolactin from the pituitary and is used to detect defective control of prolactin secretion.
Usual Dosage I.V.:
Children: 7 mcg/kg to a maximum dose of 500 mcg
Adults: 500 mcg (range: 200-500 mcg)
Dosage Forms Injection: 500 mcg/mL (1 mL)

Protopam® *see* pralidoxime chloride *on page 381*

Protostat® Oral *see* metronidazole *on page 303*

protriptyline hydrochloride (proe trip' ti leen)
Brand Names Vivactil®
Therapeutic Category Antidepressant, Tricyclic
Use Treatment of various forms of depression, often in conjunction with psychotherapy
Usual Dosage Oral:
Adolescents: 15-20 mg/day
Adults: 15-60 mg in 3-4 divided doses
Elderly: 15-20 mg/day
Dosage Forms Tablet: 5 mg, 10 mg

Protropin® Injection *see* human growth hormone *on page 226*

Provatene® [OTC] *see* beta-carotene *on page 52*

Proventil® *see* albuterol *on page 10*

Provera® Oral *see* medroxyprogesterone acetate *on page 283*

Provocholine® *see* methacholine chloride *on page 291*

Proxigel® [OTC] *see* carbamide peroxide *on page 74*

proxymetacaine *see* proparacaine hydrochloride *on page 392*

Prozac® *see* fluoxetine hydrochloride *on page 198*

prp-d *see* hemophilus b conjugate vaccine *on page 222*

Prulet® [OTC] *see* phenolphthalein *on page 362*

prymaccone *see* primaquine phosphate *on page 386*

Pseudo-Car® DM *see* carbinoxamine, pseudoephedrine, and dextromethorphan *on page 75*

Pseudo-Chlor® [OTC] *see* chlorpheniramine and pseudoephedrine *on page 94*

pseudoephedrine (soo doe e fed' rin)
Brand Names Afrinol® [OTC]; Cenafed® [OTC]; Children's Silfedrine® [OTC]; Decofed® Syrup [OTC]; Drixoral® Non-Drowsy [OTC]; Efidac/24® [OTC]; Neofed® [OTC]; Novafed®; PediaCare® Oral; Sudafed® [OTC]; Sudafed® 12 Hour [OTC]; Sufedrin® [OTC]; Triaminic® AM Decongestant Formula [OTC]
Synonyms *d*-isoephedrine hydrochloride
Therapeutic Category Adrenergic Agonist Agent; Decongestant
Use Temporary symptomatic relief of nasal congestion due to common cold, upper respiratory allergies, and sinusitis; also promotes nasal or sinus drainage
Usual Dosage Oral:
Children:
<2 years: 4 mg/kg/day in divided doses every 6 hours
2-5 years: 15 mg every 6 hours; maximum: 60 mg/24 hours
6-12 years: 30 mg every 6 hours; maximum: 120 mg/24 hours

Adults: 60 mg every 6 hours; maximum: 240 mg/24 hours
Dosage Forms
Capsule: 60 mg
Capsule, timed release, as hydrochloride: 120 mg
(Continued)

pseudoephedrine *(Continued)*

Drops, oral, as hydrochloride: 7.5 mg/0.8 mL (15 mL)
Liquid, as hydrochloride: 15 mg/5 mL (120 mL); 30 mg/5 mL (120 mL, 240 mL, 473 mL)
Syrup, as hydrochloride: 15 mg/5 mL (118 mL)
Tablet, as hydrochloride: 30 mg, 60 mg
Tablet:
    Timed release, as hydrochloride: 120 mg
    Extended release, as sulfate: 120 mg, 240 mg

pseudoephedrine and dextromethorphan

Brand Names Drixoral® Cough & Congestion Liquid Caps [OTC]; Vicks® 44D Cough & Head Congestion; Vicks® 44 Non-Drowsy Cold & Cough Liqui-Caps [OTC]
Therapeutic Category Adrenergic Agonist Agent; Antitussive; Decongestant
Use Temporary symptomatic relief of nasal congestion due to common cold, upper respiratory allergies, and sinusitis; also promotes nasal or sinus drainage; symptomatic relief of coughs caused by minor viral upper respiratory tract infections or inhaled irritants; most effective for a chronic nonproductive cough
Dosage Forms
    Capsule: Pseudoephedrine hydrochloride 60 mg and dextromethorphan hydrobromide 30 mg

pseudoephedrine and ibuprofen

Brand Names Motrin® IB Sinus [OTC]; Sine-Aid® IB [OTC]
Therapeutic Category Adrenergic Agonist Agent; Analgesic, Non-Narcotic; Decongestant
Use Temporary symptomatic relief of nasal congestion due to common cold, upper respiratory allergies, and sinusitis; also promotes nasal or sinus drainage; sinus headaches and pains
Dosage Forms Caplet: Pseudoephedrine hydrochloride 30 mg and ibuprofen 200 mg

pseudoephedrine and azatadine *see* azatadine and pseudoephedrine *on page 40*

pseudoephedrine and chlorpheniramine *see* chlorpheniramine and pseudoephedrine *on page 94*

pseudoephedrine and dexbrompheniramine *see* dexbrompheniramine and pseudoephedrine *on page 132*

pseudoephedrine and guaifenesin *see* guaifenesin and pseudoephedrine *on page 216*

pseudoephedrine and triprolidine *see* triprolidine and pseudoephedrine *on page 474*

Pseudo-gest Plus® [OTC] *see* chlorpheniramine and pseudoephedrine *on page 94*

pseudomonic acid a *see* mupirocin *on page 313*

Psorcon™ Topical *see* diflorasone diacetate *on page 143*

psoriGel® [OTC] *see* coal tar *on page 110*

Psorion® Cream *see* betamethasone *on page 52*

psp *see* phenolsulfonphthalein *on page 363*

P&S® Shampoo [OTC] *see* salicylic acid *on page 416*

psyllium *(sill' i yum)*

Brand Names Alramucil® [OTC]; Effer-Syllium® [OTC]; Fiberall® Powder [OTC]; Fiberall® Wafer [OTC]; Hydrocil® [OTC]; Konsyl® [OTC]; Konsyl-D® [OTC]; Maalox® Daily Fiber Therapy [OTC]; Metamucil® [OTC]; Metamucil® Instant Mix [OTC]; Modane® Bulk [OTC]; Mylanta® Natural Fiber Supplement [OTC]; Perdiem® Plain [OTC]; Reguloid® [OTC]; Restore® [OTC]; Serutan® [OTC]; Siblin® [OTC]; Syllact® [OTC]; V-Lax® [OTC]

Synonyms plantago seed; plantain seed

Therapeutic Category Laxative, Bulk-Producing

Use Treatment of chronic atonic or spastic constipation and in constipation associated with rectal disorders; management of irritable bowel syndrome

Usual Dosage Oral:

Children 6-11 years: $\frac{1}{2}$ to 1 rounded teaspoonful 1-3 times/day

Adults: 1-2 rounded teaspoonfuls or 1-2 packets 1-4 times/day

Dosage Forms

Granules: 4.03 g per rounded teaspoon (100 g, 250 g); 2.5 g per rounded teaspoon

Powder: Psyllium 50% and dextrose 50% (6.5 g, 325 g, 420 g, 480 g, 500 g)

Powder:

Effervescent: 3 g/dose (270 g, 480 g); 3.4 g/dose (single-dose packets)

Psyllium hydrophilic: 3.4 g/per rounded teaspoon (210 g, 300 g, 420 g, 630 g)

Squares, chewable: 1.7 g, 3.4 g

Wafers: 3.4 g

P.T.E.-4® *see* trace metals *on page 465*

P.T.E.-5® *see* trace metals *on page 465*

pteroylglutamic acid *see* folic acid *on page 201*

ptu *see* propylthiouracil *on page 395*

Pulmozyme® *see* dornase alfa *on page 156*

Purge® [OTC] *see* castor oil *on page 78*

Puri-Clens™ [OTC] *see* methylbenzethonium chloride *on page 298*

purified protein derivative *see* tuberculin tests *on page 477*

Purinethol® *see* mercaptopurine *on page 288*

P-V-Tussin® *see* hydrocodone, phenylephrine, pyrilamine, phenindamine, chlorpheniramine, and ammonium chloride *on page 231*

P$_x$E$_x$® Ophthalmic *see* pilocarpine and epinephrine *on page 369*

Pyocidin-Otic® *see* polymyxin b and hydrocortisone *on page 375*

pyrantel pamoate (pi ran' tel pam' oh ate)

Brand Names Antiminth® [OTC]; Pin-Rid® [OTC]; Pin-X® [OTC]; Reese's® Pinworm Medicine [OTC]

Therapeutic Category Anthelmintic

Use Roundworm, pinworm, and hookworm infestations, and trichostrongyliasis

Usual Dosage Children and Adults: Oral:

Roundworm, pinworm, or trichostrongyliasis: 11 mg/kg administered as a single dose; maximum dose is 1 g; dosage should be repeated in 2 weeks for pinworm infection

Hookworm: 11 mg/kg/day once daily for 3 days

Dosage Forms

Capsule: 180 mg

Liquid: 50 mg/mL (30 mL); 144 mg/mL (30 mL)

Suspension, oral (caramel-currant flavor): 50 mg/mL (60 mL)

pyrazinamide (peer a zin' a mide)

Synonyms pyrazinoic acid amide

Therapeutic Category Antitubercular Agent

Use Adjunctive treatment of tuberculosis when primary and secondary agents cannot be used or have failed

Usual Dosage Oral:

Children: 15-30 mg/kg/day in divided doses every 12-24 hours; daily dose not to exceed 2 g

Adults: 15-30 mg/kg/day in 3-4 divided doses; maximum daily dose: 2 g/day

Dosage Forms Tablet: 500 mg

pyrazinoic acid amide *see* pyrazinamide *on previous page*

pyrethrins (pye ree' thrins)
Brand Names A-200™ Pyrinate [OTC]; End Lice® [OTC]; Lice-Enz® [OTC]; Pyrinyl II® [OTC]; RID® [OTC]; Tisit® [OTC]
Therapeutic Category Antiparasitic Agent, Topical; Pediculocide
Use Treatment of *Pediculus humanus* infestations
Usual Dosage Application of pyrethrins:
Apply enough solution to completely wet infested area, including hair
Allow to remain on area for 10 minutes
Wash and rinse with large amounts of warm water
Use fine-toothed comb to remove lice and eggs from hair
Shampoo hair to restore body and luster
Treatment may be repeated if necessary once in a 24-hours period
Repeat treatment in 7-10 days to kill newly hatched lice
Dosage Forms
Gel, topical: 0.3% (30 g, 480 g)
Liquid, topical: 0.18% (60 mL); 0.2% (60 mL, 120 mL); 0.3% (60 mL, 120 mL, 240 mL)
Shampoo: 0.3% (60 mL, 118 mL); 0.33% (60 mL, 120 mL)

Pyribenzamine® *see* tripelennamine *on page 474*

Pyridiate® *see* phenazopyridine hydrochloride *on page 360*

2-pyridine aldoxime methochloride *see* pralidoxime chloride *on page 381*

Pyridium® *see* phenazopyridine hydrochloride *on page 360*

pyridostigmine bromide (peer id oh stig' meen)
Brand Names Mestinon® Injection; Mestinon® Oral; Regonol® Injection
Therapeutic Category Antidote, Neuromuscular Blocking Agent; Cholinergic Agent
Use Symptomatic treatment of myasthenia gravis; also used as an antidote for nondepolarizing neuromuscular blockers
Usual Dosage Normally, sustained release dosage form is used at bedtime for patients who complain of morning weakness

Myasthenia gravis:
Oral:
Children: 7 mg/kg/day in 5-6 divided doses
Adults: Initial: 60 mg 3 times/day with maintenance dose ranging from 60 mg to 1.5 g/day; sustained release formulation should be dosed at least every 6 hours (usually 12-24 hours)
I.M., I.V.:
Children: 0.05-0.15 mg/kg/dose (maximum single dose: 10 mg)
Adults: 2 mg every 2-3 hours or 1/30th of oral dose

Reversal of nondepolarizing neuromuscular blocker: I.M., I.V.:
Children: 0.1-0.25 mg/kg/dose preceded by atropine
Adults: 10-20 mg preceded by atropine
Dosage Forms
Injection: 5 mg/mL (2 mL, 5 mL)
Syrup (raspberry flavor): 60 mg/5 mL (480 mL)
Tablet: 60 mg
Tablet, sustained release: 180 mg

pyridoxine hydrochloride (peer i dox' een)
Brand Names Nestrex®
Synonyms vitamin b₆
Therapeutic Category Antidote, Cycloserine Toxicity; Antidote, Hydralazine Toxicity; Antidote, Isoniazid Toxicity; Vitamin, Water Soluble

Use Prevent and treat vitamin B₆ deficiency, pyridoxine-dependent seizures in infants, adjunct to treatment of acute toxicity from isoniazid, cycloserine, or hydralazine overdose

Usual Dosage
Pyridoxine-dependent Infants:
    Oral: 2-100 mg/day
    I.M., I.V.: 10-100 mg

Dietary deficiency: Oral:
    Children: 5-10 mg/24 hours for 3 weeks
    Adults: 10-20 mg/day for 3 weeks

Drug induced neuritis (eg, isoniazid, hydralazine, penicillamine, cycloserine): Oral treatment:
    Children: 10-50 mg/24 hours; prophylaxis: 1-2 mg/kg/24 hours
    Adults: 100-200 mg/24 hours; prophylaxis: 10-100 mg/24 hours

For the treatment of seizures and/or coma from acute isoniazid toxicity, a dose of pyridoxine hydrochloride equal to the amount of INH ingested can be given I.M./I.V. in divided doses together with other anticonvulsants

Dosage Forms
Injection: 100 mg/mL (10 mL, 30 mL)
Tablet: 25 mg, 50 mg, 100 mg
Tablet, extended release: 100 mg

pyrimethamine (peer i meth' a meen)
Brand Names Daraprim®
Therapeutic Category Antimalarial Agent
Use Prophylaxis of malaria due to susceptible strains of plasmodia; used in conjunction with quinine and sulfadiazine for the treatment of uncomplicated attacks of chloroquine-resistant *P. falciparum* malaria; used in conjunction with fast-acting schizonticide to initiate transmission control and suppression cure; synergistic combination with sulfonamide in treatment of toxoplasmosis

Usual Dosage Oral:
Malaria chemoprophylaxis:
    Children: 0.5 mg/kg once weekly; not to exceed 25 mg/dose **or**
    Children:
        <4 years: 6.25 mg once weekly
        4-10 years: 12.5 mg once weekly
    Children >10 years and Adults: 25 mg once weekly
    Dosage should be continued for all age groups for at least 6-10 weeks after leaving endemic areas

Chloroquine-resistant *P. falciparum* malaria (when used in conjunction with quinine and sulfadiazine):
    Children:
        <10 kg: 6.25 mg/day once daily for 3 days
        10-20 kg: 12.5 mg/day once daily for 3 days
        20-40 kg: 25 mg/day once daily for 3 days
    Adults: 25 mg twice daily for 3 days

Toxoplasmosis (with sulfadiazine or trisulfapyrimidines):
    Children: 1 mg/kg/day divided into 2 equal daily doses; decrease dose after 2-4 days by 50%, continue for about 1 month; used with 100 mg sulfadiazine/kg/day divided every 6 hours; **or** 2 mg/kg/day divided every 12 hours for 3 days followed by 1 mg/kg/day once daily for 4 weeks
    Adults: 50-75 mg/day together with 1-4 g of a sulfonamide for 1-3 weeks depending on patient's tolerance and response

Dosage Forms Tablet: 25 mg

Pyrinyl II® [OTC] *see pyrethrins on previous page*

pyrithione zinc (peer i thye' one)
Brand Names DHS Zinc® [OTC]; Head & Shoulders® [OTC]; Sebulon® [OTC]; Theraplex Z® [OTC]; Zincon® Shampoo [OTC]; ZNP® Bar [OTC]
Therapeutic Category Antiseborrheic Agent, Topical
(Continued)

pyrithione zinc *(Continued)*

Use Relieves itching, irritation, and scalp flaking associated with dandruff and/or seborrheal dermatitis of the scalp

Usual Dosage Shampoo hair twice weekly, wet hair, apply to scalp and massage vigorously, rinse and repeat

Dosage Forms
Bar: 2% (119 g)
Shampoo: 1% (120 mL); 2% (120 mL, 180 mL, 240 mL, 360 mL)

Quadra-Hist® *see* chlorpheniramine, phenyltoloxamine, phenylpropanolamine and phenylephrine *on page 96*

quazepam (kway' ze pam)

Brand Names Doral®
Therapeutic Category Benzodiazepine; Hypnotic; Sedative
Use Short-term treatment of insomnia
Usual Dosage Adults: Oral: Initial: 15 mg at bedtime, in some patients the dose may be reduced to 7.5 mg after a few nights
Dosage Forms Tablet: 7.5 mg, 15 mg

Quelicin® Injection *see* succinylcholine chloride *on page 437*

Queltuss® [OTC] *see* guaifenesin and dextromethorphan *on page 214*

Questran® *see* cholestyramine resin *on page 100*

Questran® Light *see* cholestyramine resin *on page 100*

Quibron® *see* theophylline and guaifenesin *on page 454*

Quibron®-T *see* theophylline *on page 453*

Quibron®-T/SR *see* theophylline *on page 453*

Quiess® *see* hydroxyzine *on page 237*

Quinaglute® Dura-Tabs® *see* quinidine *on next page*

Quinalan® *see* quinidine *on next page*

quinalbarbitone sodium *see* secobarbital sodium *on page 419*

Quinamm® *see* quinine sulfate *on next page*

quinapril hydrochloride (kwin' a pril)

Brand Names Accupril®
Therapeutic Category Angiotensin-Converting Enzyme (ACE) Inhibitors
Use Treatment of hypertension, either alone or in combination with other antihypertensive agents
Usual Dosage Adults: Oral: Initial: 10 mg once daily, adjust according to blood pressure response at peak and trough blood levels; in general, the normal dosage range is 40-80 mg/day
Dosage Forms Tablet: 5 mg, 10 mg, 20 mg, 40 mg

quinestrol (kwin ess' trole)

Brand Names Estrovis®
Therapeutic Category Estrogen Derivative
Use Atrophic vaginitis; hypogonadism; primary ovarian failure; vasomotor symptoms of menopause; prostatic carcinoma; osteoporosis prophylactic
Usual Dosage Adults: Oral: 100 mcg once daily for 7 days; followed by 100 mcg/week beginning 2 weeks after inception of treatment; may increase to 200 mcg/week if necessary
Dosage Forms Tablet: 100 mcg

quinethazone (kwin eth' a zone)
Brand Names Hydromox®
Therapeutic Category Diuretic, Thiazide
Use Adjunctive therapy in treatment of edema and hypertension
Usual Dosage Adults: Oral: 50-100 mg once daily up to a maximum of 200 mg daily
Dosage Forms Tablet: 50 mg

Quinidex® Extentabs® *see* quinidine *on this page*

quinidine (kwin' i deen)
Brand Names Cardioquin®; Quinaglute® Dura-Tabs®; Quinalan®; Quinidex® Extentabs®; Quinora®
Therapeutic Category Antiarrhythmic Agent, Class Ia
Use Prophylaxis after cardioversion of atrial fibrillation and/or flutter to maintain normal sinus rhythm; also used to prevent reoccurrence of paroxysmal supraventricular tachycardia, paroxysmal A-V junctional rhythm, paroxysmal ventricular tachycardia, paroxysmal atrial fibrillation, and atrial or ventricular premature contractions; also has activity against *Plasmodium falciparum* malaria
Usual Dosage Note: Dosage expressed in terms of the salt: 267 mg of quinidine gluconate = 275 mg of quinidine polygalacturonate = 200 mg of quinidine sulfate

Children: Test dose for idiosyncratic reaction (sulfate, oral or gluconate, I.M.): 2 mg/kg or 60 mg/m^2
   Oral (quinidine sulfate): 15-60 mg/kg/day in 4-5 divided doses or 6 mg/kg every 4-6 hours (AMA 1991); usual 30 mg/kg/day or 900 mg/m^2/day given in 5 daily doses
   I.V. **not** recommended (quinidine gluconate): 2-10 mg/kg/dose every 3-6 hours as needed

Adults: Test dose: 200 mg administered several hours before full dosage (to determine possibility of idiosyncratic reaction)
   Oral (sulfate): 100-600 mg/dose every 4-6 hours; begin at 200 mg/dose and titrate to desired effect
   Oral (gluconate): 324-972 mg every 8-12 hours
   Oral (polygalacturonate): 275 mg every 8-12 hours
   I.M.: 400 mg/dose every 4-6 hours
   I.V.: 200-400 mg/dose diluted and given at a rate ≤10 mg/minute
Dosage Forms
Injection, as gluconate: 80 mg/mL (10 mL)
Tablet, as polygalacturonate: 275 mg
Tablet, as sulfate: 200 mg, 300 mg
Tablet:
   Sustained action, as sulfate: 300 mg
   Sustained release, as gluconate: 324 mg

quinine sulfate (kwye' nine)
Brand Names Legatrin® [OTC]; Quinamm®; Quiphile®; Q-vel®
Therapeutic Category Antimalarial Agent; Skeletal Muscle Relaxant
Use Suppression or treatment of chloroquine-resistant *P. falciparum* malaria; treatment of *Babesia microti* infection; prevention and treatment of nocturnal recumbency leg muscle cramps
Usual Dosage Oral (parenteral dosage form may be obtained from Centers for Disease Control if needed):

Children: Chloroquine-resistant malaria and babesiosis: 25 mg/kg/day in divided doses every 8 hours for 7 days; maximum: 650 mg/dose

Adults:
   Chloroquine-resistant malaria: 650 mg every 8 hours for 7 days in conjunction with another agent
   Babesiosis: 650 mg every 6-8 hours for 7 days
   Leg cramps: 200-300 mg at bedtime
(Continued)

quinine sulfate (Continued)
Dosage Forms
Capsule: 64.8 mg, 65 mg, 200 mg, 300 mg, 325 mg
Tablet: 162.5 mg, 260 mg

Quinora® see quinidine on previous page
Quinsana® Plus Topical [OTC] see undecylenic acid and derivatives
on page 479
Quiphile® see quinine sulfate on previous page
Q-vel® see quinine sulfate on previous page

rabies immune globulin, human
Brand Names Hyperab®; Imogam®
Synonyms rig
Therapeutic Category Immune Globulin
Use Passive immunity to rabies for postexposure prophylaxis of individuals exposed to the
virus
Usual Dosage Children and Adults: I.M.: 20 units/kg in a single dose (RIG should always be
administered in conjunction with rabies vaccine (HDCV)) (Infiltrate $^1/_2$ of the dose locally
around the wound; give the remainder I.M.)
Dosage Forms Injection: 150 units/mL (2 mL, 10 mL)

rabies virus vaccine, human diploid
Brand Names Imovax® Rabies I.D. Vaccine; Imovax® Rabies Vaccine
Synonyms hdcv; hdrs
Therapeutic Category Vaccine, Inactivated Virus
Use Pre-exposure rabies immunization for high risk persons; postexposure antirabies immuni-
zation along with local treatment and immune globulin
Usual Dosage
Pre-exposure prophylaxis: Two 1 mL doses I.M. or I.D. 1 week apart, third dose 3 weeks after
second. If exposure continues, booster doses can be given every 2 years, or an antibody
titer determined and a booster dose given if the titer is inadequate.

Postexposure prophylaxis: All postexposure treatment should begin with immediate cleansing of the wound with soap and water. Persons not previously immunized as above: Rabies
immune globulin 20 units/kg body weight, half infiltrated at bite site if possible, remainder
I.M.; and 5 doses of rabies vaccine, 1 mL I.M., one each on days 0, 3, 7, 14, 28.

Persons who have previously received postexposure prophylaxis with rabies vaccine, received a recommended I.M. or I.D. pre-exposure series of rabies vaccine or have a previously documented rabies antibody titer considered adequate: Two doses of rabies vaccine, 1 mL I.M., one each on days 0 and 3
Dosage Forms Injection:
I.M. (HDCV): Rabies antigen 2.5 units/mL (1 mL)
Intradermal: Rabies antigen 0.25 units/mL (1 mL)

racemic amphetamine sulfate see amphetamine sulfate on page 25
Racet® Topical see clioquinol and hydrocortisone on page 106

radiological/contrast media (ionic)
Brand Names Anatrast®; Angio Conray®; Angiovist®; Baricon®; Barobag®; Baro-CAT®; Baro-
flave®; Barosperse®; Bar-Test®; Bilopaque®; Cholebrine®; Cholografin® Meglumine; Con-
ray®; Cystografin®; Dionosil Oily®; Enecat®; Entrobar®; Epi-C®; Ethiodol®; Flo-Coat®; Gastro-
grafin®; HD 85®; HD 200 Plus®; Hexabrix™; Hypaque-Cysto®; Hypaque® Meglumine; Hy-
paque® Sodium; Liquid Barosperse®; Liquipake®; Lymphazurin®; Magnevist®; MD-
Gastroview®; Oragrafin® Calcium; Oragrafin® Sodium; Perchloracap®; Prepcat®; Reno-M-
30®; Reno-M-60®; Reno-M-Dip®; Renovue®-65; Renovue®-DIP; Sinografin®; Telepaque®;

Tomocat®; Tonopaque®; Urovist Cysto®; Urovist® Meglumine; Urovist® Sodium 300; Vascoray®

Synonyms barium sulfate; diatrizoate meglumine; diatrizoate meglumine and diatrizoate sodium; diatrizoate meglumine and iodipamide meglumine; diatrizoate sodium; ethiodized oil; gadopentetate dimeglumine; iocetamic acid; iodamide meglumine; iodipamide meglumine; iopanoic acid; iothalamate meglumine and iothalamate sodium; iothalamate sodium; ipodate calcium; ipodate sodium; isosulfan blue; potassium perchlorate; propyliodone; tyropanoate sodium

Therapeutic Category Radiopaque Agents

Dosage Forms

Oral cholecystographic agents:
  Iocetamic acid: Tablet (Cholebrine®): 750 mg
  Iopanoic acid: Tablet (Telepaque®): 500 mg
  Ipodate calcium: Granules for oral suspension (Oragrafin® Calcium): 3 g
  Ipodate sodium: Capsule (Bilivist®, Oragrafin® Sodium): 500 mg
  Tyropanoate sodium: Capsule (Bilopaque®): 750 mg

GI contrast agents: **Barium sulfate**
  Paste (Anatrast®): 100% (500 g)
  Powder:
    Baroflave®: 100%
    Baricon®, HD 200 Plus®: 98%
    Barosperse®, Tonopaque®: 95%
  Suspension:
    Baro-CAT®, Prepcat®: 1.5%
    Enecat®, Tomocat®: 5%
    Entrobar®: 50%
    Liquid Barasperse®: 60%
    HD 85®: 85%
    Barobag®: 97%
    Flo-Coat®, Liquipake®: 100%
    Epi-C®: 150%
  Tablet (Bar-Test®): 650 mg

Parenteral agents: Injection:
  Diatrizoate meglumine:
    Hypaque® Meglumine
    Reno-M-DIP®
    Urovist® Meglumine
    Angiovist® 282
    Hypaque® Meglumine
    Reno-M-60®
  Diatrizoate sodium:
    Hypaque® Sodium
    Hypaque® Sodium
    Urovist® Sodium 300
  Gadopentetate dimeglumine: Magnevist®
  Iodamide meglumine:
    Renovue®-DIP
    Renovue®-65
  Iodipamide meglumine: Cholografin® meglumine
  Iothalamate meglumine:
    Conray® 30
    Conray® 43
    Conray®
  Iothalamate sodium
    Angio Conray®
    Conray® 325
    Conray® 400
  Diatrizoate meglumine and diatrizoate sodium
    Angiovist® 292
    Angiovist® 370
    Hypaque-76®
    Hypaque-M®, 75%

(Continued)

radiological/contrast media (ionic) *(Continued)*

Hypaque-M®, 90%
MD-60®
MD-76®
Renografin-60®
Renografin-76®
Renovist® II
Renovist®

Iothalamate meglumine and iothalamate sodium:
Vascoray®
Hexabrix™

Miscellaneous agents: (**NOT** for intravascular use, for instillation into various cavities)
Diatrizoate meglumine:
Urogenital solution, sterile:
Crystografin®
Crystografin® Dilute
Hypaque-Cysto®
Reno-M-30®
Urovist Cysto®

Diatrizoate meglumine and diatrizoate sodium Solution, oral or rectal:
Gastrografin®
MD-Gastroview®

Diatrizoate sodium:
Solution, oral or rectal (Hypaque® Sodium Oral)
Solution, urogenital (Hypaque® Sodium 20%)

Iothalamate meglumine: Solution, urogenital:
Cysto-Conray®
Cysto-Conray® II

Diatrizoate meglumine and iodipamide meglumine:
Injection, urogenital for intrauterine instillation (Sinografin®)

Ethiodized oil: Injection (Ethiodol®)
Propyliodone: Suspension (Dionosil Oily®)
Isosulfan blue: Injection (Lymphazurin® 1%)
Potassium perchlorate: Capsule (Perchloracap®): 200 mg

radiological/contrast media (non-ionic)
Brand Names Amnipaque®; Isovue®; Omnipaque®; Optiray®
Synonyms iohexol; iopamidol; ioversol; metrizamide
Therapeutic Category Radiopaque Agents
Dosage Forms
Parenteral agents: Injection:
Iohexol: Omnipaque®: 140 mg/mL; 180 mg/mL; 210 mg/mL; 240 mg/mL; 300 mg/mL; 350 mg/mL
Iopamidol:
Isovue-128®
Isovue-200®
Isovue-M 200®
Isovue-300®
Isovue-M 300®
Isovue-370®
Ioversol:
Optiray® 160
Optiray® 240
Optiray® 320
Metrizamide: Amnipaque®

ramipril *(ra mi' prill)*
Brand Names Altace™ Oral
Therapeutic Category Angiotensin-Converting Enzyme (ACE) Inhibitors
Use Treatment of hypertension, alone or in combination with thiazide diuretics

Usual Dosage Adults: Oral: 2.5-5 mg once daily
Dosage Forms Capsule: 1.25 mg, 2.5 mg, 5 mg, 10 mg

Ramses® [OTC] *see* nonoxynol 9 *on page 331*

ranitidine hydrochloride (ra nye' te deen)
Brand Names Zantac® Injection; Zantac® Oral
Therapeutic Category Histamine-2 Antagonist
Use Short-term treatment of active duodenal ulcers and benign gastric ulcers; long-term prophylaxis of duodenal ulcer and gastric hypersecretory states, gastroesophageal reflux, recurrent postoperative ulcer, upper GI bleeding, prevention of acid-aspiration pneumonitis during surgery, and prevention of stress-induced ulcers
Usual Dosage
Children:
Oral: 1.5-2 mg/kg/dose every 12 hours
I.M., I.V.: 0.75-1.5 mg/kg/dose every 6-8 hours, maximum daily dose: 400 mg
Continuous infusion: 0.1-0.25 mg/kg/hour (preferred for stress ulcer prophylaxis in patients with concurrent maintenance I.V.s or TPNs)

Adults:
Short-term treatment of ulceration: 150 mg/dose twice daily or 300 mg at bedtime
Prophylaxis of recurrent duodenal ulcer: 150 mg at bedtime
Gastric hypersecretory conditions: Oral: 150 mg twice daily, up to 6 g/day
I.M., I.V.: 50 mg/dose every 6-8 hours (dose not to exceed 400 mg/day)
Dosage Forms
Capsule (GELdose™): 150 mg, 300 mg
Granules, effervescent (EFFERdose™): 150 mg
Infusion, preservative free, in NaCl 0.45%: 1 mg/mL (50 mL)
Injection: 25 mg/mL (2 mL, 10 mL, 40 mL)
Syrup (peppermint flavor): 15 mg/mL (473 mL)
Tablet: 150 mg, 300 mg
Tablet, effervescent (EFFERdose™): 150 mg

RapidTest® Strep *see* diagnostic aids (*in vitro*), other *on page 137*
Raudixin® *see* rauwolfia serpentina *on this page*
Rauverid® *see* rauwolfia serpentina *on this page*

rauwolfia serpentina (rah wool' fee a)
Brand Names Raudixin®; Rauverid®; Wolfina®
Synonyms whole root rauwolfia
Therapeutic Category Antihypertensive; Rauwolfia Alkaloid
Use Mild essential hypertension; relief of agitated psychotic states
Usual Dosage Adults: Oral: 200-400 mg/day in 2 divided doses
Dosage Forms Tablet: 50 mg, 100 mg

rauwolfia serpentina and bendroflumethiazide
Brand Names Rauzide®
Therapeutic Category Antihypertensive, Combination

Rauzide® *see* rauwolfia serpentina and bendroflumethiazide *on this page*
Rea-Lo® [OTC] *see* urea *on page 480*
Recombigen® HIV-1 LA *see* diagnostic aids (*in vitro*), blood *on page 136*
recombinant human deoxyribonuclease *see* dornase alfa *on page 156*
Recombinate® *see* antihemophilic factor (recombinant) *on page 29*

Recombivax HB® *see* hepatitis b vaccine *on page 224*

Redisol® *see* cyanocobalamin *on page 119*

Redutemp® [OTC] *see* acetaminophen *on page 2*

Reese's® Pinworm Medicine [OTC] *see* pyrantel pamoate *on page 399*

Regitine® *see* phentolamine mesylate *on page 363*

Reglan® *see* metoclopramide *on page 302*

Regonol® Injection *see* pyridostigmine bromide *on page 400*

Regulace® [OTC] *see* docusate and casanthranol *on page 154*

Regular (Concentrated) Iletin® II U-500 *see* insulin preparations *on page 245*

Regular Iletin® I *see* insulin preparations *on page 245*

Regular Insulin *see* insulin preparations *on page 245*

Regular Purified Pork Insulin *see* insulin preparations *on page 245*

Regulax SS® [OTC] *see* docusate *on page 153*

Reguloid® [OTC] *see* psyllium *on page 398*

Regutol® [OTC] *see* docusate *on page 153*

Rela® *see* carisoprodol *on page 77*

Relafen® *see* nabumetone *on page 315*

Relaxadon® *see* hyoscyamine, atropine, scopolamine, and phenobarbital
on page 238

Relefact® TRH Injection *see* protirelin *on page 396*

Relief® Ophthalmic Solution *see* phenylephrine hydrochloride *on page 364*

Remular-S® *see* chlorzoxazone *on page 99*

Renacidin® *see* citric acid bladder mixture *on page 103*

Renese® *see* polythiazide *on page 377*

Reno-M-30® *see* radiological/contrast media (ionic) *on page 404*

Reno-M-60® *see* radiological/contrast media (ionic) *on page 404*

Reno-M-Dip® *see* radiological/contrast media (ionic) *on page 404*

Renoquid® *see* sulfacytine *on page 439*

Renormax® *see* spirapril *on page 434*

Renovue®-65 *see* radiological/contrast media (ionic) *on page 404*

Renovue®-DIP *see* radiological/contrast media (ionic) *on page 404*

Rentamine® *see* chlorpheniramine, ephedrine, phenylephrine, and carbetapentane
on page 94

ReoPro™ *see* abciximab *on page 2*

Repan *see* butalbital compound *on page 63*

Reposans-10® Oral *see* chlordiazepoxide *on page 89*

Resaid® *see* chlorpheniramine and phenylpropanolamine *on page 94*

Rescaps-D® S.R. Capsule *see* caramiphen and phenylpropanolamine
on page 73

Rescon *see* chlorpheniramine and pseudoephedrine *on page 94*

Rescon-ED® *see* chlorpheniramine and pseudoephedrine *on page 94*

Rescon Jr *see* chlorpheniramine and pseudoephedrine *on page 94*

Rescon Liquid [OTC] *see* chlorpheniramine and phenylpropanolamine
on page 94

Resectisol® Irrigation Solution *see* mannitol *on page 279*

reserpine (re ser' peen)
Brand Names Serpalan®
Therapeutic Category Rauwolfia Alkaloid
Use Management of mild to moderate hypertension
Usual Dosage Adults: Oral: 0.1-0.5 mg/day in 1-2 doses
Dosage Forms Tablet: 0.1 mg, 0.25 mg, 1 mg

reserpine and chlorothiazide *see* chlorothiazide and reserpine *on page 92*

reserpine and hydrochlorothiazide *see* hydrochlorothiazide and reserpine *on page 229*

Respa-1st® *see* guaifenesin and pseudoephedrine *on page 216*

Respa-DM® *see* guaifenesin and dextromethorphan *on page 214*

Respa-GF® *see* guaifenesin *on page 213*

Respahist® *see* brompheniramine and pseudoephedrine *on page 59*

Respaire®-60 SR *see* guaifenesin and pseudoephedrine *on page 216*

Respaire®-120 SR *see* guaifenesin and pseudoephedrine *on page 216*

Respbid® *see* theophylline *on page 453*

Respinol-G® *see* guaifenesin, phenylpropanolamine, and phenylephrine *on page 217*

Respiracult-Strep® *see* diagnostic aids (*in vitro*), other *on page 137*

Respiralex® *see* diagnostic aids (*in vitro*), other *on page 137*

Resporal® [OTC] *see* dexbrompheniramine and pseudoephedrine *on page 132*

Restore® [OTC] *see* psyllium *on page 398*

Restoril® *see* temazepam *on page 446*

Retin-A™ Topical *see* tretinoin *on page 466*

retinoic acid *see* tretinoin *on page 466*

Retrovir® Injection *see* zidovudine *on page 494*

Retrovir® Oral *see* zidovudine *on page 494*

Reversol® *see* edrophonium chloride *on page 163*

Rev-Eyes™ *see* dapiprazole hydrochloride *on page 125*

Rezine® *see* hydroxyzine *on page 237*

R-Gel® [OTC] *see* capsaicin *on page 72*

R-Gen® *see* iodinated glycerol *on page 248*

R-Gene® *see* arginine hydrochloride *on page 33*

rgm-csf *see* sargramostim *on page 418*

Rheaban® [OTC] *see* attapulgite *on page 39*

Rheomacrodex® *see* dextran *on page 133*

Rhesonativ® *see* Rh₀(D) immune globulin *on this page*

Rheumanosticon® Dri-Dot® *see* diagnostic aids (*in vitro*), blood *on page 136*

Rheumatrex® *see* methotrexate *on page 295*

Rhinall® Nasal Solution [OTC] *see* phenylephrine hydrochloride *on page 364*

Rhinocort® *see* budesonide *on page 61*

Rhinolar-EX® 12 *see* chlorpheniramine and phenylpropanolamine *on page 94*

Rhinosyn-DMX® [OTC] *see* guaifenesin and dextromethorphan *on page 214*

Rh₀(D) immune globulin

Brand Names HypRho®-D; HypRho®-D Mini-Dose; MICRhoGAM™; Mini-Gamulin® Rh; Rhesonativ®; RhoGAM™
Therapeutic Category Immune Globulin
(Continued)

Rh₀(D) immune globulin *(Continued)*

Use Prevent isoimmunization in Rh-negative individuals exposed to Rh-positive blood during delivery of an Rh-positive infant, as a result of an abortion, following amniocentesis or abdominal trauma, or following a transfusion accident; to prevent hemolytic disease of the newborn if there is a subsequent pregnancy with an Rh-positive fetus

Usual Dosage Adults: I.M.:

Obstetrical usage: 1 vial (300 mcg) prevents maternal sensitization if fetal packed red blood cell volume that has entered the circulation is <15 mL; if it is more, give additional vials. The number of vials = RBC volume of the calculated fetomaternal hemorrhage divided by 15 mL

Postpartum prophylaxis: 300 mcg within 72 hours of delivery

Antepartum prophylaxis: 300 mcg at approximately 26-28 weeks gestation; followed by 300 mcg within 72 hours of delivery if infant is Rh-positive

Following miscarriage, abortion, or termination of ectopic pregnancy at up to 13 weeks of gestation: 50 mcg ideally within 3 hours, but may be given up to 72 hours after; if pregnancy has been terminated at 13 or more weeks of gestation, administer 300 mcg

Dosage Forms

Injection: Each package contains one single dose 300 mcg of Rh₀ (D) immune globulin

Injection, microdose: Each package contains one single dose of microdose, 50 mcg of Rh₀ (D) immune globulin

RhoGAM™ *see* Rh₀(D) immune globulin *on previous page*

rhuepo-α *see* epoetin alfa *on page 168*

Rhulicaine® [OTC] *see* benzocaine *on page 48*

ribavirin (rye ba vye' rin)

Brand Names Virazole® Aerosol

Synonyms rtca; tribavirin

Therapeutic Category Antiviral Agent, Inhalation Therapy

Use Treatment of patients with respiratory syncytial virus (RSV) infections; may also be used in other viral infections including influenza A and B and adenovirus; specially indicated for treatment of severe lower respiratory tract RSV infections in patients with an underlying compromising condition (prematurity, bronchopulmonary dysplasia, congenital heart disease, immunodeficiency, and immunosuppression)

Usual Dosage Infants, Children, and Adults: Aerosol inhalation:

Use with Viratek® small particle aerosol generator (SPAG-2) at a concentration of 20 mg/mL (6 g reconstituted with 300 mL of sterile water without preservatives)

Aerosol only: 12-18 hours/day for 3 days, up to 7 days in length

Dosage Forms Powder for aerosol: 6 g (100 mL)

riboflavin (rye' boe flay vin)

Brand Names Riobin®

Synonyms lactoflavin; vitamin b_2; vitamin g

Therapeutic Category Vitamin, Water Soluble

Use Prevent riboflavin deficiency and treat ariboflavinosis; dietary sources include liver, kidney, dairy products, green vegetables, eggs, whole grain cereals, yeast, mushrooms

Usual Dosage Oral:

Riboflavin deficiency:
Children: 2.5-10 mg/day in divided doses
Adults: 5-30 mg/day in divided doses

Required daily allowance (RDA): Adults:
Male: 1.4-4.8 mg
Female: 1.2-1.3 mg

Dosage Forms Tablet: 25 mg, 50 mg, 100 mg

Rid-A-Pain® [OTC] *see* benzocaine *on page 48*

Ridaura® *see* auranofin *on page 39*

Ridenol® [OTC] *see* acetaminophen *on page 2*

RID® [OTC] *see* pyrethrins *on page 400*

rifabutin (rif a bu' tin)

Brand Names Mycobutin® Oral

Synonyms ansamycin

Therapeutic Category Antibiotic, Miscellaneous; Antitubercular Agent

Use Prevention of disseminated *Mycobacterium avium* complex (MAC) in patients with advanced HIV infection

Usual Dosage Oral:

Children: Efficacy and safety of rifabutin have not been established in children; a limited number of HIV-positive children with MAC (n=22) have been given rifabutin for MAC prophylaxis; doses of 5 mg/kg/day have been useful

Adults: 300 mg once daily; for patients who experience gastrointestinal upset, rifabutin can be administered 150 mg twice daily with food

Dosage Forms Capsule: 150 mg

Rifadin® Injection *see* rifampin *on this page*

Rifadin® Oral *see* rifampin *on this page*

Rifamate® *see* rifampin and isoniazid *on next page*

rifampicin *see* rifampin *on this page*

rifampin (rif' am pin)

Brand Names Rifadin® Injection; Rifadin® Oral; Rimactane® Oral

Synonyms rifampicin

Therapeutic Category Antibiotic, Miscellaneous; Antitubercular Agent

Use Management of active tuberculosis; eliminate meningococci from asymptomatic carriers; prophylaxis of *Haemophilus influenzae* type B infection

Usual Dosage I.V. infusion dose is the same as for the oral route

Tuberculosis: Oral:

Children: 10-20 mg/kg/day in divided doses every 12-24 hours

Adults: 10 mg/kg/day; maximum: 600 mg/day

American Thoracic Society and CDC currently recommend twice weekly therapy as part of a short-course regimen which follows 1-2 months of daily treatment of uncomplicated pulmonary tuberculosis in the compliant patient

Children: 10-20 mg/kg/dose (up to 600 mg) twice weekly under supervision to ensure compliance

Adults: 10 mg/kg (up to 600 mg) twice weekly

H. influenza prophylaxis:

Infants and Children: 20 mg/kg/day every 24 hours for 4 days

Adults: 600 mg every 24 hours for 4 days

Meningococcal prophylaxis:

<1 month: 10 mg/kg/day in divided doses every 12 hours

Infants and Children: 20 mg/kg/day in divided doses every 12 hours for 2 days

Adults: 600 mg every 12 hours for 2 days

Nasal carriers of *Staphylococcus aureus*: Adults: 600 mg/day for 5-10 days in combination with other antibiotics

Dosage Forms

Capsule: 150 mg, 300 mg

Powder for injection: 600 mg (contains a sulfite)

rifampin and isoniazid
Brand Names Rifamate®
Therapeutic Category Antibiotic, Miscellaneous; Antitubercular Agent
Use Management of active tuberculosis; see individual monographs for additional information
Dosage Forms Capsule: Rifampin 300 mg and isoniazid 150 mg

rifampin, isoniazid, and pyrazinamide
Brand Names Rifater®
Therapeutic Category Antibiotic, Miscellaneous; Antitubercular Agent
Use Management of active tuberculosis
Dosage Forms Tablet: Rifampin 120 mg, isoniazid 50 mg, and pyrazinamide 300 mg

Rifater® *see* rifampin, isoniazid, and pyrazinamide *on this page*

rifn-a *see* interferon alfa-2a *on page 247*

rig *see* rabies immune globulin, human *on page 404*

Rimactane® Oral *see* rifampin *on previous page*

rimantadine hydrochloride (ri man' to deen)
Brand Names Flumadine® Oral
Therapeutic Category Antiviral Agent, Oral
Use Prophylaxis (adults and children) and treatment (adults) of influenza A viral infection
Usual Dosage Oral:
Prophylaxis:
Children (<10 years of age): 5 mg/kg give once daily
Children (>10 years of age) and Adults: 100 mg twice/day

Treatment: Adults: 100 mg twice/day

In patients with severe hepatic dysfunction or renal function, and in elderly nursing home patients, the dosage should be reduced to 100 mg/day
Dosage Forms
Syrup: 50 mg/5 mL (60 mL, 240 mL, 480 mL)
Tablet: 100 mg

rimexolone
Brand Names Vexol®
Therapeutic Category Corticosteroid, Ophthalmic
Use Treatment of anterior uveitis and postoperative ophthalmic inflammation
Dosage Forms Solution, ophthalmic: 1%

Rimso®-50 *see* dimethyl sulfoxide *on page 148*

Riobin® *see* riboflavin *on page 410*

Riopan Plus® [OTC] *see* magaldrate and simethicone *on page 276*

Riopan® [OTC] *see* magaldrate *on page 276*

Risperdal® Oral *see* risperidone *on this page*

risperidone (ris per' i done)
Brand Names Risperdal® Oral
Therapeutic Category Antipsychotic Agent
Use Management of psychotic disorders (eg, schizophrenia)
Usual Dosage
Recommended starting dose: 1 mg twice daily; slowly increase to the optimum range of 4-8 mg/day; daily dosages >10 mg does not appear to confer any additional benefit, and the incidence of extrapyramidal reactions is higher than with lower doses

Dosing adjustment in renal, hepatic impairment, and elderly: Starting dose of 0.5 mg twice daily is advisable
Dosage Forms Tablet: 1 mg, 2 mg, 3 mg, 4 mg

Ritalin® *see* methylphenidate hydrochloride *on page 300*

Ritalin-SR® *see* methylphenidate hydrochloride *on page 300*

ritodrine hydrochloride (ri' toe dreen)
Brand Names Pre-Par®; Yutopar®
Therapeutic Category Adrenergic Agonist Agent; Beta-2-Adrenergic Agonist Agent; Tocolytic Agent
Use Inhibit uterine contraction in preterm labor
Usual Dosage Adults:
Oral: Start 30 minutes before stopping I.V. infusion; 10 mg every 2 hours for 24 hours, then 10-20 mg every 4-6 hours up to 120 mg/day. Continue treatment as long as it is desirable to prolong pregnancy.
I.V.: 50-100 mcg/minute; increase by 50 mcg/minute every 10 minutes; continue for 12 hours after contractions have stopped
Dosage Forms
Injection: 10 mg/mL (5 mL); 15 mg/mL (10 mL)
Tablet: 10 mg

rlfn-α2 *see* interferon alfa-2b *on page 247*

rlfn-b *see* interferon beta-1b *on page 247*

RMS® Rectal *see* morphine sulfate *on page 311*

Robafen® CF [OTC] *see* guaifenesin, phenylpropanolamine, and dextromethorphan *on page 217*

Robaxin® *see* methocarbamol *on page 295*

Robaxisal® *see* methocarbamol and aspirin *on page 295*

Robicillin® VK Oral *see* penicillin v potassium *on page 354*

Robinul® *see* glycopyrrolate *on page 210*

Robinul® Forte *see* glycopyrrolate *on page 210*

Robitet® Oral *see* tetracycline *on page 451*

Robitussin® A-C *see* guaifenesin and codeine *on page 214*

Robitussin-CF® [OTC] *see* guaifenesin, phenylpropanolamine, and dextromethorphan *on page 217*

Robitussin®-DAC *see* guaifenesin, pseudoephedrine, and codeine *on page 217*

Robitussin®-DM [OTC] *see* guaifenesin and dextromethorphan *on page 214*

Robitussin-PE® [OTC] *see* guaifenesin and pseudoephedrine *on page 216*

Robitussin® Cough Calmers [OTC] *see* dextromethorphan hydrobromide *on page 135*

Robitussin® Pediatric [OTC] *see* dextromethorphan hydrobromide *on page 135*

Robitussin® [OTC] *see* guaifenesin *on page 213*

Robitussin® Severe Congestion Liqui-Gels [OTC] *see* guaifenesin and pseudoephedrine *on page 216*

Robomol® *see* methocarbamol *on page 295*

Rocaltrol® *see* calcitriol *on page 65*

Rocephin® *see* ceftriaxone sodium *on page 83*

rocky mountain spotted fever vaccine
Therapeutic Category Vaccine, Live Bacteria
Dosage Forms Injection: 3 mL

rocuronium bromide

Brand Names Zemuron®

Therapeutic Category Neuromuscular Blocker Agent, Nondepolarizing

Use Inpatient and outpatient use as an adjunct to general anesthesia to facilitate both rapid-sequence and routine tracheal intubation, and to provide skeletal muscle relaxation during surgery or mechanical ventilation

Usual Dosage

Children:

Initial: 0.6 mg/kg under halothane anesthesia produce excellent to good intubating conditions within 1 minute and will provide a median time of 41 minutes of clinical relaxation in children 3 months to 1 year of age, and 27 minutes in children 1-12 years

Maintenance: 0.075-0.125 mg/kg administered upon return of T_1 to 25% of control provides clinical relaxation for 7-10 minutes

Adults:

Tracheal intubation: I.V.:

Initial: 0.6 mg/kg is expected to provide approximately 31 minutes of clinical relaxation under opioid/nitrous oxide/oxygen anesthesia with neuromuscular block sufficient for intubation attained in 1-2 minutes; lower doses (0.45 mg/kg) may be used to provide 22 minutes of clinical relaxation with median time to neuromuscular block of 1-3 minutes; maximum blockade is achieved in <4 minutes

Maximum: 0.9-1.2 mg/kg may be given during surgery under opioid/nitrous oxide/oxygen anesthesia without adverse cardiovascular effects and is expected to provide 58-67 minutes of clinical relaxation; neuromuscular blockade sufficient for intubation is achieved in <2 minutes with maximum blockade in <3 minutes

Maintenance: 0.1, 0.15, and 0.2 mg/kg administered at 25% recovery of control T_1 (defined as 3 twitches of train-of-four) provides a median of 12, 17, and 24 minutes of clinical duration under anesthesia

Rapid sequence intubation: 0.6-1.2 mg/kg in appropriately premedicated and anesthetized patients with excellent or good intubating conditions within 2 minutes

Continuous infusion: Initial: 0.01-0.012 mg/kg/minute only after early evidence of spontaneous recovery of neuromuscular function is evident

Dosage Forms Injection: 10 mg/mL

Roferon-A® *see* interferon alfa-2a *on page 247*

Rogaine® *see* minoxidil *on page 308*

Rolaids® Calcium Rich [OTC] *see* calcium carbonate *on page 66*

Rolaids® [OTC] *see* dihydroxyaluminum sodium carbonate *on page 146*

Romazicon™ Injection *see* flumazenil *on page 195*

Romycin® *see* erythromycin, topical *on page 172*

Ronase® *see* tolazamide *on page 463*

Rondamine-DM® Drops *see* carbinoxamine, pseudoephedrine, and dextromethorphan *on page 75*

Rondec®-DM *see* carbinoxamine, pseudoephedrine, and dextromethorphan *on page 75*

Rondec® Drops *see* carbinoxamine and pseudoephedrine *on page 75*

Rondec® Filmtab® *see* carbinoxamine and pseudoephedrine *on page 75*

Rondec® Syrup *see* carbinoxamine and pseudoephedrine *on page 75*

Rondec-TR® *see* carbinoxamine and pseudoephedrine *on page 75*

Rotalex® *see* diagnostic aids (*in vitro*), feces *on page 137*

Rowasa® Rectal *see* mesalamine *on page 289*

Roxanol™ Oral *see* morphine sulfate *on page 311*

Roxanol SR™ Oral *see* morphine sulfate *on page 311*

Roxicet® 5/500 *see* oxycodone and acetaminophen *on page 342*

Roxicodone™ *see* oxycodone hydrochloride *on page 343*

Roxilox® *see* oxycodone and acetaminophen *on page 342*

Roxiprin® *see* oxycodone and aspirin *on page 343*

rtca *see* ribavirin *on page 410*

Rubacell® II *see* diagnostic aids (*in vitro*), blood *on page 136*

Rubazyme® *see* diagnostic aids (*in vitro*), blood *on page 136*

rubella and measles vaccines, combined *see* measles and rubella vaccines, combined *on page 281*

rubella and mumps vaccines, combined
Brand Names Biavax®_{II}
Therapeutic Category Vaccine, Live Virus
Use Promote active immunity to rubella and mumps by inducing production of antibodies
Usual Dosage Children >12 months and Adults: 1 vial in outer aspect of the upper arm
Dosage Forms Injection (mixture of 2 viruses):
  1. Wistar RA 27/3 strain of rubella virus
  2. Jeryl Lynn (B level) mumps strain grown cell cultures of chick embryo

rubella virus vaccine, live
Brand Names Meruvax® II
Synonyms german measles vaccine
Therapeutic Category Vaccine, Live Virus
Use Provide vaccine-induced immunity to rubella
Usual Dosage S.C.: 1000 $TCID_{50}$ of rubella
Dosage Forms Injection, single dose: 1000 $TCID_{50}$ (Wistar RA 27/3 Strain)

rubeola vaccine *see* measles virus vaccine, live, attenuated *on page 281*

Rubex® *see* doxorubicin hydrochloride *on page 157*

rubidomycin hydrochloride *see* daunorubicin hydrochloride *on page 126*

Rubramin-PC® *see* cyanocobalamin *on page 119*

Rufen® *see* ibuprofen *on page 240*

Rum-K® *see* potassium chloride *on page 378*

Ru-Tuss® DE *see* guaifenesin and pseudoephedrine *on page 216*

Ru-Tuss II® *see* chlorpheniramine and phenylpropanolamine *on page 94*

Ru-Tuss® Liquid *see* chlorpheniramine and phenylephrine *on page 93*

Ru-Vert-M® *see* meclizine hydrochloride *on page 282*

Rymed® *see* guaifenesin and pseudoephedrine *on page 216*

Rymed-TR® *see* guaifenesin and phenylpropanolamine *on page 215*

Ryna-C® Liquid *see* chlorpheniramine, pseudoephedrine, and codeine *on page 97*

Ryna-CX® *see* guaifenesin, pseudoephedrine, and codeine *on page 217*

Rynatan® Pediatric Suspension *see* chlorpheniramine, pyrilamine, and phenylephrine *on page 97*

Rynatuss® Pediatric Suspension *see* chlorpheniramine, ephedrine, phenylephrine, and carbetapentane *on page 94*

Rythmol® *see* propafenone hydrochloride *on page 392*

Sabin vaccine *see* poliovirus vaccine, live (trivalent, oral) *on page 374*

Salacid® Ointment *see* salicylic acid *on next page*

Sal-Acid® Plaster *see* salicylic acid *on next page*

Salagen® Oral *see* pilocarpine *on page 369*

salbutamol *see* albuterol *on page 10*

Saleto-200® [OTC] *see* ibuprofen *on page 240*

Saleto-400® *see* ibuprofen *on page 240*

Salflex® *see* salsalate *on next page*

Salgesic® *see* salsalate *on next page*

salicylazosulfapyridine *see* sulfasalazine *on page 441*

salicylic acid

Brand Names Clear Away™ Disc [OTC]; Freezone® Solution [OTC]; Gordofilm® Liquid; Mediplast™ Plaster [OTC]; Occlusal-HP Liquid; Panscol® Lotion [OTC]; Panscol® Ointment [OTC]; PediaPatch Transdermal Patch [OTC]; P&S™ Shampoo [OTC]; Salacid® Ointment; Sal-Acid® Plaster; Trans-Plantar™ Transdermal Patch [OTC]; Trans-Ver-Sal® Transdermal Patch [OTC] Verukan™ Solution; Vergogel™ Gel [OTC]

Therapeutic Category Keratolytic Agent

Use Topically for its keratolytic effect in controlling seborrheic dermatitis or psoriasis of body and scalp, dandruff, and other scaling dermatoses; also used to remove warts, corns and calluses

Usual Dosage

Shampoo: Apply to scalp and allow to remain for a few minutes, then rinse, initially use every day or every other day; 2 treatments/week are usually sufficient to maintain control

Topical: Apply to affected area and place under occlusion at night; hydrate skin for at least 5 minutes before use

Dosage Forms

Cream: 2% (30 g); 2.5% (30 g); 10% (60 g)

Gel: 5% (60 g); 6% (30 g); 17% (7.5 g)

Liquid: 13.6% (9.3 mL); 17% (9.3 mL, 13.5 mL, 15 mL); 16.7% (15 mL)

Lotion: 2% (177 mL)

Ointment: 25% (60 g, 454 g); 40% (454 g); 60% (60 g)

Patch, transdermal: 15% (20 mm)

Plaster: 15% (6 mm, 12 mm); 40%

Pledgets: 0.5%; 2%

Shampoo: 2% (120 mL, 240 mL); 4% (120 mL)

salicylic acid and benzoic acid *see* benzoic acid and salicylic acid *on page 49*

salicylic acid and lactic acid

Brand Names Duofilm™ Solution

Synonyms lactic acid and salicylic acid

Therapeutic Category Keratolytic Agent

Use Treatment of benign epithelial tumors such as warts

Usual Dosage Topical: Apply a thin layer directly to wart once daily (may be useful to apply at bedtime and wash off in morning)

Dosage Forms Solution, topical: Salicylic acid 16.7% and lactic acid 16.7% in flexible collodion (15 mL)

salicylic acid and podophyllin *see* podophyllin and salicylic acid *on page 374*

salicylic acid and propylene glycol

Brand Names Keralyt™ Gel

Synonyms propylene glycol and salicylic acid

Therapeutic Category Keratolytic Agent

Use Removal of excessive keratin in hyperkeratotic skin disorders, including various ichthyosis, keratosis palmaris and plantaris and psoriasis; may be used to remove excessive keratin in dorsal and plantar hyperkeratotic lesions

Usual Dosage Apply to area at night after soaking region for at least 5 minutes to hydrate area, and place under occlusion; medication is washed off in morning

Dosage Forms Gel, topical: Salicylic acid 6% and propylene glycol 60% in ethyl alcohol 19.4% with hydroxypropyl methylcellulose and water (30 g)

salicylic acid and sulfur *see* sulfur and salicylic acid *on page 442*

Salivart® [OTC] *see* saliva substitute *on this page*

saliva substitute
Brand Names Moi-Stir® [OTC]; Orex® [OTC]; Salivart® [OTC]; Xero-Lube® [OTC]
Therapeutic Category Gastrointestinal Agent, Miscellaneous
Use Relief of dry mouth and throat in xerostomia
Usual Dosage Use as needed
Dosage Forms
Solution: 60 mL, 75 mL, 120 mL, 180 mL
Swabstix: 300s

Salk vaccine *see* poliovirus vaccine, inactivated *on page 374*

salmeterol xinafoate (sal me' te role)
Brand Names Serevent®
Therapeutic Category Adrenergic Agonist Agent; Beta-2-Adrenergic Agonist Agent; Bronchodilator
Use Maintenance treatment of asthma and in prevention of bronchospasm in patients > 12 years of age with reversible obstructive airway disease, including patients with symptoms of nocturnal asthma, who require regular treatment with inhaled, short-acting beta$_2$-agonists; prevention of exercise-induced bronchospasm
Usual Dosage
Inhalation: 42 mcg (2 puffs) twice daily (12 hours apart) for maintenance and prevention of symptoms of asthma

Prevention of exercise-induced asthma: 42 mcg (2 puffs) 30-60 minutes prior to exercise; additional doses should not be used for 12 hours
Dosage Forms Aerosol, oral: 21 mcg/spray [60 inhalations] (6.5 g), [120 inhalations] (13 g)

salsalate (sal' sa late)
Brand Names Argesic®-SA; Artha-G®; Disalcid"; Marthritic"; Mono-Gesic"; Salflex"; Salgesic®; Salsitab®
Synonyms disalicylic acid
Therapeutic Category Analgesic, Non-Narcotic; Anti-inflammatory Agent; Antipyretic; Nonsteroidal Anti-Inflammatory Agent (NSAID), Oral; Salicylate
Use Treatment of minor pain or fever; rheumatoid arthritis, osteoarthritis, and related inflammatory conditions
Usual Dosage Adults: Oral: 1 g 2-4 times/day
Dosage Forms
Capsule: 500 mg
Tablet: 500 mg, 750 mg

Salsitab® *see* salsalate *on this page*

salt *see* sodium chloride *on page 426*

Saluron® *see* hydroflumethiazide *on page 234*

Salutensin® *see* hydroflumethiazide and reserpine *on page 234*

Salutensin-Demi® *see* hydroflumethiazide and reserpine *on page 234*

Sandimmune® Injection *see* cyclosporine *on page 121*

Sandimmune® Oral *see* cyclosporine *on page 121*

Sandoglobulin® *see* immune globulin, intravenous *on page 243*

Sandostatin® *see* octreotide acetate *on page 335*

Sani-Supp® Suppository [OTC] *see* glycerin *on page 210*

Sansert® *see* methysergide maleate *on page 301*

Santyl® *see* collagenase *on page 114*

sargramostim (sar gram' oh stim)

Brand Names Leukine™

Synonyms gm-csf; granulocyte-macrophage colony stimulating factor; rgm-csf

Therapeutic Category Colony Stimulating Factor

Use Myeloid reconstitution after autologous bone marrow transplantation; to accelerate myeloid recovery in patients with non-Hodgkin's lymphoma, acute lymphoblastic leukemia, and Hodgkin's lymphoma undergoing autologous BMT; to accelerate myeloid engraftment following chemotherapy

Usual Dosage

Children and Adults (may also administer S.C.):

Bone marrow transplant: I.V.: 250 mcg/m^2/day over at least 2 hours to begin 2-4 hours after the marrow infusion on day 0 of autologous bone marrow transplant or not <24 hours after chemotherapy or 12 hours after last dose of radiotherapy. If significant adverse effects or "first dose" reaction is seen at this dose, discontinue the drug until toxicity resolves, then restart at a reduced dose of 125 mcg/m^2/day

Cancer chemotherapy recovery: I.V.: 3-15 mcg/kg/day over at least 2 hours for 14-21 days; maximum daily dose is 15 mcg/kg/day due to dose-related adverse effects

Discontinue therapy if the ANC count is >20,000/mm^3.

Excessive blood counts return to normal or baseline levels within 3-7 days following cessation of therapy.

Length of therapy: Bone marrow transplant patients: GM-CSF should be administered daily for up to 30 days or until the ANC has reached 1000/mm^3 for 3 consecutive days following the expected chemotherapy-induced neutrophil-nadir.

Dosage Forms Injection: 250 mcg, 500 mcg

Sarna [OTC] *see* camphor, menthol and phenol *on page 71*

Sastid® Plain Therapeutic Shampoo and Acne Wash [OTC] *see* sulfur and salicylic acid *on page 442*

Scabene® Lotion *see* lindane *on page 269*

Scabene® Shampoo *see* lindane *on page 269*

Scalpicin® *see* hydrocortisone *on page 232*

Scleromate® *see* morrhuate sodium *on page 312*

scopolamine (skoe pol' a meen)

Brand Names Isopto® Hyoscine Ophthalmic; Transderm Scop® Patch

Synonyms hyoscine

Therapeutic Category Anticholinergic Agent; Anticholinergic Agent, Ophthalmic; Anticholinergic Agent, Transdermal; Ophthalmic Agent, Mydriatic

Use Preoperative medication to produce amnesia and decrease salivation and respiratory secretions to produce cycloplegia and mydriasis; treatment of iridocyclitis, prevention of nausea and vomiting by motion

Usual Dosage

Preoperatively:

Children: I.M., S.C.: 6 mcg/kg/dose (maximum: 0.3 mg/dose) or 0.2 mg/m^2 may be repeated every 6-8 hours **or** alternatively:

4-7 months: 0.1 mg

7 months to 3 years: 0.15 mg

3-8 years: 0.2 mg
8-12 years: 0.3 mg
Adults: I.M., I.V., S.C.: 0.3-0.65 mg; may be repeated every 4-6 hours

Motion sickness: Transdermal: Children >12 years and Adults: Apply 1 disc behind the ear at least 4 hours prior to exposure and every 3 days as needed

Ophthalmic:
  Refraction:
    Children: Instill 1 drop of 0.25% to eye(s) twice daily for 2 days before procedure
    Adults: Instill 1-2 drops of 0.25% to eye(s) 1 hour before procedure
  Iridocyclitis:
    Children: Instill 1 drop of 0.25% to eye(s) up to 3 times/day
    Adults: Instill 1-2 drops of 0.25% to eye(s) up to 4 times/day

Dosage Forms
Disc, transdermal: 1.5 mg/disc (4s)
Injection, as hydrobromide: 0.3 mg/mL (1 mL); 0.4 mg/mL (0.5 mL, 1 mL); 0.86 mg/mL (0.5 mL); 1 mg/mL (1 mL)
Solution, ophthalmic, as hydrobromide: 0.25% (5 mL, 15 mL)

scopolamine and phenylephrine *see* phenylephrine and scopolamine *on page 364*

Scot-Tussin DM® Cough Chasers [OTC] *see* dextromethorphan hydrobromide *on page 135*

Scot-Tussin® [OTC] *see* guaifenesin *on page 213*

Sebulex® [OTC] *see* sulfur and salicylic acid *on page 442*

Sebulon® [OTC] *see* pyrithione zinc *on page 401*

secobarbital and amobarbital *see* amobarbital and secobarbital *on page 23*

secobarbital sodium (see koe bar' bi tal)
Brand Names Seconal™ Injection
Synonyms quinalbarbitone sodium
Therapeutic Category Barbiturate; Hypnotic; Sedative
Use Short-term treatment of insomnia and as preanesthetic agent
Usual Dosage
Children: Hypnotic: I.M.: 3-5 mg/kg/dose; maximum: 100 mg/dose

Adults:
  Hypnotic:
    I.M.: 100-200 mg/dose
    I.V.: 50-250 mg/dose
Dosage Forms Injection: 50 mg/mL (2 mL)

Seconal™ Injection *see* secobarbital sodium *on this page*

Secran® *see* vitamin, multiple (prenatal) *on page 491*

secretin (see' cre tin)
Brand Names Secretin-Ferring Injection
Therapeutic Category Diagnostic Agent, Pancreatic Exocrine Insufficiency; Diagnostic Agent, Zollinger-Ellison Syndrome and Pancreatic Exocrine Disease
Use Diagnosis of Zollinger-Ellison syndrome and pancreatic exocrine disease, and some hepatobiliary disease such as obstructive jaundice
Usual Dosage I.V.:
Pancreatic function: 1 CU/kg slow I.V. injection over 1 minute
Zollinger-Ellison: 2 CU/kg slow I.V. injection over 1 minute
Dosage Forms Powder for injection: 75 units (10 mL)

Secretin-Ferring Injection *see* secretin *on previous page*
Sectral® *see* acebutolol hydrochloride *on page 2*
Sedapap-10® *see* butalbital compound *on page 63*
Seldane® *see* terfenadine *on page 447*
Seldane-D® *see* terfenadine and pseudoephedrine *on page 448*

selegiline hydrochloride (seh ledge' ah leen)
  Brand Names Eldepryl™
  Synonyms deprenyl; l-deprenyl
  Therapeutic Category Anti-Parkinson's Agent
  Use Adjunct in the management of Parkinsonian patients in which levodopa/carbidopa
  therapy is deteriorating. Unlabeled uses: Early Parkinson's disease; Alzheimer's disease
  Usual Dosage Adults: Oral: 5 mg twice daily
  Dosage Forms Tablet: 5 mg

selenium (se lee' nee um)
  Brand Names Selepen™
  Therapeutic Category Trace Element, Parenteral
  Use Trace metal supplement
  Usual Dosage I.V. in TPN solutions:
    Children: 3 mcg/kg/day
    Adults:
        Metabolically stable: 20-40 mcg/day
        Deficiency from prolonged TPN support: 100 mcg/day for 24 and 21 days
  Dosage Forms Injection: 40 mcg/mL (10 mL, 30 mL)

selenium sulfide (se lee' nee um)
  Brand Names Exsel™; Selsun™; Selsun Blue™ [OTC]; Selsun Gold® for Women [OTC]
  Therapeutic Category Shampoos
  Use Treat itching and flaking of the scalp associated with dandruff, to control scalp seborrheic
  dermatitis; treatment of tinea versicolor
  Usual Dosage Topical:
    Dandruff, seborrhea: Massage 5-10 mL into wet scalp, leave on scalp 2-3 minutes, rinse thor-
    oughly and repeat application; shampoo twice weekly for 2 weeks initially, then use once
    every 1-4 weeks as indicated depending upon control

    Tinea versicolor: Apply the 2.5% lotion to affected area and lather with small amounts of
    water; leave on skin for 10 minutes, then rinse thoroughly; apply every day for 7 days
  Dosage Forms Shampoo: 1% (120 mL, 210 mL, 240 mL, 330 mL); 2.5% (120 mL)

Selepen® *see* selenium *on this page*
Selestoject® *see* betamethasone *on page 52*
Selsun® *see* selenium sulfide *on this page*
Selsun Blue® **[OTC]** *see* selenium sulfide *on this page*
Selsun Gold® **for Women [OTC]** *see* selenium sulfide *on this page*
Semicid® **[OTC]** *see* nonoxynol 9 *on page 331*

senna
  Brand Names Black Draught™ [OTC]; Senna-Gen™ [OTC]; Senokot® [OTC]; Senolax® [OTC];
  X-Prep™ Liquid [OTC]
  Therapeutic Category Laxative, Stimulant
  Use Short-term treatment of constipation; evacuate the colon for bowel or rectal examinations

Usual Dosage

Children:

Oral:

>6 years: 10-20 mg/kg/dose at bedtime; maximum daily dose: 872 mg

6-12 years, >27 kg: 1 tablet at bedtime, up to 4 tablets/day **or** $^1/_2$ teaspoonful of granules (326 mg/tsp) at bedtime (up to 2 teaspoonfuls/day)

Liquid:

2-5 years: 5-10 mL at bedtime

6-15 years: 10-15 mL at bedtime

Suppository: $^1/_2$ at bedtime

Syrup:

1 month to 1 year: 1.25-2.5 mL at bedtime up to 5 mL/day

1-5 years: 2.5-5 mL at bedtime up to 10 mL/day

5-10 years: 5-10 mL at bedtime up to 20 mL/day

Adults:

Granules (326 mg/teaspoon): 1 teaspoonful at bedtime, not to exceed 2 teaspoonfuls twice daily

Liquid: 15-30 mL with meals and at bedtime

Suppository: 1 at bedtime, may repeat once in 2 hours

Syrup: 2-3 teaspoonfuls at bedtime, not to exceed 30 mL/day

Tablet: 187 mg: 2 tablets at bedtime, not to exceed 8 tablets/day

Tablet: 374 mg: 1 at bedtime, up to 4/day; 600 mg: 2 tablets at bedtime, up to 3 tablets/day

Dosage Forms

Granules: 326 mg/teaspoonful

Liquid: 7% [70 mg/mL] (130 mL, 360 mL); 6.5% [65 mg/mL] (75 mL, 150 mL)

Suppository, rectal: 652 mg

Syrup: 218 mg/5 mL (60 mL, 240 mL)

Tablet: 187 mg, 217 mg, 600 mg

Senna-Gen® [OTC] *see* senna *on previous page*

Senokot® [OTC] *see* senna *on previous page*

Senolax® [OTC] *see* senna *on previous page*

Sensorcaine® *see* bupivacaine hydrochloride *on page 61*

Sensorcaine-MPF® *see* bupivacaine hydrochloride *on page 61*

Septa® Ointment [OTC] *see* bacitracin, neomycin, and polymyxin b *on page 43*

Septisol® *see* hexachlorophene *on page 224*

Septra® *see* co-trimoxazole *on page 117*

Septra® DS *see* co-trimoxazole *on page 117*

Ser-A-Gen® *see* hydralazine, hydrochlorothiazide, and reserpine *on page 228*

Ser-Ap-Es® *see* hydralazine, hydrochlorothiazide, and reserpine *on page 228*

Serathide® *see* hydralazine, hydrochlorothiazide, and reserpine *on page 228*

Serax® *see* oxazepam *on page 341*

Serentil® *see* mesoridazine besylate *on page 289*

Serevent® *see* salmeterol xinafoate *on page 417*

sermorelin acetate (ser moe rel' in)

Brand Names Geref® Injection

Therapeutic Category Diagnostic Agent, Pituitary Function

Use Evaluate ability of the somatotroph of the pituitary gland to secrete growth hormone

Dosage Forms Powder for injection, lyophilized: 50 mcg

Seromycin® Pulvules® *see* cycloserine *on page 121*

Serophene® *see* clomiphene citrate *on page 107*

Serpalan® *see* reserpine *on page 409*

sertraline hydrochloride (ser' tra leen)
Brand Names Zoloft™
Therapeutic Category Antidepressant; Serotonin Antagonist
Use Treatment of major depression; also being studied for use in obesity and obsessive-compulsive disorder
Usual Dosage Oral: Initial: 50 mg/day as a single dose, dosage may be increased at intervals of at least 1 week to a maximum recommended dosage of 200 mg/day
Dosage Forms Tablet: 50 mg, 100 mg

Serutan® [OTC] *see* psyllium *on page 398*

Serzone® *see* nefazodone *on page 321*

Shohl's solution *see* sodium citrate and citric acid *on page 427*

Shur-Seal® [OTC] *see* nonoxynol 9 *on page 331*

Siblin® [OTC] *see* psyllium *on page 398*

Sickledex™ *see* diagnostic aids (*in vitro*), blood *on page 136*

Silace-C® [OTC] *see* docusate and casanthranol *on page 154*

Silace® [OTC] *see* docusate *on page 153*

Silafed® [OTC] *see* triprolidine and pseudoephedrine *on page 474*

Silain® [OTC] *see* simethicone *on next page*

Silaminic® Expectorant [OTC] *see* guaifenesin and phenylpropanolamine *on page 215*

Sildicon-E® [OTC] *see* guaifenesin and phenylpropanolamine *on page 215*

Silphen DM® [OTC] *see* dextromethorphan hydrobromide *on page 135*

Silphen® Cough [OTC] *see* diphenhydramine hydrochloride *on page 149*

Siltussin-CF® [OTC] *see* guaifenesin, phenylpropanolamine, and dextromethorphan *on page 217*

Siltussin DM® [OTC] *see* guaifenesin and dextromethorphan *on page 214*

Siltussin® [OTC] *see* guaifenesin *on page 213*

Silvadene® *see* silver sulfadiazine *on next page*

silver nitrate
Brand Names Dey-Drop" Ophthalmic Solution
Synonyms AgNO₃
Therapeutic Category Topical Skin Product
Use Prevention of gonococcal ophthalmia neonatorum; cauterization of wounds and sluggish ulcers, removal of granulation tissue and warts; aseptic prophylaxis of burns
Usual Dosage
Neonates: Ophthalmic: Instill 2 drops immediately after birth into conjunctival sac of each eye as a single dose; do not irrigate eyes following instillation of eye drops
Children and Adults:
Sticks: Apply to mucous membranes and other moist skin surfaces only on area to be treated 2-3 times/week for 2-3 weeks
Topical solution: Apply a cotton applicator dipped in solution on the affected area 2-3 times/week for 2-3 weeks
Dosage Forms
Applicator, topical: 75% with potassium nitrate 25% (6")
Ointment, topical: 10% (30 g)
Solution:
Ophthalmic: 1% (wax ampuls)
Topical: 10% (30 mL); 25% (30 mL); 50% (30 mL)

silver protein, mild
Brand Names Argyrol® S.S. 20%
Therapeutic Category Antibiotic, Topical
Use Stain and coagulate mucus in eye surgery which is then removed by irrigation; eye infections
Usual Dosage
Preop in eye surgery: Place 2-3 drops into eye(s), then rinse out with sterile irrigating solution

Eye infections: 1-3 drops into the affected eye(s) every 3-4 hours for several days
Dosage Forms Solution, ophthalmic: 20% (15 mL, 30 mL)

silver sulfadiazine (sul fa dye' a zeen)
Brand Names Silvadene®; SSD® AF; SSD® Cream; Thermazene®
Therapeutic Category Antibacterial, Topical
Use Adjunct in the prevention and treatment of infection in second and third degree burns
Usual Dosage Children and Adults: Topical: Apply once or twice daily with a sterile gloved hand; apply to a thickness of $^1/_{16}$"; burned area should be covered with cream at all times
Dosage Forms Cream, topical: 1% [10 mg/g] (20 g, 50 g, 100 g, 400 g, 1000 g)

simethicone (sye meth' i kone)
Brand Names Flatulex [OTC]; Gas-X® [OTC]; Maalox Anti-Gas® [OTC]; Mylanta Gas® [OTC]; Mylicon® [OTC]; Phazyme® [OTC]; Silain® [OTC]
Synonyms activated dimethicone; activated methylpolysiloxane
Therapeutic Category Antiflatulent
Use Relieve flatulence and functional gastric bloating, and postoperative gas pains
Usual Dosage Oral:
Infants: 20 mg 4 times/day

Children <12 years: 40 mg 4 times/day

Children >12 years and Adults: 40-120 mg after meals and at bedtime as needed, not to exceed 500 mg/day
Dosage Forms
Capsule: 125 mg
Drops, oral: 40 mg/0.6 mL (30 mL)
Tablet: 50 mg, 60 mg, 95 mg
Tablet, chewable: 40 mg, 80 mg, 125 mg

simethicone and calcium carbonate *see* calcium carbonate and simethicone *on page 67*

simethicone and magaldrate *see* magaldrate and simethicone *on page 276*

Simron® [OTC] *see* ferrous gluconate *on page 189*

simvastatin (sim' va stat in)
Brand Names Zocor™
Therapeutic Category Antilipemic Agent; HMG-CoA Reductase Inhibitor
Use Adjunct to dietary therapy to decrease elevated serum total and LDL cholesterol concentrations in primary hypercholesterolemia
Usual Dosage Adults: Oral: 20-40 mg once or twice daily
Dosage Forms Tablet: 5 mg, 10 mg, 20 mg, 40 mg

Sinarest® 12 Hour Nasal Solution *see* oxymetazoline hydrochloride *on page 343*

Sinarest® Nasal Solution [OTC] *see* phenylephrine hydrochloride *on page 364*

sincalide (sin' ka lide)
Brand Names Kinevac®
Synonyms c8-cck; op-cck
Therapeutic Category Diagnostic Agent, Gallbladder Function
(Continued)

sincalide *(Continued)*

Use Postevacuation cholecystography; gallbladder bile sampling; stimulate pancreatic secretion for analysis

Usual Dosage Adults: I.V.:

Contraction of gallbladder: 0.02 mcg/kg over 30 seconds to 1 minute, may repeat in 15 minutes a 0.04 mcg/kg dose

Pancreatic function: 0.02 mcg/kg over 30 minutes

Dosage Forms Injection: 5 mcg

Sine-Aid® IB [OTC] *see* pseudoephedrine and ibuprofen *on page 398*

Sinemet® *see* levodopa and carbidopa *on page 265*

Sinequan® Oral *see* doxepin hydrochloride *on page 157*

Sinografin® *see* radiological/contrast media (ionic) *on page 404*

Sinubid® *see* phenyltoloxamine, phenylpropanolamine, and acetaminophen *on page 366*

Sinufed® Timecelles® *see* guaifenesin and pseudoephedrine *on page 216*

Sinumist®-SR Capsulets® [OTC] *see* guaifenesin *on page 213*

Sinusol-B® Injection *see* brompheniramine maleate *on page 59*

Sinutab® Tablets [OTC] *see* acetaminophen, chlorpheniramine, and pseudoephedrine *on page 4*

sk *see* streptokinase *on page 436*

Skelaxin® *see* metaxalone *on page 291*

skin test antigens, multiple

Brand Names Multitest CMI"

Therapeutic Category Diagnostic Agent, Skin Test

Use Detection of nonresponsiveness to antigens by means of delayed hypersensitivity skin testing

Usual Dosage Select only test sites that permit sufficient surface area and subcutaneous tissue to allow adequate penetration of all 8 points, avoid hairy areas

Press loaded unit into the skin with sufficient pressure to puncture the skin and allow adequate penetration of all points, maintain firm contact for at least five seconds, during application the device should not be "rocked" back and forth and side to side without removing any of the test heads from the skin sites

If adequate pressure is applied it will be possible to observe:
1. The puncture marks of the nine tines on each of the eight test heads
2. An imprint of the circular platform surrounding each test head
3. Residual antigen and glycerin at each of the eight sites

If any of the above three criteria are not fully followed, the test results may not be reliable

Reading should be done in good light, read the test sites at both 24 and 48 hours, the largest reaction recorded from the two readings at each test site should be used; if two readings are not possible, a single 48 hour is recommended

A positive reaction from any of the seven delayed hypersensitivity skin test antigens is **induration of ≥2 mm** providing there is no induration at the negative control site; the size of the induration reactions with this test may be smaller than those obtained with other intradermal procedures

Dosage Forms Individual carton containing one preloaded skin test antigen for cellular hypersensitivity

Sleep-eze 3® Oral [OTC] *see* diphenhydramine hydrochloride *on page 149*

Sleepinal® [OTC] *see* diphenhydramine hydrochloride *on page 149*

Slo-bid™ *see* theophylline *on page 453*

Slo-Niacin® [OTC] *see* niacin *on page 326*

Slo-Phyllin® *see* theophylline *on page 453*
Slo-Phyllin GG® *see* theophylline and guaifenesin *on page 454*
Slow FE® [OTC] *see* ferrous sulfate *on page 189*
Slow-K® *see* potassium chloride *on page 378*
Slow-Mag® [OTC] *see* magnesium chloride *on page 276*

smallpox vaccine
Therapeutic Category Vaccine, Inactivated Virus
Use There are no indications for the use of smallpox vaccine in the general civilian population. Laboratory workers involved with Orthopoxvirus or in the production and testing of smallpox vaccines should receive regular smallpox vaccinations. For advice on vaccine administration and contraindications, contact the Division of Immunization, CDC, Atlanta, GA 30333 (404-639-3356).

snake (pit vipers) antivenin *see* antivenin polyvalent (*Crotalidae*) *on page 31*
Snaplets-EX® [OTC] *see* guaifenesin and phenylpropanolamine *on page 215*
Snaplets-FR® Granules [OTC] *see* acetaminophen *on page 2*
sodium 2-mercaptoethane sulfonate *see* mesna *on page 289*

sodium acetate
Therapeutic Category Alkalinizing Agent, Parenteral; Electrolyte Supplement, Parenteral; Sodium Salt
Use Sodium source in large volume I.V. fluids to prevent or correct hyponatremia in patients with restricted intake; used to counter acidosis
Usual Dosage Sodium acetate is metabolized to bicarbonate on an equimolar basis outside the liver; administer in large volume I.V. fluids as a sodium source. Refer to sodium bicarbonate monograph.

Maintenance electrolyte requirements of sodium in parenteral nutrition solutions:
    Daily requirements: 3-4 mEq/kg/24 hours or 25-40 mEq/1000 kcal/24 hours
    Maximum: 100-150 mEq/24 hours
Dosage Forms Injection: 2 mEq/mL (20 mL, 50 mL); 4 mEq/mL (50 mL)

sodium acid carbonate *see* sodium bicarbonate *on next page*

sodium ascorbate
Brand Names Cenolate®
Therapeutic Category Urinary Acidifying Agent; Vitamin, Water Soluble
Use Prevention and treatment of scurvy and to acidify the urine; large doses may decrease the severity of "colds"
Usual Dosage Oral, I.V.:
Children:
    Scurvy: 100-300 mg/day in divided doses for at least 2 weeks
    Urinary acidification: 500 mg every 6-8 hours
    Dietary supplement: 35-45 mg/day

Adults:
    Scurvy: 100-250 mg 1-2 times/day for at least 2 weeks
    Urinary acidification: 4-12 g/day in divided doses
    Dietary supplement: 50-60 mg/day
    Prevention and treatment of cold: 1-3 g/day
Dosage Forms
    Crystals: 1020 mg per $1/4$ teaspoonful [ascorbic acid 900 mg]
    Injection: 250 mg/mL [ascorbic acid 222 mg/mL] (30 mL); 562.5 mg/mL [ascorbic acid 500 mg/mL] (1 mL, 2 mL)
    Tablet: 585 mg [ascorbic acid 500 mg]

sodium benzoate and caffeine *see* caffeine and sodium benzoate *on page 64*

sodium bicarbonate
Brand Names Neut® Injection
Synonyms baking soda; NaHCO₃; sodium acid carbonate; sodium hydrogen carbonate
Therapeutic Category Alkalinizing Agent Oral; Alkalinizing Agent, Parenteral; Antacid; Electrolyte Supplement, Oral; Electrolyte Supplement, Parenteral; Sodium Salt
Use Management of metabolic acidosis; antacid; alkalinize urine; severe diarrhea
Usual Dosage
Cardiac arrest (patient should be adequately ventilated before administering $NaHCO_3$):
Infants: Use 1:1 dilution of 1 mEq/mL $NaHCO_3$ or use 0.5 mEq/mL $NaHCO_3$ at a dose of 1 mEq/kg slow IVP initially; may repeat with 0.5 mEq/kg in 10 minutes one time or as indicated by the patient's acid-base status. Rate of administration should not exceed 10 mEq/minute.
Children and Adults: IVP: 1 mEq/kg initially; may repeat with 0.5 mEq/kg in 10 minutes one time or as indicated by the patient's acid-base status

Metabolic acidosis: Dosage should be based on the following formula if blood gases and pH measurements are available:
Infants and Children: HCO_3-(mEq) = 0.3 x weight (kg) x base deficit (mEq/L) **or** HCO_3-(mEq) = 0.5 x weight (kg) x (24 - serum HCO_3-) (mEq/L)

Adults: HCO_3-(mEq) = 0.2 x weight (kg) x base deficit (mEq/L) **or** HCO_3-(mEq) = 0.5 x weight (kg) x (24 - serum HCO_3-) (mEq/L)
If acid-base status is not available: Dose for older Children and Adults: 2-5 mEq/kg I.V. infusion over 4-8 hours; subsequent doses should be based on patient's acid-base status

Chronic renal failure: Oral: Children: 1-3 mEq/kg/day

Renal tubular acidosis: Oral:
Distal:
Children: 2-3 mEq/kg/day
Adults: 1 mEq/kg/day
Proximal: Children: Initial: 5-10 mEq/kg/day; maintenance: Increase as required to maintain serum bicarbonate in the normal range

Urine alkalinization: Oral:
Children: 1-10 mEq (84-840 mg)/kg/day in divided doses; dose should be titrated to desired urinary pH
Adults: 48 mEq (4 g) initially, then 12-24 mEq (1-2 g) every 4 hours; dose should be titrated to desired urinary pH; doses up to 16 g/day have been used
Dosage Forms
Injection: 4% [40 mg/mL = 2.4 mEq/5 mL] (5 mL); 4.2% [42 mg/mL = 5 mEq/10 mL] (10 mL); 7.5% [75 mg/mL = 8.92 mEq/10 mL] (10 mL, 50 mL); 8.4% [84 mg/mL = 10 mEq/10 mL] (10 mL, 50 mL)
Tablet: 300 mg [3.6 mEq]; 325 mg [3.8 mEq]; 520 mg [6.3 mEq]; 600 mg [7.3 mEq]; 650 mg [7.6 mEq]

sodium cellulose phosphate *see* cellulose sodium phosphate *on page 84*

sodium chloride
Brand Names Adsorbonac® Ophthalmic [OTC]; Ayr® Nasal [OTC]; Muro 128® Ophthalmic [OTC]; Ocean Nasal Mist [OTC]
Synonyms NaCl; normal saline; salt
Therapeutic Category Electrolyte Supplement, Oral; Electrolyte Supplement, Parenteral; Lubricant, Ocular; Sodium Salt
Use Prevention of muscle cramps and heat prostration; restoration of sodium ion in hyponatremia; induce abortion; restore moisture to nasal membranes; GU irrigant; reduction of corneal edema; source of electrolytes and water for expansion of the extracellular fluid compartment
Usual Dosage
Newborn electrolyte requirement:
Premature: 2-8 mEq/kg/24 hours

Term:
    0-48 hours: 0-2 mEq/kg/24 hours
    >48 hours: 1-4 mEq/kg/24 hours

Children: I.V.: Hypertonic solutions (>0.9%) should only be used for the initial treatment of acute serious symptomatic hyponatremia; maintenance: 3-4 mEq/kg/day; maximum: 100-150 mEq/day; dosage varies widely depending on clinical condition
    Replacement: Determined by laboratory determinations mEq
        Sodium deficiency (mEq/kg) = [% dehydration (L/kg)/100 x 70 (mEq/L) = [0.6 (L/kg) x (140 - serum sodium) (mEq/L)]
    Nasal: Use as often as needed

Adults:
    GI irrigant: 1-3 L/day by intermittent irrigation
    Heat cramps: Oral: 0.5-1 g with full glass of water, up to 4.8 g/day
    Replacement I.V.: Determined by laboratory determinations mEq
        Sodium deficiency (mEq/kg) = [% dehydration (L/kg)/100 x 70 (mEq/L)] + [0.6 (L/kg) x (140 - Serum sodium) (mEq/L)]

To correct acute, serious hyponatremia: mEq sodium = (desired sodium (mEq/L) - actual sodium (mEq/L) x 0.6 x wt (kg)); for acute correction use 125 mEq/L as the desired serum sodium; acutely correct serum sodium in 5 mEq/L/dose increments; more gradual correction in increments of 10 mEq/L/day is indicated in the asymptomatic patient
    Chloride maintenance electrolyte requirement in parenteral nutrition: 2-4 mEq/kg/24 hours or 25-40 mEq/1000 kcals/24 hours; maximum: 100-150 mEq/24 hours
    Sodium maintenance electrolyte requirement in parenteral nutrition: 3-4 mEq/kg/24 hours or 25-40 mEq/1000 kcals/24 hours; maximum: 100-150 mEq/24 hours.
    Nasal: Use as often as needed
    Ophthalmic:
        Ointment: Apply once daily or more often
        Solution: Instill 1-2 drops into affected eye(s) every 3-4 hours
    Abortifacient: 20% (250 mL) administered by transabdominal intra-amniotic instillation

Dosage Forms
Drops, nasal: 0.9% with dropper
Injection: 0.45% [4.5 mg/mL] (500 mL, 1000 mL); 0.9% [9 mg/mL] (10 mL, 20 mL, 50 mL, 100 mL, 150 mL, 250 mL, 500 mL, 1000 mL); 3% [30 mg/mL] (500 mL); 5% [50 mg/mL] (500 mL); 14.6% [146 mg/mL] , 20% [200 mg/mL] (250 mL); 23.4% [234 mg/mL] (30 mL, 100 mL)
Injection:
    Admixtures: 50 mEq, 100 mEq, 625 mEq
    Bacteriostatic: 0.9% [9 mg/mL] (30 mL)
Irrigation: 0.9% [9 mg/mL] (250 mL, 500 mL, 1000 mL, 3000 mL)
Ointment, ophthalmic (Muro 128®): 5% (3.5 g)
Solution:
    Nasal: 0.65% (45 mL)
    Ophthalmic (Adsorbonac®): 2% (15 mL); 5% (15 mL)
Tablet: 650 mg, 1 g
Tablet, enteric coated: 1 g

sodium citrate and citric acid
Brand Names Bicitra®; Oracit®
Synonyms modified Shohl's solution; Shohl's solution
Therapeutic Category Alkalinizing Agent Oral
Use Treatment of metabolic acidosis; alkalinizing agent in conditions where long-term maintenance of an alkaline urine is desirable
Usual Dosage Oral:
    Infants and Children: 2-3 mEq/kg/day in divided doses 3-4 times/day **or** 5-15 mL with water after meals and at bedtime

    Adults: 15-30 mL with water after meals and at bedtime
Dosage Forms Solution, oral:
    Bicitra®: Sodium citrate 500 mg and citric acid 334 mg per 5 mL (15 mL unit dose, 480 mL)
    Oracit®: Sodium citrate 490 mg and citric acid 640 mg per 5 mL
(Continued)

sodium citrate and citric acid *(Continued)*

Polycitra" : Sodium citrate 500 mg and citric acid 334 mg with potassium citrate 550 mg per 5 mL

sodium citrate and potassium citrate mixture

Brand Names Polycitra®

Therapeutic Category Alkalinizing Agent Oral

Use Conditions where long-term maintenance of an alkaline urine is desirable as in control and dissolution of uric acid and cystine calculi of the urinary tract

Usual Dosage Oral:

Children: 5-15 mL diluted in water after meals and at bedtime

Adults: 15-30 mL diluted in water after meals and at bedtime

Dosage Forms Syrup: Sodium citrate 500 mg, potassium citrate 550 mg, with citric acid 334 mg per 5 mL [sodium 1 mEq, potassium 1 mEq, bicarbonate 2 mEq]

sodium edetate *see* edetate disodium *on page 163*

sodium ethacrynate *see* ethacrynic acid *on page 176*

sodium etidronate *see* etidronate disodium *on page 182*

sodium hyaluronate (hye al yoor on' nate)

Brand Names Amvisc®; Healon®; Healon® GV; Healon® Yellow

Synonyms hyaluronic acid

Therapeutic Category Ophthalmic Agent, Viscoeleastic

Use Surgical aid in cataract extraction, intraocular implantation, corneal transplant, glaucoma filtration, and retinal attachment surgery

Usual Dosage Depends upon procedure (slowly introduce a sufficient quantity into eye)

Dosage Forms Injection, intraocular: 10 mg/mL (0.25 mL, 0.4 mL, 0.5 mL, 0.75 mL, 0.8 mL, 2 mL, 4 mL); 14 mg/mL (0.55 mL, 0.85 mL); 16 mg/mL (0.25 mL, 0.5 mL, 8 mL)

sodium hyaluronate-chrondroitin sulfate *see* chondroitin sulfate-sodium hyaluronate *on page 100*

sodium hydrogen carbonate *see* sodium bicarbonate *on page 426*

sodium hypochlorite solution (hye poe klor' ite)

Synonyms Dakin's solution; modified Dakin's solution

Therapeutic Category Disinfectant

Use Treatment of athlete's foot (0.5%); wound irrigation (0.5%); to disinfect utensils and equipment (5%)

Dosage Forms

Solution: 5% (4000 mL)

Solution (modified Dakin's solution):

Full strength: 0.5% (1000 mL)

Half strength: 0.25% (1000 mL)

Quarter strength: 0.125% (1000 mL)

sodium lactate

Therapeutic Category Alkalinizing Agent, Parenteral

Use Source of bicarbonate for prevention and treatment of mild to moderate metabolic acidosis

Usual Dosage Dosage depends on degree of acidosis

Dosage Forms Injection:

1.87 g/100 mL [sodium 16.7 mEq and lactate 16.7 mEq per 100 mL] (1000 mL)

560 mg/mL [sodium 5 mEq sodium and lactate 5 mEq per mL] (10 mL)

sodium *l*-tri-iodothyronine *see* liothyronine sodium *on page 269*

sodium methicillin *see* methicillin sodium *on page 294*

sodium nitroferricyanide *see* nitroprusside sodium *on page 330*

sodium nitroprusside *see* nitroprusside sodium *on page 330*

sodium oxacillin *see* oxacillin sodium *on page 340*

Sodium P.A.S. *see* aminosalicylate sodium *on page 20*

sodium-pca and lactic acid *see* lactic acid and sodium-PCA *on page 261*

sodium phenylacetate and sodium benzoate

Brand Names Ucephan® Oral

Therapeutic Category Hyperammonemia Agent

Use Adjunctive therapy to prevent/treat hyperammonemia in patients with urea cycle enzymopathy involving partial or complete deficiencies of carbamoylphosphate synthetase, ornithine transcarbamylase or argininosuccinate synthetase

Usual Dosage Infants and Children: Oral: 2.5 mL (250 mg sodium benzoate and 250 mg sodium phenylacetate)/kg/day divided 3-6 times/day; total daily dose should not exceed 100 mL

Dosage Forms Solution: Sodium phenylacetate 100 mg and sodium benzoate 100 mg per mL (100 mL)

sodium phosphate

Brand Names Fleet® Enema [OTC]; Fleet® Phospho®-Soda [OTC]

Therapeutic Category Electrolyte Supplement, Parenteral; Laxative, Saline; Phosphate Salt; Sodium Salt

Use Source of phosphate in large volume I.V. fluids; short-term treatment of constipation and to evacuate the colon for rectal and bowel exams; source of sodium and phosphorus in parenteral nutrition

Usual Dosage

Normal requirements elemental phosphate: Oral:

0-6 months: 240 mg

6-12 months: 360 mg

1-10 years: 800 mg

>10 years: 1200 mg

Pregnancy lactation: Additional 400 mg/day

Treatment:

It is difficult to provide concrete guidelines for the treatment of severe hypophosphatemia because the extent of total body deficits and response to therapy are difficult to predict. Aggressive doses of phosphate may result in a transient serum elevation followed by redistribution into intracellular compartments or bone tissue. It is recommended that repletion of severe hypophosphatemia (<1 mg/dL in adults) be done I.V. because large doses of oral phosphate may cause diarrhea and intestinal absorption may be unreliable

Pediatric I.V. phosphate repletion:

Neonates: 0.5 mmol/kg/dose up to 1-2 mmol/kg/day

Children: 0.25-0.5 mmol/kg **administer over 4-6 hours and repeat if symptomatic hypophosphatemia persists**; to assess the need for further phosphate administration: obtain serum inorganic phosphate after administration of the first dose and base further doses on serum levels and clinical status

Adult I.V. phosphate repletion:

Initial dose: 0.08 mmol/kg if recent uncomplicated hypophosphatemia

Initial dose: 0.16 mmol/kg if prolonged hypophosphatemia with presumed total body deficits; increase dose by 25% to 50% if patient symptomatic with severe hypophosphatemia

Severe hypophosphatemia:

High-dose = 0.36 mmol/kg over 6 hours; use if serum PO_4 <0.5 mg/dL

Adults: 0.15-0.3 mmol/kg/dose over 12 hours, may repeat as needed to achieve desired serum level

(Continued)

sodium phosphate *(Continued)*

With orders for I.V. phosphate, there is considerable confusion associated with the use of millimoles (mmol) versus milliequivalents (mEq) to express the phosphate requirement. Because inorganic phosphate exists as monobasic and dibasic anions, with the mixture of valences is dependent on pH, ordering by mEq amounts is unreliable and may lead to large dosing errors. In addition, I.V. phosphate is available in the sodium and potassium salt; therefore, the content of these cations must be considered when ordering phosphate. The most reliable method of ordering I.V. phosphate is by millimoles, then specifying the potassium or sodium salt. For example, an order for 15 mmol of phosphate as potassium phosphate in one liter of normal saline would also provide 22 mEq of potassium.

Phosphate maintenance electrolyte requirement in parenteral nutrition: 2 mmol/kg/24 hours or 35 mmol/kcal/24 hours; Maximum: 15-30 mmol/24 hours

Maintenance:
Children: 0.5-1.5 mmol/kg/24 hours I.V. **or** 2-3 mmol/kg/24 hours orally in divided doses
Adults: 15-30 mmol/24 hours I.V. **or** 50-150 mmol/24 hours orally in divided doses

Laxative (Fleet™): Rectal:
Children 2-12 years: 67.5 mL ($^1/_2$ bottle) as a single dose, may repeat
Children ≥12 years and Adults: 133 mL enema as a single dose, may repeat

Laxative (Fleet™ Phospho®-Soda): Oral:
Children:
5-9 years: 5 mL as a single dose
10-12 years: 10 mL as a single dose
Children ≥12 years and Adults: 20-30 mL as a single dose

Dosage Forms
Enema: Sodium phosphate 6 g and sodium biphosphate 16 g per 100 mL (135 mL adult enema unit, 67.5 mL pediatric enema unit)
Injection: Phosphate 3 mmol and sodium 4 mEq sodium per mL (15 mL)
Solution, oral: Sodium phosphate 18 g and sodium biphosphate 48 g per 100 mL (30 mL, 45 mL, 90 mL, 237 mL)

sodium phosphate and potassium phosphate *see* potassium phosphate and sodium phosphate *on page 380*

sodium polystyrene sulfonate (pol ee stye' reen)
Brand Names Kayexalate™; SPS®
Therapeutic Category Antidote, Hyperkalemia; Antidote, Potassium
Use Treatment of hyperkalemia
Usual Dosage
Children:
Oral: 1 g/kg/dose every 6 hours
Rectal: 1 g/kg/dose every 2-6 hours (In small children and infants employ lower doses by using the practical exchange ratio of 1 mEq potassium/g of resin as the basis for calculation)

Adults:
Oral: 15 g (60 mL) 1-4 times/day
Rectal: 30-50 g every 6 hours
Dosage Forms Oral or rectal:
Powder for suspension: 454 g
Suspension: 1.25 g/5 mL with sorbitol 33% and alcohol 0.3% (60 mL, 120 mL, 200 mL, 500 mL)

sodium salicylate
Brand Names Uracel™
Therapeutic Category Analgesic, Non-Narcotic
Use Treatment of minor pain or fever; arthritis

Usual Dosage Adults: Oral: 325-650 mg every 4 hours
Dosage Forms Tablet, enteric coated: 325 mg, 650 mg

Sodium Sulamyd® Ophthalmic *see* sodium sulfacetamide *on this page*

sodium sulfacetamide (sul fa see' ta mide)

Brand Names AK-Sulf® Ophthalmic; Bleph®-10 Ophthalmic; Cetamide® Ophthalmic; I-Sulfacet® Ophthalmic; Ophthacet® Ophthalmic; Sodium Sulamyd® Ophthalmic; Sulf-10® Ophthalmic; Sulfair® Ophthalmic

Synonyms sulfacetamide sodium

Therapeutic Category Antibiotic, Ophthalmic

Use Treatment and prophylaxis of conjunctivitis due to susceptible organisms; corneal ulcers; adjunctive treatment with systemic sulfonamides for therapy of trachoma

Usual Dosage Children >2 months and Adults: Ophthalmic:
Ointment: Apply to lower conjunctival sac 1-4 times/day and at bedtime
Solution: 1-2 drops every 2-3 hours in the lower conjunctival sac during the waking hours and less frequently at night

Dosage Forms
Ointment, ophthalmic: 10% (3.5 g, 3.75 g)
Solution, ophthalmic: 10% (1 mL, 2 mL, 2.5 mL, 3.75 mL, 5 mL, 15 mL); 15% (2 mL, 5 mL, 15 mL); 30% (5 mL, 15 mL)

sodium sulfacetamide and fluoromethalone

Brand Names FML-S®

Therapeutic Category Antibiotic, Ophthalmic; Anti-inflammatory Agent, Ophthalmic

Use Steroid-responsive inflammatory ocular conditions where infection is present or there is a risk of infection

Dosage Forms Suspension, ophthalmic: Sodium sulfacetamide 10% and fluoromethalone 0.1% (5 mL, 10 mL)

sodium sulfacetamide and phenylephrine

Brand Names Vasosulf®

Therapeutic Category Antibiotic, Ophthalmic; Ophthalmic Agent, Vasoconstrictor

Usual Dosage Ophthalmic: Instill 1-3 drops in lower conjunctival sac every 3-4 hours

Dosage Forms Solution, ophthalmic: Sodium sulfacetamide 15% and phenylephrine hydrochloride 0.125% (5 mL, 15 mL)

sodium sulfacetamide and prednisolone

Brand Names Blephamide®; Cetapred®; Metimyd®; Vasocidin®

Synonyms prednisolone acetate and sodium sulfacetamide

Therapeutic Category Antibiotic, Ophthalmic; Corticosteroid, Ophthalmic

Use Steroid-responsive inflammatory ocular conditions where infection is present or there is a risk of infection; ophthalmic suspension may be used as an otic preparation

Usual Dosage Children >2 and Adults: Ophthalmic:
Ointment: Apply to lower conjunctival sac 1-4 times/day
Solution: Instill 1-3 drops every 2-3 hours while awake

Dosage Forms
Ointment, ophthalmic: Sodium sulfacetamide 10% and prednisolone acetate 0.2% (3.5 g)
Ointment, ophthalmic:
Cetapred®: Sodium sulfacetamide 10% and prednisolone acetate 0.25% (3.5 g)
Metimyd®: Sodium sulfacetamide 10% and prednisolone acetate 0.5% (3.5 g)
Suspension, ophthalmic: Sodium sulfacetamide 10% and prednisolone sodium phosphate 0.5% (5 mL)
Suspension, ophthalmic:
Blephamide®: Sodium sulfacetamide 10% and prednisolone acetate 0.2% (2.5 mL, 5 mL, 10 mL)
Vasocidin®: Sodium sulfacetamide 10% and prednisolone acetate 0.25% (5 mL, 10 mL)

sodium sulfacetamide and sulfur *see* sulfur and sodium sulfacetamide
on page 442

sodium tetradecyl sulfate
Brand Names Sotradecol" Injection
Therapeutic Category Sclerosing Agent
Use Treatment of small, uncomplicated varicose veins of the lower extremities; endoscopic sclerotherapy in the management of bleeding esophageal varices
Usual Dosage I.V.: 0.5-2 mL of 1% (5-20 mg) for small veins; 0.5-2 mL of 3% (15-60 mg) for medium or large veins
Dosage Forms Injection: 1% [10 mg/mL] (2 mL); 3% [30 mg/mL] (2 mL)

sodium thiosulfate (thye oh sul' fate)
Brand Names Tinver" Lotion
Therapeutic Category Antidote, Cyanide; Antifungal Agent, Topical
Use Alone or with sodium nitrite or amyl nitrite in cyanide poisoning; used to reduce the risk of nephrotoxicity associated with cisplatin therapy; used topically in the treatment of tinea versicolor
Usual Dosage I.V.:
Cyanide and nitroprusside antidote:
Children <25 kg: 50 mg/kg after receiving 4.5-10 mg/kg sodium nitrite; a half dose of each may be repeated if necessary
Children >25 kg and Adults: 12.5 g after 300 mg of sodium nitrite; a half dose of each may be repeated if necessary

Cyanide poisoning: Dose should be based on determination as with nitrite, at rate of 2.5-5 mL/minute to maximum of 50 mL.
Dosage Forms
Injection: 100 mg/mL (10 mL); 250 mg/mL (50 mL)
Lotion: 25% with salicylic acid 1% and isopropyl alcohol 10% (120 mL, 180 mL)

sodium thiosulfate and resorcinol
Therapeutic Category Acne Products
Use Treatment of acne associated with oily skin
Dosage Forms Lotion, topical: 60 g

Sodol® *see* carisoprodol *on page 77*
Sofarin® *see* warfarin sodium *on page 492*
Solaquin Forte® *see* hydroquinone *on page 235*
Solaquin® [OTC] *see* hydroquinone *on page 235*
Solarcaine® [OTC] *see* benzocaine *on page 48*
Solatene® *see* beta-carotene *on page 52*
Solfoton® *see* phenobarbital *on page 361*
Solganal® *see* aurothioglucose *on page 40*
soluble fluorescein *see* fluorescein sodium *on page 196*
Solu-Cortef® *see* hydrocortisone *on page 232*
Solu-Medrol® Injection *see* methylprednisolone *on page 300*
Solurex® *see* dexamethasone *on page 131*
Solurex L.A.® *see* dexamethasone *on page 131*
Soma® *see* carisoprodol *on page 77*
Soma® Compound *see* carisoprodol *on page 77*
somatrem *see* human growth hormone *on page 226*

somatropin *see* human growth hormone *on page 226*

Sominex® Oral [OTC] *see* diphenhydramine hydrochloride *on page 149*

Somophyllin® *see* aminophylline *on page 20*

Soothe® Ophthalmic [OTC] *see* tetrahydrozoline hydrochloride *on page 452*

Soprodol® *see* carisoprodol *on page 77*

sorbitol

Therapeutic Category Genitourinary Irrigant
Use Genitourinary irrigant in transurethral prostatic resection or other transurethral resection or other transurethral surgical procedures; diuretic; humectant; sweetening agent; hyperosmotic laxative; facilitate the passage of sodium polystyrene sulfonate through the intestinal tract
Usual Dosage Hyperosmotic laxative (as single dose, at infrequent intervals):
Children 2-11 years:
Oral: 2 mL/kg (as 70% solution)
Rectal enema: 30-60 mL as 25% to 30% solution

Children >12 years and Adults:
Oral: 30-150 mL (as 70% solution)
Rectal enema: 120 mL as 25% to 30% solution
Adjunct to sodium polystyrene sulfonate: 15 mL as 70% solution orally until diarrhea occurs (10-20 mL/2 hours) or 20-100 mL as an oral vehicle for the sodium polystyrene sulfonate resin

When administered with charcoal: Oral:
Children: 4.3 mL/kg of 35% sorbitol with 1 g/kg of activated charcoal
Adults: 4.3 mL/kg of 70% sorbitol with 1·g/kg of activated charcoal
Dosage Forms
Solution: 70%
Solution, genitourinary irrigation: 3% (1500 mL, 3000 mL); 3.3% (2000 mL)

Sorbitrate® *see* isosorbide dinitrate *on page 254*

Soridol® *see* carisoprodol *on page 77*

sotalol hydrochloride (soe' ta lole)

Brand Names Betapace® Oral
Therapeutic Category Antiarrhythmic Agent, Class II; Antiarrhythmic Agent, Class III
Use Treatment of ventricular arrhythmias
Usual Dosage Adults: Oral: Initial: 80 mg twice daily; may be increased to 240-320 mg/day and up to 480-640 mg/day in patients with life-threatening refractory ventricular arrhythmias
Dosage Forms Tablet: 80 mg, 160 mg, 240 mg

Sotradecol® Injection *see* sodium tetradecyl sulfate *on previous page*

Span-FF® [OTC] *see* ferrous fumarate *on page 189*

Sparine® *see* promazine hydrochloride *on page 389*

Spasmoject® Injection *see* dicyclomine hydrochloride *on page 142*

Spasmolin® *see* hyoscyamine, atropine, scopolamine, and phenobarbital *on page 238*

Spasmophen® *see* hyoscyamine, atropine, scopolamine, and phenobarbital *on page 238*

Spasquid® *see* hyoscyamine, atropine, scopolamine, and phenobarbital *on page 238*

Spectam® Injection *see* spectinomycin hydrochloride *on next page*

Spectazole™ Topical *see* econazole nitrate *on page 162*

spectinomycin hydrochloride (spek ti noe mye' sin)
Brand Names Spectam^(®) Injection; Trobicin^(®) Injection
Therapeutic Category Antibiotic, Miscellaneous
Use Treatment of uncomplicated gonorrhea (ineffective against syphilis)
Usual Dosage I.M.:
  Children:
     <45 kg: 40 mg/kg/dose 1 time
     ≥45 kg: See adult dose
     Children >8 years who are allergic to PCNS/cephalosporins may be treated with oral tetracycline

  Adults: 2 g deep I.M. or 4 g where antibiotic resistance is prevalent 1 time; 4 g (10 mL) dose should be given as 2-5 mL injections
Dosage Forms Injection: 2 g, 4 g

Spectrobid® see bacampicillin hydrochloride on page 42

Spherulin® see coccidioidin skin test on page 111

spirapril
Brand Names Renormax^(®)
Therapeutic Category Angiotensin-Converting Enzyme (ACE) Inhibitors
Use Management of mild to severe hypertension
Usual Dosage Oral: Adults: 12 mg per day, in one or two divided doses
Dosage Forms Tablet: 3 mg, 6 mg, 12 mg, 24 mg

Spironazide® see hydrochlorothiazide and spironolactone on page 229

spironolactone (speer on oh lak' tone)
Brand Names Aldactone^(®)
Therapeutic Category Diuretic, Potassium Sparing
Use Management of edema associated with excessive aldosterone excretion; hypertension; primary hyperaldosteronism; hypokalemia; treatment of hirsutism, cirrhosis of the liver accompanied by edema or ascites (unlabeled)
Usual Dosage Oral:
  Children: 1.5-3.5 mg/kg/day in divided doses every 6-24 hours
    Diagnosis of primary aldosteronism: 125-375 mg/m^2/day in divided doses
    Vaso-occlusive disease: 7.5 mg/kg/day in divided doses twice daily (non-FDA approved dose)

  Adults:
    Edema, hypertension, hypokalemia: 25-200 mg/day in 1-2 divided doses
    Diagnosis of primary aldosteronism: 100-400 mg/day in 1-2 divided doses
Dosage Forms Tablet: 25 mg, 50 mg, 100 mg

spironolactone and hydrochlorothiazide see hydrochlorothiazide and spironolactone on page 229

Spirozide® see hydrochlorothiazide and spironolactone on page 229

Sporanox® Oral see itraconazole on page 255

Sportscreme® [OTC] see triethanolamine salicylate on page 470

SPS® see sodium polystyrene sulfonate on page 430

S-P-T see thyroid on page 459

SRC® Expectorant see hydrocodone, pseudoephedrine, and guaifenesin on page 231

SSD® AF see silver sulfadiazine on page 423

SSD® Cream see silver sulfadiazine on page 423

SSKI® *see* potassium iodide *on page 379*

Stadol® *see* butorphanol tartrate *on page 64*

Stadol® NS *see* butorphanol tartrate *on page 64*

Stagesic® *see* hydrocodone and acetaminophen *on page 230*

stanozolol (stan oh' zoe lole)
Brand Names Winstrol®
Therapeutic Category Anabolic Steroid
Use Prophylactic use against angioedema
Usual Dosage
Children: Acute attacks:
<6 years: 1 mg/day
6-12 years: 2 mg/day

Adults: Oral: Initial: 2 mg 3 times/day, may then reduce to a maintenance dose of 2 mg/day or 2 mg every other day after 1-3 months
Dosage Forms Tablet: 2 mg

Staphcillin® *see* methicillin sodium *on page 294*

Staticin® *see* erythromycin, topical *on page 172*

stavudine (stav' yoo deen)
Brand Names Zerit® Oral
Synonyms d4T
Therapeutic Category Antiviral Agent, Oral
Use Treatment of adults with advanced HIV infection who are intolerant to approved therapies with proven clinical benefit or who have experienced significant clinical or immunologic deterioration while receiving these therapies, or for whom such therapies are contraindicated
Usual Dosage Adults: Oral:
≥60 kg: 40 mg every 12 hours
<60 kg: 30 mg every 12 hours

Dosing adjustment in renal impairment:
Cl_{cr} >50 mL/minute: ≥60 kg: 40 mg every 12 hours
Cl_{cr} >50 mL/minute: <60 kg: 30 mg every 12 hours
Cl_{cr} 26-50 mL/minute: ≥60 kg: 20 mg every 12 hours
Cl_{cr} 26-50 mL/minute: <60 kg: 15 mg every 12 hours
Cl_{cr} 10-25 mL/minute: ≥60 kg: 20 mg every 12 hours
Cl_{cr} 10-25 mL/minute: <60 kg: 15 mg every 12 hours
Dosage Forms Capsule: 15 mg, 20 mg, 30 mg, 40 mg

Stay Trim® Diet Gum [OTC] *see* phenylpropanolamine hydrochloride *on page 365*

S-T Cort® *see* hydrocortisone *on page 232*

Stelazine® Injection *see* trifluoperazine hydrochloride *on page 470*

Stelazine® Oral *see* trifluoperazine hydrochloride *on page 470*

Sterapred® Oral *see* prednisone *on page 384*

stilbestrol *see* diethylstilbestrol *on page 143*

Stilphostrol® *see* diethylstilbestrol *on page 143*

St. Joseph® Adult Chewable Aspirin [OTC] *see* aspirin *on page 35*

St. Joseph® Cough Suppressant [OTC] *see* dextromethorphan hydrobromide *on page 135*

St. Joseph® Measured Dose Nasal Solution [OTC] *see* phenylephrine hydrochloride *on page 364*

Stop® **[OTC]** *see* fluoride *on page 196*

Streptase® *see* streptokinase *on this page*

streptokinase (strep toe kye' nase)

Brand Names Kabikinase®; Streptase®

Synonyms sk

Therapeutic Category Thrombolytic Agent

Use Thrombolytic agent used in treatment of recent severe or massive deep vein thrombosis, pulmonary emboli, myocardial infarction, and occluded arteriovenous cannulas

Usual Dosage I.V.:

Children: Safety and efficacy not established; limited studies have used: 3500-4000 units/kg over 30 minutes followed by 1000-1500 units/kg/hour; clotted catheter: 25,000 units, clamp for 2 hours then aspirate contents and flush with normal saline

Adults (best results are realized if used within 5-6 hours of myocardial infarction; antibodies to streptokinase remain for 3-6 months after initial dose, use another thrombolytic enzyme, ie, urokinase, if thrombolytic therapy is indicated):

Guidelines for acute myocardial infarction (AMI):

1.5 million units infused over 60 minutes. Monitor for the first few hours for signs of anaphylaxis or allergic reaction. **Infusion should be slowed if lowering of 25 mm Hg in blood pressure or terminated if asthmatic symptoms appear.** Begin heparin 5000-10,000 unit bolus followed by 1000 unit/hour approximately 3-4 hours after completion of streptokinase infusion or when PTT is <100 seconds.

Guidelines for acute pulmonary embolism (APE):

3 million unit dose; administer 250,000 units over 30 minutes followed by 100,000 units/hour for 24 hours. Monitor for the first few hours for signs of anaphylaxis or allergic reaction. **Infusion should be slowed if blood pressure is lowered by 25 mm Hg or if asthmatic symptoms appear.** Begin heparin 1000 units/hour approximately 3-4 hours after completion of streptokinase infusion or when PTT is <100 seconds.

Thromboses: 250,000 units to start, then 100,000 units/hour for 24-72 hours depending on location

Cannula occlusion: 250,000 units into cannula, clamp for 2 hours, then aspirate contents and flush with normal saline

Dosage Forms Powder for injection: 250,000 units (5 mL, 6.5 mL); 600,000 units (5 mL); 750,000 units (6 mL, 6.5 mL); 1,500,000 units (6.5 mL, 10 mL, 50 mL)

streptomycin sulfate (strep toe mye' sin)

Therapeutic Category Antibiotic, Aminoglycoside; Antitubercular Agent

Use Combination therapy of active tuberculosis; used in combination with other agents for treatment of streptococcal or enterococcal endocarditis, mycobacterial infections, plague, tularemia, and brucellosis

Usual Dosage I.M.:

Infants: 20-30 mg/kg/day in divided doses every 12 hours

Children: Tuberculosis: 20-40 mg/kg/day in divided doses every 12-24 hours, not to exceed 2 g/day; usually discontinued after 2-3 months of therapy or sooner if cultures become negative

Adults:

Tuberculosis: 15 mg/kg/day in divided doses every 12 hours, not to exceed 2 g/day

Enterococcal endocarditis: 1 g every 12 hours for 2 weeks, 500 mg every 12 hours for 4 weeks in combination with penicillin

Streptococcal endocarditis: 1 g every 12 hours for 1 week, 500 mg every 12 hours for 1 week

Tularemia: 1-2 g/day in divided doses for 7-10 days or until patient is afebrile for 5-7 days

Plague: 2-4 g/day in divided doses until the patient is afebrile for at least 3 days

Dosage Forms Injection: 400 mg/mL (12.5 mL)

Streptonase-B® *see* diagnostic aids (*in vitro*), other *on page 137*

Strepto-Sac® *see* diagnostic aids (*in vitro*), other *on page 137*

streptozocin (strep toe zoe' sin)
Brand Names Zanosar®
Therapeutic Category Antineoplastic Agent, Alkylating Agent (Nitrosourea)
Use Treat metastatic islet cell carcinoma of the pancreas, carcinoid tumor and syndrome, Hodgkin's disease, palliative treatment of colorectal cancer
Usual Dosage Children and Adults: I.V.: 500 mg/m² for 5 days every 6 weeks until optimal benefit or toxicity occurs; or may be given in single dose 1000 mg/m² at weekly intervals for 2 doses, then increased to 1500 mg/m² weekly; the median total dose to onset of response is about 2000 mg/m² and the median total dose to maximum response is about 4000 mg/m²
Dosage Forms Injection: 1 g

strong iodine solution *see* potassium iodide *on page 379*

strontium-89 chloride (stron' shee um)
Brand Names Metastron® Injection
Therapeutic Category Radiopharmaceutical
Use Relief of bone pain in patients with skeletal metastases
Usual Dosage Adults: I.V.: 148 megabecquerel (4 millicurrie) administered by slow I.V. injection over 1-2 minutes or 1.5-2.2 megabecquerel (40-60 microcurrie)/kg; repeated doses are generally not recommended at intervals <90 days
Dosage Forms Injection: 10.9-22.6 mg/mL [148 megabecquerel, 4 millicurrie] (10 mL)

Stuartnatal® 1+1 *see* vitamin, multiple (prenatal) *on page 491*

Stuart Prenatal® [OTC] *see* vitamin, multiple (prenatal) *on page 491*

Sublimaze® Injection *see* fentanyl citrate *on page 188*

succimer (sux' sim mer)
Brand Names Chemet®
Therapeutic Category Antidote, Lead Toxicity
Use Treatment of lead poisoning in children with blood levels >45 mcg/dL. It is not indicated for prophylaxis of lead poisoning in a lead-containing environment.
Usual Dosage Children and Adults: Oral: 30 mg/kg/day in divided doses every 8 hours for an additional 5 days followed by 20 mg/kg/day for 14 days
Dosage Forms Capsule: 100 mg

succinylcholine chloride (suk sin ill koe' leen)
Brand Names Anectine® Chloride Injection; Anectine® Flo-Pack®; Quelicin® Injection; Sucostrin® Injection
Synonyms suxamethonium chloride
Therapeutic Category Neuromuscular Blocker Agent, Depolarizing; Skeletal Muscle Relaxant
Use Produce skeletal muscle relaxation in procedures of short duration such as endotracheal intubation or endoscopic exams
Usual Dosage I.M., I.V.:
Neonates: Intermittent: Initial: 2 mg/kg/dose one time; maintenance: 0.3-0.6 mg/kg/dose at intervals of 5-10 minutes as necessary

Children: 1-2 mg/kg
Intermittent: Initial: 1 mg/kg/dose one time; maintenance: 0.3-0.6 mg/kg every 5-10 minutes as needed

Adults: 0.6 mg/kg (range: 0.3-1.1 mg/kg) over 10-30 seconds, up to 150 mg total dose
Maintenance: 0.04-0.07 mg/kg every 5-10 minutes as needed
Continuous infusion: 2.5 mg/minute (or 0.5-10 mg/minute); dilute to concentration of 1-2 mg/mL in D₅W or NS

(Continued)

succinylcholine chloride *(Continued)*

Note: Pretreatment with atropine may reduce occurrence of bradycardia

Dosage Forms
Injection: 20 mg/mL (10 mL); 50 mg/mL (10 mL); 100 mg/mL (5 mL, 10 mL, 20 mL)
Powder for injection: 100 mg, 500 mg, 1 g

Sucostrin® Injection *see* succinylcholine chloride *on previous page*

sucralfate *(soo kral' fate)*

Brand Names Carafate®

Synonyms aluminum sucrose sulfate, basic

Therapeutic Category Gastrointestinal Agent, Miscellaneous

Use Short-term management of duodenal ulcers; maintenance for duodenal ulcers; suspension may be used topically for treatment of stomatitis due to cancer chemotherapy and other causes of esophageal and gastric erosions

Usual Dosage
Children: Dose not established, doses of 40-80 mg/kg/day divided every 6 hours have been used
Stomatitis: Oral: 2.5-5 mL (1 g/15 mL suspension), swish and spit or swish and swallow 4 times/day

Adults:
Duodenal ulcer treatment: Oral: 1 g 4 times/day, 1 hour before meals or food and at bedtime for 4-8 weeks, or alternatively 2 g twice daily
Duodenal ulcer maintenance therapy: Oral: 1 g twice daily
Stomatitis: Oral: 1 g/15 mL suspension, swish and spit or swish and swallow 4 times/day

Dosage Forms
Suspension, oral: 1 g/10 mL (420 mL)
Tablet: 1 g

Sucrets® Cough Calmers [OTC] *see* dextromethorphan hydrobromide *on page 135*

Sucrets® [OTC] *see* dyclonine hydrochloride *on page 161*

Sudafed® 12 Hour [OTC] *see* pseudoephedrine *on page 397*

Sudafed Plus® Tablet *see* chlorpheniramine and pseudoephedrine *on page 94*

Sudafed® [OTC] *see* pseudoephedrine *on page 397*

Sudex® *see* guaifenesin and pseudoephedrine *on page 216*

Sufedrin® [OTC] *see* pseudoephedrine *on page 397*

Sufenta® Injection *see* sufentanil citrate *on this page*

sufentanil citrate *(soo fen' ta nil)*

Brand Names Sufenta® Injection

Therapeutic Category Analgesic, Narcotic

Use Analgesic supplement in maintenance of balanced general anesthesia

Usual Dosage I.V.:
Children <12 years: 10-25 mcg/kg with 100% O_2, maintenance: 25-50 mcg as needed (total dose of up to 1-2 mcg/kg)

Adults: Dose should be based on body weight. **Note:** In obese patients (ie, >20% above ideal body weight), use lean body weight to determine dosage
1-2 mcg/kg with NO_2/O_2 for endotracheal intubation; maintenance: 10-25 mcg as needed
2-8 mcg/kg with NO_2/O_2 more complicated major surgical procedures; maintenance: 10-50 mcg as needed
8-30 mcg/kg with 100% O_2 and muscle relaxant produces sleep; at doses of ≥8 mcg/kg maintains a deep level of anesthesia; maintenance: 10-50 mcg as needed

Dosage Forms Injection: 50 mcg/mL (1 mL, 2 mL, 5 mL)

sulbactam and ampicillin *see* ampicillin sodium and sulbactam sodium
   on page 26

sulconazole nitrate (sul kon' a zole)
   Brand Names Exelderm® Topical; Sulcosyn® Topical
   Therapeutic Category Antifungal Agent, Topical
   Use Treatment of superficial fungal infections of the skin, including tinea cruris, tinea corporis, tinea versicolor and possibly tinea pedis
   Usual Dosage Topical: Apply once or twice daily for 4-6 weeks
   Dosage Forms
     Cream: 1% (15 g, 30 g, 60 g)
     Solution, topical: 1% (30 mL)

Sulcosyn® Topical *see* sulconazole nitrate *on this page*

Sulf-10® Ophthalmic *see* sodium sulfacetamide *on page 431*

sulfabenzamide, sulfacetamide, and sulfathiazole
   Brand Names Gyne-Sulf®; Sultrin™; Trysul®; V.V.S.®
   Synonyms triple sulfa
   Therapeutic Category Antibiotic, Vaginal
   Use Treatment of *Haemophilus vaginalis* vaginitis
   Usual Dosage Adults:
     Cream: Insert one applicatorful in vagina twice daily for 4-6 days; dosage may then be decreased to $\frac{1}{2}$ to $\frac{1}{4}$ of an applicatorful twice daily
     Tablet: Insert one intravaginally twice daily for 10 days
   Dosage Forms
     Cream, vaginal: Sulfabenzamide 3.7%, sulfacetamide 2.86%, and sulfathiazole 3.42% (78 g with applicator, 90 g, 120 g)
     Tablet, vaginal: Sulfabenzamide 184 mg, sulfacetamide 143.75 mg, and sulfathiazole 172.5 mg (20 tablets/box with vaginal applicator)

sulfacetamide sodium *see* sodium sulfacetamide *on page 431*

Sulfacet-R® Topical *see* sulfur and sodium sulfacetamide *on page 442*

sulfacytine (sul fa sye' teen)
   Brand Names Renoquid®
   Therapeutic Category Antibiotic, Sulfonamide Derivative
   Use Treatment of urinary tract infections
   Usual Dosage Adults: Oral: Initial: 500 mg, then 250 mg every 4 hours for 10 days
   Dosage Forms Tablet: 250 mg

sulfadiazine (sul fa dye' a zeen)
   Therapeutic Category Antibiotic, Sulfonamide Derivative
   Use Treatment of urinary tract infections and nocardiosis, rheumatic fever prophylaxis; adjunctive treatment in toxoplasmosis; uncomplicated attack of malaria; asymptomatic meningococcal carriers
   Usual Dosage Oral:
     Congenital toxoplasmosis:
       Newborns and Children <2 months: 100 mg/kg/day divided every 6 hours in conjunction with pyrimethamine 1 mg/kg/day once daily and supplemental folinic acid 5 mg every 3 days for 6 months
       Children >2 months: 25-50 mg/kg/dose 4 times/day

     Toxoplasmosis:
       Children: 120-150 mg/kg/day, maximum dose: 6 g/day; divided every 6 hours in conjunction with pyrimethamine 2 mg/kg/day divided every 12 hours for 3 days followed by 1 mg/kg/day once daily (maximum: 25 mg/day) with supplemental folinic acid
   (Continued)

sulfadiazine *(Continued)*

Adults: 2-8 g/day divided every 6 hours in conjunction with pyrimethamine 25 mg/day and with supplemental folinic acid
Dosage Forms Tablet: 500 mg

sulfadiazine, sulfamethazine, and sulfamerazine (sul fa dye' a zeen)

Synonyms multiple sulfonamides; trisulfapyrimidines
Therapeutic Category Antibiotic, Sulfonamide Derivative; Antibiotic, Vaginal
Use Treatment of toxoplasmosis
Usual Dosage Adults: Oral: 2-4 g to start, then 2-4 g/day in 3-6 divided doses
Dosage Forms Tablet: Sulfadiazine 167 mg, sulfamethazine 167 mg, and sulfamerazine 167 mg

sulfadoxine and pyrimethamine

Brand Names Fansidar®
Therapeutic Category Antimalarial Agent
Use Treatment of *Plasmodium falciparum* malaria in patients in whom chloroquine resistance is suspected; malaria prophylaxis for travelers to areas where chloroquine-resistant malaria is endemic
Usual Dosage Children and Adults: Oral:
Treatment of acute attack of malaria: A single dose of the following number of Fansidar® tablets is used in sequence with quinine or alone:
2-11 months: $1/4$ tablet
1-3 years: $1/2$ tablet
4-8 years: 1 tablet
9-14 years: 2 tablets
>14 years: 2-3 tablets

Malaria prophylaxis:
The first dose of Fansidar® should be taken 1-2 days before departure to an endemic area (CDC recommends that therapy be initiated 1-2 weeks before such travel), administration should be continued during the stay and for 4-6 weeks after return. Dose = pyrimethamine 0.5 mg/kg/dose and sulfadoxine 10 mg/kg/dose up to a maximum of 25 mg pyrimethamine and 500 mg sulfadoxine/dose weekly.
2-11 months: $1/8$ tablet weekly **or** $1/4$ tablet once every 2 weeks
1-3 years: $1/4$ tablet once weekly **or** $1/2$ tablet once every 2 weeks
4-8 years: $1/2$ tablet once weekly **or** 1 tablet once every 2 weeks
9-14 years: $3/4$ tablet once weekly **or** $1 1/2$ tablets once every 2 weeks
>14 years: 1 tablet once weekly **or** 2 tablets once every 2 weeks
Dosage Forms Tablet: Sulfadoxine 500 mg and pyrimethamine 25 mg (25s)

Sulfair® Ophthalmic *see* sodium sulfacetamide *on page 431*

Sulfalax® [OTC] *see* docusate *on page 153*

Sulfamethoprim® *see* co-trimoxazole *on page 117*

sulfamethoxazole (sul fa meth ox' a zole)

Brand Names Gantanol®; Urobak®
Therapeutic Category Antibiotic, Sulfonamide Derivative
Use Treatment of urinary tract infections, nocardiosis, toxoplasmosis, acute otitis media, and acute exacerbations of chronic bronchitis due to susceptible organisms
Usual Dosage Oral:
Children >2 months: 50-60 mg/kg/day divided every 12 hours; maximum: 3 g/24 hours or 75 mg/kg/day

Adults: 2 g stat, 1 g 2-3 times/day; maximum: 3 g/24 hours
Dosage Forms
Suspension, oral (cherry flavor): 500 mg/5 mL (480 mL)
Tablet: 500 mg

sulfamethoxazole and phenazopyridine
Brand Names Azo Gantanol®
Therapeutic Category Antibiotic, Sulfonamide Derivative
Use Treatment of urinary tract infections complicated with pain
Usual Dosage Oral: 4 tablets to start, then 2 tablets twice daily for up to 2 days, then switch to sulfamethoxazole only
Dosage Forms Tablet: Sulfamethoxazole 500 mg and phenazopyridine 100 mg

sulfamethoxazole and trimethoprim see co-trimoxazole on page 117
Sulfamylon® Topical see mafenide acetate on page 276

sulfanilamide (sul fa nill' a mide)
Brand Names AVC™ Vaginal Cream; AVC™ Vaginal Suppository; Vagitrol® Vaginal
Therapeutic Category Antifungal Agent, Vaginal
Use Treatment of vulvovaginitis caused by Candida albicans
Usual Dosage One applicatorful once or twice daily continued through 1 complete menstrual cycle
Dosage Forms
Cream, vaginal (AVC™, Vagitrol®): 15% [150 mg/g] (120 g with applicator)
Suppository, vaginal (AVC™): 1.05 g (16s)

sulfasalazine (sul fa sal' a zeen)
Brand Names Azulfidine®; Azulfidine® EN-tabs®
Synonyms salicylazosulfapyridine
Therapeutic Category 5-Aminosalicylic Acid Derivative; Anti-inflammatory Agent
Use Management of ulcerative colitis
Usual Dosage Oral:
Children >2 years:
Initial: 40-60 mg/kg/day divided every 4-6 hour
Maintenance dose: 20-30 mg/kg/day divided every 6 hours, up to a maximum of 2 g/day
Adults:
Initial: 3-4 g/day divided every 4-6 hours;
Maintenance dose: 2 g/day divided every 6 hours
Dosage Forms
Suspension, oral: 250 mg/5 mL (480 mL)
Tablet: 500 mg
Tablet, enteric coated: 500 mg

Sulfatrim® see co-trimoxazole on page 117
Sulfatrim® DS see co-trimoxazole on page 117

sulfinpyrazone (sul fin peer' a zone)
Brand Names Anturane®
Therapeutic Category Uric Acid Lowering Agent
Use Treatment of chronic gouty arthritis and intermittent gouty arthritis
Usual Dosage Oral: 200 mg twice daily
Dosage Forms
Capsule: 200 mg
Tablet: 100 mg

sulfisoxazole (sul fi sox' a zole)
Brand Names Gantrisin® Ophthalmic; Gantrisin® Oral
Synonyms sulfisoxazole acetyl; sulphafurazole
Therapeutic Category Antibiotic, Sulfonamide Derivative
(Continued)

441

sulfisoxazole *(Continued)*

Use Treatment of urinary tract infections, otitis media, *Chlamydia*; nocardiosis; treatment of acute pelvic inflammatory disease in prepubertal children

Usual Dosage

Children >2 months: Oral: 75 mg/kg stat, 120-150 mg/kg/day in divided doses every 4-6 hours; not to exceed 6 g/day

Pelvic inflammatory disease: 100 mg/kg/day in divided doses every 6 hours; used in combination with ceftriaxone

Chlamydia trachomatis: 100 mg/kg/day divided every 6 hours

Children and Adults: Ophthalmic:

Solution: 1-2 drops to affected eye every 2-3 hours

Ointment: Small amount to affected eye 1-3 times/day and at bedtime

Adults: Oral: 2-4 g stat, 4-8 g/day in divided doses every 4-6 hours

Dosage Forms

Ointment, ophthalmic, as diolamine: 4% [40 mg/mL] (3.75 g)

Solution, ophthalmic, as diolamine: 4% [40 mg/mL] (15 mL)

Suspension, oral, pediatric, as acetyl (raspberry flavor): 500 mg/5 mL (480 mL)

Tablet: 500 mg

sulfisoxazole acetyl *see* sulfisoxazole *on previous page*

sulfisoxazole and erythromycin *see* erythromycin and sulfisoxazole *on page 171*

sulfisoxazole and phenazopyridine

Brand Names Azo Gantrisin®

Therapeutic Category Antibiotic, Sulfonamide Derivative; Local Anesthetic, Urinary

Use Treatment of urinary tract infections and nocardiosis

Usual Dosage Oral: 4-6 tablets to start, then 2 tablets 4 times/day for 2 days, then continue with sulfisoxazole only

Dosage Forms Tablet: Sulfisoxazole 500 mg and phenazopyridine 50 mg

sulfur and salicylic acid

Brand Names Aveeno® Cleansing Bar [OTC]; Fostex® [OTC]; Pernox® [OTC]; Sastid® Plain Therapeutic Shampoo and Acne Wash [OTC]; Sebulex® [OTC]

Synonyms salicylic acid and sulfur

Therapeutic Category Antiseborrheic Agent, Topical

Use Therapeutic shampoo for dandruff and seborrheal dermatitis; acne skin cleanser

Usual Dosage Children and Adults:

Shampoo: Initial: Use daily or every other day; 1-2 treatments/week will usually maintain control

Soap: Use daily or every other day

Dosage Forms

Cake: Sulfur 2% and salicylic acid 2% (123 g)

Cleanser: Sulfur 2% and salicylic acid 1.5% (60 mL, 120 mL)

Shampoo: Micropulverized sulfur 2% and salicylic acid 2% (120 mL, 240 mL)

Soap: Micropulverized sulfur 2% and salicylic acid 2% (113 g)

Wash: Sulfur 1.6% and salicylic acid 1.6% (75 mL)

sulfur and sodium sulfacetamide

Brand Names Novacet® Topical; Sulfacet-R® Topical

Synonyms sodium sulfacetamide and sulfur

Therapeutic Category Acne Products

Use Aid in the treatment of acne vulgaris, acne rosacea and seborrheic dermatitis

Usual Dosage Topical: Apply in a thin film 1-3 times/day

Dosage Forms Lotion, topical: Sulfur colloid 5% and sodium sulfacetamide 10% (30 mL)

sulindac (sul in' dak)
Brand Names Clinoril®
Therapeutic Category Analgesic, Non-Narcotic; Anti-inflammatory Agent; Nonsteroidal Anti-Inflammatory Agent (NSAID), Oral
Use Management of inflammatory disease, rheumatoid disorders; acute gouty arthritis; structurally similar to indomethacin but acts like aspirin; safest NSAID for use in mild renal impairment
Usual Dosage Oral:
Children: Dose not established
Adults: 150-200 mg twice daily; not to exceed 400 mg/day
Dosage Forms Tablet: 150 mg, 200 mg

sulphafurazole see sulfisoxazole on page 441

Sultrin™ see sulfabenzamide, sulfacetamide, and sulfathiazole on page 439

Sumacal® **[OTC]** see glucose polymers on page 209

sumatriptan succinate (soo' ma trip tan)
Brand Names Imitrex® Injection; Imitrex® Oral
Therapeutic Category Antimigraine Agent
Use Serotonin agonist for acute treatment of migraine
Usual Dosage Adults:
S.C.: 6 mg; a second injection may be administered at least 1 hour after the initial dose, but not more than 2 injections in a 24-hour period
Oral: Maximum dose 300 mg every 24 hours
Dosage Forms
Injection: 12 mg/mL (0.5 mL, 2 mL)
Tablet: 100 mg

Sumycin® **Oral** see tetracycline on page 451

sunscreen (paba-free) see methoxycinnamate and oxybenzone on page 297

Supprelin™ Injection see histrelin on page 225

Suppress® **[OTC]** see dextromethorphan hydrobromide on page 135

Suprane® see desflurane on page 129

Suprax® see cefixime on page 80

suprofen (soo proe' fen)
Brand Names Profenal® Ophthalmic
Therapeutic Category Nonsteroidal Anti-Inflammatory Agent (NSAID), Ophthalmic
Use Inhibition of intraoperative miosis
Usual Dosage On day of surgery, instill 2 drops in conjunctival sac at 3, 2, and 1 hour prior to surgery; or 2 drops in sac every 4 hours, while awake, the day preceding surgery
Dosage Forms Solution, ophthalmic: 1% (2.5 mL)

Surbex® **[OTC]** see vitamin b complex on page 490

Surbex® **with C Filmtabs®** **[OTC]** see vitamin b complex with vitamin c on page 490

Surbex-T® **Filmtabs®** **[OTC]** see vitamin b complex with vitamin c on page 490

Surfak® **[OTC]** see docusate on page 153

Surgicel® see cellulose, oxidized on page 84

Surmontil® see trimipramine maleate on page 473

Survanta® see beractant on page 51

Susano® see hyoscyamine, atropine, scopolamine, and phenobarbital on page 238

Sus-Phrine® *see* epinephrine *on page 167*
Sustaire® *see* theophylline *on page 453*

sutilains (soo' ti lains)
　Brand Names Travase℠ Topical
　Therapeutic Category Enzyme, Topical Debridement
　Use Promote debridement of necrotic debris, as an adjunct in the treatment of second and third degree burns, decubitus ulcers
　Usual Dosage Thoroughly cleanse and irrigate wound then apply ointment in a thin layer extending $1/4$" to $1/2$" beyond the tissue being debrided; apply loose moist dressing; repeat 3-4 times/day
　Dosage Forms Ointment: 82,000 casein units/g (14.2 g)

suxamethonium chloride *see* succinylcholine chloride *on page 437*
Sween Cream® **[OTC]** *see* methylbenzethonium chloride *on page 298*
Swim-Ear® **Otic [OTC]** *see* boric acid *on page 57*
Syllact® **[OTC]** *see* psyllium *on page 398*
Symadine® *see* amantadine hydrochloride *on page 17*
Symmetrel® *see* amantadine hydrochloride *on page 17*
Synacort® *see* hydrocortisone *on page 232*
synacthen *see* cosyntropin *on page 116*
Synalar-HP® **Topical** *see* fluocinolone acetonide *on page 195*
Synalar® **Topical** *see* fluocinolone acetonide *on page 195*
Synalgos®**-DC** *see* dihydrocodeine compound *on page 145*
Synarel® *see* nafarelin acetate *on page 316*
Synemol® **Topical** *see* fluocinolone acetonide *on page 195*
Synkayvite® *see* menadiol sodium diphosphate *on page 285*
synthetic lung surfactant *see* colfosceril palmitate *on page 113*
Synthroid® *see* levothyroxine sodium *on page 266*
Syntocinon® **Injection** *see* oxytocin *on page 345*
Syntocinon® **Nasal Spray** *see* oxytocin *on page 345*
Syprine® *see* trientine hydrochloride *on page 470*
Syracol-CF® **[OTC]** *see* guaifenesin and dextromethorphan *on page 214*
Sytobex® *see* cyanocobalamin *on page 119*
t_3/t_4 liotrix *see* liotrix *on page 270*
t_3 thyronine sodium *see* liothyronine sodium *on page 269*
t_4 thyroxine sodium *see* levothyroxine sodium *on page 266*
Tac™-3 *see* triamcinolone *on page 467*
Tacaryl® *see* methdilazine hydrochloride *on page 293*
TACE® *see* chlorotrianisene *on page 92*

tacrine hydrochloride (tak' reen)
　Brand Names Cognex℠ Oral
　Synonyms tetrahydroaminoacrine; tha
　Therapeutic Category Cholinergic Agent
　Use Treatment of Alzheimer's disease
　Usual Dosage Adults: Oral: 40 mg/day
　Dosage Forms Capsule: 10 mg, 20 mg, 30 mg, 40 mg

tacrolimus (ta kroe' li mus)
Brand Names Prograf®
Therapeutic Category Immunosuppressant Agent
Use Potent immunosuppressive drug used in liver, kidney, heart, lung, or small bowel transplant recipients
Usual Dosage
Initial: I.V. continuous infusion: 0.1 mg/kg/day until the tolerance of oral intake
Oral: Usually 3-4 times the I.V. dose, or 0.3 mg/kg/day in divided doses every 12 hours
Dosage Forms
Capsule: 1 mg, 5 mg
Injection, with alcohol and surfactant: 5 mg/mL (1 mL)

Tagamet® *see* cimetidine *on page 101*

Talacen® *see* pentazocine compound *on page 356*

talc for pleurodesis
Therapeutic Category Antidote, Malignant Pleural Effusion
Use Insufflation via thoracoscopy for management of malignant pleural effusion
Dosage Forms Aerosol 4 g can (delivering 0.4 g/sec)

Talwin® *see* pentazocine *on page 356*

Talwin® Compound *see* pentazocine compound *on page 356*

Talwin® NX *see* pentazocine *on page 356*

Tambocor® *see* flecainide acetate *on page 192*

Tamine® [OTC] *see* brompheniramine and phenylpropanolamine *on page 59*

tamoxifen citrate (ta mox' i fen)
Brand Names Nolvadex® Oral
Therapeutic Category Antineoplastic Agent, Hormone (Antiestrogen)
Use Palliative or adjunctive treatment of advanced breast cancer in postmenopausal women
Usual Dosage Oral: 10-20 mg twice daily
Dosage Forms Tablet: 10 mg

Tao® *see* troleandomycin *on page 475*

Tapazole® *see* methimazole *on page 294*

Tarabine® PFS *see* cytarabine hydrochloride *on page 123*

tat *see* tetanus antitoxin *on page 449*

Tavist® *see* clemastine fumarate *on page 104*

Tavist®-1 [OTC] *see* clemastine fumarate *on page 104*

Tavist-D® *see* clemastine and phenylpropanolamine *on page 104*

Taxol® *see* paclitaxel *on page 345*

Tazicef® *see* ceftazidime *on page 82*

Tazidime® *see* ceftazidime *on page 82*

tcn *see* tetracycline *on page 451*

td *see* diphtheria and tetanus toxoid *on page 150*

Tearisol® [OTC] *see* artificial tears *on page 34*

Tebamide® *see* trimethobenzamide hydrochloride *on page 472*

Tedral® *see* theophylline, ephedrine, and phenobarbital *on page 455*

Tega-Vert® Oral *see* dimenhydrinate *on page 147*

Tegison® *see* etretinate *on page 183*

Tegopen® *see* cloxacillin sodium *on page 109*
Tegretol® *see* carbamazepine *on page 73*
Tegrin®**-HC [OTC]** *see* hydrocortisone *on page 232*
T.E.H.® *see* theophylline, ephedrine, and hydroxyzine *on page 454*
Telachlor® **Oral** *see* chlorpheniramine maleate *on page 95*
Telador® *see* betamethasone *on page 52*
Teldrin® **Oral [OTC]** *see* chlorpheniramine maleate *on page 95*
Telepaque® *see* radiological/contrast media (ionic) *on page 404*
Teline® **Oral** *see* tetracycline *on page 451*
Temaril® *see* trimeprazine tartrate *on page 472*

temazepam (te maz' e pam)
  Brand Names Restoril®
  Therapeutic Category Benzodiazepine; Hypnotic; Sedative
  Use Treatment of anxiety and as an adjunct in the treatment of depression; also may be used in the management of panic attacks; transient insomnia and sleep latency
  Usual Dosage Adults: Oral: 15-30 mg at bedtime
  Dosage Forms Capsule: 7.5 mg, 15 mg, 30 mg

Temovate® **Topical** *see* clobetasol dipropionate *on page 106*
Tempra® **[OTC]** *see* acetaminophen *on page 2*
Tencet™ *see* butalbital compound *on page 63*
Tencon® *see* butalbital compound *on page 63*
Tenex® *see* guanfacine hydrochloride *on page 218*

teniposide (ten i poe' side)
  Brand Names Vumon Injection
  Synonyms ept; vm-26
  Therapeutic Category Antineoplastic Agent, Miscellaneous
  Use Treatment of Hodgkin's and non-Hodgkin's lymphomas, acute lymphocytic leukemia, bladder carcinoma and neuroblastoma
  Usual Dosage I.V.:
    Children: 130 mg/m^2/week, increasing to 150 mg/m^2 after 3 weeks and to 180 mg/m^2 after 6 weeks
    Adults: 50-180 mg/m^2 once or twice weekly for 4-6 weeks
  Dosage Forms Injection: 10 mg/mL (5 mL)

Tenoretic® *see* atenolol and chlorthalidone *on page 37*
Tenormin® *see* atenolol *on page 37*
Tensilon® *see* edrophonium chloride *on page 163*
Tenuate® *see* diethylpropion hydrochloride *on page 143*
Tepanil® *see* diethylpropion hydrochloride *on page 143*
Terazol® **Vaginal** *see* terconazole *on next page*

terazosin (ter ay' zoe sin)
  Brand Names Hytrin®
  Therapeutic Category Alpha-Adrenergic Blocking Agent, Oral
  Use Management of mild to moderate hypertension; considered a step 2 drug in stepped approach to hypertension; benign prostate hypertrophy
  Usual Dosage Adults: Oral: 1 mg; slowly increase dose to achieve desired blood pressure, up to 20 mg/day
  Dosage Forms Tablet: 1 mg, 2 mg, 5 mg, 10 mg

(Continued)

C.:
: 1500 units
ults >30 kg: 3000-5000 units

and Adults: Inject 10,000-40,000 units into wound; give 40,000-100,000

tion, equine: Not less than 400 units/mL (12.5 mL, 50 mL)

globulin, human
-Tet"

ry Immune Globulin
ation against tetanus; tetanus immune globulin is preferred over tetanus
nt of active tetanus; part of the management of an unclean, nonminor
hose history of previous receipt of tetanus toxoid is unknown or who has
hree doses of tetanus toxoid

us:
/kg; some recommend administering 250 units to small children

s:
0 units; some should infiltrate locally around the wound
0 units
ion: 250 units/mL

dsorbed
ry Toxoid
against tetanus
: I.M.:
: 0.5 mL; repeat 0.5 mL at 4-8 weeks after first dose and at 6-12 months

es are recommended only every 5-10 years
ion:
5 mL dose (0.5 mL, 5 mL)
2.5 mL dose (5 mL)

uid
xoid plain
ry Toxoid
on against tetanus in adults and children
3 doses of 0.5 mL I.M. or S.C. at 4- to 8-week intervals with fourth dose
hs after third dose
on:
5 mL dose (7.5 mL)
5 mL dose (0.5 mL, 7.5 mL)

see tetanus toxoid, fluid *on this page*

hloride (tet' ra kane)
aine" Injection; Pontocaine" Topical
ne hydrochloride
ry Local Anesthetic, Injectable; Local Anesthetic, Ophthalmic; Local
al Anesthetic, Topical
local anesthesia in the eye for various diagnostic and examination pur-
ed to nose and throat for various diagnostic procedures

efficacy have not been established

450

---

terbinafine hydrochloride (ter' bin a feen)
Brand Names Lamisil® Topical
Therapeutic Category Antifungal Agent, Topical
Use Topical antifungal for the treatment of tinea pedis, tinea cruris and tinea corporis
Usual Dosage Adults: Topical:
  Athlete's foot: Apply twice daily for at least 1 week, not to exceed 4 weeks
  Ringworm and jock itch: Apply once or twice daily for at least 1 week, not to exceed 4 weeks
Dosage Forms Cream: 1% (15 g, 30 g)

terbutaline sulfate (ter byoo' ta leen)
Brand Names Brethaire® Inhalation Aerosol; Brethine® Injection; Brethine® Oral; Bricanyl® Injection; Bricanyl® Oral
Therapeutic Category Adrenergic Agonist Agent; Beta-2-Adrenergic Agonist Agent; Bronchodilator; Tocolytic Agent
Use Bronchodilator in reversible airway obstruction and bronchial asthma; management of preterm labor
Usual Dosage
  Children <12 years:
    Oral: Initial: 0.05 mg/kg/dose 3 times/day, increased gradually as required; maximum: 0.15 mg/kg/dose 3-4 times/day or a total of 5 mg/24 hours
    S.C.: 0.005-0.01 mg/kg/dose to a maximum of 0.3 mg/dose every 15-20 minutes for 3 doses
    Inhalation nebulization dose: 0.06 mg/kg; maximum: 8 mg
    Inhalation: 0.3 mg/kg/dose up to maximum of 10 mg/dose every 4-6 hours

  Children >12 years and Adults:
    Oral:
      12-15 years: 2.5 mg every 6 hours 3 times/day; not to exceed 7.5 mg in 24 hours
      >15 years: 5 mg/dose every 6 hours 3 times/day; if side effects occur, reduce dose to 2.5 mg every 6 hours; not to exceed 15 mg in 24 hours
    S.C.: 0.25 mg/dose repeated in 15-30 minutes for one time only; a total dose of 0.5 mg should not be exceeded within a 4-hour period
    Nebulization: 0.01-0.03 mL/kg (1 mg = 1 mL); minimum dose: 0.1 mL; maximum dose: 2.5 mL diluted with 1-2 mL normal saline
    Inhalation: 2 inhalations every 4-6 hours; wait 1 minute between inhalations
Dosage Forms
  Aerosol, oral: 0.2 mg/actuation (10.5 g)
  Injection: 1 mg/mL (1 mL)
  Tablet: 2.5 mg, 5 mg

terconazole (ter kone' a zole)
Brand Names Terazol® Vaginal
Synonyms triaconazole
Therapeutic Category Antifungal Agent, Vaginal
Use Local treatment of vulvovaginal candidiasis
Usual Dosage One applicatorful in vagina at bedtime for 7 consecutive days
Dosage Forms
  Cream, vaginal: 0.4% (45 g); 0.8% (20 g)
  Suppository, vaginal: 80 mg (3s)

terfenadine (ter fen' a deen)
Brand Names Seldane®
Therapeutic Category Antihistamine
Use Perennial and seasonal allergic rhinitis and other allergic symptoms including urticaria
Usual Dosage Oral:
  Children:
    3-6 years: 15 mg twice daily
    6-12 years: 30 mg twice daily
(Continued)

447

terfenadine (Continued)

Children >12 years and Adults: 60 mg twice daily
Dosage Forms Tablet: 60 mg

terfenadine and pseudoephedrine

Brand Names Seldane-D®
Therapeutic Category Antihistamine/Decongestant Combination
Use Perennial and seasonal allergic rhinitis and other allergic symptoms including urticaria; has drying effect in patients with asthma
Usual Dosage Oral: Adults: One tablet every morning and at bedtime
Dosage Forms Tablet: Terfenadine 60 mg and pseudoephedrine hydrochloride 120 mg

teriparatide (ter i par' a tide)

Brand Names Parathar™ Injection
Therapeutic Category Diagnostic Agent, Hypothyroidism
Use Diagnosis of hypocalcemia in either hypoparathyroidism or pseudohypoparathyroidism
Usual Dosage I.V.:
Children ≥3 years: 3 units/kg up to 200 units
Adults: 200 units over 10 minutes
Dosage Forms Powder for injection: 200 units hPTH activity (10 mL)

terpin hydrate

Therapeutic Category Cough Preparation; Expectorant
Dosage Forms Elixir: 85 mg/5 mL (120 mL)

terpin hydrate and codeine

Synonyms eth and c
Therapeutic Category Cough Preparation; Expectorant
Use Symptomatic relief of cough
Usual Dosage Based on codeine content
Children (not recommended): 1-1.5 mg/kg/24 hours divided every 4 hours; maximum: 30 mg/24 hours
2-6 years: 1.25-2.5 mL every 4-6 hours as needed
6-12 years: 2.5-5 mL every 4-6 hours as needed <pdj[Adults: 10-20 mg/dose every 4-6 hours as needed
Dosage Forms Elixir: Terpin hydrate 85 mg and codeine 10 mg per 5 mL with alcohol 42.5%

Terramycin® I.M. Injection see oxytetracycline hydrochloride on page 345

Terramycin® Ophthalmic Ointment see oxytetracycline and polymyxin b on page 344

Terramycin® Oral see oxytetracycline hydrochloride on page 345

Terramycin® w/ Polymyxin B Sulfate see oxytetracycline and polymyxin b on page 344

Teslac® see testolactone on this page

tespa see thiotepa on page 458

Tessalon® Perles see benzonatate on page 49

Tes-Tape® [OTC] see diagnostic aids (in vitro), urine on page 137

Testoderm® Transdermal System see testosterone on next page

testolactone (tess toe lak' tone)

Brand Names Teslac™
Therapeutic Category Androgen
Use Palliative treatment of advanced disseminated breast carcinoma

Usual Dosage Adults: Females: Oral: 2[sponse may take as long as 3 months
Dosage Forms Tablet: 50 mg

Testopel® Pellet see testosterone on

testosterone (tess toss' ter one)

Brand Names Andro-Cyp® Injection; Ar jection; Andropository® Injection; Delate tion; Depo®-Testosterone Injection; Du jection; Histerone® Injection; Testoderr
Therapeutic Category Androgen
Use Androgen replacement therapy in breast pain and engorgement; inopera
Usual Dosage I.M.:
Delayed puberty: Children: 40-50 mg/m

Male hypogonadism: 50-400 mg every
Initiation of pubertal growth: 40-50 n
growth rate falls to prepubertal
During terminal growth phase: 10C
growth ceases
Maintenance virilizing dose: 100 m
50-400 mg/dose every 2-4 week

Inoperable breast cancer: Adults: 200-

Hypogonadism: Adults:
Testosterone or testosterone propi
Testosterone cypionate or enantha
Postpubertal cryptorchism: Testost
week

Transdermal system: Males: Place the
hair for optimal skin contact, do n
therapy with 6 mg/day system applie
system; the system should be worn

Dosing adjustment/comments in he
Dosage Forms
Injection:
Aqueous suspension: 25 mg/mL (1
(10 mL, 30 mL)
In oil, as cypionate: 100 mg/mL (1
In oil, as enanthate: 100 mg/mL (5
In oil, as propionate: 50 mg/mL (10
Pellet: 75 mg (1 pellet per vial)
Transdermal system: 4 mg/day; 6 mg/

testosterone and estradiol see estr

Testred® see methyltestosterone on ρ

tetanus and diphtheria toxoid see

tetanus antitoxin

Synonyms tat
Therapeutic Category Antitoxin
Use Tetanus prophylaxis or treatment
(TIG) is not available
(Continued)

tetanus antitoxi

Usual Dosage
Prophylaxis: I.M., S
Children <30 kg
Children and Ac

Treatment: Childrer
units I.V.

Dosage Forms Injec

tetanus immune

Brand Names Hype
Synonyms tig
Therapeutic Categc
Use Passive immuniz
antitoxin for treatme
wound in a person w
received less than t
Usual Dosage I.M.:
Prophylaxis of tetan
Children: 4 units
Adults: 250 units

Treatment of tetanu
Children: 500-30
Adults: 3000-600
Dosage Forms Injec

tetanus toxoid, a

Therapeutic Categc
Use Active immunity
Usual Dosage Adult
Primary immunizatio
after second dose
Routine booster dos
Dosage Forms Inject
Tetanus 5 Lf units/0
Tetanus 10 Lf units/

tetanus toxoid, fl

Synonyms tetanus tc
Therapeutic Categc
Use Active immunizat
Usual Dosage Inject
given only 6-12 mon
Dosage Forms Inject
Tetanus 4 Lf units/0
Tetanus 5 Lf units/0

tetanus toxoid plair

tetracaine hydroc

Brand Names Ponto
Synonyms amethoca
Therapeutic Categc
Anesthetic, Oral; Lo
Use Spinal anesthesia
poses; topically app
Usual Dosage
Children: Safety and

Adults:
  Ophthalmic (not for prolonged use):
    Ointment: Apply ½" to 1" to lower conjunctival fornix
    Solution: Instill 1-2 drops
  Spinal anesthesia 1% solution:
    Subarachnoid injection: 5-20 mg
    Saddle block: 2-5 mg; a 1% solution should be diluted with equal volume of CSF before administration
  Topical mucous membranes (2% solution): Apply as needed; dose should not exceed 20 mg
  Topical for skin: Apply to affected areas as needed

Dosage Forms
Cream: 1% (28 g)
Injection: 1% [10 mg/mL] (2 mL)
Injection, with dextrose 6%: 0.2% [2 mg/mL] (2 mL); 0.3% [3 mg/mL] (5 mL)
Ointment:
  Ophthalmic: 0.5% [5 mg/mL] (3.75 g)
  Topical: 0.5% [5 mg/mL] (28 g)
Solution:
  Ophthalmic: 0.5% [5 mg/mL] (1 mL, 2 mL, 15 mL, 59 mL)
  Topical: 2% [20 mg/mL] (30 mL, 118 mL)

tetracaine with dextrose

Brand Names Pontocaine® With Dextrose Injection
Therapeutic Category Local Anesthetic, Injectable
Use Spinal anesthesia (saddle block)
Usual Dosage Dose varies with procedure, depth of anesthesia, duration desired and physical condition of patient
Dosage Forms Injection: Tetracaine hydrochloride 0.2% with dextrose 6% (2 mL); tetracaine hydrochloride 0.3% with dextrose 6% (5 mL)

Tetracap® Oral *see* tetracycline *on this page*

tetracosactide *see* cosyntropin *on page 116*

tetracycline (tet ra sye' kleen)

Brand Names Achromycin® Ophthalmic; Achromycin® Topical; Achromycin® V Oral; Nor-tet® Oral; Panmycin® Oral; Robitet® Oral; Sumycin® Oral; Teline® Oral; Tetracap® Oral; Tetralan® Oral; Tetram® Oral; Topicycline® Topical
Synonyms tcn
Therapeutic Category Acne Products; Antibiotic, Ophthalmic; Antibiotic, Tetracycline Derivative; Antibiotic, Topical
Use Treatment of susceptible bacterial infections of both gram-positive and gram-negative organisms; also some unusual organisms including *Mycoplasma*, *Chlamydia*, and *Rickettsia*; may also be used for acne, exacerbations of chronic bronchitis, and treatment of gonorrhea and syphilis in patients that are allergic to penicillin
Usual Dosage
Children >8 years:
  Oral: 25-50 mg/kg/day in divided doses every 6 hours; not to exceed 3 g/day
  Ophthalmic:
    Suspension: Instill 1-2 drops 2-4 times/day or more often as needed
    Ointment: Instill every 2-12 hours

Adults:
  Oral: 250-500 mg/dose every 6 hours
  Ophthalmic:
    Suspension: Instill 1-2 drops 2-4 times/day or more often as needed
    Ointment: Instill every 2-12 hours
  Topical: Apply to affected areas 1-4 times/day
Dosage Forms
Capsule: 100 mg, 250 mg, 500 mg
(Continued)

tetracycline *(Continued)*
Ointment:
Ophthalmic: 1% [10 mg/mL] (3.5 g)
Topical: 3% [30 mg/mL] (14.2 g, 30 g)
Solution, topical: 2.2 mg/mL (70 mL)
Suspension:
Ophthalmic: 1% [10 mg/mL] (0.5 mL, 1 mL, 4 mL)
Oral: 125 mg/5 mL (60 mL, 480 mL)
Tablet: 250 mg, 500 mg

tetrahydroaminoacrine *see* tacrine hydrochloride *on page 444*

tetrahydrocannabinol *see* dronabinol *on page 159*

tetrahydrozoline hydrochloride (tet ra hye drozz' a leen)
Brand Names Collyrium Fresh® Ophthalmic [OTC]; Eyesine® Ophthalmic [OTC]; Eye-Zine® Ophthalmic [OTC]; Mallazine® Eye Drops [OTC]; Murine® Plus Ophthalmic [OTC]; Optigene® Ophthalmic [OTC]; Soothe® Ophthalmic [OTC]; Tetra-Ide® Ophthalmic [OTC]; Tyzine® Nasal; Visine® Ophthalmic [OTC]
Synonyms tetryzoline
Therapeutic Category Adrenergic Agonist Agent; Adrenergic Agonist Agent, Ophthalmic; Nasal Agent, Vasoconstrictor; Ophthalmic Agent, Vasoconstrictor
Use Symptomatic relief of nasal congestion and conjunctival congestion
Usual Dosage
Nasal congestion:
Children 2-6 years: Instill 2-3 drops of 0.05% solution every 4-6 hours as needed
Children >6 years and Adults: Instill 2-4 drops or 0.1% spray nasal mucosa every 4-6 hours as needed

Conjunctival congestion: Adults: Instill 1-2 drops in each eye 2-3 times/day
Dosage Forms Solution:
Nasal: (Tyzine®): 0.05% (15 mL), 0.1% (30 mL, 473 mL)
Ophthalmic:
Visine®: 0.05% (15 mL)
Visine A.C.®: 0.05% and zinc sulfate 0.25% (15 mL)

Tetra-Ide® Ophthalmic [OTC] *see* tetrahydrozoline hydrochloride *on this page*

Tetralan® Oral *see* tetracycline *on previous page*

Tetram® Oral *see* tetracycline *on previous page*

Tetramune® *see* diphtheria, tetanus toxoids, and whole-cell pertussis vaccine and hemophilus b conjugate vaccine *on page 151*

tetryzoline *see* tetrahydrozoline hydrochloride *on this page*

tg *see* thioguanine *on page 456*

6-tg *see* thioguanine *on page 456*

T/Gel® [OTC] *see* coal tar *on page 110*

T-Gen® *see* trimethobenzamide hydrochloride *on page 472*

T-Gesic® *see* hydrocodone and acetaminophen *on page 230*

tha *see* tacrine hydrochloride *on page 444*

Thalitone® *see* chlorthalidone *on page 99*

THAM-E® Injection *see* tromethamine *on page 476*

THAM® Injection *see* tromethamine *on page 476*

thc *see* dronabinol *on page 159*

Theelin® *see* estrone *on page 175*

Theo-24® *see* theophylline *on next page*

Theobid® *see* theophylline *on next page*

Theochron® *see* theophylline *on this page*

Theoclear® L.A. *see* theophylline *on this page*

Theo-Dur® *see* theophylline *on this page*

Theo-G® *see* theophylline and guaifenesin *on next page*

Theolair™ *see* theophylline *on this page*

Theolate® *see* theophylline and guaifenesin *on next page*

theophylline (thee off' i lin)

Brand Names Aerolate III®; Aerolate JR®; Aerolate SR® S; Aquaphyllin®; Asmalix®; Bronkodyl®; Elixicon®; Elixophyllin®; Quibron®-T; Quibron®-T/SR; Respbid®; Slo-bid™; Slo-Phyllin®; Sustaire®; Theo-24®; Theobid®; Theochron®; Theoclear® L.A.; Theo-Dur®; Theolair™; Theospan®-SR; Theovent®; Theo-X®; Uniphyl®

Therapeutic Category Antiasthmatic; Bronchodilator; Theophylline Derivative

Use Bronchodilator in reversible airway obstruction due to asthma or COPD; for neonatal apnea/bradycardia

Usual Dosage

Apnea: Dosage should be determined by plasma level monitoring; each 0.5 mg/kg of theophylline administered as a loading dose will result in a 1 mcg/mL increase in serum theophylline concentration

  Loading dose: 5 mg/kg; dilute dose in 1 hour I.V. fluid via syringe pump over one hour

  Maintenance: 2 mg/kg every 8-12 hours or 1-3 mg/kg/dose every 8-12 hours; administer I.V. push 1 mL/minute (2 mg/minute)

Treatment of acute bronchospasm in older patients: (>6 months of age): Loading dose (in patients not currently receiving theophylline): 6 mg/kg (based on aminophylline) given I.V. over 20-30 minutes; 4.7 mg/kg (based on theophylline) given I.V. over 20-30 minutes; administration rate should not exceed 20 mg (1 mL)/minute (theophylline) or 25 mg (1 mL)/minute (aminophylline)

Approximate maintenance dosage for treatment of acute bronchospasm:

  Children: 6 months to 9 years of age: 1.2 mg/kg/hour (aminophylline); 0.95 mg/kg/hour (theophylline); 9-16 years and young adult smokers: 1 mg/kg/hour (aminophylline); 0.79 mg/kg/hour (theophylline)

  Adult (healthy, nonsmoking): 0.7 mg/kg/hour (aminophylline); 0.55 mg/kg/hour (theophylline)

  Older patients and patients with cor pulmonale: 0.6 mg/kg/hour (aminophylline); 0.47 mg/kg/hour (theophylline)

  Patients with CHF or liver failure: 0.5 mg/kg/hour (aminophylline); 0.39 mg/kg/hour (theophylline)

  Chronic therapy: Slow clinical titration is generally preferred. Initial dose: 16 mg/kg/24 hours or 400 mg/24 hours, whichever is less; increasing dose: the above dosage may be increased in approximately 25% increments at 2- to 3-day intervals so long as the drug is tolerated or until the maximum dose is reached. Monitor serum levels.

Exercise caution in younger children who cannot complain of minor side effects. Older adults and those with cor pulmonale. CHF or liver disease may have unusually low dosage requirements.

Dosage Forms

Capsule:

  Immediate release (Bronkodyl®, Elixophyllin®): 100 mg, 200 mg

  Timed release:

    8-12 hours (Aerolate®): 65 mg [III]; 130 mg [JR], 260 mg [SR]

    8-12 hours (Slo-Bid™): 50 mg, 75 mg, 100 mg, 125 mg, 200 mg, 300 mg

    8-12 hours (Slo-Phyllin® Gyrocaps®): 60 mg, 125 mg, 250 mg

    12 hours (Theobid® Jr. Duracaps®): 130 mg

    12 hours (Theobid® Duracaps®): 260 mg

    12 hours (Theoclear® L.A.): 130 mg, 260 mg

    12 hours (Theo-Dur® Sprinkle®): 50 mg, 75 mg, 125 mg, 200 mg

    12 hours (Theospan®-SR): 130 mg, 260 mg

(Continued)

theophylline *(Continued)*

 12 hours (Theovent"): 125 mg, 250 mg
 24 hours (Theo-24'"): 100 mg, 200 mg, 300 mg
Elixir (Asmalix'", Elixomin'"', Elixophyllin'"', Lanophyllin'"): 80 mg/15 mL (15 mL, 30 mL, 480 mL, 4000 mL)
Infusion, in D₅W: 0.4 mg/mL (1000 mL); 0.8 mg/mL (500 mL, 1000 mL); 1.6 mg/mL (250 mL, 500 mL); 2 mg/mL (100 mL); 3.2 mg/mL (250 mL); 4 mg/mL (50 mL, 100 mL);
Solution, oral:
 Theolair™: 80 mg/15 mL (15 mL, 18.75 mL, 30 mL, 480 mL)
Syrup:
 Aquaphyllin'", Slo-Phyllin'", Theoclear-80'"', Theostat-80'"': 80 mg/15 mL (15 mL, 30 mL, 500 mL)
 Accurbron'": 150 mg/15 mL (480 mL)
Tablet: Immediate release:
 Slo-Phyllin'": 100 mg, 200 mg
 Theolair™: 125 mg, 250 mg
 Quibron'"-T: 300 mg
Tablet:
 Controlled release (Theo-X'"): 100 mg, 200 mg, 300 mg
 Timed release:
  12-24 hours: 100 mg, 200 mg, 300 mg
  8-12 hours (Quibron'"-T/SR): 300 mg
  8-12 hours (Respbid"): 250 mg, 500 mg
  8-12 hours (Sustaire"): 100 mg, 300 mg
  8-12 hours (T-Phyl"): 200 mg
  12-24 hours (Theochron'"): 100 mg, 200 mg, 300 mg
  8-24 hours (Theo-Dur'"): 100 mg, 200 mg, 300 mg, 450 mg
  8-24 hours (Theo-Sav"): 100 mg, 200 mg, 300 mg
  24 hours (Theolair™-SR): 200 mg, 250 mg, 300 mg, 500 mg
  24 hours (Uniphyl'"): 400 mg

theophylline and guaifenesin

Brand Names Bronchial'"; Glycerol-T'"; Lanophyllin-GG®; Quibron®; Slo-Phyllin GG®; Theo-G"; Theolate"
Therapeutic Category Antiasthmatic; Bronchodilator; Expectorant; Theophylline Derivative
Use Symptomatic treatment of bronchospasm associated with bronchial asthma, chronic bronchitis and pulmonary emphysema
Usual Dosage Adults: Oral: 1 or 2 capsules every 6-8 hours
Dosage Forms
 Capsule: Theophylline 150 mg and guaifenesin 90 mg; theophylline 300 mg and guaifenesin 180 mg
 Elixir: Theophylline 150 mg and guaifenesin 90 mg per 15 mL (480 mL)

theophylline, ephedrine, and hydroxyzine

Brand Names Hydrophen'"; Marax'"; T.E.H.'"
Therapeutic Category Antiasthmatic; Bronchodilator; Theophylline Derivative
Use Possibly effective for controlling bronchospastic disorders
Usual Dosage
 Children:
  2-5 years: $\frac{1}{2}$ tablet 2-4 times/day or 2.5 mL 3-4 times/day
  >5 years: $\frac{1}{2}$ tablet 2-4 times/day or 5 mL 3-4 times/day

 Adults: 1 tablet 2-4 times/day
Dosage Forms
 Syrup, dye free: Theophylline 32.5 mg, ephedrine 6.25 mg, and hydroxyzine 2.5 mg per 5 mL
 Tablet: Theophylline 130 mg, ephedrine 25 mg, and hydroxyzine 10 mg

theophylline, ephedrine, and phenobarbital
Brand Names Tedral®
Therapeutic Category Antiasthmatic; Bronchodilator; Theophylline Derivative
Use Prevention and symptomatic treatment of bronchial asthma; relief of asthmatic bronchitis and other bronchospastic disorders
Usual Dosage
Children >60 lb: 1 tablet or 5 mL every 4 hours
Adults: 1-2 tablets or 10-20 mL every 4 hours
Dosage Forms
Suspension: Theophylline 65 mg, ephedrine sulfate 12 mg, and phenobarbital 4 mg per 5 mL
Tablet: Theophylline 118 mg, ephedrine sulfate 25 mg, and phenobarbital 11 mg; theophylline 130 mg, ephedrine sulfate 24 mg, and phenobarbital 8 mg

theophylline ethylenediamine *see* aminophylline *on page 20*

Theospan®-SR *see* theophylline *on page 453*

Theovent® *see* theophylline *on page 453*

Theo-X® *see* theophylline *on page 453*

Thera-Combex® H-P Kapseals® [OTC] *see* vitamin b complex with vitamin c *on page 490*

TheraCys™ *see* BCG *on page 45*

Theramin® Expectorant [OTC] *see* guaifenesin and phenylpropanolamine *on page 215*

Theramycin Z® *see* erythromycin, topical *on page 172*

Theraplex Z® [OTC] *see* pyrithione zinc *on page 401*

Thermazene® *see* silver sulfadiazine *on page 423*

Theroxide® Wash [OTC] *see* benzoyl peroxide *on page 50*

thiabendazole (thye a ben' da zole)
Brand Names Mintezol®
Synonyms tiabendazole
Therapeutic Category Anthelmintic
Use Treatment of strongyloidiasis, cutaneous larva migrans, visceral larva migrans, dracunculiasis, trichinosis, and mixed helminthic infections
Usual Dosage Children and Adults: Oral: 50 mg/kg/day divided every 12 hours (maximum dose: 3 g/day)
Strongyloidiasis: For 2 consecutive days
Cutaneous larva migrans: For 2-5 consecutive days
Visceral larva migrans: For 5-7 consecutive days
Trichinosis: For 2-4 consecutive days
Dracunculosis: 50-75 mg/kg/day divided every 12 hours for 3 days
Dosage Forms
Suspension, oral: 500 mg/5 mL (120 mL)
Tablet, chewable (orange flavor): 500 mg

thiamazole *see* methimazole *on page 294*

thiamine hydrochloride (thye' a min)
Brand Names Betalin® S
Synonyms aneurine hydrochloride; thiaminium chloride hydrochloride; vitamin b₁
Therapeutic Category Vitamin, Water Soluble
Use Treatment of thiamine deficiency including beriberi, Wernicke's encephalopathy syndrome, and peripheral neuritis associated with pellagra, alcoholic patients with altered sensorium; various genetic metabolic disorders
(Continued)

thiamine hydrochloride *(Continued)*
Usual Dosage Dietary supplement (depends on caloric or carbohydrate content of the diet):
Infants: 0.3-0.5 mg/day
Children: 0.5-1 mg/day
Adults: 1-2 mg/day
Note: The above doses can be found as a combination in multivitamin preparations
Children:
Noncritically ill thiamine deficiency: Oral: 10-50 mg/day in divided doses every day for 2 weeks followed by 5-10 mg/day for one month
Beriberi: I.M.: 10-25 mg/day for 2 weeks, then 5-10 mg orally every day for one month (oral as therapeutic multivitamin)
Adults:
Wernicke's encephalopathy: I.M., I.V.: 50 mg as a single dose, then 50 mg I.M. every day until normal diet resumed
Noncritically ill thiamine deficiency: Oral: 10-50 mg/day in divided doses
Beriberi: I.M., I.V.: 10-30 mg 3 times/day for 2 weeks, then switch to 5-10 mg orally every day for one month (oral as therapeutic multivitamin)
Dosage Forms
Injection: 100 mg/mL (1 mL, 2 mL, 10 mL, 30 mL); 200 mg/mL (30 mL)
Tablet: 50 mg, 100 mg, 250 mg, 500 mg
Tablet, enteric coated: 20 mg

thiaminium chloride hydrochloride *see* thiamine hydrochloride *on previous page*

thiethylperazine maleate (thye eth il per' a zeen)
Brand Names Norzine"; Torecan"
Therapeutic Category Antiemetic
Use Relief of nausea and vomiting
Usual Dosage Children >12 years and Adults:
Oral, I.M., rectal: 10 mg 1-3 times/day as needed
I.V. and S.C. routes of administration are not recommended
Dosage Forms
Injection: 5 mg/mL (2 mL)
Suppository, rectal: 10 mg
Tablet: 10 mg

thimerosal (thye mer' oh sal)
Brand Names Aeroaid" [OTC]; Mersol" [OTC]; Merthiolate® [OTC]
Therapeutic Category Antibacterial, Topical
Use Organomercurial antiseptic with sustained bacteriostatic and fungistatic activity
Usual Dosage Apply 1-3 times/day
Dosage Forms
Ointment, ophthalmic: 0.02% [0.2 mg/mL] (3.5 g)
Solution, topical: 0.1% [1 mg/mL = 1:1000] (120 mL, 480 mL, 4000 mL)
Spray, antiseptic: 0.1% [1 mg/mL = 1:1000] with alcohol 2% (90 mL)
Tincture: 0.1% [1 mg/mL = 1:1000] with alcohol 50% (120 mL, 480 mL, 4000 mL)

thioguanine (thye oh gwah' neen)
Synonyms 2-amino-6-mercaptopurine; tg; 6-tg; 6-thioguanine; tioguanine
Therapeutic Category Antineoplastic Agent, Antimetabolite
Use Remission induction consolidation and maintenance therapy of acute nonlymphocytic leukemia; treatment of chronic myelogenous leukemia
Usual Dosage Oral (refer to individual protocols):
Infants <3 years: Combination drug therapy for acute nonlymphocytic leukemia: 3.3 mg/kg/day in divided doses twice daily for 4 days
Children and Adults: 2-3 mg/kg/day calculated to nearest 20 mg or 75-200 mg/m^2/day in 1-2 divided doses for 5-7 days or until remission is attained
Dosage Forms Tablet, scored: 40 mg

6-thioguanine *see* thioguanine *on previous page*

Thiola™ *see* tiopronin *on page 461*

thiopental sodium (thye oh pen' tal)
Brand Names Pentothal® Sodium
Therapeutic Category Barbiturate; General Anesthetic; Sedative
Use Induction of anesthesia; adjunct for intubation in head injury patients; control of convulsive states; treatment of elevated intracranial pressure
Usual Dosage I.V.:
Induction anesthesia:
Neonates: 3-4 mg/kg
Infants: 5-8 mg/kg
Children 1-12 years: 5-6 mg/kg
Adults: 3-5 mg/kg

Maintenance anesthesia:
Children: 1 mg/kg as needed
Adults: 25-100 mg as needed

Increased intracranial pressure: Children and Adults: 1.5-5 mg/kg/dose; repeat as needed to control intracranial pressure

Seizures:
Children: 2-3 mg/kg/dose, repeat as needed
Adults: 75-250 mg/dose, repeat as needed

Rectal administration: (Patient should be NPO for no less than 3 hours prior to administration)
Suggested initial doses of thiopental rectal suspension are:
<3 months: 15 mg/kg/dose
>3 months: 25 mg/kg/dose
Note: The age of a premature infant should be adjusted to reflect the age that the infant would have been if full-term (eg, an infant, now age 4 months, who was 2 months premature should be considered to be a 2-month old infant).
Doses should be rounded downward to the nearest 50 mg increment to allow for accurate measurement of the dose
Inactive or debilitated patients and patients recently medicated with other sedatives, (eg, chloral hydrate, meperidine, chlorpromazine, and promethazine), may require smaller doses than usual

If the patient is not sedated within 15-20 minutes, a single repeat dose of thiopental can be given. The single repeat doses are:
<3 months of age: <7.5 mg/kg/dose
>3 months of age: 15 mg/kg/dose
Children weighing >34 kg should not receive >1 g as a total dose (initial plus repeat doses)
Adults weighing >90 kg should not receive >3 g as a total dose (initial plus repeat doses)
Neither adults nor children should receive more than one course of thiopental rectal suspension (initial dose plus repeat dose) per 24-hour period
Dosage Forms
Injection: 250 mg, 400 mg, 500 mg, 1 g, 2.5 g, 5 g
Suspension, rectal: 400 mg/g (2 g)

thioridazine (thye oh rid' a zeen)
Brand Names Mellaril®; Mellaril-S®
Therapeutic Category Antipsychotic Agent; Phenothiazine Derivative
Use Management of manifestations of psychotic disorders; depressive neurosis; alcohol withdrawal; dementia in elderly; behavioral problems in children
Usual Dosage Oral:
Children >2 years: Range: 0.5-3 mg/kg/day in 2-3 divided doses; usual: 1 mg/kg/day; maximum: 3 mg/kg/day
(Continued)

457

thioridazine (Continued)

Behavior problems: Initial: 10 mg 2-3 times/day, increase gradually
Severe psychoses: Initial: 25 mg 2-3 times/day, increase gradually

Adults:
Psychoses: Initial: 50-100 mg 3 times/day with gradual increments as needed and tolerated; maximum daily dose: 800 mg/day in 2-4 divided doses
Depressive disorders, dementia: Initial: 25 mg 3 times/day; maintenance dose: 20-200 mg/day

Dosage Forms
Concentrate, oral: 30 mg/mL (120 mL); 100 mg/mL (3.4 mL, 120 mL)
Suspension, oral: 25 mg/5 mL (480 mL); 100 mg/5 mL (480 mL)
Tablet: 10 mg, 15 mg, 25 mg, 50 mg, 100 mg, 150 mg, 200 mg

thiotepa (thye oh tep' a)

Synonyms tespa; triethylenethiophosphoramide; tspa
Therapeutic Category Antineoplastic Agent, Alkylating Agent
Use Treatment of superficial tumors of the bladder; palliative treatment of adenocarcinoma of breast or ovary; lymphomas and sarcomas; controlling intracavitary effusions caused by metastatic tumors
Usual Dosage Refer to individual protocols
Children: Sarcomas: I.V.: 25-65 mg/m^2 as a single dose every 21 days

Adults:
I.M., I.V., S.C.: 8 mg/m^2 daily for 5 days or 30-60 mg/m^2 once per week
High dose therapy for bone marrow transplant: I.V.: 500 mg/m^2
Intracavitary: 0.6-0.8 mg/kg or 60 mg in 60 mL SWI instilled into the bladder at 1- to 4-week intervals
Intrathecal: Doses of 1-10 mg/m^2 administered 1-2 times/week in concentrations of 1 mg/mL diluted with preservative free sterile water for injection
Dosage Forms Powder for injection: 15 mg

thiothixene (thye oh thix' een)

Brand Names Navane®
Synonyms tiotixene
Therapeutic Category Antipsychotic Agent; Phenothiazine Derivative
Use Management of psychotic disorders
Usual Dosage
Children <12 years: Oral: Not well established; 0.25 mg/kg/24 hours in divided doses

Children >12 years and Adults:
Oral: Initial: 2 mg 3 times/day, up to 20-30 mg/day; maximum: 60 mg/day
I.M. (give undiluted injection): 4 mg 2-4 times/day, increase dose gradually; usual: 16-20 mg/day; maximum: 30 mg/day; change to oral dose as soon as able
Dosage Forms
Capsule: 1 mg, 2 mg, 5 mg, 10 mg, 20 mg
Concentrate, oral, as hydrochloride: 5 mg/mL (30 mL, 120 mL)
Injection, as hydrochloride: 2 mg/mL (2 mL)
Powder for injection, as hydrochloride: 5 mg/mL (2 mL)

Thorazine® see chlorpromazine hydrochloride on page 97
Thrombate® III see antithrombin III on page 30
Thrombinar® see thrombin, topical on this page

thrombin, topical

Brand Names Thrombinar®; Thrombogen®; Thrombostat®
Therapeutic Category Hemostatic Agent
Use Hemostasis whenever minor bleeding from capillaries and small venules is accessible

Usual Dosage Use 1000-2000 units/mL of solution where bleeding is profuse; apply powder directly to the site of bleeding or on oozing surfaces; use 100 units/mL for bleeding from skin or mucosal surfaces

Dosage Forms Powder: 1000 units, 5000 units, 10,000 units, 20,000 units, 50,000 units

Thrombogen® *see* thrombin, topical *on previous page*

Thrombostat® *see* thrombin, topical *on previous page*

thymopentin (thye' moe pen tin)
  Brand Names Timunox®
  Synonyms thymopoietin; tp5
  Therapeutic Category Immune Modulator
  Use Immunomodulator
  Dosage Forms Injection: 10 mg/mL (10 mL)

thymopoietin *see* thymopentin *on this page*

Thypinone® Injection *see* protirelin *on page 396*

Thyrar® *see* thyroid *on this page*

Thyro-Block® *see* potassium iodide *on page 379*

thyroid (thye' roid)
  Brand Names Armour® Thyroid; S-P-T; Thyrar®; Westhroid®
  Synonyms desiccated thyroid; thyroid extract
  Therapeutic Category Thyroid Product
  Use Replacement or supplemental therapy in hypothyroidism
  Usual Dosage Oral: Adults: Start at 30 mg/day and titrate by 30 mg/day in increments of 2- to 3-week intervals; usual maintenance dose: 60-120 mg/day
  Dosage Forms
    Capsule; 60 mg, 120 mg, 180 mg, 300 mg
    Tablet: 15 mg, 30 mg, 60 mg, 90 mg, 120 mg, 180 mg, 240 mg, 300 mg

thyroid extract *see* thyroid *on this page*

thyroid-stimulating hormone *see* thyrotropin *on this page*

Thyrolar® *see* liotrix *on page 270*

thyrotropin (thye roe troe' pin)
  Brand Names Thytropar®
  Synonyms thyroid-stimulating hormone; tsh
  Therapeutic Category Diagnostic Agent, Hypothyroidism; Diagnostic Agent, Thyroid Function
  Use Diagnostic aid to determine subclinical hypothyroidism or decreased thyroid reserve, to differentiate between primary and secondary hypothyroidism and between primary hypothyroidism and euthyroidism in patients receiving thyroid replacement
  Usual Dosage I.M., S.C.: 10 units/day for 1-3 days; follow by a radioiodine study 24 hours past last injection, no response in thyroid failure, substantial response in pituitary failure
  Dosage Forms Injection: 10 units

Thytropar® *see* thyrotropin *on this page*

tiabendazole *see* thiabendazole *on page 455*

Ticar® *see* ticarcillin disodium *on next page*

ticarcillin and clavulanate potassium
  Brand Names Timentin®
  Synonyms ticarcillin and clavulanic acid
  Therapeutic Category Antibiotic, Penicillin
  (Continued)

ticarcillin and clavulanate potassium *(Continued)*

Use Treat infections of lower respiratory tract, urinary tract, skin and skin structures, bone and joint, and septicemia caused by susceptible organisms. Clavulanate expands activity of ticarcillin to include beta-lactamase producing strains of *S. aureus*, *H. influenzae*, *Enterobacteriaceae*, *Pseudomonas*, *Klebsiella*, *Citrobacter*, and *Serratia*

Usual Dosage I.V.:

Children: 200-300 mg of ticarcillin/kg/day in divided doses every 4-6 hours

Adults: 3.1 g (ticarcillin 3 g plus clavulanic acid 0.1 g) every 4-6 hours; maximum: 18-24 g/day; for urinary tract infections: 3.1 g every 6-8 hours

Dosage Forms

Infusion, premixed (frozen): Ticarcillin disodium 3 g and clavulanic acid 0.1 g (100 mL)
Powder for injection: Ticarcillin disodium 3 g and clavulanic acid 0.1 g (3.1 g, 31 g)

ticarcillin and clavulanic acid *see* ticarcillin and clavulanate potassium *on previous page*

ticarcillin disodium (tye kar sill' in)

Brand Names Ticar®
Therapeutic Category Antibiotic, Penicillin
Use Treatment of susceptible infections such as septicemia, acute and chronic respiratory tract infections, skin and soft tissue infections, and urinary tract infections due to susceptible strains of *Pseudomonas*, *Proteus*, and *Escherichia coli* and *Enterobacter*
Usual Dosage I.V. (ticarcillin is generally given I.M. only for the treatment of uncomplicated urinary tract infections):

Neonates:
Postnatal age <7 days:
<2000 g: 150 mg/kg/day in divided doses every 12 hours
>2000 g: 225 mg/kg/day in divided doses every 8 hours
Postnatal age >7 days:
<1200 g: 150 mg/kg/day in divided doses every 12 hours
1200-2000 g: 225 mg/kg/day in divided doses every 8 hours
>2000 g: 300 mg/kg/day in divided doses every 6 hours

Infants and Children: 200-300 mg/kg/day in divided doses every 4-6 hours; maximum dose: 24 g/day

Adults: 1-4 g every 4-6 hours
Dosage Forms Powder for injection: 1 g, 3 g, 6 g, 20 g, 30 g

TICE® BCG *see* BCG *on page 45*

Ticlid® *see* ticlopidine hydrochloride *on this page*

ticlopidine hydrochloride (tye kloe' pi deen)

Brand Names Ticlid®
Therapeutic Category Antiplatelet Agent
Use Platelet aggregation inhibitor that reduces the risk of thrombotic stroke in patients who have had a stroke or stroke precursors
Usual Dosage Adults: Oral: 1 tablet twice daily with food
Dosage Forms Tablet: 250 mg

Ticon® *see* trimethobenzamide hydrochloride *on page 472*

tig *see* tetanus immune globulin, human *on page 450*

Tigan® *see* trimethobenzamide hydrochloride *on page 472*

Tilade® Inhalation Aerosol *see* nedocromil sodium *on page 321*

Timentin® *see* ticarcillin and clavulanate potassium *on previous page*

timolol maleate (tye' moe lole)
Brand Names Blocadren® Oral; Timoptic® Ophthalmic; Timoptic-XE® Ophthalmic
Therapeutic Category Beta-Adrenergic Blocker; Beta-Adrenergic Blocker, Ophthalmic
Use Ophthalmic dosage form used to treat elevated intraocular pressure such as glaucoma or ocular hypertension; orally for treatment of hypertension and angina and reduce mortality following myocardial infarction and prophylaxis of migraine
Usual Dosage
Children and Adults: Ophthalmic: Initial: 0.25% solution, instill 1 drop twice daily; increase to 0.5% solution if response not adequate; decrease to 1 drop/day if controlled; do not exceed 1 drop twice daily of 0.5% solution

Adults: Oral:
Hypertension: Initial: 10 mg twice daily, increase gradually every 7 days, usual dosage: 20-40 mg/day in 2 divided doses; maximum: 60 mg/day
Prevention of myocardial infarction: 10 mg twice daily initiated within 1-4 weeks after infarction
Migraine headache: Initial: 10 mg twice daily, increase to maximum of 30 mg/day
Dosage Forms
Gel, ophthalmic (Timoptic-XE®): 0.25% (2.5 mL, 5 mL); 0.5% (2.5 mL, 5 mL)
Solution, ophthalmic (Timoptic®): 0.25% (2.5 mL, 5 mL, 10 mL, 15 mL); 0.5% (2.5 mL, 5 mL, 10 mL, 15 mL)
Solution, ophthalmic, preservative free, single use (Timoptic® OcuDose®): 0.25%, 0.5%
Tablet (Blocadren®): 5 mg, 10 mg, 20 mg

Timoptic® Ophthalmic see timolol maleate on this page

Timoptic-XE® Ophthalmic see timolol maleate on this page

Timunox® see thymopentin on page 459

Tinactin® [OTC] see tolnaftate on page 464

TinBen® [OTC] see benzoin on page 49

TinCoBen® [OTC] see benzoin on page 49

Tindal® see acetophenazine maleate on page 6

Tinver® Lotion see sodium thiosulfate on page 432

tioconazole (tye oh kone' a zole)
Brand Names Vagistat® Vaginal
Therapeutic Category Antifungal Agent, Vaginal
Use Local treatment of vulvovaginal candidiasis
Usual Dosage Vaginal: Insert 1 applicatorful in vagina, just prior to bedtime, as a single dose
Dosage Forms Cream, vaginal: 6.5% with applicator (4.6 g)

tioguanine see thioguanine on page 456

tiopronin (tyo proe' nin)
Brand Names Thiola™
Therapeutic Category Urinary Tract Product
Use Prevention of kidney stone (cystine) formation in patients with severe homozygous cystinuric who have urinary cystine >500 mg/day who are resistant to treatment with high fluid intake, alkali, and diet modification, or who have had adverse reactions to penicillamine
Usual Dosage Adults: Initial dose is 800 mg/day, average dose is 1000 mg/day
Dosage Forms Tablet: 100 mg

tiotixene see thiothixene on page 458

Ti-Screen® [OTC] see methoxycinnamate and oxybenzone on page 297

Tisit® [OTC] see pyrethrins on page 400

tissue plasminogen activator, recombinant *see* alteplase, recombinant
on page 14

Titralac® Plus Liquid [OTC] *see* calcium carbonate and simethicone
on page 67

tmp *see* trimethoprim *on page 473*

tmp-smx *see* co-trimoxazole *on page 117*

TobraDex® Ophthalmic *see* tobramycin and dexamethasone *on this page*

tobramycin (toe bra mye' sin)

Brand Names AKTob Ophthalmic; Nebcin Injection; Tobrex Ophthalmic
Therapeutic Category Antibiotic, Aminoglycoside; Antibiotic, Ophthalmic
Use Treatment of documented or suspected *Pseudomonas aeruginosa* infection; infection with a nonpseudomonal enteric bacillus which is more sensitive to tobramycin than gentamicin based on susceptibility tests; susceptible organisms in lower respiratory tract infections, CNS infections, intra-abdominal, skin, bone, and urinary tract infections; empiric therapy in cystic fibrosis and immunocompromised patients; topically used to treat superficial ophthalmic infections caused by susceptible bacteria
Usual Dosage Dosage should be based on an estimate of ideal body weight
Neonates: I.M., I.V.:
  Postnatal age <7 days:
    <1000 g, <28 weeks gestational age: 3 mg/kg/dose every 24 hours
    <1500 g, <34 weeks gestational age: 2.5 mg/kg/dose every 18 hours
    >1500 g, >34 weeks gestational age: 2.5 mg/kg/dose every 12 hours
  Postnatal age >7 days:
    <2000 g: 2.5 mg/kg/dose every 12 hours
    >2000 g: 2.5 mg/kg/dose every 8 hours
Infants and Children: I.M., I.V.: 2.5 mg/kg/dose every 8 hours
  Note: Some patients may require larger or more frequent doses if serum levels document the need (ie, cystic fibrosis or febrile granulocytopenic patients)
Adults: I.M., I.V.: 3-5 mg/kg/day in 3 divided doses
Children and Adults: Renal dysfunction: 2.5 mg/kg (2-3 serum level measurements should be obtained after the initial dose to measure the half-life in order to determine the frequency of subsequent doses)
Children and Adults: Ophthalmic: 1-2 drops every 4 hours; apply ointment 2-3 times/day; for severe infections apply ointment every 3-4 hours, or 2 drops every 30-60 minutes initially, then reduce to less frequent intervals
Dosage Forms
Injection, as sulfate: 10 mg/mL (2 mL); 40 mg/mL (1.5 mL, 2 mL)
Ointment, ophthalmic: 0.3% (3.5 g)
Powder for injection: 40 mg/mL (1.2 g vials)
Solution, ophthalmic: 0.3% (5 mL)

tobramycin and dexamethasone

Brand Names TobraDex Ophthalmic
Synonyms dexamethasone and tobramycin
Therapeutic Category Antibiotic, Ophthalmic; Corticosteroid, Ophthalmic
Use Treatment of external ocular infection caused by susceptible gram-negative bacteria and steroid responsive inflammatory conditions of the palpebral and bulbar conjunctiva, lid, cornea, and anterior segment of the globe
Usual Dosage Ophthalmic: Adults:
Ointment: Apply 1.25 cm ($\frac{1}{2}$") every 3-4 hours to 2-3 times/day
Suspension: Instill 1-2 drops every 4-6 hours (first 24-48 hours may increase frequency to every 2 hours until signs of clinical improvement are seen); apply every 30-60 minutes for severe infections
Dosage Forms
Ointment, ophthalmic: Tobramycin 0.3% and dexamethasone 0.1% (3.5 g)
Suspension, ophthalmic: Tobramycin 0.3% and dexamethasone 0.1% (2.5 mL, 5 mL)

Tobrex® Ophthalmic *see* tobramycin *on previous page*

tocainide hydrochloride (toe kay' nide)
Brand Names Tonocard®
Therapeutic Category Antiarrhythmic Agent, Class Ib
Use Suppress and prevent symptomatic ventricular arrhythmias
Usual Dosage Adults: Oral: 1200-1800 mg/day in 3 divided doses
Dosage Forms Tablet: 400 mg, 600 mg

tocophersolan (toe koff er soe' lan)
Brand Names Liqui-E®
Therapeutic Category Vitamin, Fat Soluble
Use Approved for the treatment of vitamin E deficiency resulting from malabsorption due to prolonged cholestatic hepatobiliary disease.
Usual Dosage Dietary supplement: Oral: 15 mg (400 units) every day
Dosage Forms Liquid: 26.6 units/mL

Tofranil® Injection *see* imipramine *on page 242*
Tofranil® Oral *see* imipramine *on page 242*
Tofranil-PM® Oral *see* imipramine *on page 242*

tolazamide (tole az' a mide)
Brand Names Ronase®; Tolinase®
Therapeutic Category Antidiabetic Agent; Hypoglycemic Agent, Oral; Sulfonylurea Agent
Use Adjunct to diet for the management of mild to moderately severe, stable, noninsulin-dependent (type II) diabetes mellitus
Usual Dosage Adults: Oral: 100-1000 mg/day
Dosage Forms Tablet: 100 mg, 250 mg, 500 mg

tolazoline hydrochloride (tole az' oh leen)
Brand Names Priscoline® Injection
Synonyms benzazoline hydrochloride
Therapeutic Category Alpha-Adrenergic Blocking Agent, Parenteral; Vasodilator, Coronary
Use Persistent pulmonary vasoconstriction and hypertension of the newborn (persistent fetal circulation), peripheral vasospastic disorders
Usual Dosage
Neonates: Initial: I.V.: 1-2 mg/kg over 10-15 minutes via scalp vein or upper extremity; maintenance: 1-2 mg/kg/hour; use lower maintenance doses in patients with decreased renal function. Also used in neonates for acute vasospasm "cath toes" at 0.25 mg/kg/hour (no load)

Adults: Peripheral vasospastic disorder: I.M., I.V., S.C.: 10-50 mg 4 times/day
Dosage Forms Injection: 25 mg/mL (4 mL)

tolbutamide (tole byoo' ta mide)
Brand Names Orinase® Diagnostic Injection; Orinase® Oral
Therapeutic Category Antidiabetic Agent; Hypoglycemic Agent, Oral; Sulfonylurea Agent
Use Adjunct to diet for the management of mild to moderately severe, stable, noninsulin-dependent (type II) diabetes mellitus
Usual Dosage Adults:
Oral: 250-2000 mg/day
I.V. bolus: 20 mg/kg
Dosage Forms
Injection, diagnostic, as sodium: 1 g (20 mL)
Tablet: 250 mg, 500 mg

Tolectin® *see* tolmetin sodium *on this page*

Tolectin® DS *see* tolmetin sodium *on this page*

Tolinase® *see* tolazamide *on previous page*

tolmetin sodium (tole' met in)
Brand Names Tolectin®; Tolectin® DS
Therapeutic Category Analgesic, Non-Narcotic; Nonsteroidal Anti-Inflammatory Agent (NSAID), Oral
Use Treatment of rheumatoid arthritis and osteoarthritis, juvenile rheumatoid arthritis
Usual Dosage Oral:
Children ≥2 years: Anti-inflammatory: Initial: 20 mg/kg/day in 3 divided doses, then 15-30 mg/kg/day in 3 divided doses; maximum dose: 30 mg/kg/day

Adults: 400 mg 3 times/day; usual dose: 600-1.8 g/day; maximum: 2 g/day
Dosage Forms
Capsule (Tolectin® DS): 400 mg
Tablet (Tolectin®): 200 mg, 600 mg

tolnaftate (tole naf' tate)
Brand Names Absorbine® Antifungal [OTC]; Absorbine® Jock Itch [OTC]; Absorbine Jr.® Antifungal [OTC]; Aftate® [OTC]; Desenex® [OTC]; Dr Scholl's® Athlete's Foot [OTC]; Dr Scholl's® Maximum Strength Tritin [OTC]; Genaspor® [OTC]; NP-27® [OTC]; Tinactin® [OTC]; Zeasorb-AF® [OTC]
Therapeutic Category Antifungal Agent, Topical
Use Treatment of tinea pedis, tinea cruris, tinea corporis; due to *Trichophyton rubrum, T. mentagrophytes, T. tonsurans, Microsporum canis, M. audouinii,* and *Epidermophyton floccosum,* and for tinea versicolor due to *Malassezia furfur*
Usual Dosage Children and Adults: Topical: Wash and dry affected area; apply 1-2 drops of solution or a small amount of cream or powder and rub into the affected areas twice daily for 2-4 weeks
Dosage Forms
Aerosol, topical:
Liquid: 1% (59.2 mL, 90 mL, 120 mL)
Powder: 1% (56.7 g, 100 g, 105 g, 150 g)
Cream: 1% (0.7 g, 15 g, 21.3 g, 30 g)
Gel, topical: 1% (15 g)
Powder, topical: 1% (45 g, 90 g)
Solution, topical: 1% (10 mL)

Tolu-Sed® DM [OTC] *see* guaifenesin and dextromethorphan *on page 214*

Tomocat® *see* radiological/contrast media (ionic) *on page 404*

Tonocard® *see* tocainide hydrochloride *on previous page*

Tonopaque® *see* radiological/contrast media (ionic) *on page 404*

Topicort® *see* desoximetasone *on page 131*

Topicort®-LP *see* desoximetasone *on page 131*

Topicycline® Topical *see* tetracycline *on page 451*

Toprol XL® *see* metoprolol *on page 303*

topv *see* poliovirus vaccine, live (trivalent, oral) *on page 374*

Toradol® Injection *see* ketorolac tromethamine *on page 258*

Toradol® Oral *see* ketorolac tromethamine *on page 258*

Torecan® *see* thiethylperazine maleate *on page 456*

Tornalate® *see* bitolterol mesylate *on page 56*

torsemide (tore' se mide)
Brand Names Demadex® Injection; Demadex® Oral
Therapeutic Category Diuretic, Loop
Use Management of edema associated with congestive heart failure and hepatic or renal disease; used alone or in combination with antihypertensives in treatment of hypertension
Usual Dosage Adults:
Oral: 5-10 mg once daily; if ineffective, may double dose until desired effect is achieved
I.V.: 10-20 mg/dose repeated in 2 hours as needed with a doubling of the dose with each succeeding dose until desired diuresis is achieved
Continues to be effective in patients with cirrhosis, no apparent change in dose is necessary
Dosage Forms
Injection: 10 mg/mL (2 mL, 5 mL)
Tablet: 5 mg, 10 mg, 20 mg, 100 mg

Totacillin® *see* ampicillin *on page 26*

Totacillin®-N *see* ampicillin *on page 26*

Touro Ex® *see* guaifenesin *on page 213*

Touro LA® *see* guaifenesin and pseudoephedrine *on page 216*

tp5 *see* thymopentin *on page 459*

t-pa *see* alteplase, recombinant *on page 14*

TPM® Test *see* diagnostic aids (*in vitro*), blood *on page 136*

Trace-4® *see* trace metals *on this page*

trace metals
Brand Names Chroma-Pak®; Iodopen®; Molypen®; M.T.E.-4®; M.T.E.-5®; M.T.E.-6®; Multe-Pak-4®; Neotrace-4®; Pedte-Pak-5®; Pedtrace-4®; P.T.E.-4®; P.T.E.-5®; Trace-4®; Zinca-Pak®
Synonyms chromium; copper; manganese; molybdenum; neonatal trace metals; zinc
Therapeutic Category Trace Element, Parenteral
Use Supplement to TPN solutions
Dosage Forms
Chromium: Injection: 4 mcg/mL, 20 mcg/mL
Copper: Injection: 0.4 mg/mL, 2 mg/mL
Manganese: Injection: 0.1 mg/mL (as chloride or sulfate salt)
Molybdenum: Injection: 25 mcg/mL
Selenium: Injection: 40 mcg/mL
Zinc:
Capsule: 110 mg (25 mg elemental zinc); 220 mg (50 mg elemental zinc)
Injection: 1 mg/mL (sulfate); 1 mg/mL (chloride); 5 mg/mL (sulfate)
Liquid, as carbonate: 15 mg/mL
Tablet, as gluconate: 10 mg (1.4 mg elemental zinc); 15 mg (2 mg elemental zinc); 50 mg (7 mg elemental zinc); 78 mg (11 mg elemental zinc)
Tablet, as sulfate: 66 mg (15 mg elemental zinc); 200 mg (45 mg elemental zinc)

Tracer bG® [OTC] *see* diagnostic aids (*in vitro*), blood *on page 136*

Tracrium® *see* atracurium besylate *on page 38*

Trandate® Injection *see* labetalol hydrochloride *on page 260*

Trandate® Oral *see* labetalol hydrochloride *on page 260*

tranexamic acid (tran ex am' ik)
Brand Names Cyklokapron® Injection; Cyklokapron® Oral
Therapeutic Category Antihemophilic Agent
Use Short-term use (2-8 days) in hemophilia patients during and following tooth extraction to reduce or prevent hemorrhage
Usual Dosage Children and Adults: I.V.: 10 mg/kg immediately before surgery, then 25 mg/kg/dose orally 3-4 times/day for 2-8 days
(Continued)
465

tranexamic acid *(Continued)*

Alternatively:
Oral: 25 mg/kg 3-4 times/day beginning 1 day prior to surgery
I.V.: 10 mg/kg 3-4 times/day in patients who are unable to take oral
Dosage Forms
Injection: 100 mg/mL (10 mL)
Tablet: 500 mg

transamine sulphate *see* tranylcypromine sulfate *on this page*
Transdermal-NTG® Patch *see* nitroglycerin *on page 329*
Transderm-Nitro® Patch *see* nitroglycerin *on page 329*
Transderm Scop® Patch *see* scopolamine *on page 418*
Trans-Plantar® Transdermal Patch [OTC] *see* salicylic acid *on page 416*
Trans-Ver-Sal® Transdermal Patch [OTC] Verukan® Solution *see* salicylic acid *on page 416*
Tranxene® *see* clorazepate dipotassium *on page 108*

tranyicypromine sulfate (tran ill sip' roe meen)

Brand Names Parnate®
Synonyms transamine sulphate
Therapeutic Category Antidepressant, Monoamine Oxidase Inhibitor
Use Symptomatic treatment of depressed patients refractory to or intolerant to tricyclic antidepressants or electroconvulsive therapy; has a more rapid onset of therapeutic effect than other MAO inhibitors, but causes more severe hypertensive reactions
Usual Dosage Adults: Oral: 10 mg twice daily, increase by 10 mg increments at 1- to 3-week intervals; maximum: 60 mg/day
Dosage Forms Tablet: 10 mg

Trasylol® *see* aprotinin *on page 32*
Travase® Topical *see* sutilains *on page 444*

trazodone hydrochloride (traz' oh done)

Brand Names Desyrel®
Therapeutic Category Antidepressant
Use Treatment of depression
Usual Dosage Oral:
Adolescents: Initial: 25-50 mg/day; increase to 100-150 mg/day in divided doses

Adults: Initial: 150 mg/day in 3 divided doses (may increase by 50 mg/day every 3-7 days); maximum: 600 mg/day
Dosage Forms Tablet: 50 mg, 100 mg, 150 mg, 300 mg

Trecator®-SC *see* ethionamide *on page 180*
Trendar® [OTC] *see* ibuprofen *on page 240*
Trental® *see* pentoxifylline *on page 357*

tretinoin (tret' i noyn)

Brand Names Retin-A™ Topical; Vesanoid® Injection
Synonyms retinoic acid; vitamin a acid
Therapeutic Category Acne Products; Retinoic Acid Derivative; Vitamin, Topical
Use
Injection: Indection of remission of acute promyelocytic leukemia
Topical: Treatment of acne vulgaris, photodamaged skin, and some skin cancers
Usual Dosage Children >12 years and Adults: Topical: Apply once daily before retiring; if stinging or irritation develop, decrease frequency of application

Dosage Forms
Cream: 0.025% (20 g, 45 g); 0.05% (20 g, 45 g); 0.1% (20 g, 45 g)
Gel, topical: 0.01% (15 g, 45 g); 0.025% (15 g, 45 g)
Injection:
Liquid, topical: 0.05% (28 mL)

Trexan™ Oral *see* naltrexone hydrochloride *on page 318*

triacetin (trye a see' tin)
Brand Names Fungoid®; Ony-Clear® Nail
Synonyms glycerol triacetate
Therapeutic Category Antifungal Agent, Topical
Use Fungistat for athlete's foot and other superficial fungal infections
Usual Dosage Apply twice daily, cleanse areas with dilute alcohol or mild soap and water before application; continue treatment for 7 days after symptoms have disappeared
Dosage Forms
Cream: With cetylpyridinium chloride and chloroxylenol (30 g)
Liquid: With cetylpyridinium chloride and chloroxylenol (30 mL)
Solution: With cetylpyridinium chloride, chloroxylenol, and benzalkonium chloride in an oil base (15 mL)
Spray, aerosol: With cetylpyridinium chloride, chloroxylenol, and benzalkonium chloride (45 mL, 60 mL)

triacetyloleandomycin *see* troleandomycin *on page 475*

Triacin-C® *see* triprolidine, pseudoephedrine, and codeine *on page 475*

triaconazole *see* terconazole *on page 447*

Triad® *see* butalbital compound *on page 63*

Triam-A® *see* triamcinolone *on this page*

triamcinolone (trye am sin' oh lone)
Brand Names Amcort®; Aristocort® Forte; Aristocort® Intralesional Suspension; Aristocort® Tablet; Aristospan®; Azmacort™; Delta-Tritex®; Kenacort® Syrup; Kenacort® Tablet; Kenalog® Injection; Kenalog® in Orabase®; Kenonel®; Nasacort®; Tac™-3; Triam-A®; Triamolone®; Tri-Kort®; Trilog®; Trilone®; Trisoject®
Therapeutic Category Anti-inflammatory Agent; Corticosteroid, Inhalant; Corticosteroid, Systemic; Corticosteroid, Topical (Medium Potency)
Use For severe inflammation or immunosuppression
Usual Dosage In general, single I.M. dose of 4-7 times oral dose will control patient from 4-7 days up to 3-4 weeks.

Children 6-12 years:
Inhalation: 1-2 inhalations 3-4 times/day, not to exceed 12 inhalations/day
I.M.: Acetonide or hexacetonide: 0.03-0.2 mg/kg at 1- to 7-day intervals

Children >12 years and Adults:
Intranasal: 2 sprays in each nostril once daily; may increase after 4-7 days up to 4 sprays once daily or 1 spray 4 times/day in each nostril
Topical: Apply a thin film 2-3 times/day
Oral: 4-100 mg/day
I.M.: Acetonide or hexacetonide: 60 mg (of 40 mg/mL), additional 20-100 mg doses (usual: 40-80 mg) may be given when signs and symptoms recur, best at 6-week intervals to minimize HPA suppression
Oral inhalation: 2 inhalations 3-4 times/day, not to exceed 16 inhalations/day
Intra-articularly, intrasynovially, intralesionally: 2.5-40 mg as diacetate salt or acetonide salt, dose may be repeated when signs and symptoms recur
Intra-articularly: Hexacetonide: 2-20 mg every 3-4 weeks as hexacetonide salt
Intralesional (use 10 mg/mL): Diacetate or acetonide: 1 mg/injection site, may be repeated one or more times/week depending upon patients response; maximum; 30 mg at any one time; may use multiple injections if they are more than 1 cm apart
(Continued)

triamcinolone *(Continued)*

Intra-articular, intrasynovial, and soft-tissue injection (use 10 mg/mL or 40 mg/mL): Diacetate or acetonide: 2.5-40 mg depending upon location, size of joints, and degree of inflammation; repeat when signs and symptoms recur

Sublesionally (as acetonide): Up to 1 mg per injection site and may be repeated one or more times weekly; multiple sites may be injected if they are 1 cm or more apart, not to exceed 30 mg

Dosage Forms

Aerosol:

Oral inhalation: 100 mcg/metered spray (2 oz)

Nasal: 55 mcg per actuation (15 mL)

Topical, as acetonide: 0.2 mg/2 second spray (23 g, 63 g)

Cream, as acetonide: 0.025% (15 g, 60 g, 80 g, 240 g, 454 g); 0.1% (15 g, 30 g, 60 g, 80 g, 90 g, 120 g, 240 g); 0.5% (15 g, 20 g, 30 g, 240 g)

Injection, as acetonide: 10 mg/mL (5 mL); 40 mg/mL (1 mL, 5 mL, 10 mL)

Injection, as diacetate: 25 mg/mL (5 mL); 40 mg/mL (1 mL, 5 mL, 10 mL)

Injection, as hexacetonide: 5 mg/mL (5 mL); 20 mg/mL (1 mL, 5 mL)

Lotion, as acetonide: 0.025% (60 mL); 0.1% (15 mL, 60 mL)

Ointment:

Oral: 0.1% (5 g)

Topical, as acetonide: 0.025% (15 g, 30 g, 60 g, 80 g, 120 g, 454 g); 0.1% (15 g, 30 g, 60 g, 80 g, 120 g, 240 g, 454 g); 0.5% (15 g, 20 g, 30 g, 240 g)

Syrup: 2 mg/5 mL (120 mL); 4 mg/5 mL (120 mL)

Tablet: 1 mg, 2 mg, 4 mg, 8 mg

triamcinolone and nystatin *see* nystatin and triamcinolone *on page 335*

Triaminic-12® [OTC] *see* chlorpheniramine and phenylpropanolamine *on page 94*

Triaminicol® Multi-Symptom Cold Syrup [OTC] *see* chlorpheniramine, phenylpropanolamine, and dextromethorphan *on page 96*

Triaminic® Oral Infant Drops *see* pheniramine, phenylpropanolamine, and pyrilamine *on page 361*

Triaminic® Syrup [OTC] *see* chlorpheniramine and phenylpropanolamine *on page 94*

Triaminic® Expectorant [OTC] *see* guaifenesin and phenylpropanolamine *on page 215*

Triaminic® AM Decongestant Formula [OTC] *see* pseudoephedrine *on page 397*

Triamolone® *see* triamcinolone *on previous page*

triamterene (trye am' ter een)

Brand Names Dyrenium®

Therapeutic Category Diuretic, Potassium Sparing

Use Alone or in combination with other diuretics to treat edema and hypertension; decreases potassium excretion caused by kaliuretic diuretics

Usual Dosage Oral:

Children: 2-4 mg/kg/day in 1-2 divided doses; maximum: 300 mg/day

Adults: 100-300 mg/day in 1-2 divided doses; maximum dose: 300 mg/day

Dosage Forms Capsule: 50 mg, 100 mg

triamterene and hydrochlorothiazide *see* hydrochlorothiazide and triamterene *on page 229*

Triaprin® *see* butalbital compound *on page 63*

Triavil® *see* amitriptyline and perphenazine *on page 21*

triazolam (trye ay' zoe lam)
Brand Names Halcion®
Therapeutic Category Benzodiazepine; Hypnotic; Sedative
Use Short-term treatment of insomnia
Usual Dosage Oral (onset of action is rapid, patient should be in bed when taking medication):
Children <18 years: Dosage not established
Adults: 0.125-0.25 mg at bedtime
Dosage Forms Tablet: 0.125 mg, 0.25 mg

Triban® *see* trimethobenzamide hydrochloride *on page 472*

tribavirin *see* ribavirin *on page 410*

Tri-Chlor® *see* trichloroacetic acid *on this page*

trichlormethiazide (trye klor meth eye' a zide)
Brand Names Metahydrin®; Naqua®
Therapeutic Category Diuretic, Thiazide
Use Management of mild to moderate hypertension; treatment of edema in congestive heart failure and nephrotic syndrome
Usual Dosage Oral:
Children >6 months: 0.07 mg/kg/24 hours or 2 mg/m^2/24 hours
Adults: 1-4 mg/day
Dosage Forms Tablet: 2 mg, 4 mg

trichloroacetaldehyde monohydrate *see* chloral hydrate *on page 87*

trichloroacetic acid
Brand Names Tri-Chlor®
Therapeutic Category Keratolytic Agent
Use Debride callous tissue
Usual Dosage Apply to verruca, cover with bandage for 5-6 days, remove verruca, reapply as needed
Dosage Forms Liquid: 80% (15 mL)

***Trichophyton* skin test** (try ko fi' ton)
Brand Names Dermatophytin®
Therapeutic Category Diagnostic Agent, Skin Test
Use Assess cell-mediated immunity
Usual Dosage 0.1 mL intradermally, examine reaction site in 24-48 hours; induration of ≥5 mm in diameter is a positive reaction
Dosage Forms Injection:
Diluted: 1:30 V/V (5 mL)
Undiluted: 5 mL

Tri-Clear® Expectorant [OTC] *see* guaifenesin and phenylpropanolamine *on page 215*

Tricosal® *see* choline magnesium trisalicylate *on page 100*

Tridesilon® Topical *see* desonide *on page 130*

tridihexethyl chloride (trye dye hex e' thill)
Brand Names Pathilon®
Therapeutic Category Anticholinergic Agent; Antispasmodic Agent, Gastrointestinal
Use Adjunctive therapy in peptic ulcer treatment
(Continued)

tridihexethyl chloride (Continued)
Usual Dosage Adults: Oral: 1-2 tablets 3-4 times/day before meals and 2 tablets at bedtime
Dosage Forms Tablet: 25 mg

Tridil® Injection see nitroglycerin on page 329

Tridione® see trimethadione on page 472

trientine hydrochloride (trye' en teen)
Brand Names Syprine®
Therapeutic Category Antidote, Copper Toxicity; Chelating Agent, Oral
Use Treatment of Wilson's disease in patients intolerant to penicillamine
Usual Dosage Oral (administer on an empty stomach):
  Children <12 years: 500-750 mg/day in divided doses 2-4 times/day; maximum: 1.5 g/day
  Adults: 750-1250 mg/day in divided doses 2-4 times/day; maximum daily dose: 2 g
Dosage Forms Capsule: 250 mg

triethanolamine polypeptide oleate-condensate (trye eth a nole' a meen)
Brand Names Cerumenex® Otic
Therapeutic Category Otic Agent, Cerumenolytic
Use Removal of ear wax (cerumen)
Usual Dosage Children and Adults: Otic: Fill ear canal, insert cotton plug; allow to remain
  15-30 minutes; flush ear with lukewarm water
Dosage Forms Solution, otic: 6 mL, 12 mL

triethanolamine salicylate
Brand Names Myoflex® [OTC]; Sportscreme® [OTC]
Therapeutic Category Analgesic, Topical
Use Relief of pain of muscular aches, rheumatism, neuralgia, sprains, arthritis on intact skin
Usual Dosage Apply to area as needed
Dosage Forms Cream: 10% in a nongreasy base

triethylenethiophosphoramide see thiotepa on page 458

Trifed-C® see triprolidine, pseudoephedrine, and codeine on page 475

Trifed® [OTC] see triprolidine and pseudoephedrine on page 474

trifluoperazine hydrochloride (trye floo oh per' a zeen)
Brand Names Stelazine® Injection; Stelazine® Oral
Therapeutic Category Antianxiety Agent; Antipsychotic Agent; Phenothiazine Derivative
Use Treatment of psychoses and management of anxiety
Usual Dosage
  Children 6-12 years: Psychoses:
    Oral: Hospitalized or well supervised patients: Initial dose: 1 mg 1-2 times/day, gradually
      increase until symptoms are controlled or adverse effects become troublesome; max-
      imum: 15 mg/day
    I.M.: 1 mg twice daily

  Adults:
    Psychoses:
      Outpatients: Oral: 1-2 mg twice daily
      Hospitalized or well supervised patients: Initial dose: 2-5 mg twice daily with optimum
        response in the 15-20 mg/day range; do not exceed 40 mg/day
      I.M.: 1-2 mg every 4-6 hours as needed up to 10 mg/24 hours maximum
    Nonpsychotic anxiety: Oral: 1-2 mg twice daily; maximum: 6 mg/day; therapy for anxiety
      should not exceed 12 weeks; do not exceed 6 mg/day for longer than 12 weeks when
      treating anxiety; agitation, jitteriness or insomnia may be confused with original neu-
      rotic or psychotic symptoms

Dosage Forms
Concentrate, oral: 10 mg/mL (60 mL)
Injection: 2 mg/mL (10 mL)
Tablet: 1 mg, 2 mg, 5 mg, 10 mg

trifluorothymidine *see* trifluridine *on this page*

triflupromazine hydrochloride (trye floo proe' ma zeen)
Brand Names Vesprin®
Therapeutic Category Phenothiazine Derivative
Use Treatment of psychoses, nausea, vomiting, and intractable hiccups
Usual Dosage
Children: I.M.: 0.2-0.25 mg/kg

Adults:
I.M.: 5-15 mg every 4 hours
I.V.: 1 mg
Dosage Forms Injection: 20 mg/mL (1 mL)

trifluridine (trye flure' i deen)
Brand Names Viroptic® Ophthalmic
Synonyms f$_3$t; trifluorothymidine
Therapeutic Category Antiviral Agent, Ophthalmic
Use Treatment of primary keratoconjunctivitis and recurrent epithelial keratitis caused by herpes simplex virus types I and II
Usual Dosage Adults: Instill 1 drop into affected eye every 2 hours while awake, to a maximum of 9 drops/day, until re-epithelialization of corneal ulcer occurs; then use 1 drop every 4 hours for another 7 days; do **not** exceed 21 days of treatment
Dosage Forms Solution, ophthalmic: 1% (7.5 mL)

triglycerides, medium chain *see* medium chain triglycerides *on page 283*
Trihexy® *see* trihexyphenidyl hydrochloride *on this page*

trihexyphenidyl hydrochloride (trye hex ee fen' i dill)
Brand Names Artane®; Trihexy®
Synonyms benzhexol hydrochloride
Therapeutic Category Anticholinergic Agent; Anti-Parkinson's Agent
Use Adjunctive treatment of Parkinson's disease; also used in treatment of drug-induced extrapyramidal effects and acute dystonic reactions
Usual Dosage
Parkinsonism: Initial: Administer 1-2 mg the first day; increase by 2 mg increments at intervals of 3-5 days, until a total of 6-10 mg is given daily. Many patients derive maximum benefit from a total daily dose of 6-10 mg; however, postencephalitic patients may require a total daily dose of 12-15 mg in 3-4 divided doses

Concomitant use with levodopa: 3-6 mg/day in divided doses is usually adequate

Drug-induced extrapyramidal disorders: Start with a single 1 mg dose; daily dosage usually ranges between 5-15 mg in 3-4 divided doses
Dosage Forms
Capsule, sustained release: 5 mg
Elixir: 2 mg/5 mL (480 mL)
Tablet: 2 mg, 5 mg

Tri-Hydroserpine® *see* hydralazine, hydrochlorothiazide, and reserpine *on page 228*

471

Tri-Immunol® *see* diphtheria and tetanus toxoids and pertussis vaccine, adsorbed *on page 150*

Tri-Kort® *see* triamcinolone *on page 467*

Trilafon® *see* perphenazine *on page 359*

Tri-Levlen® *see* ethinyl estradiol and levonorgestrel *on page 178*

Trilisate® *see* choline magnesium trisalicylate *on page 100*

Trilog® *see* triamcinolone *on page 467*

Trilone® *see* triamcinolone *on page 467*

Trimazide® *see* trimethobenzamide hydrochloride *on this page*

trimeprazine tartrate (trye mep' ra zeen)
Brand Names Temaril®
Synonyms alimenazine tartrate
Therapeutic Category Antihistamine; Phenothiazine Derivative
Use Perennial and seasonal allergic rhinitis and other allergic symptoms including urticaria
Usual Dosage Oral:
   Children:
       6 months to 3 years: 1.25 mg at bedtime or 3 times/day if needed
       >3 years: 2.5 mg at bedtime or 3 times/day if needed
       >6 years: Sustained release: 5 mg/day

   Adults: 2.5 mg 4 times/day (5 mg every 12-hour sustained release)
Dosage Forms
   Capsule, extended release: 5 mg
   Syrup: 2.5 mg/5 mL
   Tablet: 2.5 mg

trimethadione (trye meth a dye' one)
Brand Names Tridione®
Synonyms troxidone
Therapeutic Category Anticonvulsant, Oxazolidinedione
Use Control absence (petit mal) seizures refractory to other drugs
Usual Dosage Oral:
   Children: Initial: 25-50 mg/kg/24 hours in 3-4 equally divided doses every 6-8 hours

   Adults: Initial: 900 mg/day in 3-4 equally divided doses, increase by 300 mg/day at weekly intervals until therapeutic results or toxic symptoms appear
Dosage Forms
   Capsule: 300 mg
   Solution: 40 mg/mL (473 mL)
   Tablet, chewable: 150 mg

trimethaphan camsylate (trye meth' a fan)
Brand Names Arfonad® Injection
Therapeutic Category Adrenergic Blocking Agent; Anticholinergic Agent; Ganglionic Blocking Agent
Use Immediate and temporary reduction of blood pressure in patients with hypertensive emergencies; controlled hypotension during surgery
Usual Dosage I.V.:
   Children: 50-150 mcg/kg/minute
   Adults: Initial: 0.5-2 mg/minute; titrate to effect; usual dose: 0.3-6 mg/minute
Dosage Forms Injection: 50 mg/mL (10 mL)

trimethobenzamide hydrochloride (trye meth oh ben' za mide)
Brand Names Arrestin®; Pediatric Triban®; Tebamide®; T-Gen®; Ticon®; Tigan®; Triban®; Trimazide®
Therapeutic Category Antiemetic

Use Control of nausea and vomiting (especially for long-term antiemetic therapy)
Usual Dosage Rectal use: Contraindicated in neonates and premature infants
Children:
Oral, rectal: 15-20 mg/kg/day or 400-500 mg/m^2/day divided into 3-4 doses
I.M.: Not recommended

Adults:
Oral: 250 mg 3-4 times/day
I.M., rectal: 200 mg 3-4 times/day
Dosage Forms
Capsule: 100 mg, 250 mg
Injection: 100 mg/mL (2 mL, 20 mL)
Suppository, rectal: 100 mg, 200 mg

trimethoprim (trye meth' oh prim)
Brand Names Proloprim®; Trimpex®
Synonyms tmp
Therapeutic Category Antibiotic, Miscellaneous
Use Treatment of urinary tract infections; acute otitis media in children; acute exacerbations of chronic bronchitis in adults
Usual Dosage Adults: Oral: 100 mg every 12 hours or 200 mg every 24 hours
Dosage Forms Tablet: 100 mg, 200 mg

trimethoprim and polymyxin b
Brand Names Polytrim® Ophthalmic
Synonyms polymyxin b and trimethoprim
Therapeutic Category Antibiotic, Ophthalmic
Use Treatment of surface ocular bacterial conjunctivitis and blepharoconjunctivitis
Usual Dosage Ophthalmic: Instill 1-2 drops in eye(s) every 4-6 hours
Dosage Forms Solution, ophthalmic: Trimethoprim sulfate 1 mg and polymyxin b sulfate 10,000 units per mL (10 mL)

trimethoprim and sulfamethoxazole smx-tmp *see* co-trimoxazole
on page 117

trimethylpsoralen *see* trioxsalen *on next page*

trimetrexate glucuronate (tri me trex' ate)
Brand Names Neutrexin™ Injection
Therapeutic Category Antibiotic, Miscellaneous
Use Alternative therapy for the treatment of moderate-to-severe *Pneumocystis carinii* pneumonia (PCP) in immunocompromised patients, including patients with acquired immunodeficiency syndrome (AIDS), who are intolerant of, or are refractory to, co-trimoxazole therapy or for whom co-trimoxazole is contraindicated
Usual Dosage Adults: I.V.: 45 mg/m^2 once daily over 60 minutes for 21 days; it is necessary to reduce the dose in patients with liver dysfunction, although no specific recommendations exist
Dosage Forms Powder for injection: 25 mg

trimipramine maleate (trye mi' pra meen)
Brand Names Surmontil®
Therapeutic Category Antidepressant, Tricyclic
Use Treatment of various forms of depression, often in conjunction with psychotherapy
Usual Dosage Oral: 50-150 mg/day as a single bedtime dose
Dosage Forms Capsule: 25 mg, 50 mg, 100 mg

Trimox® *see* amoxicillin trihydrate *on page 24*

Trimpex® see trimethoprim on previous page

Trinalin® see azatadine and pseudoephedrine on page 40

Trind® Liquid [OTC] see chlorpheniramine and phenylpropanolamine
on page 94

Tri-Norinyl® see ethinyl estradiol and norethindrone on page 178

Triofed® [OTC] see triprolidine and pseudoephedrine on this page

Triostat™ Injection see liothyronine sodium on page 269

trioxsalen (trye ox' sa len)
Brand Names Trisoralen™ Oral
Synonyms trimethylpsoralen
Therapeutic Category Psoralen
Use In conjunction with controlled exposure to ultraviolet light or sunlight for repigmentation
of idiopathic vitiligo; increasing tolerance to sunlight with albinism; enhance pigmentation
Usual Dosage Children >12 years and Adults: Oral: 10 mg/day as a single dose, 2-4 hours
before controlled exposure to UVA or sunlight
Dosage Forms Tablet: 5 mg

Tripalgen® Cold [OTC] see chlorpheniramine and phenylpropanolamine
on page 94

Tripedia® see diphtheria, tetanus toxoids, and acellular pertussis vaccine
on page 151

tripelennamine (tri pel enn' a meen)
Brand Names PBZ™; PBZ-SR™; Pyribenzamine®
Therapeutic Category Antihistamine
Use Perennial and seasonal allergic rhinitis and other allergic symptoms including urticaria
Usual Dosage Oral:
Infants and Children: 5 mg/kg/day in 4-6 divided doses, up to 300 mg/day maximum

Adults: 25-50 mg every 4-6 hours, extended release tablets 100 mg morning and evening up
to 100 mg every 8 hours
Dosage Forms
Elixir, as citrate: 37.5 mg/5 mL (473 mL)
Tablet, as hydrochloride: 25 mg, 50 mg
Tablet, extended release, as hydrochloride: 100 mg

Triphasil® see ethinyl estradiol and levonorgestrel on page 178

Tri-Phen-Chlor® see chlorpheniramine, phenyltoloxamine, phenylpropanolamine and
phenylephrine on page 96

Triphenyl® Syrup [OTC] see chlorpheniramine and phenylpropanolamine
on page 94

Triphenyl® Expectorant [OTC] see guaifenesin and phenylpropanolamine
on page 215

Triple Antibiotic® see bacitracin, neomycin, and polymyxin b on page 43

triple sulfa see sulfabenzamide, sulfacetamide, and sulfathiazole on page 439

Triposed® [OTC] see triprolidine and pseudoephedrine on this page

triprolidine and pseudoephedrine (trye proe' li deen)
Brand Names Actagen™ [OTC]; Actifed™ [OTC]; Allerfrin® [OTC]; Allerphed® [OTC]; Apro-
dine™ [OTC]; Cenafed™ Plus [OTC]; Genac™ [OTC]; Silafed® [OTC]; Trifed® [OTC]; Triofed®
[OTC]; Triposed™ [OTC]
Synonyms pseudoephedrine and triprolidine
Therapeutic Category Antihistamine/Decongestant Combination

Use Temporary relief of nasal congestion, running nose, sneezing, itching of nose or throat and itchy, watery eyes due to common cold, hay fever or other upper respiratory allergies

Usual Dosage May dose according to **pseudoephedrine** component (4 mg/kg/day in divided doses 3-4 times/day) Oral:

Children:
> 4 months to 2 years: 1.25 mL 3-4 times/day
> 2-4 years: 2.5 mL 3-4 times/day
> 4-6 years: 3.75 mL 3-4 times/day
> 6-12 years: 5 mL or $^1/_2$ tablet 3-4 times/day, not to exceed 2 tablets/day

Children >12 years and Adults: 10 mL or 1 tablet 3-4 times/day, not to exceed 4 tablets/day

Dosage Forms
Capsule: Triprolidine hydrochloride 2.5 mg and pseudoephedrine hydrochloride 60 mg
Capsule, extended release: Triprolidine hydrochloride 5 mg and pseudoephedrine hydrochloride 120 mg
Syrup: Triprolidine hydrochloride 1.25 mg and pseudoephedrine hydrochloride 30 mg per 5 mL
Tablet: Triprolidine hydrochloride 2.5 mg and pseudoephedrine hydrochloride 60 mg

triprolidine, pseudoephedrine, and codeine

Brand Names Actagen-C®; Actifed® With Codeine; Allerfrin® w/Codeine; Aprodine® w/C; Triacin-C®; Trifed-C®
Therapeutic Category Antihistamine/Decongestant Combination; Cough Preparation
Use Symptomatic relief of cough
Usual Dosage Oral:
Children:
> 2-6 years: 2.5 mL 4 times/day
> 7-12 years: 5 mL 4 times/day

Children >12 years and Adults: 10 mL 4 times/day

Dosage Forms Syrup: Triprolidine hydrochloride 1.25 mg, pseudoephedrine hydrochloride 30 mg, and codeine phosphate 10 mg per 5 mL with alcohol 4.3%

TripTone® Caplets® [OTC] *see* dimenhydrinate *on page 147*

tris buffer *see* tromethamine *on next page*

tris(hydroxymethyl)aminomethane *see* tromethamine *on next page*

Trisoject® *see* triamcinolone *on page 467*

Trisoralen® Oral *see* trioxsalen *on previous page*

Tri-Statin® II Topical *see* nystatin and triamcinolone *on page 335*

trisulfapyrimidines *see* sulfadiazine, sulfamethazine, and sulfamerazine *on page 440*

Tritan® *see* chlorpheniramine, pyrilamine, and phenylephrine *on page 97*

Tri-Tannate Plus® *see* chlorpheniramine, ephedrine, phenylephrine, and carbetapentane *on page 94*

Tritann® Pediatric *see* chlorpheniramine, pyrilamine, and phenylephrine *on page 97*

Tri-Thalmic® Ophthalmic Solution *see* neomycin, polymyxin b, and gramicidin *on page 322*

Tri-Vi-Flor® *see* vitamin, multiple (pediatric) *on page 491*

Trobicin® Injection *see* spectinomycin hydrochloride *on page 434*

Trocal® [OTC] *see* dextromethorphan hydrobromide *on page 135*

troleandomycin (troe lee an doe mye' sin)

Brand Names Tao®
Synonyms triacetyloleandomycin
Therapeutic Category Antibiotic, Macrolide
(Continued)

troleandomycin *(Continued)*

Use Adjunct in the treatment of corticosteroid-dependent asthma due to its steroid sparing properties; obsolete antibiotic with spectrum of activity similar to erythromycin

Usual Dosage Oral:

Children: 25-40 mg/kg/day divided every 6 hours

Adjunct in corticosteroid-dependent asthma: 14 mg/kg/day in divided doses every 6-12 hours not to exceed 250 mg every 6 hours; dose is tapered to once daily then alternate day dosing

Adults: 250-500 mg 4 times/day

Dosage Forms Capsule: 250 mg

tromethamine (troe meth' a meen)

Brand Names THAM-E® Injection; THAM® Injection

Synonyms tris buffer; tris(hydroxymethyl)aminomethane

Therapeutic Category Alkalinizing Agent, Parenteral

Use Correction of metabolic acidosis associated with cardiac bypass surgery or cardiac arrest; to correct excess acidity of stored blood that is preserved with acid citrate dextrose; to prime the pump-oxygenator during cardiac bypass surgery; indicated in infants needing alkalinization after receiving maximum sodium bicarbonate (8-10 mEq/kg/24 hours); (advantage of THAM® is that it alkalinizes without increasing pCO_2 and sodium)

Usual Dosage Dose depends on buffer base deficit; when deficit is known: tromethamine mL of 0.3 M solution = body weight (kg) x base deficit (mEq/L); when base deficit is not known: 3-6 mL/kg/dose I.V. (1-2 mEq/kg/dose)

Metabolic acidosis with cardiac arrest:

I.V.: 3.5-6 mL/kg (1-2 mEq/kg/dose) into large peripheral vein

I.V.: 500-1000 mL if needed in adults

I.V. continuous drip: Infuse slowly by syringe pump over 3-6 hours

Excess acidity of ACD priming blood: 14-70 mL of 0.3 molar solution added to each 500 mL of blood

Dosage Forms Injection:

Tham®: 18 g [0.3 molar] (500 mL)

Tham-E®: 36 g with sodium 30 mEq, potassium 5 mEq, and chloride 35 mEq (1000 mL)

Tronolane® [OTC] *see* pramoxine hydrochloride *on page 381*

Tronothane® [OTC] *see* pramoxine hydrochloride *on page 381*

Tropicacyl® Ophthalmic *see* tropicamide *on this page*

tropicamide (troe pik' a mide)

Brand Names I-Picamide® Ophthalmic; Mydriacyl® Ophthalmic; Tropicacyl® Ophthalmic

Synonyms bistropamide

Therapeutic Category Ophthalmic Agent, Mydriatic

Use Short-acting mydriatic used in diagnostic procedures; as well as preoperatively and postoperatively; treatment of some cases of acute iritis, iridocyclitis, and keratitis

Usual Dosage Children and Adults:

Cycloplegia: 1-2 drops (1%); may repeat in 5 minutes

Mydriasis: 1-2 drops (0.5%) 15-20 minutes before exam; may repeat every 30 minutes as needed

Dosage Forms Solution, ophthalmic: 0.5% (2 mL, 15 mL); 1% (2 mL, 3 mL, 15 mL)

troxidone *see* trimethadione *on page 472*

Truphylline® *see* aminophylline *on page 20*

Trusopt® *see* dorzolamide *on page 156*

trypsin, balsam peru, and castor oil
Brand Names Granulex
Therapeutic Category Protectant, Topical; Topical Skin Product
Use Treatment of decubitus ulcers, varicose ulcers, debridement of eschar, dehiscent wounds and sunburn
Usual Dosage Topical: Apply a minimum of twice daily or as often as necessary
Dosage Forms Aerosol, topical: Trypsin 0.1 mg, balsam Peru 72.5 mg, and castor oil 650 mg per 0.82 mL (60 g, 120 g)

Trysul® *see* sulfabenzamide, sulfacetamide, and sulfathiazole *on page 439*

tsh *see* thyrotropin *on page 459*

tspa *see* thiotepa *on page 458*

T-Stat® *see* erythromycin, topical *on page 172*

tuberculin tests
Brand Names Aplisol®; Tubersol®
Synonyms Mantoux; old tuberculin; ppd; purified protein derivative
Therapeutic Category Diagnostic Agent, Skin Test
Use Skin test in diagnosis of tuberculosis, to aid in assessment of cell-mediated immunity; routine tuberculin testing is recommended at 12 months of age and at every 1-2 years thereafter, before the measles vaccination
Usual Dosage Children and Adults: Intradermally: 0.1 mL approximately 4" below elbow; use $\frac{1}{4}$" to $\frac{1}{2}$" or 26- or 27-gauge needle; significant reactions are ≥5 mm in diameter
Dosage Forms Injection:
First test strength: 1 TU/0.1 mL
Intermediate test strength: 5 TU/0.1 mL
Second test strength: 250 TU/0.1 mL
Tine: 5 TU each test

Tubersol® *see* tuberculin tests *on this page*

tubocurarine chloride (too boe kyoor ar' een)
Synonyms *d*-tubocurarine chloride
Therapeutic Category Neuromuscular Blocker Agent, Nondepolarizing; Skeletal Muscle Relaxant
Use Adjunct to anesthesia to induce skeletal muscle relaxation
Usual Dosage I.V.:
Neonates <1 month: 0.3 mg/kg as a single dose; maintenance: 0.15 mg/kg/dose as needed to maintain paralysis

Children and Adults: 0.2-0.4 mg/kg as a single dose; maintenance: 0.04-0.2 mg/kg/dose as needed to maintain paralysis
Alternative adult dose: 6-9 mg once daily, then 3-4.5 mg as needed to maintain paralysis
Dosage Forms Injection: 3 mg/mL [3 units/mL] (5 mL, 10 mL, 20 mL)

Tucks® [OTC] *see* witch hazel *on page 492*

Tuinal® *see* amobarbital and secobarbital *on page 23*

Tums® E-X Extra Strength Tablet [OTC] *see* calcium carbonate *on page 66*

Tums® [OTC] *see* calcium carbonate *on page 66*

Tums® Extra Strength Liquid [OTC] *see* calcium carbonate *on page 66*

Tussafed® Drops *see* carbinoxamine, pseudoephedrine, and dextromethorphan *on page 75*

Tussafin® Expectorant *see* hydrocodone, pseudoephedrine, and guaifenesin *on page 231*

Tuss-Allergine® Modified T.D. Capsule *see* caramiphen and phenylpropanolamine *on page 73*

Tuss-DM® [OTC] *see* guaifenesin and dextromethorphan *on page 214*

Tuss-Genade® Modified Capsule *see* caramiphen and phenylpropanolamine *on page 73*

Tussigon® *see* hydrocodone and homatropine *on page 231*

Tussionex® *see* hydrocodone and chlorpheniramine *on page 230*

Tussi-Organidin® *see* iodinated glycerol and codeine *on page 248*

Tussi-Organidin® DM *see* iodinated glycerol and dextromethorphan *on page 249*

Tussi-R-Gen® *see* iodinated glycerol and codeine *on page 248*

Tussi-R-Gen DM® *see* iodinated glycerol and dextromethorphan *on page 249*

Tuss-LA® *see* guaifenesin and pseudoephedrine *on page 216*

Tusso-DM® *see* iodinated glycerol and dextromethorphan *on page 249*

Tussogest® Extended Release Capsule *see* caramiphen and phenylpropanolamine *on page 73*

Tuss-Ornade® Liquid *see* caramiphen and phenylpropanolamine *on page 73*

Tuss-Ornade® Spansule® *see* caramiphen and phenylpropanolamine *on page 73*

Tusstat® Syrup *see* diphenhydramine hydrochloride *on page 149*

Twilite® Oral [OTC] *see* diphenhydramine hydrochloride *on page 149*

Two-Dyne® *see* butalbital compound *on page 63*

Tylenol® [OTC] *see* acetaminophen *on page 2*

Tylenol® Cold Effervescent Medication Tablet [OTC] *see* chlorpheniramine, phenylpropanolamine, and acetaminophen *on page 96*

Tylenol® With Codeine *see* acetaminophen and codeine *on page 3*

Tylox® *see* oxycodone and acetaminophen *on page 342*

typhoid vaccine
Brand Names Vivotif Berna™ Oral
Synonyms typhoid vaccine live oral ty21a
Therapeutic Category Vaccine, Inactivated Bacteria
Use Promotes active immunity to typhoid fever for patients exposed to typhoid carrier or foreign travel to typhoid fever endemic area
Usual Dosage
S.C.:
   Children 6 months to 10 years: 0.25 mL; repeat in ≥4 weeks (total immunization is 2 doses)
   Adults and Children >10 years: 0.5 mL; repeat dose in ≥4 weeks (total immunization is 2 doses)
   Booster: 0.25 mL every 3 years for children 6 months to 10 years and 0.5 mL every 3 years for adults and children >10 years

Oral: Adults:
   Primary immunization: 1 capsule on alternate days (day 1, 3, 5, and 7)
   Booster immunization: Repeat full course of primary immunization every 5 years
Dosage Forms
Capsule, enteric coated: Viable *S. typhi* Ty21a Colony-forming units 2-6 x 10^9 and nonviable *S. typhi* Ty21a Colony-forming units 50 x 10^9 with sucrose, ascorbic acid, amino acid mixture, lactose and magnesium stearate
Injection: 1.5 mL

typhoid vaccine live oral ty21a *see* typhoid vaccine *on this page*

tyropanoate sodium *see* radiological/contrast media (ionic) *on page 404*

Tyzine® Nasal *see* tetrahydrozoline hydrochloride *on page 452*

UAD® Topical *see* clioquinol and hydrocortisone *on page 106*

Ucephan® Oral *see* sodium phenylacetate and sodium benzoate *on page 429*

UCG-Slide® Test *see* diagnostic aids (*in vitro*), urine *on page 137*

U-Cort™ *see* hydrocortisone *on page 232*

uk *see* urokinase *on page 481*

ULR® *see* guaifenesin, phenylpropanolamine, and phenylephrine *on page 217*

ULR-LA® *see* guaifenesin and phenylpropanolamine *on page 215*

ULTRAbrom® PD *see* brompheniramine and pseudoephedrine *on page 59*

Ultracef® *see* cefadroxil monohydrate *on page 79*

Ultralente® U *see* insulin preparations *on page 245*

Ultra Mide® Topical *see* urea *on next page*

Ultrase® MT12 *see* pancrelipase *on page 346*

Ultrase® MT20 *see* pancrelipase *on page 346*

Ultrase® MT24 *see* pancrelipase *on page 346*

Ultravate™ Topical *see* halobetasol propionate *on page 220*

Unasyn® *see* ampicillin sodium and sulbactam sodium *on page 26*

undecylenic acid and derivatives (un de sill enn' ik)

Brand Names Caldesene® Topical [OTC]; Cruex® Topical [OTC]; Fungoid® Topical Solution; Merlenate® Topical [OTC]; Pedi-Dri Topical; Pedi-Pro Topical [OTC]; Quinsana® Plus Topical [OTC]; Undoguent® Topical [OTC]

Synonyms zinc undecylenate

Therapeutic Category Antifungal Agent, Topical

Use Antifungal/antibacterial agents for athlete's foot and ringworm exclusive of nails and hairy areas; relief of diaper rash, jock itch, and other minor skin irritation; excessive perspiration and irritation in the groin area

Usual Dosage Children and Adults: Topical: Apply as needed twice daily after cleansing the affected area for 2-4 weeks

Dosage Forms
Cream: Total undecylenate 20% (15 g, 82.5 g)
Foam, topical: Undecylenic acid 10% (42.5 g)
Liquid, topical: Undecylenic acid 10% (42.5 g)
Ointment, topical: Total undecylenate 22% (30 g, 60 g, 454 g); total undecylenate 25% (60 g, 454 g)
Powder, topical: Calcium undecylenate 10% (45 g, 60 g, 120 g); total undecylenate 22% (45 g, 54 g, 81 g, 90 g, 105 g, 165 g, 454 g)
Solution, topical: Undecylenic acid 25% (29.57 mL)

Undoguent® Topical [OTC] *see* undecylenic acid and derivatives *on this page*

Unguentine® [OTC] *see* benzocaine *on page 48*

Uni-Ace® [OTC] *see* acetaminophen *on page 2*

Uni-Bent® Cough Syrup *see* diphenhydramine hydrochloride *on page 149*

Uni-Decon® *see* chlorpheniramine, phenyltoloxamine, phenylpropanolamine and phenylephrine *on page 96*

Unilax® [OTC] *see* docusate and phenolphthalein *on page 154*

Unipen® Injection *see* nafcillin sodium *on page 316*

Unipen® Oral *see* nafcillin sodium *on page 316*

Uniphyl® *see* theophylline *on page 453*

Unipres® *see* hydralazine, hydrochlorothiazide, and reserpine *on page 228*
Uni-Pro® [OTC] *see* ibuprofen *on page 240*
Uni-Tussin® [OTC] *see* guaifenesin *on page 213*
Uni-Tussin® DM [OTC] *see* guaifenesin and dextromethorphan *on page 214*
Unna's boot *see* zinc gelatin *on page 495*
Unna's paste *see* zinc gelatin *on page 495*
Uracel® *see* sodium salicylate *on page 430*

uracil mustard

Therapeutic Category Antineoplastic Agent, Alkylating Agent (Nitrogen Mustard)
Use Palliative treatment in symptomatic chronic lymphocytic leukemia; non-Hodgkin's lymphomas
Usual Dosage Oral:
Children: 0.3 mg/kg in a single weekly dose for 4 weeks

Adults: 0.15 mg/kg in a single weekly dose for 4 weeks
Thrombocytosis: 1-2 mg/day for 14 days
Dosage Forms Capsule: 1 mg

urea

Brand Names Amino-Cerv™ Vaginal Cream; Aquacare® Topical [OTC]; Carmol® Topical [OTC]; Gormel" Creme [OTC]; Lanaphilic" Topical [OTC]; Nutraplus® Topical [OTC]; Rea-Lo" [OTC]; Ultra Mide" Topical; Ureacin®-20 Topical [OTC]; Ureacin®-40 Topical; Ureaphil® Injection
Synonyms carbamide
Therapeutic Category Diuretic, Osmotic; Topical Skin Product
Use Reduce intracranial pressure and intraocular pressure (30%); promotes hydration and removal of excess keratin in hyperkeratotic conditions and dry skin; mild cervicitis
Usual Dosage
Children: I.V. slow infusion:
<2 years: 0.1-0.5 g/kg
>2 years: 0.5-1.5 g/kg

Adults:
I.V. infusion: 1-1.5 g/kg by slow infusion (1-2½ hours); maximum: 120 g/24 hours
Topical: Apply 1-3 times/day
Vaginal: 1 applicatorful in vagina at bedtime for 2-4 weeks
Dosage Forms
Cream:
Topical: 2% [20 mg/mL] (75 g); 10% [100 mg/mL] (75 g, 90 g, 454 g); 20% [200 mg/mL] (45 g, 75 g, 90 g, 454 g); 30% [300 mg/mL] (60 g, 454 g); 40% (30 g)
Vaginal: 8.34% [83.4 mg/g] (82.5 g)
Injection: 40 g/150 mL
Lotion: 2% (240 mL); 10% (180 mL, 240 mL, 480 mL); 15% (120 mL, 480 mL); 25% (180 mL)

urea and hydrocortisone

Brand Names Carmol-HC" Topical
Synonyms hydrocortisone and urea
Therapeutic Category Corticosteroid, Topical (Low Potency); Topical Skin Product
Use Inflammation of corticosteroid-responsive dermatoses
Usual Dosage Topical: Apply thin film and rub in well 1-4 times/day
Dosage Forms Cream, topical: Urea 10% and hydrocortisone acetate 1% in a water-washable vanishing cream base (30 g)

Ureacin®-20 Topical [OTC] *see* urea *on this page*
Ureacin®-40 Topical *see* urea *on this page*

urea peroxide *see* carbamide peroxide *on page 74*
Ureaphil® Injection *see* urea *on previous page*
Urecholine® *see* bethanechol chloride *on page 53*
Urex® *see* methenamine *on page 293*
Uricult® *see* diagnostic aids (*in vitro*), urine *on page 137*
Urispas® *see* flavoxate hydrochloride *on page 192*
Uristix® *see* diagnostic aids (*in vitro*), urine *on page 137*
Uri-Tet® Oral *see* oxytetracycline hydrochloride *on page 345*
Urobak® *see* sulfamethoxazole *on page 440*
Urocit®-K *see* potassium citrate *on page 378*

urofollitropin (yoor oh fol li troe' pin)
Brand Names Metrodin® Injection
Therapeutic Category Ovulation Stimulator
Use Induction of ovulation in patients with polycystic ovarian disease and to stimulate the development of multiple oocytes
Usual Dosage Adults: Female: I.M.: 75 units/day for 7-12 days, used with hCG may repeat course of treatment 2 more times
Dosage Forms Injection: 0.83 mg [75 units FSH activity] (2 mL)

urokinase (yoor oh kin' ase)
Brand Names Abbokinase® Injection
Synonyms uk
Therapeutic Category Thrombolytic Agent
Use Thrombolytic agent used in treatment of recent severe or massive deep vein thrombosis, pulmonary emboli, myocardial infarction, and occluded arteriovenous cannulas
Usual Dosage
Children and Adults: Deep vein thrombosis: I.V.: Loading: 4400 units/kg over 10 minutes, then 4400 units/kg/hour for 12 hours

Adults:
Myocardial infarction: Intracoronary: 750,000 units over 2 hours (6000 units/minute over up to 2 hours)
Occluded I.V. catheters:
5000 units (use only Abbokinase® Open Cath) in each lumen over 1-2 minutes, leave in lumen for 1-4 hours, then aspirate; may repeat with 10,000 units in each lumen if 5000 units fails to clear the catheter; **do not infuse into the patient**; volume to instill into catheter is equal to the volume of the catheter
I.V. infusion: 200 units/kg/hour in each lumen for 12-48 hours at a rate of at least 20 mL/hour
Dialysis patients: 5000 units is administered in each lumen over 1-2 minutes; leave urokinase in lumen for 1-2 days, then aspirate
Clot lysis (large vessel thrombi): Loading: I.V.: 4400 units/kg over 10 minutes, increase to 6000 units/kg/hour; maintenance: 4400-6000 units/kg/hour adjusted to achieve clot lysis or patency of affected vessel; doses up to 50,000 units/kg/hour have been used. **Note:** Therapy should be initiated as soon as possible after diagnosis of thrombi and continued until clot is dissolved (usually 24-72 hours).

Acute pulmonary embolism: Three treatment alternatives: 3 million unit dosage
Alternative 1: 12-hour infusion: 4400 units/kg (2000 units/lb) bolus over 10 minutes followed by 4400 units/kg/hour (2000 units/lb); begin heparin 1000 units/hour approximately 3-4 hours after completion of urokinase infusion or when PTT is <100 seconds
Alternative 2: 2-hour infusion: 1 million unit bolus over 10 minutes followed by 2 million units over 110 minutes; begin heparin 1000 units/hour approximately 3-4 hours after completion of urokinase infusion or when PTT is <100 seconds
Alternative 3: Bolus dose only: 15,000 units/kg over 10 minutes; begin heparin 1000 units/hour approximately 3-4 hours after completion of urokinase infusion or when PTT is <100 seconds
(Continued)
481

urokinase *(Continued)*
Dosage Forms
Powder for injection: 250,000 units (5 mL)
Powder for injection, catheter clear: 5000 units (1 mL)

Uro-KP-Neutral® *see* potassium phosphate and sodium phosphate *on page 380*
Urolene Blue® Oral *see* methylene blue *on page 299*
Uroplus® DS *see* co-trimoxazole *on page 117*
Uroplus® SS *see* co-trimoxazole *on page 117*
Urovist Cysto® *see* radiological/contrast media (ionic) *on page 404*
Urovist® Meglumine *see* radiological/contrast media (ionic) *on page 404*
Urovist® Sodium 300 *see* radiological/contrast media (ionic) *on page 404*
ursodeoxycholic acid *see* ursodiol *on this page*

ursodiol (er' soe dye ole)
Brand Names Actigall™
Synonyms ursodeoxycholic acid
Therapeutic Category Gallstone Dissolution Agent
Use Gallbladder stone dissolution
Usual Dosage Oral: 8-10 mg/kg/day in 2-3 divided doses
Dosage Forms Capsule: 300 mg

Uticort® *see* betamethasone *on page 52*
Vagistat® Vaginal *see* tioconazole *on page 461*
Vagitrol® Vaginal *see* sulfanilamide *on page 441*
Valergen® Injection *see* estradiol *on page 173*
Valertest No.1® Injection *see* estradiol and testosterone *on page 174*
Valisone® *see* betamethasone *on page 52*
Valium® *see* diazepam *on page 139*

valproic acid and derivatives (val proe' ik)
Brand Names Depakene®; Depakote®
Synonyms dipropylacetic acid; divalproex sodium; dpa; 2-propylpentanoic acid; 2-propylvaleric acid
Therapeutic Category Anticonvulsant, Miscellaneous
Use Management of simple and complex absence seizures; mixed seizure types; myoclonic and generalized tonic-clonic (grand mal) seizures; may be effective in partial seizures and infantile spasms
Usual Dosage Children and Adults:
Oral: Initial: 10-15 mg/kg/day in 1-3 divided doses; increase by 5-10 mg/kg/day at weekly intervals until therapeutic levels are achieved; maintenance: 30-60 mg/kg/day in 2-3 divided doses
  Children receiving more than 1 anticonvulsant (ie, polytherapy) may require doses up to 100 mg/kg/day in 3-4 divided doses
Rectal: Dilute syrup 1:1 with water for use as a retention enema; loading dose: 20 mg/kg one time; maintenance: 10-15 mg/kg/dose every 8 hours beginning 8 hours after administration of the loading dose
Dosage Forms
Capsule, sprinkle, as divalproex sodium (Depakote® Sprinkle®): 125 mg
Capsule, as valproic acid (Depakene®): 250 mg
Syrup, as sodium valproate (Depakene®): 250 mg/5mL (5 mL, 50 mL, 480 mL)
Tablet, delayed release, as divalproex sodium (Depakote®): 125 mg, 250 mg, 500 mg

Valrelease® *see* diazepam *on page 139*
Vamate® *see* hydroxyzine *on page 237*
Vancenase® AQ Inhaler *see* beclomethasone dipropionate *on page 45*
Vancenase® Nasal Inhaler *see* beclomethasone dipropionate *on page 45*
Vanceril® Oral Inhaler *see* beclomethasone dipropionate *on page 45*
Vancocin® Injection *see* vancomycin hydrochloride *on this page*
Vancocin® Oral *see* vancomycin hydrochloride *on this page*
Vancoled® Injection *see* vancomycin hydrochloride *on this page*

vancomycin hydrochloride (van koe mye' sin)

Brand Names Lyphocin® Injection; Vancocin® Injection; Vancocin® Oral; Vancoled® Injection
Therapeutic Category Antibiotic, Miscellaneous
Use Used in the treatment of patients with the following infections or conditions: treatment of infections due to documented or suspected methicillin-resistant *S. aureus* or beta-lactam resistant coagulase negative *Staphylococcus*; treatment of serious or life-threatening infections (ie, endocarditis, meningitis) due to documented or suspected staphylococcal or streptococcal infections in patients who are allergic to penicillins and/or cephalosporins; empiric therapy of infections associated with central lines, VP shunts, vascular grafts, prosthetic heart valves; treatment of febrile granulocytopenic patient who has not responded after 48 hours to antibiotic treatment directed at gram-negative rod infections; used orally for staphylococcal enterocolitis or for antibiotic-associated pseudomembranous colitis produced by *C. difficile*
Usual Dosage I.V. (initial dosage recommendation):
Neonates:
Preterm (postconception age <27 weeks):
<800 g: 27 mg/kg/dose every 36 hours
800-1200 g (postconception age 27-30 weeks): 24 mg/kg/dose every 24 hours
1200-2000 g (postconception age 31-36 weeks): 27 mg/kg/dose every 18 hours **or** 18 mg/kg/dose every 12 hours
>2000 g (postconception age ≥37 weeks): 22.5 mg/kg/dose every 12 hours
Term:
<7 days: 22.5 mg/kg/dose every 12 hours
7-30 days: 15 mg/kg/dose every 8 hours

Infants >1 month and Children: 40 mg/kg/day in divided doses every 6 hours

Infants >1 month and Children with staphylococcal central nervous system infection: 60 mg/kg/day in divided doses every 6 hours

Adults: With normal renal function: 0.5 g every 6 hours or 1 g every 12 hours
Intrathecal:
Neonates: 5-10 mg/day
Children: 5-20 mg/day
Adults: 20 mg/day

Oral:
Children: 10-50 mg/kg/day in divided doses every 6-8 hours; not to exceed 2 g/day
Adults: 0.5-2 g/day in divided doses every 6-8 hours
Pseudomembranous colitis produced by *C. difficile*:
Neonates: 10 mg/kg/day in divided doses
Children: 40 mg/kg/day in divided doses, added to fluids
Adults: 500 mg to 2 g/day given in 3 or 4 divided doses for 7-10 days
Dosage Forms
Capsule: 125 mg, 250 mg
Powder for oral solution: 1 g, 10 g
Powder for injection: 500 mg, 1 g, 2 g, 5 g, 10 g

Vanex-LA® *see* guaifenesin and phenylpropanolamine *on page 215*
Vanoxide-HC® *see* benzoyl peroxide and hydrocortisone *on page 50*

Vanoxide® [OTC] *see* benzoyl peroxide *on page 50*
Vansil™ *see* oxamniquine *on page 340*
Vantin® *see* cefpodoxime proxetil *on page 81*
Vaponefrin® *see* epinephrine *on page 167*

varicella-zoster immune globulin (human) (veer i sel' a- zos' ter)

Synonyms vzig
Therapeutic Category Immune Globulin
Use Passive immunization of susceptible immunodeficient patients after exposure to varicella; most effective if begun within 96 hours of exposure

VZIG supplies are limited, restrict administration to those meeting the following criteria:
One of the following underlying illnesses or conditions:
Neoplastic disease (eg, leukemia or lymphoma)
Congenital or acquired immunodeficiency
Immunosuppressive therapy with steroids, antimetabolites or other immunosuppressive treatment regimens
Newborn of mother who had onset of chickenpox within 5 days before delivery or within 48 hours after delivery
Premature ($\geq$28 weeks gestation) whose mother has no history of chickenpox
Premature (<28 weeks gestation or $\leq$1000 g VZIG) regardless of maternal history
One of the following types of exposure to chickenpox or zoster patient(s):
Continuous household contact
Playmate contact (>1 hour play indoors)
Hospital contact (in same 2-4 bedroom or adjacent beds in a large ward or prolonged face-to-face contact with an infectious staff member or patient)
Susceptible to varicella-zoster
Age of <15 years; administer to immunocompromised adolescents and adults and to other older patients on an individual basis

An acceptable alternative to VZIG prophylaxis is to treat varicella, if it occurs, with high-dose I.V. acyclovir
Usual Dosage High risk susceptible patients who are exposed again more than 3 weeks after a prior dose of VZIG should receive another full dose; there is no evidence VZIG modifies established varicella-zoster infections.

I.M.: Administer by deep injection in the gluteal muscle or in another large muscle mass. Inject 125 units/10 kg (22 lb); maximum dose: 625 units (5 vials); minimum dose: 125 units; do not give fractional doses. Do not inject I.V.
Dosage Forms Injection: 125 units of antibody in single-dose vials

Vascor® *see* bepridil hydrochloride *on page 51*
Vascoray® *see* radiological/contrast media (ionic) *on page 404*
Vaseretic® 10-25 *see* enalapril and hydrochlorothiazide *on page 165*
Vasocidin® *see* sodium sulfacetamide and prednisolone *on page 431*
VasoClear® Ophthalmic [OTC] *see* naphazoline hydrochloride *on page 319*
Vasocon-A® Ophthalmic *see* naphazoline and antazoline *on page 318*
Vasocon Regular® Ophthalmic *see* naphazoline hydrochloride *on page 319*
Vasodilan® *see* isoxsuprine hydrochloride *on page 255*

vasopressin (vay soe press' in)

Brand Names Pitressin" Injection
Synonyms antidiuretic hormone; 8-arginine vasopressin
Therapeutic Category Antidiuretic Hormone Analog; Hormone, Posterior Pituitary
Use Treatment of diabetes insipidus; prevention and treatment of postoperative abdominal distention; differential diagnosis of diabetes insipidus; [unlabeled] adjunct in the treatment of GI hemorrhage and esophageal varices

Usual Dosage
Diabetes insipidus:
  I.M., S.C.:
    Children: 2.5-5 units 2-4 times/day as needed
    Adults: 5-10 units 2-4 times/day as needed (dosage range 5-60 units/day)
    Intranasal: Administer on cotton pledget or nasal spray

Abdominal distention Adults: I.M.: 5 mg stat, 10 mg every 3-4 hours

GI hemorrhage: I.V.: Administer in a peripheral vein; dilute aqueous in NS or D_5W to 0.1-1 unit/mL and infuse at 0.2-0.4 units/minute and progressively increase to 0.9 units/minute if necessary; I.V. infusion administration requires the use of an infusion pump and should be administered in a peripheral line to minimize adverse reactions on coronary arteries

Dosage Forms Injection, aqueous: 20 pressor units/mL (0.5 mL, 1 mL)

Vasosulf® see sodium sulfacetamide and phenylephrine on page 431

Vasotec® I.V. see enalapril on page 165

Vasotec® Oral see enalapril on page 165

Vasoxyl® see methoxamine hydrochloride on page 296

V-Cillin K® Oral see penicillin v potassium on page 354

vcr see vincristine sulfate on page 488

V-Dec-M® see guaifenesin and pseudoephedrine on page 216

vecuronium (ve kyoo' roe ni um)
Brand Names Norcuron®
Therapeutic Category Neuromuscular Blocker Agent, Nondepolarizing; Skeletal Muscle Relaxant
Use Adjunct to anesthesia, to facilitate intubation, and provide skeletal muscle relaxation during surgery or mechanical ventilation
Usual Dosage I.V.:
Infants >7 weeks to 1 year: Initial: 0.08-0.1 mg/kg/dose; maintenance: 0.05-0.1 mg/kg/every hour as needed

Children >1 year and Adults: Initial: 0.08-0.1 mg/kg/dose; maintenance: 0.05-0.1 mg/kg/every hour as needed; may be administered as a continuous infusion at 0.1 mg/kg/hour

Note: Children may require slightly higher initial doses and slightly more frequent supplementation

Dosage Forms Powder for injection: 10 mg (5 mL, 10 mL)

Veetids® Oral see penicillin v potassium on page 354

Velban® see vinblastine sulfate on page 487

Velosef® see cephradine on page 85

Velosulin® Human see insulin preparations on page 245

Veltane® Tablet see brompheniramine maleate on page 59

venlafaxine (ven' la fax een)
Brand Names Effexor®
Therapeutic Category Antidepressant, Monoamine Oxidase Inhibitor
Use Treatment of depression
Usual Dosage Geriatrics and Adults: Oral: 75 mg/day, administered in 2 or 3 divided doses, taken with food; dose may be increased to 150 mg/day up to 225-375 mg/day

Dosing adjustment in renal impairment: Cl_{cr} 10-70 mL/minute: Decrease dose by 25%; decrease total daily dose by 50% if dialysis patients; dialysis patients should receive dosing after completion of dialysis

Dosing adjustment in moderate hepatic impairment: Reduce total dosage by
Dosage Forms Tablet: 25 mg, 37.5 mg, 50 mg, 75 mg, 100 mg

Venoglobulin®-I *see* immune globulin, intravenous *on page 243*

Venoglobulin®-S *see* immune globulin, intravenous *on page 243*

Ventolin® *see* albuterol *on page 10*

VePesid® Injection *see* etoposide *on page 183*

VePesid® Oral *see* etoposide *on page 183*

verapamil hydrochloride (ver ap' a mill)

Brand Names Calan®; Isoptin®; Verelan®

Synonyms iproveratril hydrochloride

Therapeutic Category Antianginal Agent; Antiarrhythmic Agent, Class IV; Calcium Channel Blocker

Use Angina, hypertension; I.V. for supraventricular tachyarrhythmias (PSVT, atrial fibrillation, atrial flutter); hypertrophic cardiomyopathy

Usual Dosage

Children: I.V.:

0-1 year: 0.1-0.2 mg/kg/dose, repeated after 30 minutes as needed

1-16 years: 0.1-0.3 mg/kg over 2-3 minutes; maximum: 5 mg/dose, may repeat dose once in 30 minutes if adequate response not achieved; maximum for second dose: 10 mg/dose

Children: Oral (dose not well established):

4-8 mg/kg/day in 3 divided doses **or** 1-5 years: 40-80 mg every 8 hours

>5 years: 80 mg every 6-8 hours

Adults:

Oral: 240-480 mg/24 hours divided 3-4 times/day

I.V.: 5-10 mg (0.075-0.15 mg/kg); may repeat 10 mg (0.15 mg/kg) 15-30 minutes after the initial dose if needed and if patient tolerated initial dose

Dosage Forms

Capsule, sustained release: 120 mg, 180 mg, 240 mg

Injection: 2.5 mg/mL (2 mL, 4 mL)

Tablet: 40 mg, 80 mg, 120 mg

Tablet, sustained release: 120 mg, 180 mg, 240 mg

Verazinc® Oral [OTC] *see* zinc sulfate *on page 496*

Vercyte® *see* pipobroman *on page 371*

Verelan® *see* verapamil hydrochloride *on this page*

Vergogel® Gel [OTC] *see* salicylic acid *on page 416*

Vergon® [OTC] *see* meclizine hydrochloride *on page 282*

Vermizine® *see* piperazine citrate *on page 371*

Vermox® *see* mebendazole *on page 281*

Verr-Canth™ *see* cantharidin *on page 71*

Verrex-C&M® *see* podophyllin and salicylic acid *on page 374*

Versacaps® *see* guaifenesin and pseudoephedrine *on page 216*

Versed® *see* midazolam hydrochloride *on page 306*

Vesanoid® Injection *see* tretinoin *on page 466*

Vesprin® *see* triflupromazine hydrochloride *on page 471*

Vexol® *see* rimexolone *on page 412*

V-Gan® Injection *see* promethazine hydrochloride *on page 390*

Vibramycin® Injection *see* doxycycline *on page 158*

Vibramycin® Oral *see* doxycycline *on page 158*

Vibra-Tabs® *see* doxycycline *on page 158*

Vicks® 44D Cough & Head Congestion *see* pseudoephedrine and dextromethorphan *on page 398*

Vicks® 44E *see* guaifenesin and dextromethorphan *on page 214*

Vicks® 44 Non-Drowsy Cold & Cough Liqui-Caps [OTC] *see* pseudoephedrine and dextromethorphan *on page 398*

Vicks® DayQuil® Allergy Relief 12 Hour [OTC] *see* brompheniramine and phenylpropanolamine *on page 59*

Vicks® DayQuil® Sinus Pressure & Congestion Relief [OTC] *see* guaifenesin and phenylpropanolamine *on page 215*

Vicks® Formula 44® [OTC] *see* dextromethorphan hydrobromide *on page 135*

Vicks Formula 44® Pediatric Formula [OTC] *see* dextromethorphan hydrobromide *on page 135*

Vicks® Sinex® Nasal Solution [OTC] *see* phenylephrine hydrochloride *on page 364*

Vicks® Sinex® Long-Acting Nasal Solution [OTC] *see* oxymetazoline hydrochloride *on page 343*

Vicodin® *see* hydrocodone and acetaminophen *on page 230*

Vicodin® ES *see* hydrocodone and acetaminophen *on page 230*

Vicon-C® [OTC] *see* vitamin b complex with vitamin c *on page 490*

vidarabine (vye dare' a been)
Brand Names Vira-A® Injection; Vira-A® Ophthalmic Ointment
Synonyms adenine arabinoside; ara-a
Therapeutic Category Antiviral Agent, Ophthalmic; Antiviral Agent, Parenteral
Use Treatment of acute keratoconjunctivitis and epithelial keratitis due to herpes simplex virus; herpes simplex encephalitis; neonatal herpes simplex virus infections; herpes zoster in immunosuppressed patients; reduces mortality from herpes simplex encephalitis from 70% to 28%; definitive diagnosis of herpes simplex conjunctivitis should be made before instituting ophthalmic therapy
Usual Dosage
Neonates: I.V.: 15-30 mg/kg/day as an 18- to 24-hour infusion

Children and Adults:
 I.V.: 10-15 mg/kg/day as a 12-hour or longer infusion
 Ophthalmic: Keratoconjunctivitis: $\frac{1}{2}$" of ointment in lower conjunctival sac 5 times/day every 3 hours while awake until complete re-epithelialization has occurred, then twice daily for an additional 7 days
Dosage Forms
Injection, suspension: 200 mg/mL [base 187.4 mg] (5 mL)
Ointment, ophthalmic, as monohydrate: 3% [30 mg/mL = 28 mg/mL base] (3.5 g)

Vi-Daylin/F® *see* vitamin, multiple (pediatric) *on page 491*

Vi-Daylin® [OTC] *see* vitamin, multiple (pediatric) *on page 491*

Videx® Oral *see* didanosine *on page 142*

vinblastine sulfate (vin blas' teen)
Brand Names Alkaban-AQ®; Velban®
Synonyms vincaleukoblastine; vlb
Therapeutic Category Antineoplastic Agent, Miotic Inhibitor
Use Palliative treatment of Hodgkin's disease and other lymphomas; breast cancer, advanced testicular germinal-cell cancers; mycosis fungoides; Kaposi's sarcoma
Usual Dosage Refer to individual protocol. Varies depending upon clinical and hematological response. Give at intervals of at least 7 days and only after leukocyte count has returned to at least 4000/mm^3; maintenance therapy should be titrated according to leukocyte count.
(Continued)

vinblastine sulfate (Continued)

Dosage should be reduced in patients with recent exposure to radiation therapy or chemotherapy; single doses in these patients should not exceed 5.5 mg/m^2.

Children and Adults: I.V.: 4-12 mg/m^2 every 7-10 days **or** 5-day continuous infusion of 1.4-1.8 mg/m^2/day **or** 0.1-0.5 mg/kg/week

Dosage Forms
Injection: 1 mg/mL (10 mL)
Powder for injection: 10 mg

vincaleukoblastine see vinblastine sulfate on previous page

Vincasar® PFS Injection see vincristine sulfate on this page

vincristine sulfate (vin kris' teen)

Brand Names Oncovin™ Injection; Vincasar® PFS Injection
Synonyms lcr; leurocristine; vcr
Therapeutic Category Antineoplastic Agent, Miotic Inhibitor
Use Treatment of leukemias, Hodgkin's disease, neuroblastoma, malignant lymphomas, Wilms' tumor, and rhabdomyosarcoma
Usual Dosage Refer to individual protocol as dosages vary with protocol used. Adjustments are made depending upon clinical and hematological response and upon adverse reactions

Children: I.V.:
$\leq$10 kg or BSA <1 m^2: 0.05 mg/kg once weekly
2 mg/m^2; may repeat every week

Adults: I.V.: 0.4-1.4 mg/m^2, up to 2 mg maximum; may repeat every week
Dosage Forms Injection: 1 mg/mL (1 mL, 2 mL, 5 mL)

Vioform® Topical [OTC] see clioquinol on page 106

Viokase® see pancrelipase on page 346

viosterol see ergocalciferol on page 169

Vira-A® Injection see vidarabine on previous page

Vira-A® Ophthalmic Ointment see vidarabine on previous page

Virazole® Aerosol see ribavirin on page 410

Virilon® see methyltestosterone on page 301

Virogen® Herpes Slide Test see diagnostic aids (in vitro), other on page 137

Virogen® Rotatest® see diagnostic aids (in vitro), feces on page 137

Virogen® Rubella Microlatex® see diagnostic aids (in vitro), blood on page 136

Virogen® Rubella Slide Test see diagnostic aids (in vitro), blood on page 136

Viroptic® Ophthalmic see trifluridine on page 471

Viscoat® see chondroitin sulfate-sodium hyaluronate on page 100

Visine® Ophthalmic [OTC] see tetrahydrozoline hydrochloride on page 452

Visken® see pindolol on page 370

Vistacon-50® see hydroxyzine on page 237

Vistaject-25® see hydroxyzine on page 237

Vistaject-50® see hydroxyzine on page 237

Vistaquel® see hydroxyzine on page 237

Vistaril® see hydroxyzine on page 237

Vistazine® see hydroxyzine on page 237

Vitacarn® Oral see levocarnitine on page 265

Vita-C® [OTC] *see* ascorbic acid *on page 34*

vitamin a
Brand Names Aquasol A® [OTC]; Palmitate-A® 5000 [OTC]
Synonyms oleovitamin a
Therapeutic Category Vitamin, Fat Soluble
Use Treatment and prevention of vitamin A deficiency
Usual Dosage
RDA:
- 0-3 years: 400 mcg*
- 4-6 years: 500 mcg*
- 7-10 years: 700 mcg*
- >10 years: 800-1000 mcg*

*mcg retinol equivalent (0.3 mcg retinol = 1 unit vitamin A)

Supplementation in measles: Children: Oral:
- <1 year: 100,000 units/day for 2 days
- >1 year: 200,000 units/day for 2 days

Severe deficiency with xerophthalmia:
Children 1-8 years:
Oral: 5000-10,000 units/kg/day for 5 days or until recovery occurs
I.M.: 5000-15,000 units/day for 10 days
Children >8 years and Adults:
Oral: 500,000 units/day for 3 days, then 50,000 units/day for 14 days, then 10,000-20,000 units/day for 2 months
I.M.: 50,000-100,000 units/day for 3 days, 50,000 units/day for 14 days

Deficiency (without corneal changes): Oral:
Infants <1 year: 10,000 units/kg/day for 5 days, then 7500-15,000 units/day for 10 days
Children 1-8 years: 5000-10,000 units/kg/day for 5 days, then 17,000-35,000 units/day for 10 days
Children >8 years and Adults: 100,000 units/day for 3 days then 50,000 units/day for 14 days

Malabsorption syndrome (prophylaxis): Children >8 years and Adults: Oral: 10,000-50,000 units/day of water miscible product

Dietary supplement: Oral:
Infants up to 6 months: 1500 units/day
Children:
6 months to 3 years: 1500-2000 units/day
4-6 years: 2500 units/day
7-10 years: 3300-3500 units/day
Children >10 years and Adults: 4000-5000 units/day

Dosage Forms
Capsule: 10,000 units, 25,000 units, 50,000 units
Drops, oral (water miscible): 5000 units/0.1 mL (30 mL)
Injection: 50,000 units/mL (2 mL)
Tablet: 5000 units

vitamin a acid *see* tretinoin *on page 466*

vitamin a and vitamin d
Brand Names A and D™ Ointment [OTC]
Synonyms cod liver oil
Therapeutic Category Protectant, Topical; Topical Skin Product
Use Temporary relief of discomfort due to chapped skin, diaper rash, minor burns, abrasions, as well as irritations associated with ostomy skin care
Usual Dosage
Oral, oil: Dietary supplement: 2.5 mL/day
(Continued)

vitamin a and vitamin d *(Continued)*

Topical: Apply locally with gentle massage as needed
Dosage Forms Ointment, topical: In a lanolin-petrolatum base (60 g)

vitamin b₁ *see* thiamine hydrochloride *on page 455*
vitamin b₂ *see* riboflavin *on page 410*
vitamin b₃ *see* niacin *on page 326*
vitamin b₅ *see* pantothenic acid *on page 348*
vitamin b₆ *see* pyridoxine hydrochloride *on page 400*
vitamin b₁₂ *see* cyanocobalamin *on page 119*
vitamin b₁₂ₐ *see* hydroxocobalamin *on page 235*

vitamin b complex

Brand Names Apatate® [OTC]; Gevrabon® [OTC]; Lederplex® [OTC]; Lipovite® [OTC]; Mega-B" [OTC]; Megaton™ [OTC]; Mucoplex® [OTC]; NeoVadrin® B Complex [OTC]; Orexin" [OTC]; Surbex® [OTC]
Therapeutic Category Vitamin, Water Soluble
Usual Dosage Dosage is usually 1 tablet or capsule/day; please refer to package insert

vitamin b complex with vitamin c

Brand Names Allbee® With C [OTC]; Surbex-T® Filmtabs® [OTC]; Surbex® with C Filmtabs® [OTC]; Thera-Combex® H-P Kapseals® [OTC]; Vicon-C® [OTC]
Therapeutic Category Vitamin, Water Soluble
Use Supportive nutritional supplementation in conditions in which water-soluble vitamins are required like GI disorders, chronic alcoholism, pregnancy, severe burns, and recovery from surgery
Usual Dosage Adults: Oral: 1 every day

vitamin b complex with vitamin c and folic acid

Brand Names Berocca®; Folbesyn®; Nephrocaps® [OTC]
Therapeutic Category Vitamin, Water Soluble
Use Supportive nutritional supplementation in conditions in which water-soluble vitamins are required like GI disorders, chronic alcoholism, pregnancy, severe burns, and recovery from surgery
Usual Dosage Adults: Oral: 1 every day

vitamin c *see* ascorbic acid *on page 34*
vitamin d₂ *see* ergocalciferol *on page 169*

vitamin e

Brand Names Amino-Opti-E® Oral [OTC]; Aquasol E® Oral [OTC]; Vitec® Topical [OTC]
Synonyms *d*-alpha tocopherol; *dl*-alpha tocopherol
Therapeutic Category Vitamin, Fat Soluble
Use Prevention and treatment hemolytic anemia secondary to vitamin E deficiency, dietary supplement
Usual Dosage
RDA: Oral:
Premature infants ≤3 months: 25 units/day
Infants:
≤6 months: 4.5 units/day
6-12 months: 6 units/day
Children:
1-3 years: 9 units/day

4-10 years: 10.5 units/day
Adults >11 years:
Female: 12 units/day
Male: 15 units/day

Prevention of vitamin E deficiency: Neonates, premature, low birthweight (results in normal levels within 1 week): Oral: 25-50 units/24 hours until 6-10 weeks of age or 125-150 units/kg total in 4 doses on days 1, 2, 7, and 8 of life

Vitamin E deficiency treatment: Adults: Oral: 50-200 units/24 hours for 2 weeks

Topical: Apply a thin layer over affected areas as needed

Dosage Forms
Capsule: 100 units, 200 units, 400 units, 500 units, 600 units, 1000 units
Capsule, water miscible: 73.5 mg, 147 mg, 165 mg, 330 mg, 400 units
Cream: 50 mg/g (15 g, 30 g, 60 g, 75 g, 120 g, 454 g)
Drops, oral: 50 mg/mL
Liquid, topical: 10 mL, 15 mL, 30 mL, 60 mL
Oil: 15 mL, 30 mL, 60 mL
Ointment, topical: 30 mg/g (45 g, 60 g)
Tablet: 200 units, 400 units

vitamin g *see* riboflavin *on page 410*

vitamin k₁ *see* phytonadione *on page 368*

vitamin k₄ *see* menadiol sodium diphosphate *on page 285*

vitamin, multiple (injectable)
Brand Names M.V.C.® 9 + 3; M.V.I.®-12; M.V.I.® Concentrate; M.V.I.® Pediatric
Therapeutic Category Vitamin
Usual Dosage
Children:
Oral:
≤2 years: Drops: 1 mL/day (premature infants may get 0.5-1 mL/day)
>2 years: Chew 1 tablet daily
≥4 years: 5 mL/day
I.V.:
≤5 kg: 10 mL/1000 mL TPN (M.V.I.® Pediatric)
5.1 kg to 11 years: 5 mL/one TPN bag/day (M.V.I.® Pediatric)
Adults:
Oral: 1 tablet daily or 5 mL/day
I.V.: >11 years: 5 mL of vials 1 and 2 (M.V.I.®-12)/one TPN bag/day

vitamin, multiple (pediatric)
Brand Names Adeflor®; Florvite®; LKV-Drops® [OTC]; Multi Vit® Drops [OTC]; Poly-Vi-Flor®; Poly-Vi-Sol® [OTC]; Tri-Vi-Flor®; Vi-Daylin® [OTC]; Vi-Daylin/F®
Synonyms children's vitamins; multivitamins/fluoride
Therapeutic Category Vitamin
Use Nutritional supplement, vitamin deficiency
Usual Dosage Oral: 0.6 mL or 1 mL daily; please refer to package insert

vitamin, multiple (prenatal)
Brand Names Chromagen® OB [OTC]; Filibon® [OTC]; Natabec® [OTC]; Natabec® FA [OTC]; Natabec® Rx; Natalins® [OTC]; Natalins® Rx; NeoVadrin® [OTC]; Niferex®-PN; Pramet® FA; Pramilet® FA; Prenavite® [OTC]; Secran®; Stuartnatal® 1+1; Stuart Prenatal® [OTC]
Synonyms prenatal vitamins
Therapeutic Category Vitamin
Use Nutritional supplement, vitamin deficiency
Usual Dosage Oral: 1 tablet or capsule daily; please refer to package insert

Vitec® Topical [OTC] *see* vitamin e *on page 490*

Vivactil® *see* protriptyline hydrochloride *on page 397*

Vivotif Berna™ Oral *see* typhoid vaccine *on page 478*

V-Lax® [OTC] *see* psyllium *on page 398*

vlb *see* vinblastine sulfate *on page 487*

vm-26 *see* teniposide *on page 446*

Volmax® *see* albuterol *on page 10*

Voltaren® Ophthalmic *see* diclofenac sodium *on page 141*

Voltaren® Oral *see* diclofenac sodium *on page 141*

Vontrol® *see* diphenidol hydrochloride *on page 149*

VoSol® HC Otic *see* acetic acid, propanediol diacetate, and hydrocortisone *on page 6*

VoSol® Otic *see* acetic acid *on page 5*

vp-16 *see* etoposide *on page 183*

Vumon Injection *see* teniposide *on page 446*

V.V.S.® *see* sulfabenzamide, sulfacetamide, and sulfathiazole *on page 439*

Vytone® Topical *see* iodoquinol and hydrocortisone *on page 249*

vzig *see* varicella-zoster immune globulin (human) *on page 484*

warfarin sodium (war' far in)
Brand Names Coumadin®; Sofarin®
Therapeutic Category Anticoagulant
Use Prophylaxis and treatment of thromboembolic disorders
Usual Dosage Oral:
Children and Infants: 0.05-0.34 mg/kg/day; infants <12 months old may require doses at or near the high end of this range; consistent anticoagulation may be difficult to maintain in children <5 years of age

Adults: 5-15 mg/day for 2-5 days, then adjust dose according to results of prothrombin time; usual maintenance dose ranges from 2-10 mg/day
Dosage Forms Tablet: 1 mg, 2 mg, 2.5 mg, 5 mg, 7.5 mg, 10 mg

4-Way® Long Acting Nasal Solution [OTC] *see* oxymetazoline hydrochloride *on page 343*

Wehdryl® Injection *see* diphenhydramine hydrochloride *on page 149*

Wellbutrin® *see* bupropion *on page 62*

Wellcovorin® Injection *see* leucovorin calcium *on page 263*

Wellcovorin® Oral *see* leucovorin calcium *on page 263*

Westcort® *see* hydrocortisone *on page 232*

Westhroid® *see* thyroid *on page 459*

Westrim® LA [OTC] *see* phenylpropanolamine hydrochloride *on page 365*

Whitfield's Ointment [OTC] *see* benzoic acid and salicylic acid *on page 49*

whole root rauwolfia *see* rauwolfia serpentina *on page 407*

Wigraine® *see* ergotamine derivatives *on page 169*

Winstrol® *see* stanozolol *on page 435*

witch hazel
Brand Names Tucks™ [OTC]
Synonyms hamamelis water
Therapeutic Category Astringent

Use After-stool wipe to remove most causes of local irritation; temporary management of vulvitis, pruritus ani and vulva; help relieve the discomfort of simple hemorrhoids, anorectal surgical wounds, and episiotomies
Usual Dosage Apply to anorectal area as needed
Dosage Forms
Cream: 50% (40 g)
Pads: 50% with glycerine, water and methylparaben (40/jar)

Wolfina® see rauwolfia serpentina on page 407

wood sugar see d-xylose on page 161

Wyamine® Sulfate Injection see mephentermine sulfate on page 287

Wycillin® Injection see penicillin g procaine, aqueous on page 354

Wydase® Injection see hyaluronidase on page 227

Wygesic® see propoxyphene and acetaminophen on page 393

Wymox® see amoxicillin trihydrate on page 24

Wytensin® see guanabenz acetate on page 218

Xanax® see alprazolam on page 14

Xero-Lube® [OTC] see saliva substitute on page 417

X-Prep® Liquid [OTC] see senna on page 420

X-seb® T [OTC] see coal tar and salicylic acid on page 110

Xylocaine® see lidocaine hydrochloride on page 267

Xylocaine® With Epinephrine see lidocaine and epinephrine on page 267

xylometazoline hydrochloride (zye loe met az' oh leen)
Brand Names Otrivin® Nasal [OTC]
Therapeutic Category Adrenergic Agonist Agent; Nasal Agent, Vasoconstrictor
Use Symptomatic relief of nasal and nasopharyngeal mucosal congestion
Usual Dosage
Children <12 years: 2-3 drops (0.05%) in each nostril every 8-10 hours
Children >12 years and Adults: 2-3 drops or sprays (0.1%) in each nostril every 8-10 hours
Dosage Forms Solution, nasal: 0.05% [0.5 mg/mL] (20 mL); 0.1% [1 mg/mL] (15 mL, 20 mL)

Xylo-Pfan® [OTC] see d-xylose on page 161

yellow fever vaccine
Brand Names YF-VAX®
Therapeutic Category Vaccine, Live Virus
Use Active immunization against yellow fever
Usual Dosage Single-dose S.C.: 0.5 mL
Dosage Forms Injection: Not less than 5.04 Log_{10} Plaque Forming Units (PFU) per 0.5 mL

yellow mercuric oxide see mercuric oxide on page 288

YF-VAX® see yellow fever vaccine on this page

Yocon® see yohimbine hydrochloride on this page

Yodoxin® see iodoquinol on page 249

yohimbine hydrochloride (yo him' bine)
Brand Names Aphrodyne™; Dayto Himbin®; Yocon®; Yohimex™
Therapeutic Category Miscellaneous Product
Use No FDA sanctioned indications
Usual Dosage Adults: Oral: 1 tablet 3 times/day
Dosage Forms Tablet: 5.4 mg

Yohimex™ *see* yohimbine hydrochloride *on previous page*

Yutopar® *see* ritodrine hydrochloride *on page 413*

zalcitabine (zal site' a been)
Brand Names Hivid™
Synonyms ddc; dideoxycytidine
Therapeutic Category Antiviral Agent, Oral
Use The FDA has approved zalcitabine for use in the treatment of HIV infections only in combination with zidovudine in adult patients with advanced HIV disease demonstrating a significant clinical or immunological deterioration
Usual Dosage
Safety and efficacy in children <13 years of age has not been established
Adults: Oral (dosed in combination with zidovudine): Daily dose: 0.750 mg every 8 hours, given together with 200 mg of zidovudine (ie, total daily dose: 2.25 mg of zalcitabine and 600 mg of zidovudine).
Dosage Forms Tablet: 0.375 mg, 0.75 mg

Zanosar® *see* streptozocin *on page 437*

Zantac® Injection *see* ranitidine hydrochloride *on page 407*

Zantac® Oral *see* ranitidine hydrochloride *on page 407*

Zantryl® *see* phentermine hydrochloride *on page 363*

Zarontin® *see* ethosuximide *on page 181*

Zaroxolyn® *see* metolazone *on page 303*

Zartan *see* cephalexin monohydrate *on page 84*

Zeasorb-AF® Powder [OTC] *see* miconazole *on page 305*

Zeasorb-AF® [OTC] *see* tolnaftate *on page 464*

Zebeta® *see* bisoprolol fumarate *on page 56*

Zebrax® *see* clidinium and chlordiazepoxide *on page 105*

Zefazone® *see* cefmetazole sodium *on page 80*

Zemuron® *see* rocuronium bromide *on page 414*

Zephiran® [OTC] *see* benzalkonium chloride *on page 48*

Zephrex® *see* guaifenesin and pseudoephedrine *on page 216*

Zephrex LA® *see* guaifenesin and pseudoephedrine *on page 216*

Zerit® Oral *see* stavudine *on page 435*

Zestoretic® *see* lisinopril and hydrochlorothiazide *on page 270*

Zestril® *see* lisinopril *on page 270*

Zetar® [OTC] *see* coal tar *on page 110*

Zetran® Injection *see* diazepam *on page 139*

Ziac™ *see* bisoprolol and hydrochlorothiazide *on page 55*

zidovudine (zye doe' vue deen)
Brand Names Retrovir™ Injection; Retrovir™ Oral
Synonyms azidothymidine; azt; compound s
Therapeutic Category Antiviral Agent, Oral; Antiviral Agent, Parenteral
Use Management of patients with HIV infections who have had at least one episode of *Pneumocystis carinii* pneumonia or who have CD4 cell counts of ≤500/mm³; patients who have HIV-related symptoms or who are asymptomatic with abnormal laboratory values indicating HIV-related immunosuppression
Usual Dosage
Children 3 months to 12 years:
Oral: 90-180 mg/m²/dose every 6 hours; maximum: 200 mg every 6 hours

I.V. continuous infusion: 0.5-1.8 mg/kg/hour
I.V. intermittent infusion: 100 mg/m^2/dose every 6 hours
Adults:
Oral:
Asymptomatic infection: 100 mg every 4 hours while awake (500 mg/day)
Symptomatic HIV infection: Initial: 200 mg every 4 hours (1200 mg/day), then after 1 month, 100 mg every 4 hours (600 mg/day)
I.V.: 1-2 mg/kg/dose every 4 hours
Dosage Forms
Capsule: 100 mg
Injection: 10 mg/mL (20 mL)
Syrup (strawberry flavor): 50 mg/5 mL (240 mL)

Zilactin-L® [OTC] *see* lidocaine hydrochloride *on page 267*
Zinacef® Injection *see* cefuroxime *on page 83*
zinc *see* trace metals *on page 465*
Zinca-Pak® *see* trace metals *on page 465*
Zincate® Oral *see* zinc sulfate *on next page*

zinc chloride

Therapeutic Category Trace Element, Parenteral
Use Cofactor for replacement therapy to different enzymes helps maintain normal growth rates, normal skin hydration and senses of taste and smell
Usual Dosage Clinical response may not occur for up to 6-8 weeks
Supplemental to I.V. solutions:
Premature Infants <1500 g, up to 3 kg: 300 mcg/kg/day
Full-term Infants and Children ≤5 years: 100 mcg/kg/day
Adults:
Stable with fluid loss from small bowel: 12.2 mg zinc/liter TPN or 17.1 mg zinc/kg (added to 1000 mL I.V. fluids) of stool or ileostomy output
Metabolically stable: 2.5-4 mg/day, add 2 mg/day for acute catabolic states
Dosage Forms Injection: 1 mg/mL (10 mL)

Zincfrin® Ophthalmic [OTC] *see* phenylephrine and zinc sulfate *on page 364*

zinc gelatin

Brand Names Gelucast®
Synonyms Unna's boot; Unna's paste
Therapeutic Category Protectant, Topical
Use Protectant and to support varicosities and similar lesions of the lower limbs
Usual Dosage Apply externally as an occlusive boot
Dosage Forms Bandage: 3" x 10 yards, 4" x 10 yards

Zincon® Shampoo [OTC] *see* pyrithione zinc *on page 401*

zinc oxide

Synonyms Lassar's zinc paste
Therapeutic Category Topical Skin Product
Use Protective coating for mild skin irritations and abrasions, soothing and protective ointment to promote healing of chapped skin, diaper rash
Usual Dosage Infants, Children and Adults: Topical: Apply several times daily to affected area
Dosage Forms
Ointment, topical: 20% in white ointment (480 g)
Paste, topical: 25% in white petrolatum (480 g)

zinc oxide, cod liver oil, and talc
Brand Names Desitin® Topical [OTC]
Therapeutic Category Protectant, Topical
Use Relief of diaper rash, superficial wounds and burns, and other minor skin irritations
Usual Dosage Apply thin layer as needed
Dosage Forms Ointment, topical: Zinc oxide, cod liver oil and talc in a petrolatum and lanolin base (30 g, 60 g, 120 g, 240 g, 270 g)

zinc oxide paste and cold cream
Brand Names Lessadale [OTC]
Therapeutic Category Topical Skin Product
Dosage Forms Cream, topical: Zinc oxide paste (Lassar's paste) 50% and cold cream 50% (480 g)

zinc sulfate
Brand Names Eye-Sed™ Ophthalmic [OTC]; Orazinc® Oral [OTC]; Verazinc® Oral [OTC]; Zincate® Oral
Therapeutic Category Mineral, Oral; Trace Element, Parenteral
Use Zinc supplement (oral and parenteral); may improve wound healing in those who are deficient
Usual Dosage
RDA: Oral:
  Birth to 6 months: 3 mg elemental zinc/day
  6-12 months: 5 mg elemental zinc/day
  1-10 years: 10 mg elemental zinc/day
  ≥11 years: 15 mg elemental zinc/day

Zinc deficiency: Oral:
  Infants and Children: 0.5-1 mg elemental zinc/kg/day divided 1-3 times/day; somewhat larger quantities may be needed if there is impaired intestinal absorption or an excessive loss of zinc
  Adults: 110-220 mg zinc sulfate (25-50 mg elemental zinc)/dose 3 times/day
Dosage Forms
Capsule: 110 mg [elemental zinc 25 mg]; 220 mg [elemental zinc 50 mg]
Injection: 1 mg/mL (10 mL, 30 mL); 4 mg/mL (10 mL); 5 mg/mL (5 mL, 10 mL, 50 mL)
Tablet: 66 mg [elemental zinc 15 mg]; 200 mg [elemental zinc 46 mg]

zinc undecylenate *see* undecylenic acid and derivatives *on page 479*

Zinecard® *see* dexrazoxone *on page 133*

Zithromax™ *see* azithromycin dihydrate *on page 41*

ZNP® Bar [OTC] *see* pyrithione zinc *on page 401*

Zocor™ *see* simvastatin *on page 423*

Zofran® Injection *see* ondansetron hydrochloride *on page 337*

Zofran® Oral *see* ondansetron hydrochloride *on page 337*

Zoladex® Implant *see* goserelin acetate *on page 212*

Zolicef® *see* cefazolin sodium *on page 79*

Zoloft™ *see* sertraline hydrochloride *on page 422*

zolpidem tartrate (zole pi' dem)
Brand Names Ambien™
Therapeutic Category Hypnotic; Sedative
Use Short-term treatment of insomnia
Usual Dosage Adults: Oral: 10 mg immediately before bedtime
Dosage Forms Tablet: 5 mg, 10 mg

Zonalon® Topical Cream *see* doxepin hydrochloride *on page 157*

Zone-A Forte® *see* pramoxine and hydrocortisone *on page 381*

ZORprin® *see* aspirin *on page 35*

Zostrix® [OTC] *see* capsaicin *on page 72*

Zostrix® HP [OTC] *see* capsaicin *on page 72*

Zosyn™ *see* piperacillin sodium and tazobactam sodium *on page 371*

Zovirax® Injection *see* acyclovir *on page 7*

Zovirax® Oral *see* acyclovir *on page 7*

Zovirax® Topical *see* acyclovir *on page 7*

Zydone® *see* hydrocodone and acetaminophen *on page 230*

Zyloprim® *see* allopurinol *on page 13*

Zymase® *see* pancrelipase *on page 346*

APPENDIX

ABBREVIATIONS COMMONLY USED
IN MEDICAL ORDERS

Abbreviation	From	Meaning
a̅a̅, aa	ana	of each
ac	ante cibum	before meals or food
ad	ad	to, up to
a.d.	aurio dextra	right ear
ad lib	ad libitum	at pleasure
a.l.	aurio laeva	left ear
AM	ante meridiem	morning
amp		ampul
amt		amount
aq	aqua	water
aq. dest.	aqua destillata	distilled water
a.s.	aurio sinister	left ear
ASAP		as soon as possible
a.u.	aures utrae	each ear
bid	bis in die	twice daily
bm		bowel movement
bp		blood pressure
BSA		body surface area
c	cong	a gallon
c̄	cum	with
cal		calorie
cap	capsula	capsule
cc		cubic centimeter
cm		centimeter
comp	compositus	compound
cont		continue
d	dies	day
d/c		discontinue
dil	dilue	dilute
disp	dispensa	dispense
div	divide	divide
dtd	dentur tales doses	give of such a dose
elix, el	elixir	elixir
emp		as directed
et	et	and
ex aq		in water
f, ft	fac, fiat, fiant	make, let be made
FDA		Food and Drug Administration
g	gramma	gram
gr	granum	grain
gtt	gutta	a drop
h	hora	hour
hs	hora somni	at bedtime
I.M.		intramuscular
I.V.		intravenous
kcal		kilocalorie
kg		kilogram
L		liter
liq	liquor	a liquor, solution
mcg		microgram
mEq		milliequivalent
mg		milligram
mixt	mixtura	a mixture
mL		milliliter
mm		millimeter
M	misce	mix
m. dict	more dictor	as directed
NF		National Formulary

(continued)

Abbreviation	From	Meaning
no.	numerus	number
noc	nocturnal	in the night
non rep	non repetatur	do not repeat, no refills
NPO		nothing by mouth
O, Oct	octarius	a pint
o.d.	oculus dexter	right eye
o.l.	oculus laevus	left eye
o.s.	oculus sinister	left eye
o.u.	oculo uterque	each eye
pc, post cib	post cibos	after meals
per		through or by
PM	post meridiem	afternoon or evening
P.O.	per os	by mouth
P.R.	per rectum	rectally
prn	pro re nata	as needed
pulv	pulvis	a powder
q		every
qad	quoque alternis die	every other day
qd		every day
qh	quiaque hora	every hour
qid	quater in die	four times a day
qod		every other day
qs	quantum sufficiat	a sufficient quantity
qs ad		a sufficient quantity to make
qty		quantity
qv	quam volueris	as much as you wish
Rx	recipe	take, a recipe
rep	repetatur	let it be repeated
$\bar{s}$	sine	without
sa	secundum artem	according to art
sat	sataratus	saturated
S.C.		subcutaneous
sig	signa	label, or let it be printed
sol	solutio	solution
solv		dissolve
$\bar{ss}$, ss	semis	one-half
sos	si opus sit	if there is need
stat	statim	at once, immediately
supp	suppositorium	suppository
syr	syrupus	syrup
tab	tabella	tablet
tal		such
tid	ter in die	three times a day
tr, tinct	tincture	tincture
trit		triturate
tsp		teaspoonful
ung	unguentum	ointment
USAN		United States Adopted Names
USP		United States Pharmacopeia
u.d., ut dict	ut dictum	as directed
v.o.		verbal order
w.a.		while awake
x3		3 times
x4		4 times

NORMAL LABORATORY VALUES FOR ADULTS*

CHEMISTRY

Chemistry, Routine

Albumin		3.5-5.0 g/dL
Bilirubin, conjugated		0-0.2 mg/dL
Bilirubin, total		0.2-1.2 mg/dL
Blood urea nitrogen		8-23 mg/dL
Calcium		8.4-10.3 mg/dL
Creatinine		0.5-1.2 mg/dL
Glucose		65-110 mg/dL
Phosphorus		2.8-4.5 mg/dL
Protein, total		6.0-8.0 g/dL
Uric acid	male	3.5-7.2 mg/dL
	female	2.6-6.5 mg/dL

Electrolytes

Chlorides		100-110 mEq/L
CO_2		23-31 mEq/L
Potassium		3.5-5.0 mEq/L
Sodium		136-146 mEq/L
Anion gap		5-14 mEq/L

Enzymes

Alkaline phosphatase	male	34-110 units/L
	female	24-100 units/L
ALT		5-35 units/L
AST		5-35 units/L
CPK	male	0-206 units/L
	female	0-175 units/L
LDH		50-200 units/L

Thyroid Function

FTI (free thyroxine index)	4.5-12.0
T_3 resin uptake	25%-35%
T_3 (tri-iodothyronine) by RIA	70-200 ng/dL
T_4 (thyroxine) by RIA	4.0-11.0 μg/dL

Others

Ammonia, plasma		20-60 μg/dL
Amylase, serum		44-128 units/L
Calcium, ionized		4.6-5.2 mg/dL
Cholesterol		140-230 mg/dL
Iron, serum		50-170 μg/dL
Lactate, serum		1.4-3.9 mEq/L
Lipase		10-208 units/L
Magnesium		1.5-2.5 mg/dL
Oncotic pressure		22-28 mm Hg
Osmolality		280-300 mOsm/kg
Serum ferritin	male	25-400 ng/mL
	female	10-150 ng/mL
TIBC		270-390 μg/dL
Triglycerides		50-150 mg/dL

*The normal ranges for laboratory values vary with different age groups, and may change as new methodologies for the lab tests are used. These values are current for adults (age 17 years or older). **Note:** Normal laboratory values may differ according to laboratory, institution, and analytical technique.

HEMATOLOGY

Hematocrit	male	40%-52%
	female	35%-47%
Hemoglobin	male	13.5-17.5 g/dL
	female	11.5-16.0 g/dL
MCH		27-34 pg
MCV		82-100 fL
Platelet count		150-450 $10^3/mm^3$
RBC count	male	4.5-5.9 $10^6/mm^3$
	female	4.0-4.9 $10^6/mm^3$
Reticulocyte count		0.5%-1.5%
Sed rate (Westergren)	male	0-10 mm/h
	female	0-20 mm/h
WBC count		4.5-11.0 $10^3/mm^3$
WBC differential		
bands		2%-8%
basophils		0%-2%
eosinophils		0%-4%
lymphocytes		20%-45%
monocytes		2%-8%
neutrophils		40%-70%

BLOOD GASES

	Arterial	Venous
Base excess	-3.0 to +3.0 mEq/L	-5.0 to +5.0 mEq/L
HCO_3	18-25 mEq/L	18-25 mEq/L
O_2 saturation	90%-98%	60%-85%
pCO_2	34-45 mm Hg	35-52 mm Hg
pH	7.35-7.45	7.32-7.42
pO_2	80-95 mm Hg	30-48 mm Hg
TCO_2	23-29 mEq/L	24-30 mEq/L

Weight/Volume Equivalents

1 mg/dL = 10 μg/mL	1 ppm = 1 mg/L
1 mg/dL = 1 mg%	1 μg/mL = 1 mg/L

NORMAL LABORATORY VALUES FOR CHILDREN

CHEMISTRY

Albumin	0-1 y	2-4 g/dL
	1 y - adult	3.5-5.5 g/dL
Ammonia	newborn	90-150 μg/dL
	child	40-120 μg/dL
	adult	18-54 μg/dL
Amylase	newborn	0-60 units/L
	adult	30-110 units/L
Bilirubin, conjugated, direct	newborn	<1.5 mg/dL
	1 mo - adult	0-0.5 mg/dL
Bilirubin, total	0-3 d	2-10 mg/dL
	1 mo - adult	0-1.5 mg/dL
Bilirubin, unconjugated, indirect		0.6-10.5 mg/dL
Calcium	newborn	7-12 mg/dL
	0-2 y	8.8-11.2 mg/dL
	2 y - adult	9-11 mg/dL
Calcium, ionized, whole blood		4.4-5.4 mg/dL
Carbon dioxide, total		23-33 mEq/L
Chloride		95-105 mEq/L
Cholesterol	newborn	45-170 mg/dL
	0-1 y	65-175 mg/dL
	1-20 y	120-230 mg/dL
Creatinine	0-1 y	≤0.6 mg/dL
	1 y - adult	0.5-1.5 mg/dL
Glucose	newborn	30-90 mg/dL
	0-2 y	60-105 mg/dL
	child - adult	70-110 mg/dL
Iron	newborn	110-270 μg/dL
	infant	30-70 μg/dL
	child	55-120 μg/dL
	adult	70-180 μg/dL
Iron binding	newborn	59-175 μg/dL
	infant	100-400 μg/dL
	adult	250-400 μg/dL
Lactic acid, lactate		2-20 mg/dL
Lead, whole blood		<30 μg/dL
Lipase	child	20-140 units/L
	adult	0-190 units/L
Magnesium		1.5-2.5 mEq/L
Osmolality, serum		275-296 mOsm/kg
Osmolality, urine		50-1400 mOsm/kg

Chemistry *(continued)*

Phosphorus	newborn	4.2-9 mg/dL
	6 wk - 19 mo	3.8-6.7 mg/dL
	18 mo - 3 y	2.9-5.9 mg/dL
	3-15 y	3.6-5.6 mg/dL
	>15 y	2.5-5 mg/dL
Potassium, plasma	newborn	4.5-7.2 mEq/L
	2 d - 3 mo	4-6.2 mEq/L
	3 mo - 1 y	3.7-5.6 mEq/L
	1-16 y	3.5-5 mEq/L
Protein, total	0-2 y	4.2-7.4 g/dL
	>2 y	6-8 g/dL
Sodium		136-145 mEq/L
Triglycerides	infant	0-171 mg/dL
	child	20-130 mg/dL
	adult	30-200 mg/dL
Urea nitrogen, blood	0-2 y	4-15 mg/dL
	2 y - adult	5-20 mg/dL
Uric acid	male	3-7 mg/dL
	female	2-6 mg/dL

ENZYMES

Alanine aminotransferase (ALT) (SGPT)	0-2 mo	8-78 units/L
	>2 mo	8-36 units/L
Alkaline phosphatase (ALKP)	newborn	60-130 units/L
	0-16 y	85-400 units/L
	>16 y	30-115 units/L
Aspartate aminotransferase (AST) (SGOT)	infant	18-74 units/L
	child	15-46 units/L
	adult	5-35 units/L
Creatine kinase (CK)	infant	20-200 units/L
	child	10-90 units/L
	adult male	0-206 units/L
	adult female	0-175 units/L
Lactate dehydrogenase (LDH)	newborn	290-501 units/L
	1 mo - 2 y	110-144 units/L
	>16 y	60-170 units/L

BLOOD GASES

	Arterial	Capillary	Venous
pH	7.35-7.45	7.35-7.45	7.32-7.42
pCO$_2$ (mm Hg)	35-45	35-45	38-52
pO$_2$ (mm Hg)	70-100	60-80	24-48
HCO$_3$ (mEq/L)	19-25	19-25	19-25
TCO$_2$ (mEq/L)	19-29	19-29	23-33
O$_2$ saturation (%)	90-95	90-95	40-70
Base excess (mEq/L)	-5 to +5	-5 to +5	-5 to +5

THYROID FUNCTION TESTS

T$_4$ (thyroxine)	1-7 d	10.1-20.9 μg/dL
	8-14 d	9.8-16.6 μg/dL
	1 mo - 1 y	5.5-16 μg/dL
	>1 y	4-12 μg/dL
FTI	1-3 d	9.3-26.6
	1-4 wk	7.6-20.8
	1-4 mo	7.4-17.9
	4-12 mo	5.1-14.5
	1-6 y	5.7-13.3
	>6 y	4.8-14
T$_3$ by RIA	newborns	100-470 ng/dL
	1-5 y	100-260 ng/dL
	5-10 y	90-240 ng/dL
	10 y - adult	70-210 ng/dL
T$_3$ uptake		35%-45%
TSH	cord	3-22 μU/mL
	1-3 d	<40 μU/mL
	3-7 d	<25 μU/mL
	>7 d	0-10 μU/mL

HEMATOLOGY

Complete Blood Count

	Hgb (g/dL)	Hct (%)	MCV (fL)	MCH (pg)	MCHC (%)	RBC (x 10^6/mm³)	RDW	PLTS (x 10^3/mm³)
0-3 d	15-20	45-61	95-115	31-37	29-37	4-5.9	<18	250-450
1-2 wk	12.5-18.5	39-57	86-110	28-36	28-38	3.6-5.5	<17	250-450
1-6 mo	10-13	29-42	74-96	25-35	30-36	3.1-4.3	<16.5	300-700
7 mo - 2 y	10.5-13	33-38	70-84	23-30	31-37	3.7-4.9	<16	250-600
2-5 y	11.5-13	34-39	75-87	24-30	31-37	3.9-5	<15	250-550
5-8 y	11.5-14.5	35-42	77-95	25-33	31-37	4-4.9	<15	250-550
13-18 y	12-15.2	36-47	78-96	25-35	31-37	4.5-5.1	<14.5	150-450
Adult male	13.5-16.5	41-50	80-100	26-34	31-37	4.5-5.5	<14.5	150-450
Adult female	12-15	36-44	80-100	26-34	31-37	4-4.9	<14.5	150-450

WBC and Diff

	WBC (x 10³/mm³)	Segmented Neutrophils	Band Neutrophils	Eosinophils	Basophils	Lymphocytes	Atypical Lymphs	Monocytes	# of NRBCs
0-3 d	9-35	32-62	10-18	0-2	0-1	19-29	0-8	5-7	0-2
1-2 wk	5-20	14-34	6-14	0-2	0-1	36-45	0-8	6-10	0
1-6 mo	6-17.5	13-33	4-12	0-3	0-1	41-71	0-8	4-7	0
7 mo - 2 y	6-17	15-35	5-11	0-3	0-1	45-76	0-8	3-6	0
2-5 y	5.5-15.5	23-45	5-11	0-3	0-1	35-65	0-8	3-6	0
5-8 y	5-14.5	32-54	5-11	0-3	0-1	28-48	0-8	3-6	0
13-18 y	4.5-13	34-64	5-11	0-3	0-1	25-45	0-8	3-6	0
Adult	4.5-11	35-66	5-11	0-3	0-1	24-44	0-8	3-6	0

Sedimentation rate, Westergren   Children   0-20 mm/hour
   Adult male   0-15 mm/hour
   Adult female   0-20 mm/hour

Sedimentation rate, Wintrobe   Children   0-13 mm/hour
   Adult male   0-10 mm/hour
   Adult female   0-15 mm/hour

Reticulocyte count   Newborn   2-6%
   1-6 months   0-2.8%
   Adult   0.5-1.5%

APOTHECARY/METRIC CONVERSIONS

Liquid Measures

Basic equivalent: 1 fluid ounce = 30 mL

Examples:

1 gallon . . . . . 3800 mL	4 fluid ounces . . . 120 mL
1 quart . . . . 960 mL	15 minims . . . . 1 mL
1 pint . . . . 480 mL	10 minims . . . . 0.6 mL
8 fluid ounces . . 240 mL	
1 gallon . . . . . . 128 fluid ounces	
1 quart . . . . 32 fluid ounces	
1 pint . . . . 16 fluid ounces	

Approximate Household Equivalents

1 teaspoonful . . . . 5 mL   1 tablespoonful . . . . 15 mL

Weights

Basic equivalents:

1 ounce = 30 g   15 grains = 1 g

Examples:

4 ounces . . . . . . 120 g	1 grain . . . . .60 mg
2 ounces . . . . 60 g	1/100 grain . . . . . . 600 μg
10 grains . . . . . 600 mg	1/150 grain . . . . . . 400 μg
7 ½ grains . . 500 mg	1/200 grain . . . . . . 300 μg
16 ounces . . . . 1 pound	

Metric Conversions

Basic equivalents:

1 g . . . . 1000 mg   1 mg . . . . 1000 μg

Examples:

5 g . . . . 5000 mg	5 mg . . . . 5000 μg
0.5 g . . . . 500 mg	0.5 mg . . . . 500 μg
0.05 g . . . . 50 mg	0.05 mg . . . . .50 μg

Exact Equivalents

1 gram (g) = 15.43 grains	0.1 mg = 1/600 gr
1 milliliter (mL) = 16.23 minims	0.12 mg = 1/500 gr
1 minim (℥) = 0.06 milliliter	0.15 mg = 1/400 gr
1 grain (gr) = 64.8 milligrams	0.2 mg = 1/300 gr
1 ounce (℥) = 31.1 grams	0.5 mg = 1/120 gr
1 ounce (oz) = 28.35 grams	0.8 mg = 1/80 gr
1 pound (lb) = 453.6 grams	1 mg = 1/65 gr
1 kilogram (kg) = 2.2 pounds	

Solids*

¼ grain = 15 mg
½ grain = 30 mg
1½ grain = 100 mg
5 grains = 300 mg
10 grains = 600 mg

*Use exact equivalents for compounding and calculations requiring a high degree of accuracy.

POUNDS/KILOGRAMS CONVERSION

1 pound = 0.45359 kilograms
1 kilogram = 2.2 pounds

lb	=	kg	lb	=	kg	lb	=	kg
1		0.45	70		31.75	140		63.50
5		2.27	75		34.02	145		65.77
10		4.54	80		36.29	150		68.04
15		6.80	85		38.56	155		70.31
20		9.07	90		40.82	160		72.58
25		11.34	95		43.09	165		74.84
30		13.61	100		45.36	170		77.11
35		15.88	105		47.63	175		79.38
40		18.14	110		49.90	180		81.65
45		20.41	115		52.16	185		83.92
50		22.68	120		54.43	190		86.18
55		24.95	125		56.70	195		88.45
60		27.22	130		58.91	200		90.72
65		29.48	135		61.24			

TEMPERATURE CONVERSION

Centigrade to Fahrenheit = (°C x 9/5) + 32 = °F
Fahrenheit to Centigrade = (°F - 32) x 5/9 = °C

°C	=	°F	°C	=	°F	°C	=	°F
100.0		212.0	39.0		102.2	36.8		98.2
50.0		122.0	38.8		101.8	36.6		97.9
41.0		105.8	38.6		101.5	36.4		97.5
40.8		105.4	38.4		101.1	36.2		97.2
40.6		105.1	38.2		100.8	36.0		96.8
40.4		104.7	38.0		100.4	35.8		96.4
40.2		104.4	37.8		100.1	35.6		96.1
40.0		104.0	37.6		99.7	35.4		95.7
39.8		103.6	37.4		99.3	35.2		95.4
39.6		103.3	37.2		99.0	35.0		95.0
39.4		102.9	37.0		98.6	0		32.0
39.2		102.6						

ACQUIRED IMMUNODEFICIENCY SYNDROME (AIDS)

This list of tests is not intended in any way to suggest patterns of physician's orders, nor is it complete. These tests may support possible clinical diagnoses or rule out other diagnostic possibilities. Each laboratory test relevant to AIDS is listed and weighted. Two symbols (**) indicate that the test is diagnostic, that is, documents the diagnosis if the expected is found. A single symbol (*) indicates a test frequently used in the diagnosis or management of the disease. The other listed tests are useful on a selective basis with consideration of clinical factors and specific aspects of the case.

Acid-Fast Stain
Acid-Fast Stain, Modified, *Nocardia* Species
Babesiosis Serological Test
Bacteremia Detection, Buffy Coat Micromethod
Beta$_2$-Microglobulin
Biopsy or Body Fluid Anaerobic Bacterial Culture
Biopsy or Body Fluid Fungus Culture
Biopsy or Body Fluid Mycobacteria Culture
Blood and Fluid Precautions, Specimen Collection
Blood Culture, Aerobic and Anaerobic
Blood Fungus Culture
Bronchial Washings Cytology
Bronchoalveolar Lavage
Bronchoalveolar Lavage Cytology
Brushings Cytology
Candida Antigen
Candidiasis Serologic Test
Cerebrospinal Fluid Cytology
Cerebrospinal Fluid Fungus Culture
Cerebrospinal Fluid Mycobacteria Culture
Chromosome Analysis, Blood or Bone Marrow
Complete Blood Count
Cryptococcal Antigen Titer, Serum or Cerebrospinal Fluid
Cryptosporidium Diagnostic Procedures, Stool
Cytomegalic Inclusion Disease Cytology
Cytomegalovirus Antibody
Cytomegalovirus Culture
Cytomegalovirus Isolation, Rapid
Darkfield Examination, Syphilis
Electron Microscopy
Estrogen Receptor Immunocytochemical Assay
Folic Acid, Serum
Hemoglobin A$_2$
Hepatitis B Surface Antigen
Herpes Cytology
Herpes Simplex Virus Antigen Detection
Herpes Simplex Virus Culture
Herpes Simplex Virus Isolation, Rapid
Histopathology
Histoplasmosis Serology
**HIV-1/HIV-2 Serology
HTLV-I/II Antibody
*Human Immunodeficiency Virus Culture
*Human Immunodeficiency Virus DNA Amplification
India Ink Preparation
Inhibitor, Lupus, Phospholipid Type
KOH Preparation
Leishmaniasis Serological Test

*Lymphocyte Subset Enumeration
Lymphocyte Transformation Test
Migration Inhibition Test
Mycobacteria by DNA Probe
Neisseria gonorrhoeae Culture
Nocardia Culture, All Sites
*p24 Antigen
Ova and Parasites, Stool
Platelet Count
Pneumocystis carinii Preparation
Pneumocystis Fluorescence
Polymerase Chain Reaction
Red Blood Cell Indices
Risks of Transfusion
Skin Biopsies
Skin Mycobacteria Culture
Skin Test, Tuberculosis
Sputum Culture
Sputum Cytology
Sputum Fungus Culture
Sputum Mycobacteria Culture
Stool Culture
Stool Fungus Culture
Stool Mycobacteria Culture
Susceptibility Testing, Fungi
Susceptibility Testing, Mycobacteria
T- and B-Lymphocyte Subset Assay
Throat Culture
Toxoplasmosis Serology
Urine Culture, Clean Catch
Urine Fungus Culture
VDRL, Serum
Viral Culture
Viral Culture, Blood
Viral Culture, Body Fluid
Viral Culture, Dermatological Symptoms
Viral Culture, Tissue
White Blood Count

Drugs Used in the Treatment of Acquired Immunodeficiency Syndrome (AIDS) or AIDS related complex:

Currently on market:

aminosidine (Gabbromicina®)
atovaquone (Mepron®)
bovine colostrum
bovine whey protein concentrate (Immuno-C®)
bropirimine [ABPP]
carbovir
CD4, human recombinant soluble [rCD4] (Receptin®)
CD4, human truncated-369 AA polypeptide (Soluble T4®)
CD4, immunoglobulin G, recombinant human
clindamycin (Cleocin®)
co-trimoxazole (Bactrim™, Septra®, and others)
Cryptosporidium hyperimmune bovine colostrum IgC concentrate
Cryptosporidium parvum bovine immunoglobulin concentrate (Sporidin-G®)
dapsone

didanosine (Videx®)
2'-3'-dideoxyadenosine
2'-3'-dideoxycytidine
2'-3'-dideoxyinosine
dronabinol (Marinol®)
eflornithine hydrochloride (Orinidyl®)
epoetin alfa (Epogen®, Procrit®)
filgrastim (Neupogen®)-new indication
fluconazole (Diflucan®)
foscarnet (Foscavir®)
gentamicin liposome infection
L-glutathione (Cachexon®)
granulocyte marcophage colony-stimulating factor [molgramostim, GM-CSF] (Leucomax®)
HIV neutralizing antibodies (Immupath®)
HIV protease inhibitor (Vertex®)
HPA-23
human T-lymphotropic virus type III gp160 antigens, recombinant
human immunodeficiency virus (HIV-1) immune globulin
immune globulin I.V., human (Gamimune N®)
interferon alfa-2a (Roferon-A®)
interferon alfa-2b (Intron® A)
lactobin
megestrol acetate (Megace®)
mitoguazone
monoclonal antibody to CD4, 5a8
muramyl-tripeptide [MTP-PE]
oxandrolone (Oxandrin®, Hepandrin®)
pentamidine isethionate (NebuPent™, Pentam-300®)
piritrexim isethionate
poloxamer 331 (Protox®)
primaquine phosphate
rifabutin (Mycobutin™)
roquinimex (Linomide®)
SDZ MSL-109
sermorelin acetate (Geref®)
somatropin (Biotropine®, Humatrope®, Norditropine®, Nutrotropin®, Protropin® II, Saizen®)
stavudine [d4T; didehydrothymidine] (Zerit®)
sulfadiazine
trimetrexate glucuronate (Neutrexin®)
zalcitabine (Hivid®)
zidovudine [AZT] (Retrovir®)

AIDS/ARC drugs soon to be released or in development:

acemannan (Carrisyn®)
AIDS vaccine
AL-271 [AZT]
alvicept sudotox [CD4-PE40]
AR-121 (Nystatin-LF® I.V.)
AS-101
atevirdine mesylate
azidouridine (AzdU®)
AZT-P-ddi (Scriptene®)
bropirimineK [ABPP]
CD4-IgG
curdlan sulfate [CRDS]

delavirdine mesylate

deoxynojirimycin, n-butyl [DNJ]

dextran sulfate sodium

diethyldithiocarbamate [DTC] (Imuthiol®)

fiacitabine [FIAC]

fialuridine [FIAU]

FK-565

fluorothymidine [FLT]

hypericin (VIMRxyn®)

interferon alfa-NL (Wellferon®)

interferon beta, recombinant [r-IFN-beta] (R-Fone®)

interferon beta, recombinant human (Betaseron®)

interleukin-2 (Proleukin®)

interleukin-3

iscador

isoprinosine

lamivudine [3TC]

lentinan

methionine-enkephalin

molgramostim (Leucomax®)

nevirapine

oxothiazolidone carboxylate (Procysteine®)

poly I: poly C12U (Ampligen®)

PR-225 [redox-acyclovir]

PR-239 [redox-penicillin G]

TAT antagonist

thymopentin (Timunox®)

thymostimuline [TP-1]

trichosanthin [GLQ223; Compound Q]

tumor necrosis factor [TNF] binding protein I

tumor necrosis factor [TNF] binding protein II

CANCER CHEMOTHERAPY

Acronyms	Used for
7 + 3	Leukemia — acute myeloid leukemia, induction
ABP	Lymphoma — non-Hodgkin's
ABC-P	Multiple myeloma
ABDIC	Lymphoma — Hodgkin's
ABVD	Lymphoma — Hodgkin's
AC	Sarcoma — bony sarcoma
AC (DC)	Multiple myeloma
ACE	Lung cancer — small cell
ACe	Breast cancer
ACMF	Breast cancer
ACOMLA	Lymphoma — non-Hodgkin's
ADOC	Thymoma (Malignant)
AVM	Breast cancer
m-BACOD	Lymphoma — non-Hodgkin's
BACOP	Lymphoma — non-Hodgkin's
BAP	Multiple myeloma
BAPP	Thymoma (Malignant)
BCDT	Malignant melanoma
BCNU-DAG	Brain tumors
B-CMF	Head and neck cancer
BCVM	Cervical cancer
BCP	Multiple myeloma
BEP	Genitourinary cancer — testicular, induction, good risk
BHD	Malignant melanoma Breast cancer
BMC	Head and neck cancer
B-MOPP	Lymphoma — Hodgkin's
BMVL	Head and neck cancer
BOMP	Cervical cancer
BVCPP	Lymphoma — Hodgkin's
CAF	Breast cancer
CAFVP	Breast cancer
CAM	Genitourinary cancer — prostate
CAMP	Lung cancer — non-small cell
CAP	Genitourinary cancer — bladder Head and neck cancer Lung cancer — non-small cell Adrenal cortical cancer Endometrial cancer
CAP-BOP	Lymphoma — non-Hodgkin's
CAP-M	Genitourinary cancer — bladder
CBM	Head and neck cancer
CC	Ovarian cancer — epithelial
CCCP	Multiple myeloma
CCNU-VP	Lymphoma — Hodgkin's
CCVPP	Lymphoma — Hodgkin's
CD	Leukemia — acute nonlymphoblastic, consolidation Ewing's sarcoma Genitourinary cancer — prostate

APPENDIX

Acronyms	Used for
CDC	Ovarian cancer — epithelial
CDF	Genitourinary cancer — prostate
CE	Adrenal cortical cancer
CF	Head and neck cancer
CFM	Breast cancer
CFPT	Breast cancer
CHAP	Ovarian cancer — epithelial
CHL + PRED	Leukemia — chronic lymphocytic leukemia
CHOP	Lymphoma — non-Hodgkin's
CHOP-B (Yale)	Lymphoma — non-Hodgkin's
CHOP-Bleo	Lymphoma — non-Hodgkin's
CHOP (P)	Lymphoma — non-Hodgkin's
CHOR	Lung cancer — small cell
CISCA	Genitourinary cancer — bladder
Cladribine (2-CdA)	Leukemia — chronic lymphocytic leukemia
CMB	Cervical cancer
CMC-High Dose	Lung cancer — small cell
CMF	Breast cancer
CMFP	Breast cancer
CMFVP (Cooper's)	Breast cancer
C-MOPP	Lymphoma — non-Hodgkin's
CMV	Genitourinary cancer — bladder
COB	Head and neck cancer
COLP	Thymoma (Malignant)
COM	Colon cancer
COMF	Colon cancer
COP-BLAM	Lymphoma — non-Hodgkin's
COP-BLAM III	Lymphoma — non-Hodgkin's
COP-BLAM IV	Lymphoma — non-Hodgkin's
COP	Lymphoma — non-Hodgkin's
COP-BLAM	Lymphoma — non-Hodgkin's
COPP (or "C" MOPP)	Lymphoma — non-Hodgkin's
CP	Ovarian cancer — epithelial
CV	Lung cancer — non-small cell
CVB	Esophageal cancer
CVI	Lung cancer — non-small cell
CVM	Gestational trophoblastic disease
CVP	Leukemia — chronic lymphocytic leukemia Lymphoma — non-Hodgkin's
CYADIC	Sarcoma — soft tissue
CYVADIC	Sarcoma — bony sarcoma Sarcoma — soft tissue
DAFS	Carcinoid (Malignant)
DAT	Leukemia — acute myeloid leukemia, induction Breast cancer
DC	Multiple myeloma
DHAP	Lymphoma — non-Hodgkin's
DMBV	Throid cancer
DMC	Gestational trophoblastic cancer
DS	Genitourinary cancer — prostate
DTIC-ACTD	Malignant melanoma

Acronyms	Used for
DVP	Leukemia — acute lymphoblastic, induction
DVPA	Leukemia — acute lymphoblastic, induction
EMA-CO	Gestational trophoblastic disease
FAC	Breast cancer
FAC-S	Carcinoid (Malignant)
FAM	Gastric cancer Lung cancer — non-small cell Pancreatic cancer
FAME	Gastric cancer
FAMTX	Gastric cancer
FAP	Esophageal cancer Pancreatic cancer
FAP-2	Pancreatic cancer
FCE	Gastric cancer
FDC	Gastric cancer
FL	Genitourinary cancer — prostate
Fludarabine	Leukemia — chronic lymphocytic leukemia
FMS (SMF)	Pancreatic cancer
FMV	Colon cancer
FOAM	Breast cancer
FOMi	Lung cancer — non-small cell
FOMi/CAP	Lung cancer — non-small cell
5FU/LDLF	Colon cancer
FU/HU	Colon cancer
FU/LV	Colon cancer
5FU/LV (Weekly)	Colon cancer
HDAC	Leukemia — acute myeloid leukemia, induction
HDMTX	Sarcoma — bony sarcoma
IC	Leukemia — acute myeloid leukemia, induction
ID	Sarcoma — soft tissue
IMAC	Sarcoma — bony sarcoma
IMF	Breast cancer
IMVP-16	Lymphoma — non-Hodgkin's
LDAC	Leukemia — acute myeloid leukemia, induction
L-VAM	Genitourinary cancer — prostate
M-2	Multiple myeloma
MAC	Genitourinary cancer — bladder Endometrial cancer
MACC	Lung cancer — non-small cell
MACOP-B	Lymphoma — non-Hodgkin's
MAID	Sarcoma — soft tissue
MAP	Head and neck cancer
MBC (MBD)	Head and neck cancer Cervical cancer Esophageal cancer
MBD	Head and neck cancer
MC	Leukemia — acute myeloid leukemia, induction
MeCP	Multiple myeloma
MF	Head and neck cancer Esophageal cancer
MINE	Lymphoma — non-Hodgkin's
MM	Leukemia — acute lymphoblastic, maintenance
MMC (MTX + MP + CTX)	Leukemia — acute lymphoblastic, maintenance
MOF-STREP	Colon cancer
MOP-BAP	Lymphoma — Hodgkin's
MOPP	Lymphoma — Hodgkin's

APPENDIX

Acronyms	Used for
MOPP/ABV Hybrid	Lymphoma — Hodgkin's
MP	Multiple myeloma
MS	Adrenal cortical cancer
MV	Leukemia — acute myeloid leukemia, induction
MVAC	Genitourinary cancer — bladder
MVPP	Lymphoma — Hodgkin's
PAC (CAP)	Ovarian cancer — epithelial Endometrial cancer
PE	Genitourinary cancer — testicular, induction, good risk Lung cancer — small cell
PFL	Head and neck cancer
POCC	Lung cancer — small cell
Pro-MACE	Lymphoma — non-Hodgkin's
Pro-MACE-CytaBOM	Lymphoma — non-Hodgkin's
Pro-MACE-MOPP	Lymphoma — non-Hodgkin's
PT	Ovarian cancer — epithelial
SC	Carcinoid (Malignant)
SCAB	Lymphoma — Hodgkin's
SD	Pancreatic cancer
SF	Carcinoid (Malignant)
SMF	Pancreatic cancer
T-9	Ewing's sarcoma
VAB VI	Genitourinary cancer — testicular, induction, salvage
VAC	Ovarian cancer — germ cell Sarcoma — soft tissue Ewing's sarcoma
VAC (CAV) (Induction)	Lung cancer — small cell
VAD	Multiple myeloma
VADRIAC — High Dose	Sarcoma — bony sarcoma
VAIE	Sarcoma — bony sarcoma
VAM	Breast cancer
VAP	Multiple myeloma
VATH	Breast cancer
VBAP	Multiple myeloma
VBC	Malignant melanoma
VBP (PVB)	Genitourinary cancer — testicular, induction, salvage
VC	Lung cancer — small cell
VCAP	Multiple myeloma
VDCP	Endometrial cancer
VDP	Malignant melanoma
VIP	Genitourinary cancer — testicular, induction, poor risk
VIP (Einhorn)	Genitourinary cancer — testicular, induction, poor risk
VP	Leukemia — acute lymphoblastic, induction
VP-L-Asparaginase	Leukemia — acute lymphoblastic, induction

CANCER CHEMOTHERAPY REGIMENS

Breast Cancer

CAP
Cyclophosphamide
Doxorubicin (Adriamycin™)
Cisplatin (Platinol™)

MS
Mitotane
Streptozocin

Breast Cancer

ACe
Cyclophosphamide
Doxorubicin (Adriamycin™)

ACMF
Doxorubicin (Adriamycin™)
Cyclophosphamide
Methotrexate
Fluorouracil

AVM
Doxorubicin (Adriamycin™)
Vinblastine
Mitomycin

CAF
Cyclophosphamide
Doxorubicin (Adriamycin™)
Fluorouracil
G CSF

CFM
Cyclophosphamide
Fluorouracil
Mitoxantrone

CFPT
Cyclophosphamide
Fluorouracil
Prednisone
Tamoxifen

CMF
Cyclophosphamide
Methotrexate
Fluorouracil

CMFP
Cyclophosphamide
Methotrexate
Fluorouracil
Prednisone

CMFVP (Cooper's)
Cyclophosphamide
Methotrexate
Fluorouracil
Vincristine
Prednisone

DAT
Dibromodulcitol
Doxorubicin (Adriamycin®)
Tamoxifen

FAC
Fluorouracil
Doxorubicin (Adriamycin®)
Cyclophosphamide

FOAM
Fluorouracil
Vincristine (Oncovin®)
Doxorubicin (Adriamycin®)
Mitomycin

IMF
Ifosfamide
Mesna
Methotrexate
Fluorouracil

VATH
Vinblastine
Doxorubicin (Adriamycin®)
Thiotepa
Fluoxymesterone (Halotestin®)

Carcinoid (Malignant)

DAFS
Dacarbazine
Doxorubicin (Adriamycin®)
Fluorouracil
Streptozocin

FAC-S
Fluorouracil
Doxorubicin (Adriamycin®)
Cyclophosphamide
Streptozocin

SF
Streptozocin
Fluorouracil

Cervical cancer

BOMP
Bleomycin
Vincristine (Oncovin™)
Mitomycin
Cisplatin (Platinol™)

CMB
Cisplatin (Platinol™)
Methotrexate
Bleomycin

MBC
Methotrexate
Bleomycin
Cisplatin

Colon Cancer

COM
Cyclophosphamide
Vincristine (Oncovin™)
Methotrexate

COMF
Cyclophosphamide
Vincristine (Oncovin™)
Methotrexate

FU/HU
Fluorouracil
Hydroxyurea

FU/LV
Fluorouracil
Leucovorin

5FU/LV (Weekly)
Fluorouracil
Leucovorin

FMV
Fluorouracil
Methyl-CCNU
Vincristine

5FU/LDLF
Fluorouracil
Leucovorin

MOF-STREP
Semustine
Vincristine (Oncovin™)
Fluorouracil
Streptozocin

Endometrial cancer

CAP
Cyclophosphamide
Doxorubicin (Adriamycin™)
Cisplatin (Platinol™)

PAC (CAP)
Cisplatin (Platinol™)
Doxorubicin (Adriamycin™)
Cyclophosphamide

VDCF
Vincristine
Doxorubicin (Adriamycin®)
Cyclophosphamide
Fluorouracil

Esophageal Cancer

CVB
Cisplatin
Videsine
Bleomycin

FAP
Fluorouracil
Doxorubicin (Adriamycin®)
Cisplatin (Platinol®)

MBC (MBD)
Methotrexate
Bleomycin
Cisplatin

Ewing's sarcoma

CD
Cyclophosphamide
Doxorubicin (Adriamycin™)

T-9
Doxorubicin (Adriamycin®)
Methotrexate
Cyclophosphamide
Dactinomycin
Bleomycin
Vincristine

VAC
Vincristine
Dactinomycin (Actinomycin D)
Cyclophosphamide

Gastric Cancer

FAM
Fluorouracil
Doxorubicin (Adriamycin®)
Mitomycin C

FAME
Fluorouracil
Doxorubicin (Adriamycin®)
Methyl-CCNU

FAMTX
Methotrexate
Fluorouracil
Leucovorin
Doxorubicin (Adriamycin®)

FCE
Fluorouracil
Cisplatin
Etoposide

FDC
Fluorouracil
Doxorubicin
Cisplatin

Genitourinary Cancer — Bladder

CAP
Cyclophosphamide
Doxorubicin (Adriamycin™)
Cisplatin (Platinol™)

CAP-M
Cyclophosphamide
Doxorubicin (Adriamycin™.)
Cisplatin (Platinol™)
Methotrexate

CISCA
Cisplatin
Cyclophosphamide
Doxorubicin (Adriamycin™)

CMV
Cisplatin
Methotrexate
Vinblastine

MVAC
Methotrexate
Vinblastine
Doxorubicin (Adriamycin™)
Cisplatin

Genitourinary Cancer — Prostate

CAM
Cyclophosphamide
Doxorubicin (Adriamycin™)
Methotrexate

CD
Cisplatin
Doxorubicin

CDF
Cyclophosphamide
Doxorubicin
Fluorouracil

DS
Doxorubicin
Stiphostrol

FL
Flutamide
Leuprolide acetate
Leuprolide acetate depot

L-VAM
Leuprolide acetate
Vinblastine
Doxorubicin (Adriamycin™)
Mitomycin C

Genitourinary Cancer — Testicular, Induction, Good Risk

BEP
Bleomycin
Etoposide
Cisplatin (Platinol®)

PE
Cisplatin (Platinol®)
Etoposide

Genitourinary Cancer — Testicular, Induction, Poor Risk

VIP
Etoposide (VePesid®)
Ifosfamide
Cisplatin (Platinol®)
Mesna

VIP (Einhorn)
Vinblastine
Ifosfamide
Cisplatin (Platinol®)
Mesna

Genitourinary Cancer — Testicular, Induction, Salvage

VAB VI
Vinblastine
Dactinomycin (Actinomycin D)
Bleomycin
Cisplatin
Cyclophosphamide

VBP (PVB)
Vinblastine
Bleomycin
Cisplatin (Platinol®)

Gestational Trophoblastic Cancer

CVM
Cisplatin
Vincristine
Methotrexate

DMC
Dactinomycin
Methotrexate
Cyclophosphamide

EMA-CO
Etoposide
Methotrexate
Dactinomycin
Cyclophosphamide
Vincristine (Oncovin®

Head and Neck Cancer

B-CMF
Bleomycin
Cyclophosphamide
Methotrexate
Fluorouracil

BMC
Bleomycin
Methotrexate
Cisplatin

BMVL
Bleomycin
Methotrexate
Vinblastine
Lomustine

CAP
Cyclophosphamide
Doxorubicin (Adriamycin™)
Cisplatin (Platinol™)

CBM
Cisplatin
Bleomycin
Mitomycin

CF
Cisplatin
Fluorouracil

COB
Cisplatin
Vincristine (Oncovin™)
Bleomycin

MAP
Mitomycin C
Doxorubicin (Adriamycin™)
Cisplatin (Platinol™)

MBC (MBD)
Methotrexate
Bleomycin
Cisplatin

MBD
Methotrexate
Bleomycin
Cisplatin

MF
Methotrexate
Fluorouracil
Leucovorin calcium

PFL
Cisplatin (Platinol™)
Fluorouracil
Leucovorin calcium

Leukemia — Acute Lymphoblastic, Induction

DVP
Daunorubicin
Vincristine
Prednisone

DVPA
Daunorubicin
Vincristine
Prednisone
Asparaginase

VP
Vincristine
Prednisone

VP-L-Asparaginase
Vincristine
Prednisone
L-asparaginase

Leukemia — Acute Lymphoblastic, Maintenance

MM
Mercaptopurine
Methotrexate

MMC (MTX + MP + CTX)
Methotrexate
Mercaptopurine
Cyclophosphamide

Leukemia — Acute Lymphoblastic, Relapse

AVDP
Asparaginase
Vincristine
Daunorubicin
Prednisone

Leukemia — Acute Myeloid, Induction

7 + 3
Cytarabine
Daunorubicin

DAT
Daunorubicin
Cytarabine (Ara-C)
Tioguanine

HDAC
Cytarabine

IC
Idarubicin (Idamycin®)
Cytarabine

LDAC
Cytarabine

MC
Mitoxantrone
Cytarabine

MV
Mitoxantrone
Etoposide (VePesid™)

Leukemia — Acute Nonlymphoblastic, Consolidation

CD
Cytarabine
Daunorubicin

Leukemia — Chronic Lymphocytic

CHL + PRED
Chlorambucil
Prednisone

CVP
Cyclophosphamide
Vincristine (Oncovin™)
Prednisone

Fludarabine

Cladribine (2-CdA)

Lung Cancer — Small Cell

ACE
Doxorubicin (Adriamycin™)
Cyclophosphamide
Etoposide

CHOR
Cyclophosphamide
Doxorubicin (Adriamycin™)
Vincristine
Radiation

CMC-High Dose
Cyclophosphamide
Methotrexate
Lomustine (CCNU)

PE
Cisplatin (Platinol™)
Etoposide

POCC
Procarbazine
Vincristine (Oncovin™)
Cyclophosphamide
Lomustine (CCNU)

VAC (CAV) (Induction)
Vincristine
Doxorubicin (Adriamycin™)
Cyclophosphamide

VC
Etoposide (VePesid™)
Carboplatin

Lung Cancer — Non-Small Cell

CAMP
Cyclophosphamide
Doxorubicin (Adriamycin®)
Methotrexate
Procarbazine

CAP
Cyclophosphamide
Doxorubicin (Adriamycin®)
Cisplatin (Platinol®)

CV
Cisplatin
Etoposide (VePesid®)

CVI
Carboplatin
Etoposide (VePesid®)
Ifosfamide
Mesna

FAM
Fluorouracil
Doxorubicin (Adriamycin®)
Mitomycin C

FOMi
Fluorouracil
Vincristine (Oncovin®)
Mitomycin C

FOMi/CAP
Fluorouracil
Vincristine
Mitomycin C
Cyclophosphamide
Doxorubicin (Adriamycin®)
Cisplatin

MACC
Methotrexate
Doxorubicin (Adriamycin®)
Cyclophosphamide
Lomustine

Lymphoma — Hodgkin's

ABDIC
Doxorubicin (Adriamycin®)
Bleomycin
Dacarbazine
Lomustine
Prednisone

ABVD
Doxorubicin (Adriamycin®)
Bleomycin
Vinblastine
Dacarbazine

B-MOPP
Bleomycin
Mechlorethamine
Vincristine (Oncovin®)
Procarbazine
Prednisone

BVCPP
Carmustine (BCNU)
Vinblastine
Cyclophosphamide
Procarbazine
Prednisone

CCNU-VP
Lomustine (CCNU)
Vinblastine
Prednisone

CCVPP
Cyclophosphamide
Lomustine (CCNU)
Vinblastine
Procarbazine
Prednisone

MOP-BAP
Mechlorethamine
Vincristine (Oncovin™)
Procarbazine
Bleomycin
Doxorubicin (Adriamycin™)
Prednisone

MOPP
Mechlorethamine
Vincristine (Oncovin™)
Procarbazine
Prednisone

MOPP/ABV Hybrid
Mechlorethamine
Vincristine (Oncovin™)
Procarbazine
Prednisone
Doxorubicin (Adriamycin™)
Bleomycin
Vinblastine

MVPP
Mechlorethamine
Vinblastine
Procarbazine
Prednisone

SCAB
Streptozocin
Lomustine (CCNU)
Doxorubicin (Adriamycin™)
Bleomycin

Lymphoma — Non-Hodgkin's

ABP
Doxorubicin (Adriamycin®)
Bleomycin
Prednisone

ACOMLA
Doxorubicin (Adriamycin®)
Cyclophosphamide
Vincristine (Oncovin®)
Methotrexate
Cytarabine
Leucovorin

BACOP
Bleomycin
Doxorubicin (Adriamycin®)
Cyclophosphamide
Vincristine (Oncovin®)
Prednisone

CAP-BOP
Cyclophosphamide
Doxorubicin
Procarbazine
Bleomycin
Vincristine (Oncovin®)
Prednisone

CHOP
Cyclophosphamide
Doxorubicin (Hydroxydaunomycin)
Vincristine (Oncovin®)
Prednisone

CHOP-Bleo
Cyclophosphamide
Doxorubicin (Hydroxydaunomycin)
Vincristine (Oncovin®)
Prednisone
Bleomycin

CHOP (P)
Cyclophosphamide
Doxorubicin (Hydroxydaunomycin)
Vincristine (Oncovin®)
Prednisone
Procarbazine

C-MOPP
Cyclophosphamide
Vincristine (Oncovin®)
Procarbazine
Prednisone

COP
Cyclophosphamide
Vincristine (Oncovin®)
Prednisone

COP-BLAM
Cyclophosphamide
Vincristine (Oncovin®)
Prednisone
Bleomycin
Doxorubicin (Adriamycin®)
Procarbazine (Matulane®)

COPP (or "C" MOPP)
Cyclophosphamide
Vincristine (Oncovin)
Procarbazine
Prednisone

CVP
Cyclophosphamide
Vincristine
Prednisone

DHAP
Dexamethasone (Decadron)
Cytarabine
Cisplatin

IMVP-16
Ifosfamide
Mesna
Methotrexate
Etoposide (VePesid)

MACOP-B
Methotrexate
Doxorubicin (Adriamycin)
Cyclophosphamide
Vincristine (Oncovin)
Bleomycin
Prednisone
Leucovorin

m-BACOD
Methotrexate
Calcium leucovorin
Bleomycin
Doxorubicin (Adriamycin)
Cyclophosphamide
Vincristine (Oncovin)
Dexamethasone

MINE
Mesna
Ifosfamide
Mitoxantrone (Novantrone)
Etoposide

Pro-MACE
Prednisone
Methotrexate
Calcium leucovorin
Doxorubicin (Adriamycin)
Cyclophosphamide
Etoposide

Pro-MACE-CytaBOM
Prednisone
Doxorubicin (Adriamycin)
Cyclophosphamide
Etoposide
Cytarabine
Bleomycin
Vincristine (Oncovin)
Methotrexate
Leucovorin

Malignant Melanoma

BCDT
Carmustine (BCNU)
Cisplatin
Dacarbazine
Tamoxifen

BHD
Carmustine (BCNU)
Hydroxyurea
Dacarbazine

DTIC-ACTD
Dacarbazine
Dactinomycin

VBC
Vinblastine
Bleomycin
Cisplatin

VDP
Vinblastine
Dacarbazine
Cisplatin (Platinol)

Multiple Myeloma

ABC-P
Carmustine
Cyclophosphamide
Doxorubicin (Hydroxydaunomycin)
Prednisone

AC (DC)
Doxorubicin (Adriamycin)
Carmustine

BAP
Carmustine (BCNU)
Doxorubicin (Adriamycin)
Prednisone

BCP
Carmustine (BCNU)
Cyclophosphamide
Prednisone

CCCP
Cisplatin
Carmustine
Cyclophosphamide
Prednisone

DC
Doxorubicin
Carmustine

MeCP
Methyl-CCNU
Cyclophosphamide
Prednisone

MP
Melphalan
Prednisone

M-2
Vincristine
Carmustine
Cyclophosphamide
Melphalan
Prednisone

VAD
Vincristine
Doxorubicin (Adriamycin™)
Dexamethasone

VAP
Vincristine
Doxorubicin (Adriamycin™)
Prednisone

VBAP
Vincristine
Carmustine (BCNU)
Doxorubicin (Adriamycin™)
Prednisone

VCAP
Vincristine
Cyclophosphamide
Doxorubicin (Adriamycin™)
Prednisone

Ovarian Cancer — Epithelial

CC
Carboplatin
Cyclophosphamide

CDC
Carboplatin
Doxorubicin
Cyclophosphamide

CHAP
Cyclophosphamide
Hexamethylmelamine
Doxorubicin (Adriamycin™)
Cisplatin (Platinol™)

CP
Cyclophosphamide
Cisplatin (Platinol™)

PAC (CAP)
Cisplatin (Platinol™)
Doxorubicin (Adriamycin™)
Cyclophosphamide

PT
Cisplatin (Platinol™)
Taxol

Ovarian Cancer — Germ Cell

VAC
Vincristine
Dactinomycin (Actinomycin D)
Cyclophosphamide

Pancreatic Cancer

FAM
Fluorouracil
Doxorubicin (Adriamycin®)
Mitomycin C

FAP-2
Fluorouracil
Doxorubicin (Adriamycin®)
Cisplatin (Platinol®)

FMS (SMF)
Fluorouracil
Mitomycin C
Streptozocin

SD
Streptozocin
Doxorubicin

Sarcoma — Bony Sarcoma

AC
Doxorubicin (Adriamycin®)
Cisplatin

CYVADIC
Cyclophosphamide
Vincristine
Doxorubicin (Adriamycin™)
Dacarbazine (DTIC)

HDMTX
Methotrexate
Calcium leucovorin

IMAC
Ifosfamide
Mesna
Doxorubicin (Adriamycin™)
Cisplatin

VAIE
Vincristine
Doxorubicin (Adriamycin®)
Ifosfamide
Etoposide

VADRIAC — High Dose
Vincristine
Cyclophosphamide
Doxorubicin (Adriamycin®)

Sarcoma — Soft Tissue

CYADIC
Cyclophosphamide
Doxorubicin (Adriamycin™)
Dacarbazine (DTIC)

CYVADIC
Cyclophosphamide
Vincristine
Doxorubicin (Adriamycin™)
Dacarbazine (DTIC)

ID
Ifosfamide
Mesna
Doxorubicin

MAID
Mesna
Doxorubicin (Adriamycin™)
Ifosfamide
Dacarbazine

VAC
Vincristine
Dactinomycin
Cyclophosphamide

Thymoma (Malignant)

ADOC
Doxorubicin (Adriamycin®)
Vincristine (Oncovin®)
Cyclophosphamide
Cisplatin

BAPP
Bleomycin
Doxorubicin (Adriamycin®)
Cisplatin
Prednisone

COLP
Cyclophosphamide
Vincristine (Oncovin®)
Lomustine
Prednisone

Thyroid cancer

ADOC
Doxorubicin (Adriamycin®)
Melphalan
Bleomycin
Vincristine (Oncovin®)

SOUND-ALIKE COMPARISON LIST

The following list contains 952 pairs of sound-alike drugs accompanied by a subjective pronunciation of each drug name. Any such list can only suggest possible pronunciation or enunciation miscues and is by no means meant to be exhaustive.

New or rarely used drugs are likely to cause the most problems related to interpretation. Healthcare workers should be made aware of the existence of both drugs in a sound-alike pair in order to avoid (or minimize) the potential for error. Drug companies attempt to avoid naming different drugs with similar-sounding names; however, mix-ups do occur. For example, recently there was a confusion with Lasix® and a new drug, Losec®. Both of these drugs were available in a 20 mg strength and some healthcare workers who were unaware that the new drug even existed inadvertently assumed that Lasix® was being requested. This is the reason that Losec® is now known as Prilosec™. Reading current drug advertisements, professional literature, and drug handbooks is a good way to avert or surely lessen such sound-alike drug errors at all levels of the healthcare industry.

Drug Name	Pronunciation	Drug Name	Pronunciation
Accubron‴	(ak' cue bron)	AK-Mycin‴	(aye kay mye' sin)
Accutane‴	(ak' yu tane)	Akne-Mycin‴	(ak nee mye' sin)
Accutane‴	(ak' yu tane)	Akne-Mycin‴	(ak nee mye' sin)
Accubron‴	(ak' cue bron)	AK-Mycin‴	(aye kay mye' sin)
Accutane‴	(ak' yu tane)	AKTob‴	(ak' tobe)
Acutrim‴	(ak' yu trim)	AK-Trol‴	(aye' kay trol)
acetazolamide	(a set a zole' a mide)	AK-Trol‴	(aye' kay trol)
acetohexamide	(a set o heks' a mide)	AKTob‴	(ak' tobe)
acetohexamide	(a set o heks' a mide)	Alazide‴	(al' a zide)
acetazolamide	(a set a zole' a mide)	Alazine‴	(al' a zine)
Achromycin‴	(ak roe mye' sin)	Alazine‴	(al' a zine)
Adriamycin™	(ade rya mye' sin)	Alazide‴	(al' a zide)
Achromycin‴	(ak roe mye' sin)	Aldactazide‴	(al dak' ta zide)
actinomycin	(ak ti noe mye' sin)	Aldactone‴	(al' dak tone)
Actidil‴	(ak' tee dill)	Aldactone‴	(al' dak tone)
Actifed‴	(ak' tee fed)	Aldactazide‴	(al dak' ta zide)
Actifed‴	(ak' tee fed)	Aldomet‴	(al' doe met)
Actidil‴	(ak' tee dill)	Aldoril‴	(al' doe ril)
actinomycin	(ak ti noe mye' sin)	Aldoril‴	(al' doe ril)
Achromycin‴	(ak roe mye' sin)	Aldomet‴	(al' doe met)
Acutrim‴	(ak' yu trim)	Aldoril‴	(al' doe ril)
Accutane‴	(ak' yu tane)	Elavil‴	(el' a vil)
Adapin‴	(ad' da pin)	Alfenta‴	(al fen' tah)
Ativan‴	(at' tee van)	Sufenta‴	(sue fen' tah)
Adriamycin™	(ade rya mye' sin)	alfentanil	(al fen' ta nill)
Achromycin‴	(ak roe mye' sin)	Anafranil‴	(a naf' ra nil)
Adriamycin™	(ade rya mye' sin)	Allerfrin‴	(al' er frin)
Idamycin‴	(eye da mye' sin)	Allergan‴	(al' er gan)
Aerolone‴	(air' o lone)	Allergan‴	(al' er gan)
Aralen‴	(air' a len)	Allerfrin‴	(al' er frin)
Afrin‴	(aye' frin or af' rin)	Allergan‴	(al' er gan)
aspirin	(as' pir in)	Auralate‴	(ahl' a late)
Afrinol‴	(af' ree nol)	Altace™	(al' tase)
Arfonad‴	(arr' foe nad)	alteplase	(al' te place)
Agoral‴	(ag' a ral)	alteplase	(al' te place)
Argyrol‴	(ar' gee roll)	Altace™	(al' tase)

Drug Name	Pronunciation	Drug Name	Pronunciation
alteplase	(al′ te place)	Artane™	(ar′ tane)
anistreplase	(a nis′ tre place)	Anturane™	(an′ chu rane)
Alupent™	(al′ yu pent)	Artane™	(ar′ tane)
Atrovent™	(at′ troe vent)	Aramine™	(air′ a meen)
Alupent™	(al′ yu pent)	Asbron™	(as′ bron)
Atrovent™	(at′ troe vent)	aspirin	(as′ pir in)
Ambenyl™	(am′ ba nil)	aspirin	(as′ pir in)
Aventyl™	(a ven′ til)	Afrin™	(aye′ frin or af′ rin)
Ambi 10™	(am′ bee ten′)	aspirin	(as′ pir in)
Ambien™	(am′ bee en)	Asbron™	(as′ bron)
Ambien™	(am′ bee en)	Atarax™	(at′ a raks)
Ambi 10™	(am′ bee ten′)	Ativan™	(at′ tee van)
Anafranil™	(a naf′ ra nil)	Atarax™	(at′ a raks)
alfentanil	(al fen′ ta nill)	Marax™	(may′ raks)
Anafranil™	(a naf′ ra nil)	Ativan™	(at′ tee van)
enalapril	(e nal′ a pril)	Adapin™	(add′ da pin)
Anatrast™	(an′ a trast)	Ativan™	(at′ tee van)
Anatuss™	(an′ a tuss)	Atarax™	(at′ a raks)
Anatuss™	(an′ a tuss)	Ativan™	(at′ tee van)
Anatrast™	(an′ a trast)	ATnativ™	(aye tee nay′ tif)
Ancobon™	(an′ coe bon)	Ativan™	(at′ tee van)
Oncovin™	(on′ coe vin)	Avitene™	(aye′ va teen)
anistreplase	(a nis′ tre place)	ATnativ™	(aye tee nay′ tif)
alteplase	(al′ te place)	Ativan™	(at′ tee van)
Ansaid™	(an′ said)	Atrovent™	(at′ troe vent)
Axid™	(aks′ id)	Alupent™	(al′ yu pent)
Anturane™	(ann′ chu rane)	Auralate™	(ahl′ a late)
Artane™	(ar′ tane)	Allergan™	(al′ er gan)
Aplisol™	(ap′ lee sol)	Auralgan™	(a ral′ gan)
A.P.L.™	(aye pee el′)	Larylgan™	(la ril′ gan)
A.P.L.™	(aye pee el′)	Auralgan™	(a ral′ gan)
Aplisol™	(ap′ lee sol)	Ophthalgan™	(opp thal′ gan)
Apresoline™	(aye press′ sow leen)	Aventyl™	(a ven′ til)
Priscoline™	(pris′ coe leen)	Ambenyl™	(am′ ba nil)
AquaTar™	(ah′ kwa tar)	Aventyl™	(a ven′ til)
Aquatag™	(ah′ kwa tag)	Bentyl™	(ben′ till)
Aquatag™	(ah′ kwa tag)	Avitene™	(aye′ va teen)
AquaTar™	(ah′ kwa tar)	Ativan™	(at′ tee van)
Aralen™	(air′ a len)	Axid™	(aks′ id)
Aerolone™	(air′ o lone)	Ansaid™	(an′ said)
Aralen™	(air′ a len)	Aygestin™	(aye ges′ tin)
Arlidin™	(ar′ le din)	Arrestin™	(aye res′ tin)
Aramine™	(air′ a meen)	baclofen	(bak′ loe fen)
Artane™	(ar′ tane)	Bactroban™	(bak′ troe ban)
Arfonad™	(arr′ foe nad)	Bactocill™	(bak′ tow sill)
Afrinol™	(af′ ree nol)	Pathocil™	(path′ o sill)
Argyrol™	(ar′ gee roll)	Bactroban™	(bak′ troe ban)
Agoral™	(ag′ a ral)	baclofen	(bak′ loe fen)
Arlidin™	(ar′ le din)	Banophen™	(ban′ o fen)
Aralen™	(air′ a len)	Barophen™	(bear′ o fen)
Arrestin™	(aye res′ tin)	Banthine™	(ban′ theen)
Aygestin™	(aye ges′ tin)	Brethine™	(breath′ een)

Drug Name	Pronunciation	Drug Name	Pronunciation
Barophen'''	(bear' o fen)	Brevoxyl'''	(brev ox' il)
Banophen'''	(ban' o fen)	Benoxyl'''	(ben ox' ill)
Beconase'''	(beck' o nase)	Bromfed'''	(brom' fed)
Bexophene'''	(beks' o feen)	Bromphen'''	(brom' fen)
Beminal'''	(bem' eh nall)	Bromphen'''	(brom' fen)
Benemid'''	(ben' a mid)	Bromfed'''	(brom' fed)
Benadryl'''	(ben' a drill)	bumetanide	(byoo met' a nide)
Bentyl'''	(ben' till)	Buminate'''	(byoo' mi nate)
Benemid'''	(ben' a mid)	Buminate'''	(byoo' mi nate)
Beminal'''	(bem' eh nall)	bumetanide	(byoo met' a nide)
Benoxyl'''	(ben ox' ill)	bupivacaine	(byoo piv' a kane)
Brevoxyl'''	(brev ox' il)	mepivacaine	(me piv' a kane)
Bentyl'''	(ben' till)	butabarbital	(byoo ta bar' bi tal)
Aventyl'''	(a ven' til)	butalbital	(byoo tal' bi tal)
Bentyl'''	(ben' till)	butalbital	(byoo tal' bi tal)
Benadryl'''	(ben' a drill)	butabarbital	(byoo ta bar' bi tal)
Benylin'''	(ben' eh lin)	Byclomine'''	(bye' clo meen)
Ventolin'''	(ven' tow lin)	Bydramine'''	(bye' dra meen)
Benza'''	(ben' zah)	Byclomine'''	(bye' clo meen)
Benzac'''	(ben' zak)	Hycomine'''	(hye' coe meen)
Benzac'''	(ben' zak)	Bydramine'''	(bye' dra meen)
Benza'''	(ben' zah)	Byclomine'''	(bye' clo meen)
Betadine'''	(bay' ta deen)	Bydramine'''	(bye' dra meen)
Betagan'''	(bay' ta gan)	Hydramyn'''	(hye' dra min)
Betagan'''	(bay' ta gan)	Cepastat'''	(sea' pa stat)
Betadine'''	(bay' ta deen)	Capastat'''	(kap' a stat)
Betapace'''	(bay' ta pace)	Cankaid'''	(kan' kaid)
Betapen'''	(bay' ta pen)	Enkaid'''	(enn' kaid)
Betapen'''	(bay' ta pen)	Capastat'''	(kap' a stat)
Betapace'''	(bay' ta pace)	Cepastat'''	(sea' pa stat)
Bexophene'''	(beks' o feen)	Capital'''	(kap' i tal)
Beconase'''	(beck' o nase)	Capitrol'''	(kap' i trol)
Bicillin'''	(bye sil' lin)	Capitrol'''	(kap' i trol)
V-Cillin K'''	(vee sil' lin kay)	Capital'''	(kap' i tal)
Bicillin'''	(bye sil' lin)	Capitrol'''	(kap' i trol)
Wycillin'''	(wye sil' lin)	captopril	(kap' toe pril)
bleomycin	(blee o mye' sin)	captopril	(kap' toe pril)
Cleocin'''	(klee o sin)	Capitrol'''	(kap' i trol)
Bleph'''-10	(blef ten')	Cardio-Green'''	(kar' dee yo green')
Blephamide'''	(blef' a mide)	Cardioquin'''	(kar' dee yo kwin)
Blephamide'''	(blef' a mide)	Cardioquin'''	(kar' dee yo kwin)
Bleph'''-10	(blef ten')	Cardio-Green'''	(kar' dee yo green')
Borofax'''	(boroe' faks)	Cardura'''	(kar dur' ah)
Boropak'''	(boroe' pak)	Cordarone'''	(kor da rone')
Boropak'''	(boroe' pak)	Cardura'''	(kar dur' ah)
Borofax'''	(boroe' faks)	Cordran'''	(kor' dran)
Brethine'''	(breath' een)	Catapres'''	(kat' a pres)
Banthine'''	(ban' theen)	Catarase'''	(kat' a race)
Bretylol'''	(brett' tee loll)	Catapres'''	(kat' a pres)
Brevital'''	(brev' i tall)	Combipres'''	(kom' bee pres)
Brevital'''	(brev' i tall)	Catapres'''	(kat' a pres)
Bretylol'''	(brett' tee loll)	Ser-Ap-Es'''	(ser ap' ess)

Drug Name	Pronunciation	Drug Name	Pronunciation
Catarase"	(kat' a race)	clomipramine	(kloe mi' pra meen)
Catapres"'	(kat' a pres)	clomiphene	(kloe' mi feen)
cefazolin	(sef a' zoe lin)	clonidine	(kloe' ni deen)
cephalexin	(sef a leks' in)	clomiphene	(kloe' mi feen)
cefazolin	(sef a' zoe lin)	clonidine	(kloe' ni deen)
cephalothin	(sef a' loe thin)	Klonopin™	(klon' o pin)
cefotaxime	(sef o taks' eem)	clonidine	(kloe' ni deen)
cefoxitin	(se fox' i tin)	Loniten"	(lon' eh ten)
cefoxitin	(se fox' i tin)	clonidine	(kloe' ni deen)
cefotaxime	(sef o taks' eem)	quinidine	(kwin' i deen)
ceftizoxime	(sef ti zoks' eem)	clotrimazole	(kloe trim' a zole)
cefuroxime	(se fyoor ox' eem)	co-trimoxazole	(koe-trye moks' a zole)
cefuroxime	(se fyoor ox' eem)	Cloxapen"	(klox' a pen)
ceftizoxime	(sef ti zoks' eem)	clozapine	(kloe' za peen)
cephalexin	(sef a leks' in)	clozapine	(kloe' za peen)
cefazolin	(sef a' zoe lin)	Cloxapen"	(klox' a pen)
cephalothin	(sef a' loe thin)	Co-Lav"	(koe' lav)
cefazolin	(sef a' zoe lin)	Colax"	(koe' laks)
cephapirin	(sef a pye' rin)	co-trimoxazole	(koe-trye moks' a zole)
cephradine	(sef' ra deen)	clotrimazole	(kloe trim' a zole)
cephradine	(sef' ra deen)	CodAphen"	(kod' a fen)
cephapirin	(sef a pye' rin)	Codafed"	(kode' a fed)
chloroxine	(klor ox' een)	Codafed"	(kode' a fed)
Choloxin"	(koe lox' in)	CodAphen"	(kod' a fen)
Choloxin"	(koe lox' in)	codeine	(koe' deen)
chloroxine	(klor ox' een)	Cophene"	(koe' feen)
Chorex"	(ko' reks)	codeine	(koe' deen)
Chymex"	(kye' meks)	Lodine"	(low' deen)
Chymex"	(kye' meks)	Colax"	(koe' laks)
Chorex"	(ko' reks)	Co-Lav"	(koe' lav)
Citracal"	(sit' tra cal)	Colestid"	(koe les' tid)
Citrucel"	(sit' tru cel)	colistin	(koe lis' tin)
Citrucel"	(sit' tru cel)	colistin	(koe lis' tin)
Citracal"	(sit' tra cal)	Colestid"	(koe les' tid)
clarithromycin	(kla rith' roe mye sin)	Combipres"	(kom' bee pres)
erythromycin	(er ith roe mye' sin)	Catapres"'	(kat' a pres)
Cleocin"	(klee' o sin)	Congestac"	(kon ges' tin)
bleomycin	(blee o mye' sin)	Congestant"	(kon ges' tant)
Cleocin"	(klee' o sin)	Congestant"	(kon ges' tant)
Lincocin"	(link' o sin)	Congestac"	(kon ges' tin)
Clinoxide"	(klin ox' ide)	Cophene"	(koe' feen)
Clipoxide'	(kleh pox' ide)	codeine	(koe' deen)
Clipoxide'	(kleh pox' ide)	Cordarone"	(kor da rone')
Clinoxide"	(klin ox' ide)	Cardura"	(kar dur' ah)
Clocort"	(klo' kort)	Cordran"'	(kor' dran)
Cloderm"	(klo' derm)	Cardura"'	(kar dur' ah)
Cloderm"'	(klo' derm)	Cort-Dome"	(kort' dome)
Clocort"	(klo' kort)	Cortone"'	(kor' tone)
clomiphene	(kloe' mi feen)	cortisone	(kor' ti sone)
clomipramine	(kloe mi' pra meen)	Cortizone"'	(kor' ti sone)
clomiphene	(kloe' mi feen)	Cortizone"'	(kor' ti sone)
clonidine	(kloe' ni deen)	cortisone	(kor' ti sone)

APPENDIX

Drug Name	Pronunciation	Drug Name	Pronunciation
Cortone'''	(kor' tone)	Decadron'''	(dek' a dron)
Cort-Dome'''	(kort' dome)	Percodan'''	(per' coe dan)
Coumadin'''	(ku' ma din)	Decholin'''	(dek' o lin)
Kemadrin'''	(kem' a drin)	Decadron'''	(dek' a dron)
Crysticillin'''	(kris ta sil' lin)	Deconal'''	(dek' o nal)
Crystodigin'''	(kris toe dig' in)	Deconsal'''	(dek' on sal)
Crystodigin'''	(kris toe dig' in)	Deconsal'''	(dek' on sal)
Crysticillin'''	(kris ta sil' lin)	Deconal'''	(dek' o nal)
cycloserine	(sye kloe ser' een)	Delacort'''	(del' a kort)
cyclosporine	(sye' kloe spor een)	Delcort'''	(del' kort)
Cyclospasmol'''	(sye kloe spas' mol)	Delcort'''	(del' kort)
cyclosporine	(sye' kloe spor een)	Delacort'''	(del' a kort)
cyclosporine	(sye' kloe spor een)	Delfen'''	(del' fen)
Cyclospasmol'''	(sye kloe spas' mol)	Delsym'''	(del' sim)
cyclosporine	(sye' kloe spor een)	Delsym'''	(del' sim)
Cyklokapron'''	(sye kloe kay' pron)	Delfen'''	(del' fen)
cyclosporine	(sye' kloe spor een)	Demadex'''	(dem' a deks)
cycloserine	(sye kloe ser' een)	Denorex'''	(den' o reks)
Cyklokapron'''	(sye kloe kay' pron)	Demerol'''	(dem' eh rol)
cyclosporine	(sye' kloe spor een)	dicumarol	(dye koo' ma role)
cytarabine	(sye tare' a been)	Demerol'''	(dem' eh rol)
vidarabine	(vye dare' a been)	Dymelor'''	(dye' meh lo)
Cytotec'''	(sye' toe tek)	Demerol'''	(dem' eh rol)
Cytoxan'''	(sye tox' an)	Temaril'''	(tem' a ril)
Cytotec'''	(sye' toe tek)	Denorex'''	(den' o reks)
Sytobex'''	(sye' toe beks)	Demadex'''	(dem' a deks)
Cytoxan'''	(sye tox' an)	Depakene'''	(dep' a keen)
Cytotec'''	(sye' toe tek)	Depakote'''	(dep' a kote)
dacarbazine	(da kar' ba zeen)	Depakote'''	(dep' a kote)
Dicarbosil'''	(dye kar' bow sil)	Depakene'''	(dep' a keen)
dacarbazine	(da kar' ba zeen)	Depo-Testadiol'''	(dep o tes ta dye' ol)
procarbazine	(proe kar' ba zeen)	Depotestogen'''	(dep o tes' tow gen)
dactinomycin	(dak ti noe mye' sin)	Depogen'''	(dep' o gen)
daunorubicin	(daw noe roo' bi sin)	Depoject'''	(dep' o ject)
Daranide'''	(dare' a nide)	Depoject'''	(dep' o ject)
Daraprim'''	(dare' a prim)	Depogen'''	(dep' o gen)
Daraprim'''	(dare' a prim)	Depotestogen'''	(dep o tes' tow gen)
Daranide'''	(dare' a nide)	Depo-Testadiol'''	(dep o tes ta dye' ol)
Daricon'''	(dare' eh kon)	Deprol'''	(deh' prol)
Darvon'''	(dar' von)	Daypro'''	(day' pro)
Darvon'''	(dar' von)	Dermacort'''	(der' ma kort)
Daricon'''	(dare' eh kon)	DermiCort'''	(der' meh kort)
Darvon'''	(dar' von)	Dermatop'''	(der' ma top)
Devrom'''	(dev' rom)	DermiCort'''	(der' meh kort)
daunorubicin	(daw noe roo' bi sin)	DermiCort'''	(der' meh kort)
dactinomycin	(dak ti noe mye' sin)	Dermacort'''	(der' ma kort)
daunorubicin	(daw noe roo' bi sin)	DermiCort'''	(der' meh kort)
doxorubicin	(dox o roo' bi sin)	Dermatop'''	(der' ma top)
Daypro'''	(day' pro)	deserpidine	(de ser' pi deen)
Deprol'''	(deh' prol)	desipramine	(dess ip' ra meen)
Decadron'''	(dek' a dron)	Desferal'''	(des' fer al)
Decholin'''	(dek' o lin)	Disophrol'''	(dye' so frol)

532

Drug Name	Pronunciation	Drug Name	Pronunciation
Desferal"	(des' fer al)	Diprivan"	(dip' riv an)
desflurane	(des flu' rane)	Ditropan"	(di troe' pan)
desflurane	(des flu' rane)	dipyridamole	(dye peer id' a mole)
Desferal"	(des' fer al)	disopyramide	(dye soe peer' a mide)
desipramine	(dess ip' ra meen)	Disophrol"	(dye' so frol)
deserpidine	(de ser' pi deen)	Desferal"	(des' fer al)
desoximetasone	(des ox i met' a sone)	disopyramide	(dye soe peer' a mide)
dexamethasone	(deks a meth' a sone)	dipyridamole	(dye peer id' a mole)
Devrom"	(dev' rom)	Ditropan"	(di troe' pan)
Darvon"	(dar' von)	Diprivan"	(dip' riv an)
dexamethasone	(deks a meth' a sone)	Ditropan"	(di troe' pan)
desoximetasone	(des ox i met' a sone)	Intropin"	(in troe' pin)
Diaβeta"	(dye a bay' tah)	Diutensin"	(dye yu ten' sin)
Diabinese"	(dye ab' beh neese)	Salutensin"	(sal yu ten' sin)
Diabinese"	(dye ab' beh neese)	dobutamine	(doe byoo' ta meen)
Diaβeta"	(dye a bay' tah)	dopamine	(doe' pa meen)
Diamox"	(dye' a moks)	docusate	(dok' yoo sate)
Trimox"	(trye' moks)	Doxinate"	(dox' eh nate)
Dicarbosil"	(dye kar' bow sil)	Donnapine"	(don' a peen)
dacarbazine	(da kar' ba zeen)	Donnazyme"	(don' a zime)
diclofenac	(dye kloe' fen ak)	Donnazyme"	(don' a zime)
Diflucan"	(dye flu' can)	Donnapine"	(don' a peen)
dicumarol	(dye koo' ma role)	dopamine	(doe' pa meen)
Demerol"	(dem' eh rol)	dobutamine	(doe byoo' ta meen)
Diflucan"	(dye flu' can)	dopamine	(doe' pa meen)
diclofenac	(dye kloe' fen ak)	Dopram"	(doe' pram)
digitoxin	(di ji tox' in)	Dopar"	(doe' par)
digoxin	(di jox' in)	Dopram"	(doe' pram)
digoxin	(di jox' in)	Dopram"	(doe' pram)
digitoxin	(di ji tox' in)	dopamine	(doe' pa meen)
Dilantin"	(dye lan' tin)	Dopram"	(doe' pram)
Dilaudid"	(dye law' did)	Dopar"	(doe' par)
Dilantin"	(dye lan' tin)	doxepin	(dox' e pin)
diltiazem	(dil tye' a zem)	Doxidan"	(dox' e dan)
Dilantin"	(dye lan' tin)	Doxidan"	(dox' e dan)
Dipentum"	(dye pen' tum)	doxepin	(dox' e pin)
Dilaudid"	(dye law' did)	Doxinate"	(dox' eh nate)
Dilantin"	(dye lan' tin)	docusate	(dok' yoo sate)
diltiazem	(dil tye' a zem)	doxorubicin	(dox o roo' bi sin)
Dilantin"	(dye lan' tin)	daunorubicin	(daw noe roo' bi sin)
dimenhydrinate	(dye men hye' dri nate)	Duo-Cyp"	(du' o sip)
diphenhydramine	(dye fen hye' dra meen)	DuoCet™	(du' o set)
Dimetabs"	(dime' tabs)	DuoCet™	(du' o set)
Dimetapp"	(dime' tap)	Duo-Cyp"	(du' o sep)
Dimetapp"	(dime' tap)	Dura-Gest"	(dur' a gest)
Dimetabs"	(dime' tabs)	Duragen"	(dur' a gen)
Dipentum"	(dye pen' tum)	Duragen"	(dur' a gen)
Dilantin"	(dye lan' tin)	Dura-Gest"	(dur' a gest)
diphenhydramine	(dye fen hye' dra meen)	Dyazide"	(dye' a zide)
dimenhydrinate	(dye men hye' dri nate)	Dynacin"	(dye' na sin)
Diphenylan"	(dye fen' eh lan)	Dymelor"	(dye' meh lo)
dyphenylan	(dye fen' eh lan)	Demerol"	(dem' eh rol)

Drug Name	Pronunciation	Drug Name	Pronunciation
Dymelor"	(dye' meh lor)	Epinal"	(ep' eh nal)
Pamelor"	(pam' meh lor)	Epitol"	(ep' eh tol)
Dynacin"	(dye' na sin)	Epitol"	(ep' eh tol)
Dyazide"	(dye' a zide)	Epinal"	(ep' eh nal)
Dynacin"	(dye' na sin)	Equanil"	(eh' kwa nil)
Dynapen"	(dye' ne pen)	Elavil"	(el' a vil)
Dynapen"	(dye' ne pen)	erythromycin	(er ith roe mye' sin)
Dynacin"	(dye' na sin)	clarithromycin	(kla rith' roe mye sin)
dyphenylan	(dye fen' eh lan)	Esimil"	(es' eh mil)
Diphenylan"	(dye fen' eh lan)	Estinyl"	(es' teh nil)
Dyrenium"	(dye ren' e um)	Esimil"	(es' eh mil)
Pyridium"	(pye rid' dee um)	Ismelin"	(is' meh lin)
Ecotrin"	(eh' ko trin)	Esimil"	(es' eh mil)
Edecrin"	(ed' eh crin)	F.M.L."	(ef' em el)
Edecrin"	(ed' eh crin)	Estinyl"	(es' teh nil)
Ecotrin"	(eh' ko trin)	Esimil"	(es' eh mil)
Edecrin"	(ed' eh crin)	Estratab"	(es' tra tab)
Ethaquin"	(eth' a kwin)	Ethatab"	(eth' a tab)
Elavil"	(el' a vil)	Ethaquin"	(eth' a kwin)
Aldoril"	(al' doe ril)	Edecrin"	(ed' eh crin)
Elavil"	(el' a vil)	Ethatab"	(eth' a tab)
Equanil"	(eh' kwa nil)	Estratab"	(es' tra tab)
Elavil"	(el' a vil)	ethosuximide	(eth o sux' i mide)
Mellaril"	(mel' la ril)	methsuximide	(meth sux' i mide)
Elixicon"	(eh lix' i con)	etidocaine	(e ti' doe kane)
Elocon"	(ee' lo con)	etidronate	(e ti droe' nate)
Elocon"	(ee' lo con)	etidronate	(e ti droe' nate)
Elixicon"	(eh lix' i con)	etidocaine	(e ti' doe kane)
emetine	(em' eh teen)	etidronate	(e ti droe' nate)
Emetrol"	(em' eh trol)	etretinate	(e tret' i nate)
Emetrol"	(em' eh trol)	etretinate	(e tret' i nate)
emetine	(em' eh teen)	etidronate	(e ti droe' nate)
enalapril	(e nal' a pril)	Eurax"	(yoor' aks)
Anafranil"	(a naf' ra nil)	Serax"	(sear' aks)
Endal"	(en' dal)	Eurax"	(yoor' aks)
Intal"	(in' tal)	Urex"	(yu' eks)
Enduron"	(en' du ron)	Factrel"	(fak' trel)
Imuran"	(im' yu ran)	Sectral"	(sek' tral)
Enduron"	(en' du ron)	Feldene"	(fel' deen)
Inderal"	(in' der al)	Seldane"	(sel' dane)
Enduronyl"	(en dur' o nil)	fenoprofen	(fen o proe' fen)
Inderal"	(in' der al)	flurbiprofen	(flure bi' proe fen)
Enduronyl" Forte	(en dur' o nil for' tay)	Feosol"	(fee' o sol)
Inderal" 40	(in' der al for' tee)	Fer-In-Sol"	(fehr' in sol)
enflurane	(en' floo rane)	Feosol"	(fee' o sol)
isoflurane	(eye soe flure' ane)	Festal"	(fes' tal)
Enkaid"	(enn' kaid)	Feosol"	(fee' o sol)
Cankaid"	(kan' kaid)	Fluosol"	(flu' o sol)
EpiPen"	(ep' eh pen)	Fer-In-Sol"	(fehr' in sol)
Epifrin"	(ep' eh frin)	Feosol"	(fee' o sol)
Epifrin"	(ep' eh frin)	Festal"	(fes' tal)
EpiPen"	(ep' eh pen)	Feosol"	(fee' o sol)

Drug Name	Pronunciation	Drug Name	Pronunciation
Feverall™ Fiberall	(fee' ver all) (fye' ber all)	Genapax Genapap	(gen' a paks) (gen' a pap)
Fiberall Feverall™	(fye' ber all) (fee' ver all)	gentamicin kanamycin	(jen ta mye' sin) (kan a mye' sin)
Fioricet Lorcet	(fee oh' reh set) (lor' set)	Glycotuss Glytuss	(glye' co tuss) (glye' tuss)
Fiorinal Florinef	(fee or' reh nal) (flor' eh nef)	Glytuss Glycotuss	(glye' tuss) (glye' co tuss)
Flaxedil Flexeril	(flaks' eh dil) (fleks' eh ril)	gonadorelin guanadrel	(goe nad o rell' in) (gwahn' a drel)
Flexeril Flaxedil	(fleks' eh ril) (flaks' eh dil)	Gonak™ Gonic	(gon' ak) (gon' ik)
Florinef Fiorinal	(flor' eh nef) (fee or' reh nal)	Gonic Gonak™	(gon' ik) (gon' ak)
flunisolide fluocinonide	(floo nis' o lide) (floo o sin' o nide)	guaifenesin guanfacine	(gwye fen' e sin) (gwahn' fa seen)
fluocinolone fluocinonide	(floo o sin' o lone) (floo o sin' o nide)	guanadrel gonadorelin	(gwahn' a drel) (goe nad o rell' in)
fluocinonide flunisolide	(floo o sin' o nide) (floo nis' o lide)	guanethidine guanidine	(gwahn eth' i deen) (gwahn' i deen)
fluocinonide fluocinolone	(floo o sin' o nide) (floo o sin' o lone)	guanfacine guaifenesin	(gwahn' fa seen) (gwye fen' e sin)
Fluosol Feosol	(flu' o sol) (fee' o sol)	guanidine guanethidine	(gwahn' i deen) (gwahn eth' i deen)
flurbiprofen fenoprofen	(flure bi' proe fen) (fen o proe' fen)	Haldol Halenol	(hal' dol) (hal' e nol)
F.M.L. Esimil	(ef' em el) (es' eh mil)	Haldol Halog	(hal' dol) (hay' log)
Fostex pHisoHex	(fos' teks) (fye' so heks)	Halenol Haldol	(hal' e nol) (hal' dol)
Fulvicin Furacin	(ful' vi sin) (fur' a sin)	Halfan Halfprin	(hal' fan) (half' prin)
Furacin Fulvicin	(fur' a sin) (ful' vi sin)	Halfprin Halfan	(half' prin) (hal' fan)
Gamastan Garamycin	(gam' a stan) (gar a mye' sin)	Halfprin Haltran	(half' prin) (hal' tran)
Gantanol Gantrisin	(gan' ta nol) (gan' tri sin)	Halog Haldol	(hay' log) (hal' dol)
Gantrisin Gantanol	(gan' tri sin) (gan' ta nol)	Halotestin Halotex	(hay lo tes' tin) (hay' lo teks)
Gantrisin Gastrosed™	(gan' tri sin) (gas' troe sed)	Halotestin Halotussin	(hay lo tes' tin) (hay lo tus' sin)
Garamycin Gamastan	(gar a mye' sin) (gam' a stan)	Halotex Halotestin	(hay' lo teks) (hay lo tes' tin)
Garamycin kanamycin	(gar a mye' sin) (kan a mye' sin)	Halotussin Halotestin	(hay lo tus' sin) (hay lo tes' tin)
Garamycin Terramycin	(gar a mye' sin) (tehr a mye' sin)	Haltran Halfprin	(hal' tran) (half' prin)
Gastrosed™ Gantrisin	(gas' troe sed) (gan' tri sin)	Herplex Hiprex	(her' pleks) (hi' preks)
Genapap Genapax	(gen' a pap) (gen' a paks)	Hespan Histaspan	(hes' pan) (his' ta span)

Drug Name	Pronunciation	Drug Name	Pronunciation
Hexadrol"	(heks' a drol)	Idamycin"	(eye da mye' sin)
Hexalol"	(heks' a drol)	Adriamycin™	(ade rya mye' sin)
Hexalol"	(heks' a drol)	imipramine	(im ip' ra meen)
Hexadrol"	(heks' a drol)	Norpramin"	(nor pray' min)
Hiprex"	(hi' preks)	Imuran"	(im' yu ran)
Herplex"	(her' pleks)	Enduron"	(en' du ron)
Histaspan"	(his' ta span)	Inapsine"	(i nap' seen)
Hespan"	(hes' pan)	Nebcin"	(neb' sin)
Hycodan"	(hye' co dan)	Inderal"	(in' der al)
Hycomine"	(hye' co meen)	Enduron"	(en' du ron)
Hycodan"	(hye' co dan)	Inderal"	(in' der al)
Vicodin"	(vye' co din)	Enduronyl"	(en dur' o nil)
Hycomine"	(hye' coe meen)	Inderal"	(in' der al)
Byclomine"	(bye' clo meen)	Isordil"	(eye' sor dil)
Hycomine"	(hye' co meen)	Inderal"	(in' der al)
Hycodan"	(hye' co dan)	Medrol"	(meh' drol)
Hydergine"	(hye' der geen)	Inderal" 40	(in' der al for' tee)
Hydramyn"	(hye' dra min)	Enduronyl" Forte	(en dur' o nil for' tay)
hydralazine	(hye dral' a zeen)	Indocin"	(in' doe sin)
hydroxyzine	(hye drox' i zeen)	Lincocin"	(lin' coe sin)
Hydramyn"	(hye' dra min)	Indocin"	(in' doe sin)
Hydergine"	(hye' der geen)	Minocin"	(min' o sin)
Hydramyn"	(hye' dra min)	Intal"	(in' tal)
Bydramine"	(bye' dra meen)	Endal"	(en' dal)
Hydrocet"	(hye' dro set)	Intropin"	(in tro' pin)
Hydrocil"	(hye' dro sil)	Isoptin"	(eye sop' tin)
Hydrocil"	(hye' dro sil)	Intropin"	(in troe' pin)
Hydrocet"	(hye' dro set)	Ditropan"	(di troe' pan)
hydroxyurea	(hye drox ee yoor ee' a)	Ismelin"	(is' meh lin)
hydroxyzine	(hye drox' i zeen)	Esimil"	(es' eh mil)
hydroxyzine	(hye drox' i zeen)	Ismelin"	(is' meh lin)
hydralazine	(hye dral' a zeen)	Ritalin"	(ri' ta lin)
hydroxyzine	(hye drox' i zeen)	isoflurane	(eye soe flure' ane)
hydroxyurea	(hye drox ee yoor ee' a)	enflurane	(en' floo rane)
Hygroton"	(hye gro' ton)	isoflurane	(eye soe flure' ane)
Regroton"	(reg' ro ton)	isoflurophate	(eye soe flure' o fate)
Hyper-Tet"	(hye' per tet)	isoflurophate	(eye soe flure' o fate)
HyperHep"	(hye' per hep)	isoflurane	(eye soe flure' ane)
Hyper-Tet"	(hye' per tet)	Isoptin"	(eye sop' tin)
Hyperstat"	(hye' per stat)	Intropin"	(in tro' pin)
HyperHep"	(hye' per hep)	Isoptin"	(eye sop' tin)
Hyperab"	(hye' per ab)	Isopto" Tears	(eye sop' tow tears)
HyperHep"	(hye' per hep)	Isopto" Tears	(eye sop' tow tears)
Hyper-Tet"	(hye' per tet)	Isoptin"	(eye sop' tin)
Hyperab"	(hye' per ab)	Isordil"	(eye' sor dil)
HyperHep"	(hye' per hep)	Inderal"	(in' der al)
Hyperstat"	(hye' per stat)	Isordil"	(eye' sor dil)
Hyper-Tet"	(hye' per tet)	Isuprel"	(eye' sue prel)
Hyperstat"	(hye' per stat)	Isuprel"	(eye' sue prel)
Nitrostat"	(nye' troe stat)	Isordil"	(eye' sor dil)
Hytone"	(hye' tone)	K-Lor™	(kay' lor)
Vytone"	(vye' tone)	Kaochlor"	(kay' o klor)

Drug Name	Pronunciation	Drug Name	Pronunciation
kanamycin	(kan a mye′ sin)	Lincocin"	(link′ o sin)
Garamycin"	(gar a mye′ sin)	Minocin"	(min′ o sin)
kanamycin	(kan a mye′ sin)	Lioresal"	(lye or′ reh sal)
gentamicin	(jen ta mye′ sin)	lisinopril	(lyse in′ o pril)
Kaochlor"	(kay′ o klor)	liothyronine	(lye o thye′ roe neen)
K-Lor™	(kay′ lor)	levothyroxine	(lee voe thye rox′ een)
Keflex"	(keh′ fleks)	lisinopril	(lyse in′ o pril)
Keflin"	(keh′ flin)	Lioresal"	(lye or′ reh sal)
Keflin"	(keh′ flin)	Lithane"	(lith′ ane)
Keflex"	(keh′ fleks)	Lithonate"	(lith′ o nate)
Kemadrin"	(kem′ a drin)	Lithonate"	(lith′ o nate)
Coumadin"	(ku′ ma din)	Lithane"	(lith′ ane)
Klonopin™	(klon′ o pin)	Lithostat"	(lith′ o stat)
clonidine	(kloe′ ni deen)	Lithotabs"	(lith′ o tabs)
Komex"	(koe′ meks)	Lithotabs"	(lith′ o tabs)
Koromex"	(kor′ o meks)	Lithostat"	(lith′ o stat)
Koromex"	(kor′ o meks)	Lodine"	(low′ deen)
Komex"	(koe′ meks)	codeine	(koe′ deen)
Lanoxin"	(lan ox′ in)	Loniten"	(lon′ eh ten)
Levoxine"	(lev ox een)	clonidine	(kloe′ ni deen)
Lanoxin"	(lan ox′ in)	Lopressor"	(lo pres′ sor)
Levsinex"	(lev′ si neks)	Lopurin"	(lo pure′ in)
Larylgan"	(la ril′ gan)	Lopurin"	(lo pure′ in)
Auralgan"	(a ral′ gan)	Lopressor"	(lo pres′ sor)
Lasix"	(lay′ siks)	Lopurin"	(lo pure′ in)
Lidex"	(lye′ deks)	Lupron"	(lu′ pron)
leucovorin	(loo koe vor′ in)	Lorcet"	(lor′ set)
Leukeran"	(lu′ keh ran)	Fioricet"	(fee oh′ reh set)
Leukeran"	(lu′ keh ran)	Lotrimin"	(low′ tri min)
leucovorin	(loo koe vor′ in)	Otrivin"	(oh′ tri vin)
levodopa	(lee voe doe′ pa)	Luminal"	(lu′ mi nal)
methyldopa	(meth ill doe′ pa)	Tuinal"	(tu′ i nal)
levothyroxine	(lee voe thye rox′ een)	Lupron"	(lu′ pron)
liothyronine	(lye o thye′ roe neen)	Lopurin"	(lo pure′ in)
Levoxine"	(lev ox een)	Lupron"	(lu′ pron)
Lanoxin"	(lan ox′ in)	Nuprin"	(nu′ prin)
Levsinex"	(lev′ si neks)	Maalox"	(may′ loks)
Lanoxin"	(lan ox′ in)		
Lidex"	(lye′ deks)	Maalox"	(may′ loks)
Lasix"	(lay′ siks)	Maox"	(may′ oks)
		Marax"	(mare′ aks)
Lidex"	(lye′ deks)	Maalox"	(may′ loks)
Lidox"	(lye′ dox)	Monodox"	(mon′ o doks)
Lidex"	(lye′ deks)	Maltsupex"	(malt′ su peks)
Videx"	(vye′ deks)	Manoplax"	(man′ o laks)
Lidex"	(lye′ deks)	Mandol"	(man′ dole)
Wydase"	(wye′ dase)	nadolol	(nay doe′ lole)
Lidox"	(lye′ dox)	Manoplax"	(man′ o laks)
Lidex"	(lye′ deks)	Maltsupex"	(malt′ su peks)
Lincocin"	(link′ o sin)	Maox"	(may′ oks)
Cleocin"	(klee′ o sin)	Maalox"	(may′ loks)
Lincocin"	(lin′ coe sin)	Maox"	(may′ oks)
Indocin"	(in′ doe sin)	Marax"	(may′ raks)

APPENDIX

Drug Name	Pronunciation	Drug Name	Pronunciation
Marax'''	(mare' aks)	Mephyton'''	(meh fye' ton)
Maalox''	(may' loks)	mephenytoin	(me fen' i toyn)
Marax'''	(may' raks)	Mephyton'''	(meh fye' ton)
Atarax''	(at' a raks)	methadone	(meth' a done)
Marax'''	(may' raks)	mepivacaine	(me piv' a kane)
Maox''	(may' oks)	bupivacaine	(byoo piv' a kane)
Marcaine'''	(mar' kane)	Meprospan''	(meh' pro span)
Narcan''	(nar' kan)	Naprosyn''	(na' pro sin)
Marinol'''	(mare' i nole)	mesalamine	(me sal' a meen)
Marnal''	(mar' nal)	mecamylamine	(mek a mill' a meen)
Marnal''	(mar' nal)	Mesantoin''	(meh san' toyn)
Marinol'''	(mare' i nole)	mephenytoin	(me fen' i toyn)
Matulane''	(mat' chu lane)	Mesantoin''	(meh san' toyn)
Modane''	(moe' dane)	Mestinon''	(meh' sti non)
Maxidex''	(maks' i deks)	Mestinon''	(meh' sti non)
Maxzide''	(maks' zide)	Mesantoin'''	(meh san' toyn)
Maxzide''	(maks' zide)	Metahydrin''	(me ta hye' drin)
Maxidex''	(maks' i deks)	Metandren''	(me tan' dren)
Mebaral''	(meb' a ral)	Metandren''	(me tan' dren)
Medrol''	(med' role)	Metahydrin''	(me ta hye' drin)
Mebaral''	(meb' a ral)	metaproterenol	(met a proe ter' e nol)
Mellaril''	(mel' a ril)	metoprolol	(me toe' proe lole)
Mebaral''	(meb' a ral)	metaxalone	(me taks' a lone)
Tegretol''	(teg' ree tol)	metolazone	(me tole' a zone)
mecamylamine	(mek a mill' a meen)	methadone	(meth' a done)
mesalamine	(me sal' a meen)	Mephyton'''	(meh fye' ton)
Meclan'''	(me' klan)	methazolamide	(meth a zoe' la mide)
Meclomen'''	(meh' klo men)	metolazone	(me tole' a zone)
Meclan''	(me' klan)	methenamine	(meth en' a meen)
Mezlin''	(mes' lin)	methionine	(me thye' o neen)
Meclomen'''	(meh' klo men)	methicillin	(meth i sill' in)
Meclan''	(me' klan)	mezlocillin	(mez loe sill' in)
Medrol''	(med' role)	methionine	(me thye' o neen)
Mebaral''	(meb' a ral)	methenamine	(meth en' a meen)
Medrol''	(meh' drol)	methocarbamol	(meth o kar' ba mole)
Inderal''	(in' der al)	mephobarbital	(me foe bar' bi tal)
Mellaril''	(mel' la ril)	methsuximide	(meth sux' i mide)
Elavil''	(el' a vil)	ethosuximide	(eth o sux' i mide)
Mellaril''	(mel' a ril)	methyldopa	(meth ill doe' pa)
Mebaral''	(meb' a ral)	levodopa	(lee voe doe' pa)
melphalan	(mel' fa lan)	metolazone	(me tole' a zone)
Mephyton'''	(meh fye' ton)	metaxalone	(me taks' a lone)
mephenytoin	(me fen' i toyn)	metolazone	(me tole' a zone)
Mephyton'''	(meh fye' ton)	methazolamide	(meth a zoe' la mide)
mephenytoin	(me fen' i toyn)	metolazone	(me tole' a zone)
Mesantoin'''	(meh san' toyn)	minoxidil	(mi nox' i dill)
mephenytoin	(me fen' i toyn)	metoprolol	(me toe' proe lole)
phenytoin	(fen' i toyn)	metaproterenol	(met a proe ter' e nol)
mephobarbital	(me foe bar' bi tal)	metyrapone	(me teer' a pone)
methocarbamol	(meth o kar' ba mole)	metyrosine	(me tye' roe seen)
Mephyton'''	(meh fye' ton)	metyrosine	(me tye' roe seen)
melphalan	(mel' fa lan)	metyrapone	(me teer' a pone)

Drug Name	Pronunciation	Drug Name	Pronunciation
Mexitil"	(meks' i til)	Mutamycin"	(mute a mye' sin)
Mezlin"	(mes' lin)	mitomycin	(mye toe mye' sin)
Mezlin"	(mes' lin)	Myambutol"	(mya am' byoo tol)
Meclan"	(me' klan)	Nembutal"	(nem' byoo tal)
Mezlin"	(mes' lin)	Mycelex"	(mye' si leks)
Mexitil"	(meks' i til)	Myoflex"	(mye' o fleks)
mezlocillin	(mez loe sill' in)	Mydfrin"	(mid' frin)
methicillin	(meth i sill' in)	Midrin"	(mid' rin)
miconazole	(mi kon' a zole)	Mylanta"	(mye lan' tah)
Micronase"	(mye' croe nase)	Milontin"	(mi lon' tin)
Micronase"	(mye' croe nase)	Myleran"	(mye' leh ran)
Micronor"	(mye' croe nor)	Mylicon"	(mye' li kon)
Micronase"	(mye' croe nase)	Mylicon"	(mye' li kon)
miconazole	(mi kon' a zole)	Modicon"	(mod' i kon)
Micronor"	(mye' croe nor)	Mylicon"	(mye' li kon)
Micronase"	(mye' croe nase)	Myleran"	(mye' leh ran)
Midrin"	(mid' rin)	Myochrysine"	(mye o kris' seen)
Mydfrin"	(mid' frin)	vincristine	(vin kris' teen)
Milontin"	(mi lon' tin)	Myoflex"	(mye' o fleks)
Miltown"	(mil' town)	Mycelex"	(mye' si leks)
Milontin"	(mi lon' tin)	nadolol	(nay doe' lole)
Mylanta"	(mye lan' tah)	Mandol"	(man' dole)
Miltown"	(mil' town)	Naldecon"	(nal' dee kon)
Milontin"	(mi lon' tin)	Nalfon"	(nal' fon)
Minizide"	(min' i zide)	Nalfon"	(nal' fon)
Minocin"	(min' o sin)	Naldecon"	(nal' dee kon)
Minocin"	(min' o sin)	Nallpen"	(nall' pen)
Indocin"	(in' doe sin)	Nalspan"	(nal' span)
Minocin"	(min' o sin)	naloxone	(nal ox' one)
Lincocin"	(link' o sin)	naltrexone	(nal treks' one)
Minocin"	(min' o sin)	Nalspan"	(nal' span)
Minizide"	(min' i zide)	Nallpen"	(nall' pen)
Minocin"	(min' o sin)	naltrexone	(nal treks' one)
Mithracin"	(mith' ra sin)	naloxone	(nal ox' one)
Minocin"	(min' o sin)	Naprosyn"	(na' pro sin)
niacin	(nye' a sin)	Meprospan"	(meh' pro span)
minoxidil	(mi nox' i dill)	Naprosyn"	(na' pro sin)
metolazone	(me tole' a zone)	naproxen	(na prox' en)
Mithracin"	(mith' ra sin)	Naprosyn"	(na' pro sin)
Minocin"	(min' o sin)	Natacyn"	(na' ta sin)
mitomycin	(mye toe mye' sin)	Naprosyn"	(na' pro sin)
Mutamycin"	(mute a mye' sin)	Nebcin"	(neb' sin)
Moban"	(moe' ban)	naproxen	(na prox' en)
Modane"	(moe' dane)	Naprosyn"	(na' pro sin)
Modane"	(moe' dane)	Narcan"	(nar' kan)
Matulane"	(mat' chu lane)	Marcaine"	(mar' kane)
Modane"	(moe' dane)	Nardil"	(nar' dil)
Moban"	(moe' ban)	Norinyl"	(nor' eh nil)
Modicon"	(mod' i kon)	Natacyn"	(na' ta sin)
Mylicon"	(mye' li kon)	Naprosyn"	(na' pro sin)
Monodox"	(mon' o doks)	Nebcin"	(neb' sin)
Maalox"	(may' loks)	Inapsine"	(i nap' seen)

APPENDIX

Drug Name	Pronunciation	Drug Name	Pronunciation
Nebcin'''	(neb' sin)	Nutramigen''	(nu' tra gen)
Naprosyn'''	(na' pro sin)	Neupogen'''	(nu' po gen)
Nembutal'''	(nem' byoo tal)	Omnipaque''	(om' ni pak)
Myambutol'''	(mya am' byoo tol)	Omnipen''	(om' ni pen)
Neptazane''	(nep' ta zane)	Omnipen'''	(om' ni pen)
Nesacaine'''	(nes' a kane)	Omnipaque''	(om' ni pak)
Nesacaine'''	(nes' a kane)	Omnipen''	(om' ni pen)
Neptazane''	(nep' ta zane)	Unipen''	(yu' ni pen)
Neupogen'''	(nu' po gen)	Oncovin''	(on' coe vin)
Nutramigen'''	(nu' tra gen)	Ancobon''	(an' coe bon)
niacin	(nye' a sin)	Ophthaine''	(op' thane)
Minocin''	(min' o sin)	Ophthetic''	(op thet' ik)
nicardipine	(nye kar' de peen)	Ophthalgan''	(opp thal' gan)
nifedipine	(nye fed' i peen)	Auralgan''	(a ral' gan)
Nicobid''	(nye' ko bid)	Ophthetic''	(op thet' ik)
Nitro-Bid'''	(nye' troe bid)	Ophthaine''	(op' thane)
Nicorette'''	(nik' o ret)	Ophthochlor''	(op' tho klor)
Nordette'''	(nor det')	Ophthocort''	(op' tho kort)
nifedipine	(nye fed' i peen)	Ophthocort''	(op' tho kort)
nicardipine	(nye kar' de peen)	Ophthochlor''	(op' tho klor)
nifedipine	(nye fed' i peen)	Orabase'''	(or' a base)
nimodipine	(nye moe' di peen)	Orinase''	(or' in ase)
Nilstat''	(nil' stat)	Oretic''	(or et' ik)
Nitrostat'''	(nye' troe stat)	Oreton''	(or' eh ton)
Nimodipine	(nye moe' di peen)	Oreton'''	(or' eh ton)
nifedipine	(nye fed' i peen)	Oretic''	(or et' ik)
Nitro-Bid''	(nye' troe bid)	Orinase''	(or' in ase)
Nicobid'''	(nye' ko bid)	Orabase''	(or' a base)
Nitroglycerin	(nye troe gli' ser in)	Orinase''	(or' in ase)
Nitroglyn''	(nye' troe glin)	Ornade''	(or' nade)
Nitroglyn''	(nye' troe glin)	Orinase''	(or' in ase)
nitroglycerin	(nye troe gli' ser in)	Tolinase''	(tole' i nase)
Nitrostat'''	(nye' troe stat)	Ornade''	(or' nade)
Hyperstat''	(hye' per stat)	Orinase''	(or' in ase)
Nitrostat''	(nye' troe stat)	Otrivin''	(oh' tri vin)
Nilstat''	(nil' stat)	Lotrimin''	(low' tri min)
Nordette'''	(nor det')	oxymetazoline	(ox i met az' o leen)
Nicorette'''	(nik' o ret)	oxymetholone	(ox i meth' o lone)
Norinyl''	(nor' eh nil)	oxymetholone	(ox i meth' o lone)
Nardil''	(nar' dil)	oxymetazoline	(ox i met az' o leen)
Norlutate'''	(nor' lu tate)	oxymetholone	(ox i meth' o lone)
Norlutin''	(nor lu' tin)	oxymorphone	(ox i mor' fone)
Norlutin''	(nor lu' tin)	oxymorphone	(ox i mor' fone)
Norlutate'''	(nor' lu tate)	oxymetholone	(ox i meth' o lone)
Norpramin'''	(nor pray' min)	Pamelor'''	(pam' meh lor)
imipramine	(im ip' ra meen)	Dymelor'''	(dye' meh lor)
Novafed'''	(nove' a fed)	Pathilon'''	(path' i lon)
Nucofed'''	(nu' co fed)	Pathocil'''	(path' o sil)
Nucofed'''	(nu' co fed)	Pathocil'''	(path' o sil)
Novafed'''	(nove' a fed)	Pathilon'''	(path' i lon)
Nuprin'''	(nu' prin)	Pathocil'''	(path' o sil)
Lupron'''	(lu' pron)	Placidyl'''	(pla' ce dil)

Drug Name	Pronunciation	Drug Name	Pronunciation
Pathocil™	(path′ o sill)	physostigmine	(fye zoe stig′ meen)
Bactocill™	(bak′ tow sill)	pyridostigmine	(peer id o stig′ meen)
Pavabid™	(pav′ a bid)	Pitocin™	(pi toe′ sin)
Pavased™	(pav′ a sed)	Pitressin™	(ph tres′ sin)
Pavased™	(pav′ a sed)	Pitressin™	(ph tres′ sin)
Pavabid™	(pav′ a bid)	Pitocin™	(ph toe′ sin)
pentobarbital	(pen toe bar′ bi tal)	Placidyl™	(pla′ ce dil)
phenobarbital	(fee noe bar′ bi tal)	Pathocil™	(path′ o sil)
Percodan™	(per′ coe dan)	Plaquenil™	(pla′ kwe nil)
Decadron™	(dek′ a dron)	Platinol™	(pla′ tee nol)
Perdiem™	(per dee′ em)	Platinol™	(pla′ tee nol)
Pyridium™	(pye rid′ dee um)	Plaquenil™	(pla′ kwe nil)
Persantine™	(per san′ teen)	Ponstel™	(pon′ stel)
Pertofrane™	(per′ toe frane)	Pronestyl™	(pro nes′ til)
Pertofrane™	(per′ toe frane)	pralidoxime	(pra li dox′ eem)
Persantine™	(per san′ teen)	pramoxine	(pra moks′ een)
Phazyme™	(fay′ zeem)	pralidoxime	(pra li dox′ eem)
Pherazine™	(fer′ a zeen)	pyridoxine	(peer i dox′ een)
Phenergan™	(fen′ er gan)	Pramosone™	(pra′ mo sone)
Phrenilin™	(fren′ ni lin)	prednisone	(pred′ ni sone)
Phenergan™	(fen′ er gan)	pramoxine	(pra moks′ een)
Theragran™	(ther′ a gran)	pralidoxime	(pra li dox′ eem)
phenobarbital	(fee noe bar′ bi tal)	prazepam	(pra′ ze pam)
pentobarbital	(pen toe bar′ bi tal)	prazosin	(pra′ zoe sin)
phentermine	(fen′ ter meen)	prazosin	(pra′ zoe sin)
phentolamine	(fen tole′ a meen)	prazepam	(pra′ ze pam)
phentolamine	(fen tole′ a meen)	Predalone™	(pred′ a lone)
phentermine	(fen′ ter meen)	prednisone	(pred′ ni sone)
phentolamine	(fen tole′ a meen)	prednisolone	(pred nis′ o lone)
Ventolin™	(ven′ to lin)	prednisone	(pred′ ni sone)
phenytoin	(fen′ i toyn)	prednisone	(pred′ ni sone)
mephenytoin	(me fen′ i toyn)	Pramosone™	(pra′ mo sone)
Pherazine™	(fer′ a zeen)	prednisone	(pred′ ni sone)
Phazyme™	(fay′ zeem)	Predalone™	(pred′ a lone)
pHisoHex™	(fye′ so heks)	prednisone	(pred′ ni sone)
Fostex™	(fos′ teks)	prednisolone	(pred nis′ o lone)
Phos-Flur™	(fos′ flur)	prednisone	(pred′ ni sone)
PhosLo™	(fos′ lo)	primidone	(pri′ mi done)
PhosLo™	(fos′ lo)	prilocaine	(pril′ o kane)
Phos-Flur™	(fos′ flur)	Prilosec™	(pre′ lo sek)
PhosLo™	(fos′ lo)	Prilosec™	(pre′ lo sek)
ProSom™	(pro′ som)	Prozac™	(proe′ zak)
Phosphaljel™	(fos′ fal gel)	Prilosec™	(pre′ lo sek)
Phospholine™	(fos′ fo leen)	prilocaine	(pril′ o kane)
Phospholine™	(fos′ fo leen)	primidone	(pri′ mi done)
Phosphaljel™	(fos′ fal gel)	prednisone	(pred′ ni sone)
Phrenilin™	(fren′ ni lin)	Priscoline™	(pris′ coe leen)
Phenergan™	(fen′ er gan)	Apresoline™	(aye press′ sow leen)
Phrenilin™	(fren′ ni lin)	Pro-Sof™	(proe′ sof)
Trinalin™	(tri′ na lin)	ProSom™	(pro′ som)
physostigmine	(fye zoe stig′ meen)	ProSom™	(pro′ som)
Prostigmin™	(pro stig′ min)	PhosLo™	(fos′ lo)

Drug Name	Pronunciation	Drug Name	Pronunciation
ProSom™	(pro' som)	quinidine	(kwin' i deen)
Pro-Sof" Plus	(proe' sof)	quinine	(kwye' nine)
ProStep"	(proe' step)	quinine	(kwye' nine)
Prozac"	(proe' zak)	quinidine	(kwin' i deen)
procarbazine	(proe kar' ba zeen)	Reglan"	(reg' lan)
dacarbazine	(da kar' ba zeen)	Regonol"	(reg' o nol)
promazine	(proe' ma zeen)	Regonol"	(reg' o nol)
promethazine	(proe meth' a zeen)	Reglan"	(reg' lan)
Prometh"	(proe' meth)	Regonol"	(reg' o nol)
Promit"	(proe' mit)	Regutol"	(reg' yu tol)
promethazine	(proe meth' a zeen)	Regroton"	(reg' ro ton)
promazine	(proe' ma zeen)	Hygroton"	(hye gro' ton)
Promit"	(proe' mit)	Regutol"	(reg' yu tol)
Prometh"	(proe' meth)	Regonol"	(reg' o nol)
Pronestyl"	(pro nes' til)	Repan"	(ree' pan)
Ponstel"	(pon' stel)	Riopan"	(rye' o pan)
Propacet"	(proe' pa set)	Restore"	(res tore')
Propagest"	(proe' pa gest)	Restoril"	(res' tor ril)
Propagest"	(proe' pa gest)	Restoril"	(res' tor ril)
Propacet"	(proe' pa set)	Restore"	(res tore')
Prostigmin"	(pro stig' min)	Restoril"	(res' tor ril)
physostigmine	(fye zoe stig' meen)	Vistaril"	(vis' tar ril)
protamine	(proe' ta meen)	ribavirin	(rye ba vye' rin)
Protopam"	(proe' toe pam)	riboflavin	(rye' boe flay vin)
Protopam"	(proe' toe pam)	riboflavin	(rye' boe flay vin)
protamine	(proe' ta meen)	ribavirin	(rye ba vye' rin)
Protopam"	(proe' toe pam)	Rifadin"	(rif' a din)
Protropin"	(proe tro' pin)	Ritalin"	(ri' ta lin)
Protropin"	(proe tro' pin)	Rimactane"	(ri mak' tane)
Protopam"	(proe' toe pam)	rimantadine	(ri man' to deen)
Prozac"	(proe' zak)	rimantadine	(ri man' to deen)
Prilosec™	(pre' lo sek)	Rimactane"	(ri mak' tane)
Prozac"	(proe' zak)	Riobin"	(rye' o bin)
ProStep"	(proe' step)	Riopan"	(rye' o pan)
Pyridium"	(pye rid' dee um)	Riopan"	(rye' o pan)
Dyrenium"	(dye ren' e um)	Repan	(ree' pan)
Pyridium"	(pye rid' dee um)	Riopan"	(rye' o pan)
Perdiem"	(per dee' em)	Riobin"	(rye' o bin)
Pyridium"	(pye rid' dee um)	Ritalin"	(ri' ta lin)
pyridoxine	(peer i dox' een)	Ismelin"	(is' meh lin)
Pyridium"	(pye rid' dee um)	Ritalin"	(ri' ta lin)
pyrithione	(peer i thye' one)	Rifadin"	(rif' a din)
pyridostigmine	(peer id o stig' meen)	Ritalin"	(ri' ta lin)
physostigmine	(fye zoe stig' meen)	ritodrine	(ri' toe dreen)
pyridoxine	(peer i dox' een)	ritodrine	(ri' toe dreen)
Pyridium"	(pye rid' dee um)	Ritalin"	(ri' ta lin)
pyridoxine	(peer i dox' een)	Rocephin"	(roe sef' fen)
pralidoxime	(pra li dox' eem)	Roferon"	(roe fer' on)
pyrithione	(peer i thye' one)	Roferon"	(roe fer' on)
Pyridium"	(pye rid' dee um)	Rocephin"	(roe sef' fen)
quinidine	(kwin' i deen)	Rynatan"	(rye' na tan)
clonidine	(kloe' ni deen)	Rynatuss"	(rye' na tuss)

Drug Name	Pronunciation	Drug Name	Pronunciation
Rynatuss"	(rye' na tuss)	sulfisoxazole	(sul fi sox' a zole)
Rynatan"	(rye' na tan)	sulfasalazine	(sul fa sal' a zeen)
Salacid"	(sal as' sid)	Surbex"	(sur' beks)
Salagen"	(sal' a gen)	Surfak"	(sur' fak)
Salagen"	(sal' a gen)	Surfak"	(sur' fak)
Salacid"	(sal as' sid)	Surbex"	(sur' beks)
Salutensin"	(sal yu ten' sin)	Surital"	(su' ri tal)
Diutensin"	(dye yu ten' sin)	Serentil"	(su ren' til)
Seconal™	(sek' o nal)	Sytobex"	(sye' toe beks)
Sectral"	(sek' tral)	Cytotec"	(sye' toe tek)
Sectral"	(sek' tral)	Tacaryl"	(tak' a ril)
Factrel"	(fak' trel)	tacrine	(tak' reen)
Sectral"	(sek' tral)	tacrine	(tak' reen)
Seconal™	(sek' o nal)	Tacaryl"	(tak' a ril)
Seldane"	(sel' dane)	Tagamet"	(tag' a met)
Feldene"	(fel' deen)	Tegopen"	(teg' o pen)
Septa"	(sep' tah)	Talacen"	(tal' a sen)
Septra"	(sep' trah)	Tegison"	(teg' i son)
Septra"	(sep' trah)	Talacen"	(tal' a sen)
Septa"	(sep' tah)	Tinactin"	(tin ak' tin)
Ser-Ap-Es"	(ser ap' ess)	Tedral"	(ted' ral)
Catapres"	(kat' a pres)	Teldrin"	(tel' drin)
Serax"	(sear' aks)	Tegison"	(teg' i son)
Eurax"	(yoor' aks)	Talacen"	(tal' a sen)
Serax"	(sear' aks)	Tegopen"	(teg' o pen)
Urex"	(yu' eks)	Tagamet"	(tag' a met)
Serentil"	(su ren' til)	Tegopen"	(teg' o pen)
Surital"	(su' ri tal)	Tegretol"	(teg' ree tol)
Silace"	(sye' lace)	Tegopen"	(teg' o pen)
Silain"	(sye' lain)	Tegrin"	(teg' rin)
Silain"	(sye' lain)	Tegretol"	(teg' ree tol)
Silace"	(sye' lace)	Mebaral"	(meb' a ral)
Solarcaine"	(sole' ar kane)	Tegretol"	(teg' ree tol)
Solatene"	(sole' a teen)	Tegopen"	(teg' o pen)
Solatene"	(sole' a teen)	Tegrin"	(teg' rin)
Solarcaine"	(sole' ar kane)	Tegopen"	(teg' o pen)
Staphcillin"	(staf sil' lin)	Teldrin"	(tel' drin)
Staticin"	(stat' i sin)	Tedral"	(ted' ral)
Staticin"	(stat' i sin)	Temaril"	(tem' a ril)
Staphcillin"	(staf sil' lin)	Demerol"	(dem' eh rol)
streptomycin	(strep toe mye' sin)	Temaril"	(tem' a ril)
streptozocin	(strep toe zoe' sin)	Tepanil"	(tep' a nil)
streptozocin	(strep toe zoe' sin)	Tenex"	(ten' eks)
streptomycin	(strep toe mye' sin)	Xanax"	(zan' aks)
Sudafed"	(sue' da fed)	Tepanil"	(tep' a nil)
Sufenta"	(sue fen' tah)	Temaril"	(tem' a ril)
Sufenta"	(sue fen' tah)	Tepanil"	(tep' a nil)
Alfenta"	(al fen' tah)	Tofranil"	(toe fray' nil)
Sufenta"	(sue fen' tah)	terbinafine	(ter' bin a feen)
Sudafed"	(sue' da fed)	terbutaline	(ter byoo' ta leen)
sulfasalazine	(sul fa sal' a zeen)	terbutaline	(ter byoo' ta leen)
sulfisoxazole	(sul fi sox' a zole)	terbinafine	(ter' bin a feen)

Drug Name	Pronunciation	Drug Name	Pronunciation
terbutaline	(ter byoo' ta leen)	Tigan"	(tye' gan)
tolbutamide	(tole byoo' ta mide)	Ticar"	(tye' kar)
terconazole	(ter kone' a zole)	Tigan"	(tye' gan)
tioconazole	(tye o kone' a zole)	Ticon"	(tye' kon)
Terramycin"	(tehr a mye' sin)	timolol	(tye' moe lole)
Garamycin"'	(gar a mye' sin)	Tylenol"	(tye' le nole)
testolactone	(tess toe lak' tone)	Timoptic"	(tim op' tik)
testosterone	(tess toss' ter one)	Viroptic"	(vir op' tik)
testosterone	(tess toss' ter one)	Tinactin"	(tin ak' tin)
testolactone	(tess toe lak' tone)	Talacen"	(tal' a sen)
Theelin"	(thee' lin)	Tindal"	(tin' dal)
Theolair™	(thee' o lare)	Trental"	(tren' tal)
Theoclear"	(thee' o clear)	tioconazole	(tye o kone' a zole)
Theolair™	(thee' o lare)	terconazole	(ter kone' a zole)
Theolair™	(thee' o lare)	TobraDex"	(toe' bra deks)
Theelin"	(thee' lin)	Tobrex"	(toe' breks)
Theolair™	(thee' o lare)	tobramycin	(toe bra mye' sin)
Theoclear"	(thee' o clear)	Trobicin"	(troe' bi sin)
Theolair™	(thee' o lare)	Tobrex"	(toe' breks)
Thiola™	(thye oh' la)	TobraDex"	(toe' bra deks)
Theolair™	(thee' o lare)	Tofranil"	(toe fray' nil)
Thyrolar"	(thye' roe lar)	Tepanil"	(tep' a nil)
Theragran"	(ther' a gran)	tolazamide	(tole az' a mide)
Phenergan"'	(fen' er gan)	tolazoline	(tole az' o leen)
Theramin"'	(there' a min)	tolazamide	(tole az' a mide)
thiamine	(thye' a min)	tolbutamide	(tole byoo' ta mide)
thiamine	(thye' a min)	tolazoline	(tole az' o leen)
Theramin"	(there' a min)	tolazamide	(tole az' a mide)
Thiola™	(thye oh' la)	tolbutamide	(tole byoo' ta mide)
Theolair™	(thee' o lare)	terbutaline	(ter byoo' ta leen)
thioridazine	(thye o rid' a zeen)	tolbutamide	(tole byoo' ta mide)
thiothixene	(thye o thix' een)	tolazamide	(tole az' a mide)
thiothixene	(thye o thix' een)	Tolinase"'	(tole' i nase)
thioridazine	(thye o rid' a zeen)	Orinase"	(or' in ase)
Thyrar"	(thyer' are)	tolnaftate	(tole naf' tate)
Thyrolar"	(thye' roe lar)	Tornalate"	(tor' na late)
Thyrar"	(thyer' are)	Tonocard"	(ton' o kard)
Ticar"'	(tye' kar)	Torecan"	(tor' e kan)
Thyrolar"	(thye' roe lar)	Torecan"	(tor' e kan)
Theolair™	(thee' o lare)	Tonocard"	(ton' o kard)
Thyrolar"	(thye' roe lar)	Tornalate"	(tor' na late)
Thyrar"	(thyer' are)	tolnaftate	(tole naf' tate)
Thyrolar"	(thye' roe lar)	Trandate"	(tran' date)'
Thytropar"	(thye' troe par)	Trendar"	(tren' dar)
Thytropar"	(thye' troe par)	Trandate"	(tran' date)
Thyrolar"	(thye' roe lar)	Trental"	(tren' tal)
Ticar"'	(tye' kar)	Trendar"	(tren' dar)
Thyrar"	(thyer' are)	Trandate"	(tran' date)
Ticar"	(tye' kar)	Trental"	(tren' tal)
Tigan"	(tye' gan)	Tindal"'	(tin' dal)
Ticon"'	(tye' kon)	Trental"	(tren' tal)
Tigan"	(tye' gan)	Trandate"	(tran' date)

Drug Name	Pronunciation	Drug Name	Pronunciation
tretinoin	(tret' i noyn)	Tylenol"	(tye' le nole)
trientine	(trye' en teen)	timolol	(tye' moe lole)
Tri-Levlen"	(trye' lev len)	Tylenol"	(tye' le nole)
Trilafon"	(tri' la fon)	Tuinal"	(tu' i nal)
triacetin	(trye a see' tin)	Tylenol"	(tye' le nole)
Triacin"	(trye' a sin)	Tylox"	(tye' loks)
Triacin"	(trye' a sin)	Tylox"	(tye' loks)
triacetin	(trye a see' tin)	Trimox"	(trye' moks)
triamterene	(trye am' ter een)	Tylox"	(tye' loks)
trimipramine	(trye mi' pra meen)	Tylenol"	(tye' le nole)
trientine	(trye' en teen)	Tylox"	(tye' loks)
tretinoin	(tret' i noyn)	Wymox"	(wye' moks)
Trilafon"	(tri' la fon)	Unipen"	(yu' ni pen)
Tri-Levlen"	(trye' lev len)	Omnipen"	(om' ni pen)
trimeprazine	(trye mep' ra zeen)	Urex"	(yu' eks)
trimipramine	(trye mi' pra meen)	Eurax"	(yoor' aks)
trimethaphan	(trye meth' a fan)	Urex"	(yu' eks)
trimethoprim	(trye meth' o prim)	Serax"	(sear' aks)
trimethoprim	(trye meth' o prim)	V-Cillin K"	(vee sil' lin kay)
trimethaphan	(trye meth' a fan)	Bicillin"	(bye sil' lin)
trimipramine	(trye mi' pra meen)	V-Cillin K"	(vee' sil lin kay)
triamterene	(trye am' ter een)	Wycillin"	(wye sil' lin)
trimipramine	(trye mi' pra meen)	Vamate"	(vam' ate)
trimeprazine	(trye mep' ra zeen)	Vancenase"	(van' sen ase)
Trimox"	(trye' moks)	Vancenase"	(van' sen ase)
Diamox"	(dye' a moks)	Vamate"	(vam' ate)
Trimox"	(trye' moks)	Vanceril"	(van' ser il)
Tylox"	(tye' loks)	Vansil™	(van' sil)
Trinalin"	(tri' na lin)	Vansil™	(van' sil)
Phrenilin"	(fren' ni lin)	Vanceril"	(van' ser il)
Triofed"	(trye' o fed)	Vasocidin"	(vay so sye' din)
Triostat™	(tree' o stat)	Vasodilan"	(vay so di' lan)
Triostat™	(tree' o stat)	Vasodilan"	(vay so di' lan)
Triofed"	(trye' o fed)	Vasocidin"	(vay so sye' din)
Trisoralen"	(trye sore' a len)	Vasosulf"	(vay' so sulf)
Trysul"	(trye' sul)	Velosef"	(vel' o sef)
Trobicin"	(troe' bi sin)	VePesid"	(veh' pe sid)
tobramycin	(toe bra mye' sin)	Versed"	(ver' sed)
Tronolane"	(tron' o lane)	Velosef"	(vel' o sef)
Tronothane"	(tron' o thane)	Vasosulf"	(vay' so sulf)
Tronothane"	(tron' o thane)	Ventolin"	(ven' to lin)
Tronolane"	(tron' o lane)	phentolamine	(fen tole' a meen)
Trysul"	(trye' sul)	Ventolin"	(ven' tow lin)
Trisoralen"	(trye sore' a len)	Benylin"	(ben' eh lin)
Tuinal"	(tu' i nal)	Verelan"	(ver' e lan)
Luminal"	(lu' mi nal)	Voltaren"	(vo tare' en)
Tuinal"	(tu' i nal)	Versed"	(ver' sed)
Tylenol"	(tye' le nole)	VePesid"	(veh' pe sid)
Tussafed"	(tus' a fed)	Vicodin"	(vye' co din)
Tussafin"	(tus' a fin)	Hycodan"	(hye' co dan)
Tussafin"	(tus' a fin)	vidarabine	(vye dare' a been)
Tussafed"	(tus' a fed)	cytarabine	(sye tare' a been)

APPENDIX

Drug Name	Pronunciation	Drug Name	Pronunciation
Videx"	(vye' deks)	Wydase"	(wye' dase)
Lidex"	(lye' deks)	Lidex"	(lye' deks)
vinblastine	(vin blas' teen)	Wymox"	(wye' moks)
vincristine	(vin kris' teen)	Tylox"	(tye' loks)
vincristine	(vin kris' teen)	Xanax"	(zan' aks)
Myochrysine"	(mye o kris' seen)	Tenex"	(ten' eks)
vincristine	(vin kris' teen)	Xanax"	(zan' aks)
vinblastine	(vin blas' teen)	Zantac"	(zan' tak)
Viroptic"	(vir op' tik)	Xylo-Pfan"	(zye' lo fan)
Timoptic"	(tim op' tik)	Zyloprim"	(zye' lo prim)
Visine"	(vye' seen)	Zantac"	(zan' tak)
Visken"	(vis' ken)	Xanax"	(zan' aks)
Visken"	(vis' ken)	Zarontin"	(za ron' tin)
Visine"	(vye' seen)	Zaroxolyn"	(za roks' o lin)
Vistaril"	(vis' tar ril)	Zaroxolyn"	(za roks' o lin)
Restoril"	(res' tor ril)	Zarontin"	(za ron' tin)
Voltaren"	(vo tare' en)	Zerit"	(zer' it)
Verelan"	(ver' e lan)	Ziac™	(zye' ak)
Voltaren"	(vo tare' en)	Ziac™	(zye' ak)
Vontrol"	(von' trole)	Zerit"	(zer' it)
Vontrol"	(von' trole)	Zofran"	(zoe' fran)
Voltaren"	(vo tare' en)	Zosyn™	(zoe' sin)
Vytone"	(vye' tone)	Zosyn™	(zoe' sin)
Hytone"	(hye' tone)	Zofran"	(zoe' fran)
Vytone"	(vye' tone)	Zydone"	(zye' doan)
Zydone"	(zye' doan)	Vytone"	(vye' tone)
Wycillin"	(wye sil' lin)	Zyloprim"	(zye' lo prim)
Bicillin"	(bye sil' lin)	Xylo-Pfan"	(zye' lo fan)
Wycillin"	(wye sil' lin)		
V-Cillin K"	(vee' sil lin kay)		

WHAT'S NEW

New Drugs Introduced or Approved by the FDA in 1994

Brand Name	Generic Name	Use
Bactroban Nasal	mupirocin	Nasal carriage in children
Cozaar	losarton potassium	Hypertension
Cystagon	cysteamine bitartrate	Nephrotic cystinosis
Fragmin	dalteparin	Deep vein thombosis
Flonase	fluticasone	Anti-inflammatory nasal spray
Fosamax	alendronate	Osteoporosis
Havrix	hepatitis a vaccine	Vaccine for hepatitis A
Imitrex tablet	sumatriptan	Oral antimigraine agent
Kytril tablet	granisetron	Oral antinauseant
Lamcital	lamotrigine	Anticonvulsant
Luvox	fluvoxamine	Antidepressant
Prevacid	lansoprazole	Reflux esophagitis
Renormax	spirapril	ACE inhibitor
ReoPro™	abciximab	Cardiac ischemia
Serzone	nefazodone	Antidepressant
Trusopt	dorzolamide	Antiglaucoma agent
Vesanoid	trans-retinoic acid	Acute promyelocytic leukemia
Vexol	rimexolone	Ophthalmic corticosteroid
Zinecard	dexrazoxone	Drug induced cardiomyopathy

Pending Drugs or Drugs in Clinical Trials

Alredase	tolrestat	Controlling late complications of diabetes
Arkin-Z	vesnarinone	Congestive heart failure agent
Baypress	nitrendipone	Calcium channel blocker for hypertension
Berotec	fenoterol	Beta-2 agonist for asthma
Catatrol	viloxazine	Bicyclic antidepressant
Cipralan	cifeline succinate	Antiarrhythmic agent
Decabid	indecainide HCl	Antiarrhythmic agent
Delaprem	hexoprenaline sulfate	Tocolytic agent
Eldisine	vindesine sulfate	Antineoplastic
Frisium	clobazam	Benzodiazepine
Gastrozepine	pirenzepine	Antiulcer drug
Halfan	halofantrine HCl	Antimalarial
Inhibace	cilazapril	ACE inhibitor
Isoprinosine	inosiplex	Immunomodulating drug
Maxicam	isoxicam	NSAID
Mentane	velnacrine	Alzheimer's disease agent
Micturin	terodiline HCl	Agent for urinary incontinence
Mogadon	nitrazepam	Benzodiazepine
Motilium	domperidone	Antiemetic
Napa	acecainide	Antiarrhythmic agent
Navelbine	vinorelbine	Antineoplastic
Pindac	pinacidil	Antihypertensive
Prothiaden	dothiepen HCl	Tricyclic antidepressant
RU-486	mifepristone	Abortion agent
Reactine	cetirizine	Antihistamine
Rimadyl	caprofen	NSAID
Roxiam	remoxipride	Antipsychotic agent
Sabril	vigabatrin	Anticonvulsant
Selecor	celiprolol HCl	Beta-adrenergic blocker
Targocoid	teicoplanin	Antibiotic, similar to vancomycin
Unicard	dilevalol	Beta-adrenergic blocker
Zaditen	ketotifen	Antiasthmatic

INDICATION/THERAPEUTIC
CATEGORY
INDEX

ADENOSINE DEAMINASE DEFICIENCY

Enzyme, Replacement Therapy

ALCOHOLISM

Aldehyde Dehydrogenase Inhibitor Agent

Phenothiazine Derivative

Sedative

ALCOHOL WITHDRAWAL

Alpha-Adrenergic Agonist

Antianxiety Agent

Antihistamine

Antipsychotic Agent

Benzodiazepine

Beta-Adrenergic Blocker

Phenothiazine Derivative

Sedative

ALDOSTERONISM

Diuretic, Potassium Sparing

ANGIOGRAPHY (OPHTHALMIC)

Diagnostic Agent, Ophthalmic Dye

ANTERIOR UVEITIS

Corticosteroid, Ophthalmic

ANTHRAX

Antibiotic, Macrolide

Antibiotic, Miscellaneous

Antibiotic, Penicillin

Antibiotic, Tetracycline Derivative

ANTITHROMBIN III DEFICIENCY (HEREDITARY)

Blood Product Derivative

ANXIETY

Antianxiety Agent

ARTHRITIS (PSORIATIC)

Adrenal Corticosteroid

Corticosteroid, Systemic

ARTHRITIS (RHEUMATOID)

Adrenal Corticosteroid

Analgesic, Non-Narcotic

Theophylline Derivative

ASTHMA (DIAGNOSTIC)

Diagnostic Agent, Bronchial Airway Hyperactivity

ATELECTASIS

Expectorant

ATROPHIC GASTRITIS

Gastrointestinal Agent, Miscellaneous

ATTENTION DEFICIT HYPERACTIVE DISORDER (ADHD)

Central Nervous System Stimulant, Amphetamine

Central Nervous System Stimulant, Nonamphetamine

AUTISM

Antipsychotic Agent

BABESIA INFECTION

Antibiotic, Miscellaneous

BRONCHIECTASIS

Adrenergic Agonist Agent

Beta-2-Adrenergic Agonist Agent

Bronchodilator

BRONCHIOLITIS

Antiviral Agent, Inhalation Therapy

BRONCHITIS (ACUTE)

Adrenergic Agonist Agent

Antibiotic, Cephalosporin (Second Generation)

Antibiotic, Cephalosporin (Third Generation)

Antibiotic, Penicillin

Antibiotic, Sulfonamide Derivative

Antibiotic, Tetracycline Derivative

BRONCHITIS (ASTHMATIC)

Adrenal Corticosteroid

Bronchodilator

Corticosteroid, Inhalant

BRONCHITIS (CHRONIC)

Antiasthmatic

Antibiotic, Cephalosporin (Second Generation)

Antibiotic, Cephalosporin (Third Generation)

Antibiotic, Macrolide

Antibiotic, Miscellaneous

Antibiotic, Penicillin

Antibiotic, Quinolone

Antibiotic, Sulfonamide Derivative

Antibiotic, Tetracycline Derivative

Anticholinergic Agent

Beta-2-Adrenergic Agonist Agent

BRONCHOSPASM

Adrenergic Agonist Agent

BRUCELLOSIS

BULLOUS SKIN DISEASE

BURNS

BURSITIS

Nonsteroidal Anti-Inflammatory Agent (NSAID), Oral

CALYMMATOBACTERIUM GRANULOMATIS INFECTION

Antibiotic, Aminoglycoside

Antibiotic, Macrolide

Antibiotic, Penicillin

Corticosteroid, Topical (Medium Potency)

CANDIDIASIS (DISSEMINATED)

Antifungal Agent, Systemic

CANDIDIASIS (MUCOCUTANEOUS)

Antifungal Agent, Systemic

Antifungal Agent, Topical

CANDIDIASIS (OROPHARYNGEAL)

Antifungal Agent, Oral Nonabsorbed

Antifungal Agent, Systemic

CANDIDIASIS (VULVOVAGINAL)

Antifungal Agent, Topical

Antifungal Agent, Vaginal

CANKER SORE

Anti-infective Agent, Oral

Local Anesthetic, Topical

CHRONIC LUNG DISEASE

Adrenergic Agonist Agent

Antiasthmatic

Anticholinergic Agent

Bronchodilator

Expectorant

CONDYLOMA ACUMINATUM

Antineoplastic Agent, Miscellaneous

Interferon

Keratolytic Agent

CONGESTIVE HEART FAILURE

Adrenergic Agonist Agent

Alpha-Adrenergic Blocking Agent, Oral

Angiotensin-Converting Enzyme (ACE) Inhibitors

Antihypertensive, Combination

Cardiac Glycoside

Cardiovascular Agent, Other

Diuretic, Loop

Diuretic, Potassium Sparing

Nitrate

CONVULSANT DRUG POISONING

Hypnotic

CORNEAL ULCER

Antibiotic, Ophthalmic

CORYNEBACTERIUM JEIKEIUM INFECTION

Antibiotic, Aminoglycoside

Antibiotic, Miscellaneous

Antibiotic, Penicillin

CORYNEBACTERIUM INFECTION, OTHER THAN *C. JEIKEIUM*

Antibiotic, Macrolide

ENCEPHALITIS

Vaccine, Inactivated Virus

ENCEPHALITIS (HERPESVIRUS)

Antiviral Agent, Parenteral

ENDOCARDITIS, ACUTE, I.V. DRUG ABUSE

Antibiotic, Aminoglycoside

Antibiotic, Miscellaneous

ENDOCARDITIS, ACUTE NATIVE VALVE

Antibiotic, Miscellaneous

ENDOCARDITIS, PROSTHETIC VALVE, EARLY

Antibiotic, Aminoglycoside

Antibiotic, Topical

EYELID INFECTION

Antibiotic, Ophthalmic

Pharmaceutical Aid

FACTOR IX DEFICIENCY

Antihemophilic Agent

FACTOR VIII DEFICIENCY

Antihemophilic Agent

Hemophilic Agent

FATTY ACID DEFICIENCY

Caloric Agent

Intravenous Nutritional Therapy

Nutritional Supplement

FEVER, NEUTROPENIC

Antibiotic, Aminoglycoside

Corticosteroid, Systemic

Local Anesthetic, Injectable

FLUTTER (ATRIAL)

Antiarrhythmic Agent, Class II

Antiarrhythmic Agent, Class IV

Antiarrhythmic Agent, Miscellaneous

FUNGUS (DIAGNOSTIC)

Diagnostic Agent, Fungus

Diagnostic Agent, Skin Test

FURUNCULOSIS

Antibiotic, Macrolide

Antibiotic, Miscellaneous

Antibiotic, Penicillin

FUSOBACTERIUM INFECTION

Antibiotic, Anaerobic
Flagyl® Oral 303
Metro I.V.® Injection 303
metronidazole...............303
Protostat® Oral..............303

Antibiotic, Miscellaneous
chloramphenicol...............88
Chloromycetin® 88
Cleocin HCl® 105
Cleocin Pediatric® 105
Cleocin Phosphate® 105
clindamycin 105

Antibiotic, Penicillin
ampicillin...................26
ampicillin sodium and sulbactam
   sodium 26
Beepen-VK® Oral 354
Betapen®-VK Oral 354
Ledercillin® VK Oral 354
Marcillin® 26
Mezlin® 305
mezlocillin sodium 305
Omnipen® 26
Omnipen®-N 26
penicillin g, parenteral 353
penicillin v potassium 354
Pen.Vee® K Oral 354
Pfizerpen® Injection 353
piperacillin sodium 370
piperacillin sodium and
   tazobactam sodium 371
Pipracil® 370
Polycillin® 26
Polycillin-N® 26
Principen® 26
Robicillin® VK Oral 354
Ticar® 460
ticarcillin and clavulanate
   potassium................459
ticarcillin disodium 460
Timentin® 459
Totacillin® 26
Totacillin®-N 26
Unasyn® 26
V-Cillin K® Oral 354
Veetids® Oral 354
Zosyn™ 371

GAG REFLEX SUPPRESSION

Local Anesthetic, Oral
Americaine® [OTC] 48
benzocaine..................48
Dermoplast® [OTC] 48
Dyclone® 161
dyclonine hydrochloride 161
Hurricaine® 48
Pontocaine® Topical 450
Rid-A-Pain® [OTC] 48
tetracaine hydrochloride 450

GALACTORRHEA

Antihistamine
cyproheptadine hydrochloride
  122
Periactin® 122

Ergot Alkaloid
bromocriptine mesylate 58
Parlodel® 58

GALL BLADDER DISEASE (DIAGNOSTIC)

Diagnostic Agent, Gallbladder Function
Kinevac® 423
sincalide 423

GARDNERELLA VAGINALIS INFECTION

Antibiotic, Anaerobic
Flagyl® Oral 303
metronidazole...............303
Protostat® Oral..............303

Antibiotic, Penicillin
ampicillin...................26
Marcillin® 26
Omnipen® 26
Omnipen®-N 26
Polycillin® 26
Polycillin-N® 26
Principen® 26
Totacillin® 26
Totacillin®-N 26

GAS PAINS

Antiflatulent
Actidose-Aqua® [OTC] 86
Actidose® With Sorbitol [OTC] ...86
aluminum hydroxide, magnesium
   hydroxide, and simethicone
  16
calcium carbonate and
   simethicone 67
Charcoaid® [OTC] 86
charcoal 86
Charcocaps® [OTC] 86
Di-Gel® [OTC] 16
Flatulex [OTC] 423
Gas-X® [OTC] 423
Gelusil® [OTC] 16
Liqui-Char® [OTC] 86
Maalox Anti-Gas® [OTC] 423
Maalox® Plus [OTC] 16
magaldrate and simethicone
  276
Mylanta® [OTC] 16
Mylanta Gas® [OTC] 423
Mylanta®-II [OTC] 16
Mylicon® [OTC] 423
Phazyme® [OTC] 423
Riopan Plus® [OTC]..........276
Silain® [OTC] 423
simethicone 423
Titralac® Plus Liquid [OTC].....67

GASTRIC ULCER

Antacid
Aludrox® [OTC] 16
aluminum hydroxide and
   magnesium hydroxide 16

GLAUCOMA

Carbonic Anhydrase Inhibitor

GLAUCOMA (ANGLE CLOSURE)

Carbonic Anhydrase Inhibitor

Cholinergic Agent, Ophthalmic

Diuretic, Carbonic Anhydrase Inhibitor

Laxative, Hyperosmolar

Ophthalmic Agent, Miotic

Ophthalmic Agent, Osmotic

GLAUCOMA (OPEN ANGLE)

Adrenergic Agonist Agent, Ophthalmic

Beta-Adrenergic Blocker, Ophthalmic

GOODPASTURE'S SYNDROME

Antineoplastic Agent, Alkylating Agent (Nitrogen Mustard)

Corticosteroid, Systemic

GOUT

Adrenal Corticosteroid

Corticosteroid, Systemic

Nonsteroidal Anti-Inflammatory Agent (NSAID), Oral

HEPATITIS C INFECTION

Biological Response Modulator

Interferon

HERNIATED DISC

Enzyme, Proteolytic

HERPES SIMPLEX INFECTION

Antiviral Agent, Ophthalmic

Antiviral Agent, Oral

Antiviral Agent, Parenteral

Antiviral Agent, Topical

HERPES ZOSTER INFECTION

Antiviral Agent, Ophthalmic

Antiviral Agent, Oral

Antiviral Agent, Parenteral

Antiviral Agent, Topical

Topical Skin Product

HICCUPS

Phenothiazine Derivative

HISTOPLASMA CAPSULATUM INFECTION

Antifungal Agent, Systemic

HODGKIN'S DISEASE

Antineoplastic Agent, Alkylating Agent

Antineoplastic Agent, Alkylating Agent (Nitrogen Mustard)

Antineoplastic Agent, Alkylating Agent (Nitrosourea)

Antineoplastic Agent, Antibiotic

Antineoplastic Agent, Miotic Inhibitor

HYPERPIGMENTATION

Depigmenting Agent

HYPERPLASIA, VULVAR SQUAMOUS

Estrogen Derivative

HYPERPROLACTINEMIA

Ergot Alkaloid

HYPERSENSITIVITY SKIN TESTING (DIAGNOSTIC)

Diagnostic Agent, Skin Test

HYPERTENSION

Adrenergic Agonist Agent

Adrenergic Blocking Agent

Alpha-Adrenergic Agonist

Alpha-Adrenergic Blocking Agent, Oral

Alpha-Adrenergic Blocking Agent, Parenteral

Alpha-Adrenergic Inhibitors, Central

Biological Response Modulator

Colony Stimulating Factor

Corticosteroid, Systemic

MACROGLOBULINEMIA OF WALDENSTRÖM

Antineoplastic Agent, Alkylating Agent (Nitrogen Mustard)

MALABSORPTION

Trace Element, Parenteral

Vitamin, Fat Soluble

MALARIA

Antibiotic, Tetracycline Derivative

Antimalarial Agent

Corticosteroid, Systemic

MYOCARDIAL INFARCTION

Anticoagulant

Antiplatelet Agent

Beta-Adrenergic Blocker

Thrombolytic Agent

Vasodilator, Coronary

MYOCARDIAL ISCHEMIA (PROPHYLAXIS)

Blood Modifiers

MYOCARDIAL REINFARCTION

Antiplatelet Agent

Beta-Adrenergic Blocker

Vasodilator, Coronary

NARCOLEPSY

Adrenergic Agonist Agent

Central Nervous System Stimulant, Amphetamine

Central Nervous System Stimulant, Nonamphetamine

NAUSEA

Antiemetic

Phenothiazine Derivative

NEISSERIA GONORRHOEAE INFECTION

Antibiotic, Cephalosporin (Third Generation)

Otic Agent, Analgesic

OVARIAN FAILURE

Estrogen and Androgen Combination

Estrogen Derivative

OVULATION

Ovulation Stimulator

PAGET'S DISEASE OF BONE

Biphosphonate Derivative

PAIN (BONE)

Radiopharmaceutical

PAIN, DIABETIC NEUROPATHY NEURALGIA

Analgesic, Topical

PAIN (MILD TO MODERATE)

Analgesic, Narcotic

Analgesic, Non-Narcotic

PAIN (MODERATE TO SEVERE)

Analgesic, Narcotic

Analgesic, Non-Narcotic

PANCREATIC EXOCRINE DISEASE (DIAGNOSTIC)

Diagnostic Agent, Pancreatic Exocrine Insufficiency

PANCREATIC EXOCRINE INSUFFICIENCY

Pancreatic Enzyme

PSEUDOGOUT

Anti-inflammatory Agent

PSEUDOHYPOPARATHYROIDISM

Vitamin D Analog

PSEUDOMONAS AERUGINOSA INFECTION

Antibiotic, Aminoglycoside

Antibiotic, Cephalosporin (Third Generation)

Antibiotic, Miscellaneous

Antibiotic, Penicillin

Antibiotic, Quinolone

PSORIASIS

Antineoplastic Agent, Antimetabolite

Antipsoriatic Agent, Systemic

Antipsoriatic Agent, Topical

RESPIRATORY DISTRESS SYNDROME

Lung Surfactant

RESPIRATORY SYNCYTIAL VIRUS

Antiviral Agent, Inhalation Therapy

RETINOBLASTOMA

Antineoplastic Agent, Alkylating Agent (Nitrogen Mustard)

Antineoplastic Agent, Antibiotic

REYE'S SYNDROME

Corticosteroid, Systemic

Diuretic, Osmotic

Laxative, Hyperosmolar

Vitamin, Fat Soluble

RHABDOMYOSARCOMA

Antineoplastic Agent, Alkylating Agent (Nitrogen Mustard)

STAPHYLOCOCCUS SAPROPHYTICUS INFECTION

STEVENS-JOHNSON SYNDROME

TINEA (CRURIS)

Antifungal Agent, Systemic

Antifungal Agent, Topical

TINEA (PEDIS)

Antifungal Agent, Systemic

INDICATION/THERAPEUTIC CATEGORY INDEX

VON WILLEBRAND'S DISEASE

Hemophilic Agent

Vasopressin Analog, Synthetic

VULVOVAGINITIS

Antifungal Agent, Vaginal

WHIPPLE'S DISEASE

Antibiotic, Miscellaneous

Antibiotic, Tetracycline Derivative

WHIPWORM INFESTATION

Anthelmintic

WHOOPING COUGH

Antibiotic, Macrolide

Antibiotic, Sulfonamide Derivative

Immune Globulin

Toxoid

WILMS' TUMOR

Antineoplastic Agent, Antibiotic

Antineoplastic Agent, Miotic Inhibitor

WILSON'S DISEASE

Antidote, Copper Toxicity

NOTES

NOTES

NOTES

NOTES

NOTES

NOTES

NOTES